Third Edition

Appleton & Lange's Review for the

USMLE STEP 1

Thomas K. Barton, MD
Department of Pathology
Palms of Pasadena Hospital
St. Petersburg, Florida

APPLETON & LANGE
Stamford, Connecticut

Notice: The authors and the publisher of this volume have taken care to make certain that the doses of drugs and schedules of treatment are correct and compatible with the standards generally accepted at the time of publication. Nevertheless, as new information becomes available, changes in treatment and in the use of drugs become necessary. The reader is advised to carefully consult the instruction and information material included in the package insert of each drug or therapeutic agent before administration. This advice is especially important when using, administering, or recommending new or infrequently used drugs. The authors and publisher disclaim all responsibility for any liability, loss, injury, or damage incurred as a consequence, directly or indirectly, of the use and application of any of the contents of this volume.

www.appletonlange.com

99 00 01 02 03 / 10 9 8 7 6 5 4 3 2 1

Prentice Hall International (UK) Limited, *London*
Prentice Hall of Australia Pty. Limited, *Sydney*
Prentice Hall Canada, Inc., *Toronto*
Prentice Hall Hispanoamericana, S.A., *Mexico*
Prentice Hall of India Private Limited, *New Delhi*
Prentice Hall of Japan, Inc., *Tokyo*
Simon & Schuster Asia Pte. Ltd., *Singapore*
Editora Prentice Hall do Brasil Ltda., *Rio de Janeiro*
Prentice Hall, *Upper Saddle River, New Jersey*

ISBN 0-8385-0375-6

Acquisitions Editor: Jessica Hirshon
Development Editor: Deborah King
Production Editor: Elizabeth Ryan
Production Service: Rainbow Graphics, LLC
Designer: Elizabeth Schmitz

ISBN 0-8385-0375-6

90000
9 780838 503751

PRINTED IN THE UNITED STATES OF AMERICA

Table of Contents

Contributors

Thomas K. Barton, MD
Department of Pathology
Palms of Pasadena Hospital
St. Petersburg, Florida

Andreas Carl, MD, PhD
Department of Physiology and Cell Biology
Reno, Nevada
School of Medicine
University of Nevada

Michael W. King, PhD
Associate Professor
Department of Biochemistry and Molecular Biology
Indiana University School of Medicine
Terre Haute Center for Medical Education
Terre Haute, Indiana

Hoyle Leigh, MD
Professor and Vice Chair
Department of Psychiatry
University of California, San Francisco
Director, Fresno Division and
Associate Chief of Staff for Mental Health/Academic Affairs
Fresno VA Medical Center
Lecturer in Psychiatry
Yale University
New Haven, Connecticut

Martin G. Lewis, MD, MBBS, FRC (Path)
Clinical Professor
Department of Pathology and Laboratory Medicine
University of South Florida
Tampa, Florida
and
Department of Pathology
Palms of Pasadena Hospital
St. Petersburg, Florida

Gregory Mihailoff, PhD
Assistant Director of Research Affairs
Arizona College of Osteopathic Medicine
Midwestern University
Glendale, Arizona

Anthony Moore, PhD
Associate Professor of Anatomy
Department of Anatomy
University of Mississippi Medical Center
Jackson, Mississippi

John Naftel, PhD
Associate Professor of Anatomy
Department of Anatomy
University of Mississippi Medical Center
Jackson, Mississippi

Russell K. Yamazaki, PhD
Associate Professor and Associate Chair
Department of Pharmacology
Wayne State University School of Medicine
Detroit, Michigan

William W. Yotis, PhD
Professor Emeritus of Microbiology and Immunology
Loyola University
Stritch School of Medicine
Maywood, Illinois
Clinical Professor of Microbiology and Immunology
University of South Florida
College of Medicine
Tampa, FL

Preface

Success on the USMLE Step 1 requires a thorough understanding of the basic sciences covered in the first and second years of medical education. In order to offer the most complete and accurate review book, we assembled a team of authors and editors from around the country who are engaged in various specialties and involved in both academic and clinical settings.

The author team was asked to research and write test questions using the parameters set forth by the National Board of Medical Examiners. All of the subjects, types of questions, and techniques that will be encountered on the USMLE Step 1 are presented in this book.

Appleton & Lange's Review for the USMLE Step 1 is designed to provide you with a comprehensive review of the basic sciences as well as a valuable self-assessment tool for exam preparation. A total of 1,200 questions are included in this edition.

Key Features and Use:

- Approximately 150 questions are covered in the basic sciences: Anatomy, Physiology, Biochemistry, Microbiology, Pathology, Pharmacology, and Behavioral Sciences.
- Questions are followed by a section with answers and detailed explanations referenced to the most current and popular resources available.
- A subspecialty list at the end of each chapter helps assess your strengths and weaknesses, thus pinpointing areas for concentration during exam preparation.
- A Practice Test (with 300 questions) simulates the USMLE Step 1 and is included at the end of this text.

We believe that you will find the questions, explanations, and format of the text to be of great assistance to you during your review. We wish you luck on the USMLE Step 1.

The Editors and the Publisher

Review Preparation Guide

If you are planning to prepare for the United States Medical Licensing Examination Step 1, then this book is designed for you. Here, in one package, is a comprehensive review resource with 1200 examination-type basic science multiple-choice questions with referenced, paragraph-length explanations of each answer. In addition, the last section of the book offers an integrated practice test for self-assessment purposes.

This introduction provides specific information on the USMLE Step 1, information on question types, question-answering strategies, and various ways to use this review.

THE UNITED STATES MEDICAL LICENSING EXAMINATION STEP 1

The USMLE Step 1 is a two-day written examination which tests your knowledge of Anatomy, Physiology, Biochemistry, Microbiology, Pathology, Pharmacology, and Behavioral Sciences. It contains a total of about 720 multiple choice questions which have been proffered by senior academic faculty to test your comprehension of basic science concepts that they feel are relevant to your future successful practice of medicine. In order to correctly answer these test questions you may be required to recall memorized facts, to use deductive reasoning, or both. A minority of the questions will employ graphs, photographs, or line drawings that you will need to interpret.

During each day of the two-day exam you will be asked to answer about 360 questions divided into two sessions of three hours each. The application materials you receive for the USMLE Step 1 will more fully discuss the exam procedure, rules of test administration, types of questions asked, and the scope of material you may be tested on.

ORGANIZATION OF THIS BOOK

This book is organized to cover sequentially each of the basic science areas specified by the National Board of Medical Examiners (NBME). There are seven sections, one for each of the basic sciences, and an integrated practice test section at the end of the review. The sections are as follows:

1. **Anatomy** (including gross and microscopic anatomy; neuroanatomy; and development and control mechanisms).
2. **Physiology** (including general and cellular functions; major body system physiology; energy balance; and fluid and electrolyte balance).
3. **Biochemistry** (including energy metabolism; major metabolic pathways of small molecules; major tissue and cellular structures, properties, and functions; biochemical aspects of cellular and molecular biology; and special biochemistry of tissues).
4. **Microbiology** (including microbial structure and composition; cellular metabolism, physiology, and regulation; microbial and molecular genetics; immunology; bacterial pathogens; virology; and medical mycology and parasitology).

5. **Pathology** (including general and systemic pathology; and pathology of syndromes and complex reactions).
6. **Pharmacology** (including general principles; major body system agents; vitamins; chemotherapeutic agents; and poisoning and therapy of intoxication).
7. **Behavioral Sciences** (including behavioral biology; individual, interpersonal, and social behavior; and culture and society).
8. **Practice Test** (includes 300 questions from all seven basic sciences, presented in an integrated format).

Each of the eight chapters is organized in the following order:

1. Questions
2. Answers and Explanations
3. References
4. Subspecialty List

These sections and how you might use them are discussed below.

Question Formats

The style and presentation of the questions have been fully revised to conform with the United States Medical Licensing Examinations. This will enable you to familiarize yourself with the types of questions to be expected, and provide practice in recalling your knowledge in each format. Following the answers in each chapter is a list of suggested references for additional consultation.

Each of the seven basic science chapters contains multiple choice questions composed in the **Single Best Answer** query format (example question 1). This is the most frequently encountered format in the USMLE Step 1. It generally contains a brief statement, followed by five options of which only ONE is ENTIRELY correct. The answer options on the USMLE are lettered A, B, C, D, and E. Although the format for this question type is straightforward, the questions can be difficult because some of the distractors in the answer list are partially correct. An example of this question format follows.

DIRECTIONS (Question 1): Each of the numbered items or incomplete statements in this section is followed by answers or by completions of the statement. Select the ONE lettered answer or completion that is BEST in each case.

1. Liquefaction necrosis is the characteristic result of infarcts in the

(A) brain
(B) heart
(C) kidney
(D) spleen
(E) small intestine

The correct answer is A. There are two ways to attack this style of question. If after reading the query an answer immediately comes to mind, then look for it in the answer list. Alternatively, if no answer immediately comes to mind, or if the answer you thought was obvious is not a choice, then you will need to spend time examining all of the answer options to find the correct one. In this case anything you can do to eliminate an answer option will increase your odds of choosing the correct answer. With this in mind, scan all of the possible answers. Eliminate any that are clearly wrong and all that are only partially right. Even if you can eliminate one or two of the answer choices by this method you will have significantly increased your chance of guessing the right answer from the remaining choices. Always answer every question, even if you have to guess among all five answer choices, because there is no penalty for a wrong answer. Your test score is dependent only on the number of correct answers obtained.

STRATEGIES FOR ANSWERING SINGLE BEST ANSWER QUESTIONS

1. Remember that only one choice can be the correct answer.
2. Read the question carefully to be sure that you understand what is being asked.
3. If you immediately know the answer look for it in the answer choices.
4. If no answer is immediately obvious, quickly scan all the five answer choices for familiarity.
5. Eliminate any answer that is completely wrong or only partially correct. This increases your odds of picking the correct answer from a lesser number of remaining answer choices.
6. If two of the remaining choices are mutually exclusive, the correct answer is probably one of them.
7. Fill in the appropriate circle on the answer sheet.
8. Always answer every question even if you have to guess.
9. Don't spend too much time with any one question. In order to finish each three-hour session you will need to answer a question about every 50 seconds.

Practice Tests

The two 150-question practice tests at the end of the book consist of questions from each of the seven basic sciences. This format mimics the actual exam and enables you to test your skill at answering questions in all of the basic sciences under simulated examination conditions.

The practice test section is organized in the same format as the seven earlier sections: questions; answers, explanations, and references.

HOW TO USE THIS BOOK

There are two logical ways to get the most value from this book. We will call them Plan A and Plan B.

In Plan A, you go straight to the Practice Tests and complete them according to the instructions. This will be a good indicator of your initial knowledge of the subject and will help you identify specific areas for preparation and review. You can now use the first seven chapters of the book to help you improve your relative weak points.

In Plan B, you go through chapters 1 through 7 checking off your answers, and then comparing your choices with the answers and discussions in the book. Once you have completed this process, you can take the Practice Tests and see how well prepared you are. If you still have a major weakness, it should be apparent in time for you to take remedial action.

In Plan A, by taking the Practice Tests first, you get quick feedback regarding your initial areas of strength and weakness. You may find that you have a good command of the material, indicating that perhaps only a cursory review of the seven chapters is necessary. This, of course, would be good to know early on in your exam preparation. On the other hand, you may find that you have many areas of weakness. In this case, you could then focus on these areas in your review—not just with this book, but also with the cited references and with your current textbooks.

It is, however, unlikely that you will not do some studying prior to taking the USMLE (especially since you have this book). Therefore, it may be more realistic to take the Practice Tests after you have reviewed the first seven chapters (as in Plan B). This will probably give you a more realistic type of testing situation since very few of us just sit down to a test without studying. In this case, you will have done some reviewing (from superficial to in-depth), and your Practice Tests will reflect this studying time. If, after reviewing the first seven chapters and taking the Practice Tests, you still have some weaknesses, you can then go back to the first seven chapters and supplement your review with your texts.

SPECIFIC INFORMATION ON THE PART I EXAMINATION

The official source of all information with respect to the United States Medical Licensing Examination Step 1 is the National Board of Medical Examiners (NBME), 3930 Chestnut Street, Philadelphia, PA 19104. Established in 1915, the NBME is a voluntary, nonprofit, independent organization whose sole function is the design, implementation, distribution, and processing of a vast bank of question items, certifying examinations, and evaluative services in the professional medical field.

In order to sit for the Step 1 examination, a person must be either an officially enrolled medical student or a graduate of an accredited medical school. It is not necessary to complete any particular year of medical school to be a candidate for Step 1. Neither is it required to take Step 1 before Step 2.

In applying for Step 1, you must use forms supplied by NBME. Remember that registration closes *ten weeks* before the scheduled examination date. Some United States and Canadian medical schools require their students to take Step 1 even if they are noncandidates. Such students can register as noncandidates at the request of their school. A person who takes Step 1 as a noncandidate can later change to candidate status and, after payment of a fee, receive certification credit.

Scoring

Because there is no deduction for wrong answers, you should **answer every question.** Your test is scored in the following way:

1. The number of questions answered correctly is totaled. This is called the raw score.
2. The raw score is converted statistically to a "standard" score on a scale of 200 to 800, with the mean set at 500. Each 100 points away from 500 is one standard deviation.
3. Your score is compared statistically with the criteria set by the scores of the second-year

medical school candidates for certification in the June administration during the prior four years. This is what is meant by the term, "criterion referenced test."

4. A score of 500 places you around the 50th percentile. A score of 380 is the minimum passing score for Step 1; this probably represents about the 12th to 15th percentile. If you answer 50 percent or so of the questions correctly, you will probably receive a passing score.

Remember: You do not have to pass all seven basic science components, although you will receive a standard score in each of them. A score of less than 400 (about the 15th percentile) on any particular area is a real cause for concern as it will certainly drag down your overall score. Likewise, a 600 or better (85th percentile) is an area of great relative strength. (You can use the practice test included in this book to help determine your areas of strength and weakness well in advance of the actual examination.)

Physical Conditions

The NBME is very concerned that all their exams be administered under uniform conditions in the numerous centers that are used. Beginning in January 1999, the USMLE examination is administered electronically. Please visit www.nmbe.org for details, or contact your local Sylvan Learning center for scheduling and further information.

The number of candidates who fail Step 1 is quite small; however, individual students as well as entire medical school programs benefit when scores are high. No one wants to squeak by with a 380 when a little effort might raise that score to 450. That is why you have made a wise decision to use the self-assessment and review materials available in *Appleton & Lange's Review for the USMLE Step 1.*

Standard Abbreviations

ACTH: adrenocorticotropic hormone
ADH: antidiuretic hormone
ADP: adenosine diphosphate
AFP: α-fetoprotein
AMP: adenosine monophosphate
ATP: adenosine triphosphate
ATPase: adenosine triphosphatase
bid: 2 times a day
BP: blood pressure
BUN: blood urea nitrogen
CT: computed tomography
CBC: complete blood count
CCU: coronary care unit
CNS: central nervous system
CPK: creatine phosphokinase
CSF: cerebrospinal fluid
DNA: deoxyribonucleic acid
DNAse: deoxyribonuclease
ECG: electrocardiogram
EDTA: ethylenediaminetetraacetate
EEG: electroencephalogram
ER: emergency room
FSH: follicle-stimulating hormone
GI: gastrointestinal
GU: genitourinary
Hb: hemoglobin
HCG: human chorionic gonadotropin
Hct: hematocrit
IgA, etc.: immunoglobulin A, etc.
IM: intramuscular(ly)
IQ: intelligence quotient
IU: international unit
IV: intravenous(ly)
KUB: kidney, ureter, and bladder
LDH: lactic dehydrogenase
LH: luteinizing hormone
LSD: lysergic acid diethylamide
mRNA: messenger RNA
PO: oral(ly)
prn: as needed
RBC: red blood cell
RNA: ribonucleic acid
RNAse: ribonuclease
rRNA: ribosomal RNA
SC: subcutaneous(ly)
SGOT: serum glutamic oxaloacetic transaminase
SGPT: serum glutamic pyruvic transaminase
TB: tuberculosis
tRNA: transfer RNA
TSH: thyroid-stimulating hormone
WBC: white blood cell

CHAPTER 1

Anatomy
Questions

Gregory Mihailoff, PhD, Anthony Moore, PhD, and John Naftel, PhD

DIRECTIONS (Questions 1 through 155): Each of the numbered items or incomplete statements in this section is followed by answers or by completions of the statement. Select the ONE lettered answer or completion that is BEST in each case.

1. Neurons that participate in smooth pursuit eye movements are found in which of the following cell groups?

(A) fovea of the retina
(B) lateral geniculate nucleus
(C) primary visual cortex
(D) frontal eye field
(E) all of the above

Questions 2 and 3

The following observations are noted while examining a patient in the emergency room. The pupil of the left eye is dilated and both direct and consensual pupillary light reflexes are absent in that eye. The left eye also appears to be deviated laterally and downward. The patient exhibits right hemiplegia with increased deep tendon reflexes and a positive Babinski sign on the right.

2. The deficits involving the left eye suggest involvement of the

(A) left oculomotor nerve
(B) right trochlear nerve
(C) left abducens nerve
(D) left trigeminal nerve
(E) left facial nerve

3. The presence of unilateral ocular movement deficits, lateral strabismus, and mydriasis in combination with hemiplegia involving the contralateral extremities is referred to as

(A) Wallenberg's syndrome
(B) capsular hemiplegia
(C) superior alternating hemiplegia
(D) middle alternating hemiplegia
(E) syringomyelia

4. Which of the following statements concerning the lateral geniculate nucleus is correct?

(A) It contains projection-type cells whose axons synapse in layer IV of the contralateral striate cortex.
(B) It receives input from both the right and left eyes.
(C) It consists entirely of parvocellular (small) projection neurons.
(D) It contains projection neurons whose axons enter the optic tract.
(E) It receives parasympathetic input from the Edinger–Westphal nucleus.

5. Which of the following statements concerning the eye and photic stimulation are true?
   (A) Light stimuli first pass through the lens and then penetrate all of the intervening layers of the retina before striking the photoreceptors.
   (B) While in the dark, photoreceptors are depolarized due to dark current and are releasing neurotransmitter.
   (C) The optic disc is located nasally (medially) with respect to the macula.
   (D) Horizontal cells form direct synaptic connections with photoreceptors.
   (E) All of the above are true statements.

6. Microscopic examination of the brain of an aborted fetus revealed the presence of mitotic figures (condensed chromosomes visible during prophase of mitosis). During early histogenesis in the normal, developing cerebral hemisphere, you would expect all of the cells exhibiting mitotic figures to be located
   (A) in the ventricular zone
   (B) in the mantle layer
   (C) in the alar plate
   (D) at the pial surface
   (E) evenly distributed throughout the thickness of the cortical mantle

7. The neurotransmitter released from cerebellar Purkinje cells is
   (A) glutamate
   (B) gamma-aminobutyric acid
   (C) acetylcholine
   (D) serotonin
   (E) glycine

8. Which statement concerning the inverse myotatic reflex is correct?
   (A) Type Ia sensory fibers synapse with interneurons that lead to inhibition of the muscle from which the sensory fibers originated.
   (B) Sensory fibers originating in Golgi tendon organs synapse with interneurons that lead to inhibition of the muscle related to that tendon organ.
   (C) Type Ib sensory fibers do not play a role in this reflex.
   (D) A painful stimulus (i.e., pinprick) to the skin overlying a Golgi tendon organ is the typical mode of stimulation that will elicit the reflex.
   (E) Type II sensory fibers are most active in this reflex and their input excites inhibitory interneurons that synapse with gamma motor neurons.

9. Which layer of the cerebral cortex contains most of the neurons that give rise to subcortical projections such as corticospinal and corticopontine fibers?
   (A) external granular (layer 2)
   (B) external pyramidal (layer 3)
   (C) internal granular (layer 4)
   (D) internal pyramidal (layer 5)
   (E) multiform (layer 6)

10. Occlusion of the anterior spinal artery would simultaneously damage the ipsilateral corticospinal fibers in the medullary pyramid and exiting fibers of the hypoglossal nerve. This clinical entity is known as
    (A) inferior alternating hemiplegia
    (B) middle alternating hemiplegia
    (C) superior alternating hemiplegia
    (D) spina bifida
    (E) syringomyelia

11. A patient with a large ependymoma in the roof of the fourth ventricle is likely to compress a portion of the overlying cerebellar cortex against the bony wall of the posterior fossa. Beginning with the pial surface and progressing into the cerebellum, what is the correct sequence of cerebellar cortical layers that would be compressed by this tumor?
    (A) pia, molecular, Purkinje, granular
    (B) pia, Purkinje, molecular, granular
    (C) pia, granular, Purkinje, molecular
    (D) pia, molecular, granular, Purkinje
    (E) none of the above are correct

12. Which of the following structures in the medulla originates from the alar plate?

(A) hypoglossal nucleus
(B) dorsal motor nucleus of the vagus nerve
(C) cochlear nuclei
(D) nucleus ambiguus
(E) all of the above originate from the alar plate

13. Occlusion of which of the following vessels would affect the entire dorsolateral part of the rostral medulla (level of the restiform body) and produce the lateral medullary (Wallenberg's) syndrome?

(A) posterior spinal artery
(B) anterior inferior cerebellar artery
(C) anterior spinal artery
(D) posterior inferior cerebellar artery
(E) superior cerebellar artery

14. Pain and temperature signals arising from receptors on the right side of the face would pass through which of the following structures?

(A) right spinal trigeminal nucleus
(B) left ventral posterior lateral nucleus of the thalamus
(C) right principal sensory trigeminal nucleus
(D) right mesencephalic trigeminal nucleus
(E) right posterior limb of the internal capsule

15. Which statement concerning the lateral medullary syndrome is most correct?

(A) Patients usually exhibit a loss of pain and temperature sensibility on the side of the face contralateral to the lesion.
(B) Due to involvement of fibers in the medullary pyramid, patients exhibit spastic paralysis involving the contralateral upper extremity.
(C) Patients typically exhibit loss of pain and temperature sensibility over the ipsilateral upper and contralateral lower extremities.
(D) An infarct involving the anterior inferior cerebellar artery is typically the cause of this syndrome.
(E) Pain and temperature sensibility is lost over the ipsilateral face and the contralateral trunk and extremities.

16. In addition to the inability to voluntarily adduct the right eye, which of the following would you expect to see in a patient with occlusion of paramedian branches of the basilar bifurcation on the right side (Weber's syndrome)?

(A) paralysis of most movements of the left eye
(B) deviation of the tongue to the right
(C) ipsilateral hemiplegia
(D) dilation of the pupil on the right
(E) complete paralysis of facial expression musculature on the left side

17. Which of the following statements concerning Parkinson's disease is correct?

(A) It involves neuronal degeneration in the substantia nigra pars compacta.
(B) There is a reduction in the release of norepinephrine by nigrostriatal axon terminals.
(C) Tachykinesia, an increase in the speed of movement, is a characteristic of the disease.
(D) Carbidopa, an inhibitor of aromatic amino acid decarboxylase, is given because it can cross the blood–brain barrier.
(E) It is characterized by an intention-type tremor involving the hands and fingers.

18. You make the following observations during a neurological examination of your patient. Both eyes can move conjugately to the right without difficulty. On attempted horizontal gaze to the left, the left eye abducts (looks laterally) but the right eye does not adduct. Based on this information, which of the following is the most likely site of the lesion?

(A) trochlear nerve on the right
(B) abducens nerve on the right
(C) medial longitudinal fasciculus on the right
(D) abducens nerve on the left
(E) medial longitudinal fasciculus on the left

19. In a medial medullary syndrome that involves a left-sided branch of the anterior spinal artery, which of the following deficits would be seen?

(A) deviation of the tongue to the left, hemiplegia of arm and leg on left
(B) deviation of the tongue to the right, hemiplegia of arm and leg on right
(C) loss of conscious proprioception and precise tactile discrimination over the right side of the body exclusive of the face
(D) only hemiplegia on the right
(E) only deviation of the tongue to the left

20. A vascular infarct involves the left frontal lobe and includes the frontal opercular region. Such a patient would exhibit an aphasic syndrome in combination with motor dysfunction in the hand. Which of the following combinations is correct?

(A) Wernicke's aphasia—right hand
(B) Broca's aphasia—right hand
(C) conduction aphasia—right hand
(D) Wernicke's aphasia—left hand
(E) Broca's aphasia—left hand

21. You are asked to evaluate a patient in the neurology clinic. Your neurological examination reveals the following symptoms: (1) loss of pain and temperature sensation over the left side of the face; (2) loss of pain and temperature sensation in the right arm and leg; (3) normal tactile and vibratory sensations on the face, body, and extremities. Identify this clinical entity.

(A) right lateral medullary syndrome
(B) syringomyelia
(C) left Wallenberg's syndrome
(D) left capsular infarct
(E) left Weber's syndrome

22. When the stereocilia of an auditory hair cell are deflected in the appropriate direction, potassium channels open in the apical membrane of the cell and

(A) potassium ions flow out of the cell, hyperpolarizing the cell
(B) potassium ions flow out of the cell, depolarizing the cell
(C) potassium ions flow into the cell, hyperpolarizing the cell
(D) potassium ions flow into the cell, depolarizing the cell
(E) there is no net movement of potassium ions

23. A patient comes to you in the ear, nose, and throat clinic complaining of dizziness. You have a vestibular caloric test done with the following results. Warm caloric irrigation of the right ear produces right beating horizontal nystagmus. Warm caloric irrigation of the left ear produces no response. You conclude which of the following?

(A) Receptors in the right ear have been damaged.
(B) The lateral vestibulospinal tract has been destroyed on the left side.
(C) The left labyrinth or VIIIth nerve has been affected either through trauma or possibly an acoustic neuroma.
(D) The right labyrinth or VIIIth nerve has been affected either through trauma or possibly an acoustic neuroma.
(E) There is no lesion in the vestibular system.

24. Which of the following cortical areas contribute fibers to the corticospinal tract?

(A) primary motor cortex (precentral gyrus)
(B) premotor cortex
(C) supplementary motor cortex
(D) primary somatosensory cortex (postcentral gyrus)
(E) all of the above contribute fibers to the corticospinal tract

25. Which of the following statements can be correctly applied to the basal ganglia and Parkinson's disease?

(A) In Parkinson's disease, the loss of nigrostriatal dopamine projections has no influence on the indirect pathway.
(B) Typically, activity through the indirect pathway leads to a reduction in the output of thalamocortical neuron activity.

(C) Signals passing through the direct pathway lead to a decrease in motor activity elicited by the thalamocortical system.
(D) Loss of function in the direct pathway can lead to the production of involuntary movements called choreiform movements.
(E) The tremor of Parkinson's disease becomes more pronounced with attempted voluntary movement.

26. Which of the following statements can be correctly applied to the regulation of the autonomic nervous system by the hypothalamus and the amygdala?

(A) The hypothalamus regulates autonomic function on a long-term basis.
(B) The amygdaloid complex in general regulates autonomic function on a short-term basis.
(C) The cingulate cortex contains the "upper motoneurons" controlling autonomic function.
(D) The amygdaloid complex contains the "lower motoneurons" controlling autonomic function.
(E) Autonomic nuclei of the brainstem are influenced by "upper motoneurons" in both the hypothalamus and the amygdala.

27. Which of the following are symptoms of cerebellar disease?

(A) resting tremor
(B) wide-based stance or staggering gait
(C) spasticity
(D) loss of pain and temperature sensation
(E) hyperreflexia

28. Which of the following symptoms can result from interruption of the oculomotor nerve?

(A) The affected eye looks down and out
(B) The pupillary light reflex is intact
(C) Lens accommodation is not affected
(D) The affected eye looks up and out
(E) The contralateral eyelid droops (ptosis)

Questions 29 through 31

Your 28-year-old male patient reports to you in the emergency room that he fell from a pine tree while attempting to install a satellite dish. In an effort to break his fall he grabbed at a passing limb with his right arm but was unable to hold on. After a thorough examination, you suspect that he has damaged the brachial plexus on his right side at the point indicated in Figure 1–1.

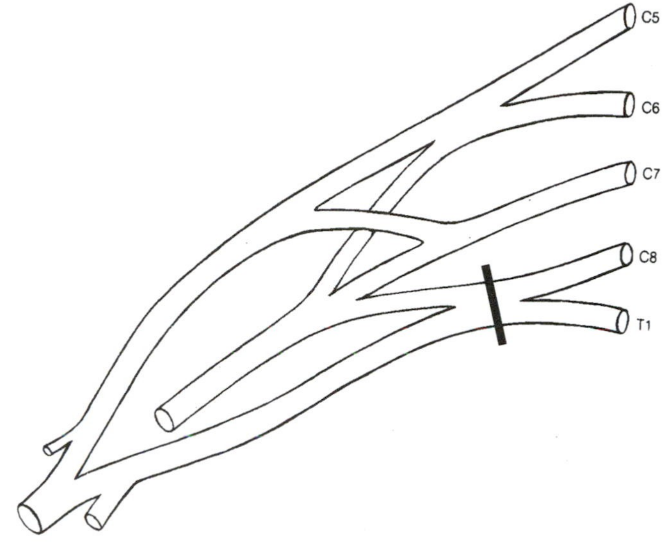

Figure 1–1

29. Which of the following muscles is likely to be the most adversely affected by this injury?

(A) supraspinatus
(B) deltoid
(C) biceps brachii
(D) pronator teres
(E) opponens pollicis

30. You would expect to observe a cutaneous sensory loss

(A) over the web between the thumb and index finger
(B) over the lateral side of the forearm
(C) over the medial palm and small finger
(D) over the deltoid muscle just above its insertion
(E) over the dorsum of the wrist and the anatomical snuffbox

31. The condition resulting from this injury is commonly known as

(A) Klumpke's paralysis
(B) Horner's syndrome
(C) waiter's tip hand
(D) Erb–Duchenne palsy
(E) wrist drop

32. Your patient presents with a complaint of difficulty in raising his right arm above his shoulder. You ask him to push against the wall with outstretched arms as shown in Figure 1–2. Your examination reveals no loss of cutaneous sensation. You conclude that the injury or disease has affected the

(A) upper roots of the brachial plexus
(B) posterior cord of the brachial plexus
(C) accessory nerve
(D) suprascapular nerve
(E) long thoracic nerve

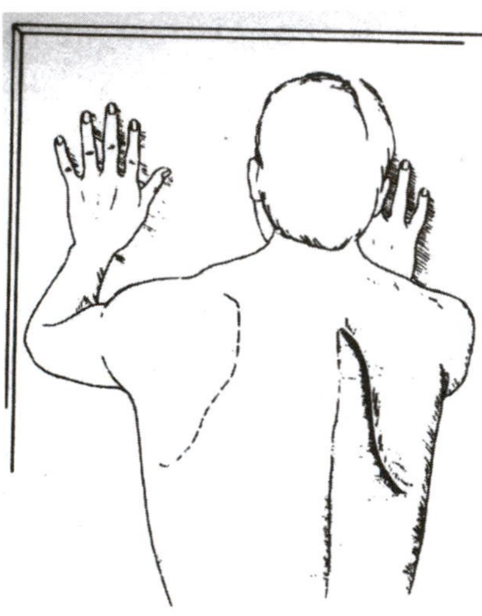

Figure 1–2

Questions 33 and 34

Your patient presents with sensory loss over the areas indicated in Figure 1–3. He has no obvious motor difficulty.

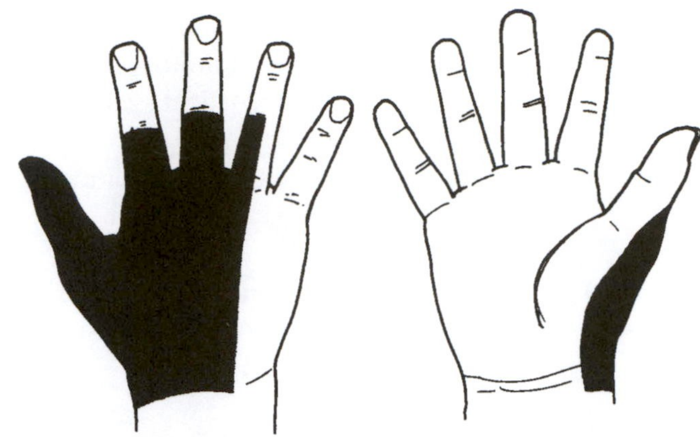

Figure 1–3

33. You suspect that he has damaged the

(A) ulnar nerve at the elbow
(B) dorsal cutaneous branch of the ulnar nerve
(C) radial nerve in the cubital fossa
(D) superficial branch of the radial nerve
(E) posterior antebrachial cutaneous nerve

34. The spinal cord segments supplying this area most likely include

(A) C5 and C6
(B) C6 and C7
(C) C7 and C8
(D) C8 and T1
(E) T1 only

35. A patient in the emergency room has been stabbed in the back of the neck and complains that he is unable to lift his shoulder. Which of the following nerves has likely been damaged?

(A) suprascapular nerve
(B) dorsal scapular nerve
(C) accessory nerve
(D) thoracodorsal nerve
(E) long thoracic nerve

36. The structure most likely to be damaged in a fracture of the surgical neck of the humerus is the

(A) radial nerve
(B) axillary nerve

(C) scapular circumflex artery
(D) profunda brachii artery
(E) brachial artery

37. A penetrating wound to the axilla which severs the posterior cord of the brachial plexus would denervate the

(A) serratus anterior
(B) pronator teres
(C) deltoid
(D) biceps brachii
(E) infraspinatus

38. Which of the following is least likely to be involved in a collateral anastomosis which bypasses an obstruction of the first part of the axillary artery?

(A) suprascapular artery
(B) subscapular artery
(C) dorsal scapular artery
(D) scapular circumflex artery
(E) posterior humeral circumflex artery

39. A young mother arrives at the emergency room with her small son who is crying inconsolably. She reports that the child's distress came on suddenly as she lifted the boy by his raised arm to assist him over the curb. You suspect a relatively common condition known as "nursemaid's elbow" that results from

(A) separation of the ulna from its articulation with the trochlea of the humerus
(B) separation of the head of the radius from its articulation with the trochlea of the humerus
(C) separation of the head of the radius from its articulation with the capitulum of the humerus and from its articulation with the ulna
(D) stretching of the radial nerve as it passes behind the medial epicondyle of the humerus
(E) compression of the median nerve as it penetrates the supinator muscle

40. A tumor in the posterior mediastinum would most likely involve the

(A) recurrent laryngeal nerves
(B) tracheal bifurcation
(C) thoracic duct
(D) phrenic nerves
(E) left atrium

41. Damaged heart muscle resulting from occlusion of the circumflex branch of the left coronary artery would most likely be found in the

(A) left atrium and left ventricle
(B) right atrium and right ventricle
(C) apex
(D) right and left ventricles
(E) right ventricle and interventricular septum

42. A radiograph of the patient's abdomen indicates a blockage in an artery running from the epigastric region to the left hypochondriac region. The vessel most likely involved is the

(A) superior epigastric artery
(B) superior mesenteric artery
(C) inferior mesenteric artery
(D) renal artery
(E) splenic artery

43. A surgeon's finger placed into the epiploic foramen (of Winslow) will be related superiorly to the

(A) first part of the duodenum
(B) caudate lobe of the liver
(C) head of the pancreas
(D) common bile duct
(E) hepatic veins

44. Cancer of the testis would most likely metastasize first to which set of nodes?

(A) superficial inguinal
(B) deep inguinal
(C) aortic
(D) internal iliac
(E) common iliac

45. Derivatives of the hindgut are typically supplied by the

(A) celiac artery
(B) superior mesenteric artery
(C) inferior mesenteric artery
(D) ductus arteriosus
(E) umbilical artery

46. As you examine a newborn in the nursery, you notice an apparent oozing of fluid in the area of the umbilicus. You suspect that the leaking fluid is urine and is the result of

(A) an incomplete obliteration of the lumen of the allantois
(B) a persistent and patent vitelline duct
(C) an omphalocele
(D) gastroschisis
(E) an umbilical hernia

47. The long head of the biceps arises from which of the following structures?

(A) coracoid process
(B) radial tuberosity
(C) supraglenoid tubercle
(D) bicipital aponeurosis
(E) lesser tubercle of the humerus

48. A "claw hand" is usually associated with injury to which of the following nerves?

(A) median
(B) radial
(C) ulnar
(D) axillary
(E) musculocutaneous

49. Several days after your teenage male patient fell on his outstretched hand he reports increasing pain on movement of his wrist. Your examination reveals particular tenderness in the area of the anatomical snuffbox. Which of the carpal bones has most likely been injured?

(A) scaphoid
(B) pisiform
(C) hamate
(D) capitate
(E) lunate

50. Your patient in the emergency room has an obvious fracture of the mid-shaft of the humerus. You support his extremity as you work and notice that with the forearm in a horizontal position his wrist drops and he is unable to extend his wrist or the metacarpophalangeal joints of the hand. Which nerve has been injured?

(A) axillary
(B) musculocutaneous
(C) radial
(D) median
(E) ulnar

51. The outflow tract leading into the pulmonary trunk through the pulmonary orifice is known as the

(A) crista terminalis
(B) infundibulum
(C) crista supraventricularis
(D) limbus fossa ovalis
(E) ostium of the coronary sinus

52. Damage to the coracobrachialis muscle and to the nerve passing through it could reasonably be expected to produce

(A) weakened extension at the elbow
(B) weakened abduction at the shoulder
(C) weakened flexion at the shoulder
(D) diminished cutaneous sensation over the medial forearm
(E) diminished cutaneous sensation over the medial palm

53. As you examine a computed tomography (CT) scan through the transpyloric plane of your patient, you would reasonably expect to find the

(A) pancreas
(B) bifurcation of the abdominal aorta
(C) celiac trunk
(D) transverse colon
(E) esophagus

54. Which label in Figure 1–4 (A through E) indicates the nucleus of a primary spermatocyte in pachytene of the first meiotic division?

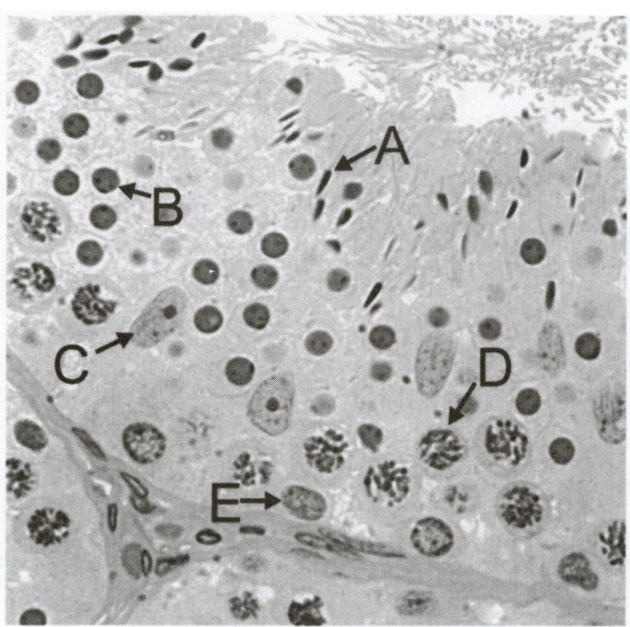

Figure 1–4

55. Which label in Figure 1–5 (A through E) indicates the tectorial membrane of the cochlea?

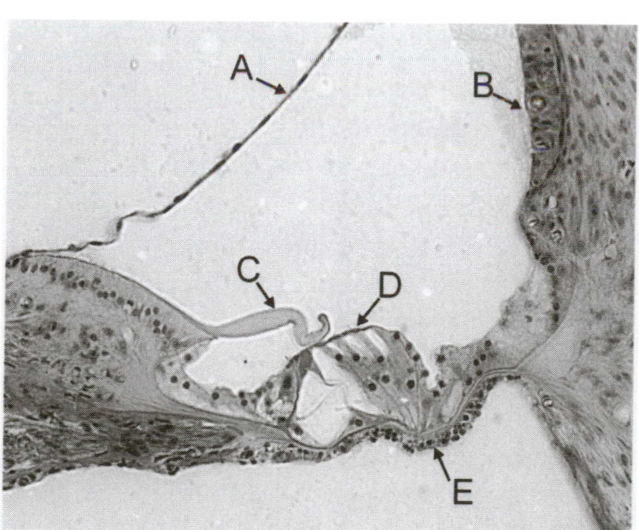

Figure 1–5

56. Which label in Figure 1–6 (A through E) indicates the typical plane of separation at which retinal detachment occurs?

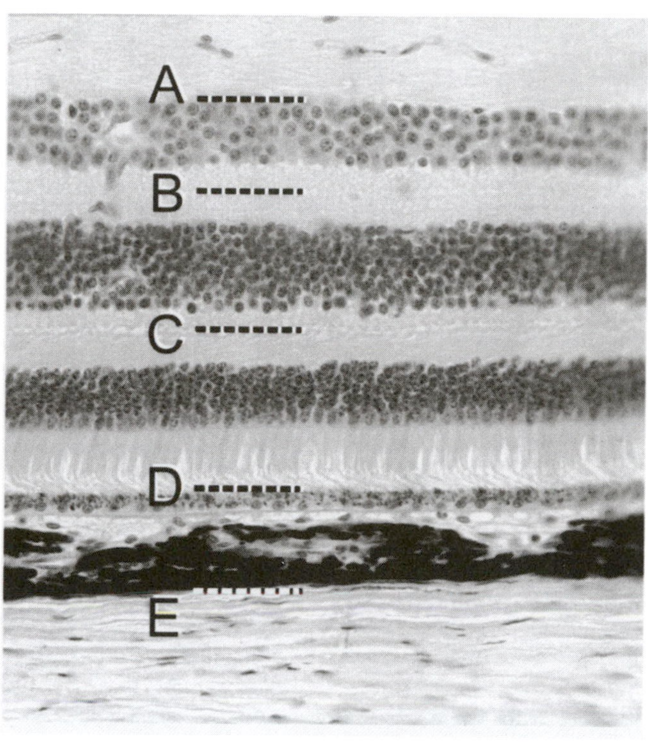

Figure 1–6

57. The principal natural targets of cytotoxic T cells are

(A) allogenic tissue transplants
(B) bacterial toxins
(C) virus-infected cells
(D) bacteria
(E) protozoans

58. Which of the following is derived from neuroectoderm of the optic cup?

(A) anterior iridal epithelium
(B) lens epithelium
(C) ciliary muscle
(D) choriocapillaris
(E) lateral rectus muscle

59. A woman has a menstrual cycle of 28 days' duration. At day 8 of her cycle, the dominant ovarian follicle contains

(A) an oogonium
(B) both a secondary oocyte and a polar body
(C) both a primary oocyte and a polar body
(D) a primary oocyte, but no polar body
(E) a secondary oocyte, but no polar body

60. Which normal cell type will be most severely affected by a chemotherapy regimen that includes an antimitotic drug such as vinblastine?

(A) intestinal epithelium
(B) epithelial cells of the lens
(C) neurons in dorsal root ganglia
(D) neurons of the cerebral cortex
(E) cardiac muscle cells

61. Which structure most effectively prevents toxic molecules from penetrating an epithelium by passing between adjacent epithelial cells?

(A) desmosome
(B) tight junction
(C) hemidesmosome
(D) gap junction
(E) terminal bar

62. Propagation of an action potential into the interior of a skeletal muscle fiber is a function of

(A) Z lines
(B) transverse (T) tubules
(C) muscle spindles
(D) the sarcoplasmic reticulum
(E) the endomysium

63. The macula densa, a component of the juxtaglomerular apparatus, is a specialization of

(A) mesangial cells
(B) the afferent arteriole
(C) Bowman's capsule
(D) the proximal tubule
(E) the distal tubule

64. Nuclei in the pars nervosa of the hypophysis predominantly belong to

(A) neurosecretory neurons
(B) basophils
(C) chromophobes
(D) pituicytes
(E) Schwann cells

65. Oxytocin is released from

(A) nerve terminals in the hypothalamus
(B) nerve terminals in the pars nervosa
(C) basophils in the pars distalis
(D) acidophils in the pars distalis
(E) pituicytes in the pars nervosa

66. Which of the following is characterized by an absence of lymphoid follicles and germinal centers?

(A) spleen
(B) axillary lymph node
(C) thymus
(D) Peyer's patch
(E) pharyngeal tonsil

67. Among the differences between thin skin and thick skin, a prominent distinction is the presence only in thin skin of

(A) hair follicles
(B) sweat glands
(C) dermal papillae
(D) stratum basale
(E) stratum spinosum

Questions 68 and 69

A 19-year-old black female is brought to the emergency room complaining of severe abdominal pain that began immediately after eating dinner. The physical examination reveals extreme tenderness in the lower right abdominal quadrant, but no abdominal masses are noted. Her temperature is 100°F. Among other tests, a complete blood count is ordered, with the following findings (normal ranges in parentheses):

Hematocrit	39% (36–46%)
Hemoglobin	14.9 g/dL (12.0–16.0 g/dL)
Total leukocyte count	24,000/mm^3 (4500–11,000/mm^3)

DIFFERENTIAL LEUKOCYTE COUNT:

Segmented neutrophils	71% (54–62%)
Band form neutrophils	16% (3–5%)
Eosinophils	4% (1–3%)
Basophils	0.2% (0–0.75%)
Lymphocytes	3% (25–33%)
Monocytes	6% (3–7%)

68. For which leukocytes is there an elevation above the normal range in absolute numbers per microliter of blood?

(A) only neutrophils
(B) only neutrophils and eosinophils
(C) only neutrophils, eosinophils, and monocytes
(D) only monocytes and lymphocytes
(E) only band form neutrophils

69. Which of the following conditions is most consistent with the laboratory findings?

(A) parasitic worm infection
(B) acute inflammation in response to bacterial infection
(C) severe allergic condition
(D) chronic lymphocytic leukemia
(E) sickle cell disease

70. The space of Disse in the liver

(A) is delimited entirely by hepatocytes
(B) contains formed elements of blood
(C) is bordered partly by microvilli of hepatocytes
(D) constitutes the initial channel for the flow of bile
(E) is a constituent of the portal triad

71. Production of specific granules occurs mainly during which stage of granulocyte development?

(A) myeloblast
(B) promyelocyte
(C) myelocyte
(D) metamyelocyte
(E) granulocyte-colony–forming unit

72. The acidophilic staining of the cytoplasm of gastric parietal (oxyntic) cells is most likely attributable to their high content of

(A) hydrochloric acid
(B) secretory granules containing intrinsic factor
(C) secretory granules containing pepsinogen
(D) rough endoplasmic reticulum
(E) mitochondria

73. Fenestrated capillaries are characteristic of

(A) the cerebral cortex
(B) skeletal muscle
(C) the renal glomerulus
(D) the splenic red pulp
(E) the epidermis

74. In the placenta, maternal blood comes in direct contact with

(A) the syncytiotrophoblast
(B) the cytotrophoblast
(C) endothelial cells of fetal capillaries
(D) connective tissue cells of secondary villi
(E) no fetally derived cells

75. Serous cells are glandular acinar cells that produce a watery, proteinaceous fluid. This cell type is most predominant in

(A) the submandibular gland
(B) the sublingual gland
(C) the parotid gland
(D) esophageal glands
(E) intestinal glands (of Lieberkün)

76. A researcher wishes to examine the role of gastric cells in the absorption of vitamin B_{12}. A relevant initial experiment could be use of immunostaining to verify that

(A) chief cells are stained using a primary antibody against pepsinogen
(B) chief cells are stained using a primary antibody against lipase
(C) parietal cells are stained using a primary antibody against intrinsic factor
(D) enteroendocrine cells are stained using a primary antibody against gastrin
(E) Paneth cells are stained using a primary antibody against lysozyme

77. Which of the following structures is located within the epidural space?

(A) external vertebral venous plexus
(B) internal vertebral venous plexus
(C) anterior spinal artery
(D) posterior spinal arteries
(E) middle cerebral artery

78. The glossopharyngeal nerve provides the parasympathetic innervation of the

(A) lacrimal gland
(B) submandibular salivary gland
(C) sublingual salivary gland
(D) parotid salivary gland
(E) nasal mucus glands

79. The epithelium illustrated in the photomicrograph in Figure 1–7 is characteristic of the lining of the

(A) esophagus
(B) colon
(C) aorta
(D) urinary bladder
(E) trachea

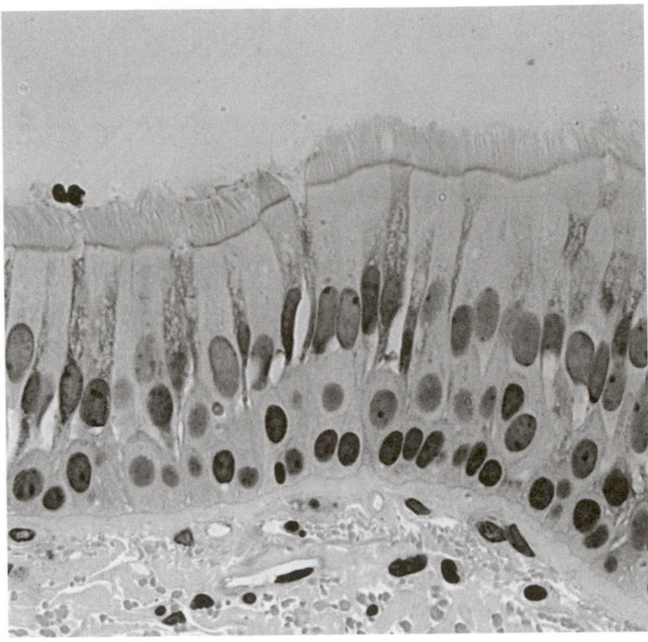

Figure 1–7

80. The photomicrograph in Figure 1–8 depicts a gland (crypt) of Lieberkühn in the ileum. What cell type is indicated by the arrow?

(A) goblet cell
(B) Paneth cell
(C) absorptive cell (enterocyte)
(D) enteroendocrine (DNES) cell
(E) stem cell

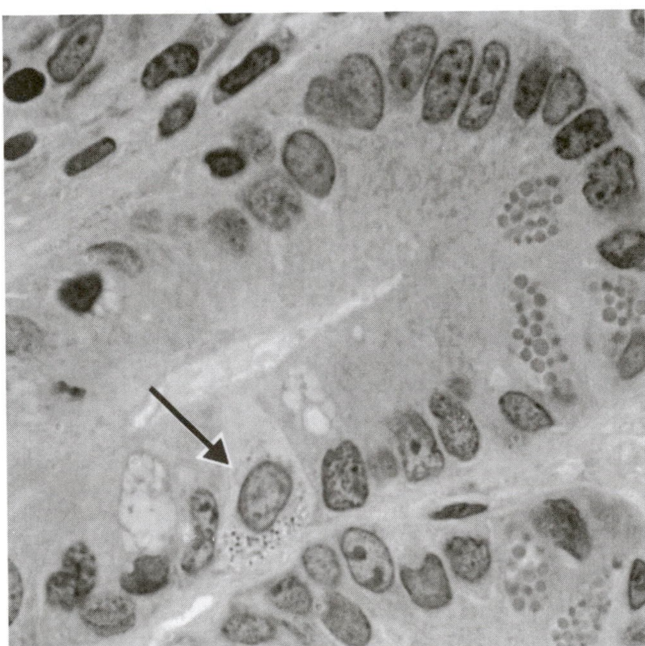

Figure 1–8

81. The photomicrograph in Figure 1–9 illustrates a section of

(A) dorsal root ganglion
(B) superior cervical ganglion
(C) pterygopalatine ganglion
(D) peripheral nerve
(E) cerebellar cortex

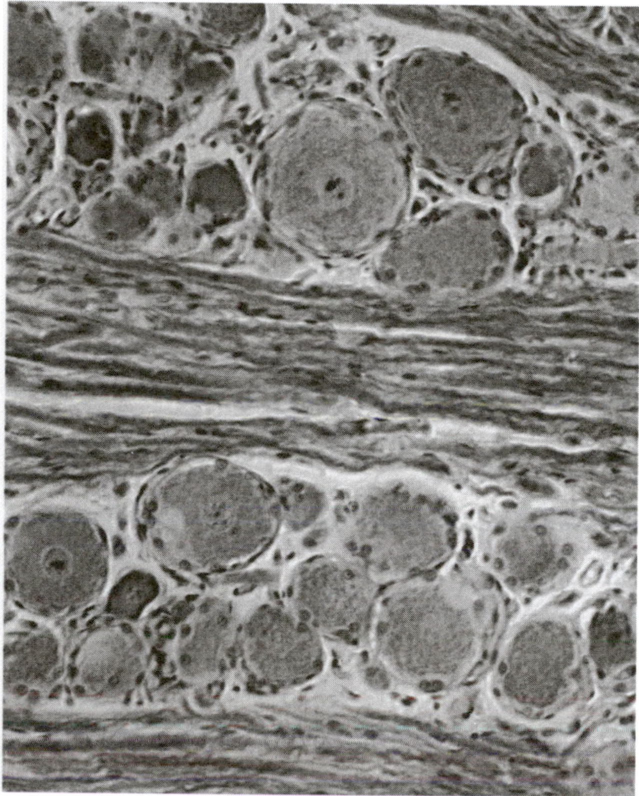

Figure 1–9

82. The dark spaces indicated by the arrows in Figure 1–10 are normally occupied by

(A) osteoclasts
(B) osteoblasts
(C) osteocytes
(D) blood vessels
(E) differentiating blood cell precursors

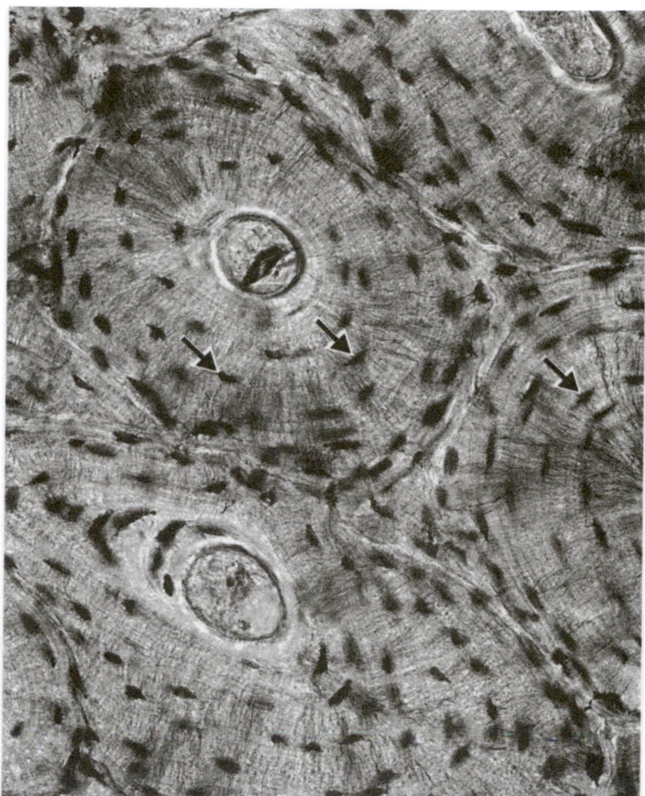

Figure 1–10

83. Which of the following muscles is innervated by the facial nerve?

(A) lateral pterygoid
(B) masseter
(C) buccinator
(D) anterior belly of the digastric
(E) temporalis

84. Which of the following statements concerning the control of reflexive ocular movements is correct?

(A) Signals originating in the right eye are directed only to the right pretectal region.
(B) Neurons in the left Edinger–Westphal nucleus receive input only from the right eye.
(C) Dilation of the pupil is the result of signals transmitted by postganglionic neurons in the ciliary ganglion.
(D) The near response or "near triad" involves activation of the ciliary, sphincter pupillae, and medial rectus muscles.
(E) The blink reflex involves the oculomotor and trigeminal cranial nerves.

85. The cell bodies of origin (first-order neurons) for the ascending somatosensory signals that reach consciousness are located in

(A) dorsal root ganglia
(B) dorsal horn of the spinal cord
(C) dorsal primary rami
(D) nucleus gracilis and cuneatus
(E) nucleus dorsalis (of Clarke)

86. The axon of the second-order neuron in the pathway for conscious awareness of fine, discriminative touch and vibratory sensation from the upper limb

(A) has its cell body in the nucleus gracilis
(B) decussates in the ventral white commissure of the spinal cord
(C) ascends the brainstem in the medial lemniscus
(D) terminates in the nucleus cuneatus
(E) all of the above are correct

87. Pathways for the conscious awareness of somatosensory signals

(A) terminate in the precentral gyrus
(B) pass through the posterior limb of the internal capsule
(C) decussate at the level of the thalamus
(D) typically involve a two-neuron sequence from receptor to cortex
(E) pass through the ventral lateral nucleus of the thalamus

88. Choose the correct statement.

(A) The lateral vestibulospinal tract originates from the medial vestibular nucleus.
(B) The medial vestibulospinal tract descends to lumbar levels of the spinal cord.
(C) The lateral vestibulospinal tract primarily influences flexor musculature.
(D) The ascending portion of the medial longitudinal fasciculus (MLF) gives off axons that terminate in the ipsilateral oculomotor nucleus.
(E) The descending portion of the medial longitudinal fasciculus (medial vestibulospinal tract) provides the vestibular system with control over extraocular musculature.

89. Ocular movements termed nystagmus

(A) are unlikely to be induced in a patient with bilateral damage in the pontine and medullary levels of the brainstem
(B) cannot be induced by caloric stimulation in a normal, conscious patient
(C) are named for the direction of the slow phase of movement
(D) when observed in a patient following caloric stimulation indicate the presence of a lesion involving some portion of the vestibular system
(E) are only observed in reference to horizontal eye movements

90. Increased excitation (depolarization) of the sensory hair cells of the crista ampullaris of the horizontal semicircular canal occurs when their stereocilia

(A) bend toward the utricle (midline)
(B) bend away from the utricle
(C) bend in any direction
(D) are motionless in a vertical position
(E) are detached from the kinocilium

91. The accommodation–convergence reflex (near response) differs from the pupillary light reflex in that it (accommodation–convergence) involves

(A) conjugate eye movements
(B) bilateral activation of lateral rectus motoneurons
(C) only the optic nerve
(D) only the oculomotor nerve
(E) the primary visual cortex

92. You are about to remove a small lesion from the mucosa of the laryngeal vestibule and want to anesthetize the nerve that supplies general sensation to the mucous membrane of that area. The nerve you are interested in is the

(A) external laryngeal nerve
(B) inferior laryngeal nerve
(C) glossopharyngeal nerve
(D) pharyngeal plexus
(E) internal laryngeal nerve

93. Which of the following statements is correct?

(A) Intrinsic spinal cord circuits can produce coordinated movement of all four extremities.
(B) Type Ia sensory fibers primarily form synapses with inhibitory interneurons and only a relatively small number of alpha motoneurons.
(C) Type Ib sensory fibers primarily form synapses with alpha motoneurons and only a relatively small number of inhibitory interneurons.
(D) Type C pain fibers do not form synapses with spinal cord interneurons.
(E) Golgi tendon organ activation excites the muscle to which it is structurally related.

94. Which statement concerning a motor unit is true?

(A) Each motor unit includes one alpha and one gamma motoneuron for each muscle fiber.
(B) A motor unit includes one alpha motoneuron and all the muscle fibers it innervates.
(C) A motor unit includes all the sensory and motor fibers that distribute to a single muscle.
(D) The smallest motor units include motoneurons with the largest cell bodies.
(E) The motor units of the extraocular muscles are among the largest (one motoneuron to hundreds of muscle fibers) in the neuromuscular system.

95. Which of the following histological or cytological features are characteristic of the basal ganglia?

(A) striosomes or patches
(B) pyramidal neurons
(C) glomeruli
(D) Renshaw cells
(E) callosal neurons

96. The efferent limb of the pupillary light reflex is interrupted along with corticospinal and corticobulbar fibers in which of the following clinical entities?

(A) superior alternating hemiplegia
(B) middle alternating hemiplegia
(C) inferior alternating hemiplegia
(D) Broca's aphasia
(E) Wallenberg's syndrome

97. Horner's syndrome is sometimes seen in patients diagnosed with the lateral medullary syndrome. Which of the following is a characteristic feature of Horner's syndrome?

(A) mydriasis
(B) profuse sweating
(C) red blushing of the skin in the affected area
(D) atrophy of tongue musculature
(E) paralysis of muscles of facial expression

98. During development of the central nervous system, the neural crest contributes cells to

(A) cranial nerve and dorsal root ganglia
(B) the cerebellum
(C) the retina
(D) the vestibular and cochlear nuclei
(E) ventral horn motoneurons

99. A large lesion involving the ventrolateral portion of the parietal lobe in the dominant hemisphere will result in

(A) Wernicke's aphasia
(B) Broca's aphasia
(C) contralateral hemineglect
(D) motor aprosodia
(E) prosopagnosia

100. With regard to the basal ganglia, which statement is correct?

(A) Patients with intention (action) tremor are likely to have degeneration of neurons in the substantia nigra.
(B) The thalamic fasciculus is primarily composed of axons that arise from cells in the subthalamic nucleus.
(C) The ansa lenticularis is primarily composed of axons that arise from cells in the globus pallidus.
(D) Most of the neurons in the pars reticulata of the substantia nigra use dopamine as a neurotransmitter agent.
(E) The term *lenticular nucleus* refers to the combination of the caudate nucleus and putamen.

101. A large vascular infarct involving the posterior limb of the internal capsule on the right side is likely to produce which of the following deficits?

(A) spastic hemiplegia involving the right side of the body
(B) deviation of the protruded tongue to the right
(C) hypertonia and hyperreflexia in the right upper limb
(D) paralysis of facial expression muscles on the lower left portion of face
(E) paraplegia involving the lower extremities

102. Which of the statements below concerning the primary somatosensory cortex (SI) is correct?

(A) Cytoarchitectural subdivisions of SI are numbered anterior to posterior as 3a, 3b, 1, and 2.
(B) A complete representation of the body surface is found only in cytoarchitectural subdivision 3b of SI cortex.
(C) The somatotopic representation of the body surface in SI is arranged in a classic "tail to tongue" sequence from ventrolateral to dorsomedial.
(D) Areas 3a and 2 receive their major input from cutaneous receptors.
(E) Areas 3b and 1 receive their major input from muscle spindle afferents and Golgi tendon organs.

103. Which of the following events is associated with vesicular release of neurotransmitter?

(A) Activation of voltage-gated Ca^{++} channels allows calcium to enter the axon terminal.
(B) "Docking proteins" are present and attach vesicles to mitochondrial membranes.
(C) Fusion of vesicles with the presynaptic membrane allows 10 quanta of neurotransmitter to be released into the synaptic cleft.
(D) Movement of neurotransmitter occurs along actin "bridges" which structurally join the pre- and postsynaptic membranes.
(E) Binding of neurotransmitter molecules to receptors on the presynaptic membrane follows vesicular release.

104. Which of the following statements concerning muscle spindles is correct?

(A) Only one type of intrafusal muscle fiber (cell) is present in most muscle spindles.
(B) Each intrafusal fiber is innervated by two different gamma motoneurons.
(C) Type Ia sensory fibers from a spindle form direct synaptic contact with alpha motoneurons in the spinal cord.
(D) Activation of type Ia sensory fibers from a given spindle leads to inhibition of the muscle in which that spindle is located.
(E) Alpha motoneurons synapse directly with intrafusal muscle fibers.

105. Which of the following is characteristic of damage to the corticospinal (pyramidal) system?

(A) flaccid paralysis and hypotonia
(B) Babinski sign
(C) loss of deep tendon reflexes

(D) immediate muscle degeneration and atrophy
(E) intention tremor

106. Which of the following is a characteristic feature of spastic paralysis?

(A) It usually involves paravertebral postural muscles most severely.
(B) The affected muscles are hypotonic.
(C) The affected muscles exhibit fibrillations and fasciculations.
(D) It is observed as an increase in the resistance to passive movement.
(E) The affected muscles exhibit decreased (hypoactive) deep tendon reflexes.

107. Which of the following signs or symptoms is associated with basal ganglia lesions?

(A) paralysis of antigravity muscles in the limbs on one side of the body
(B) muscles that exhibit a total absence of stretch reflexes
(C) ataxia and scanning speech
(D) athetosis
(E) horizontal nystagmus

108. Which of the following is directly involved with the descending modulation of pain transmission?

(A) ventral lateral thalamic nucleus
(B) medial longitudinal fasciculus
(C) nucleus raphe magnus
(D) rubrospinal fibers
(E) dopamine

109. Which of the following statements concerning taste receptors is correct?

(A) Each receptor responds best to one stimulus quality (i.e., sweet, salty, sour, bitter) but also responds less vigorously to other stimulus qualities.
(B) The receptors are arranged in a medial to lateral pattern on the tongue such that the most lateral respond best to sweet and salty stimuli.
(C) Taste receptors have a life span of approximately 3 months.
(D) Taste receptors are stimulated when a food or fluid substance diffuses through the apical pore and hyperpolarizes the cell.
(E) Taste receptors are most numerous on the sides of the tongue.

110. Your patient is unable to dorsiflex and evert his right foot. The nerve most likely damaged is the

(A) common peroneal nerve
(B) superficial peroneal nerve
(C) deep peroneal nerve
(D) tibial nerve
(E) obturator nerve

111. The nerve most likely to be injured by a fracture of the neck of the fibula is the

(A) sural nerve
(B) tibial nerve
(C) common fibular nerve
(D) deep fibular nerve
(E) femoral nerve

112. An examination of your patient's injured knee reveals excessive posterior movement of the tibia on the femur. The chief ligament preventing posterior sliding of the tibia on the femur is the

(A) tibial collateral ligament
(B) fibular collateral ligament
(C) oblique popliteal ligament
(D) anterior cruciate ligament
(E) posterior cruciate ligament

113. A failure of the truncoconal septum to follow a spiral course results in

(A) persistent truncus arteriosus
(B) tetralogy of Fallot
(C) transportation of the great vessels
(D) persistent atrioventricular canal
(E) common atrium

114. The horizontal fissure and the inferior part of the oblique fissure form the boundaries of which of the following?

(A) apex of the left lung
(B) lingula of the left lung
(C) middle lobe of the right lung
(D) upper lobe of the right lung
(E) lower lobe of the left lung

115. The bulbourethral glands of the male are embedded in the fibers of the

(A) sphincter urethrae muscle
(B) ischiocavernosus muscles
(C) superficial transverse perineal muscles
(D) bulbospongiosus muscles
(E) corpora cavernosa

116. The digastric muscle is a two-bellied muscle that forms two sides of the submandibular triangle of the neck. The two bellies attach by an intermediate tendon to the

(A) sixth cervical vertebra
(B) mandible
(C) mastoid process
(D) cricoid cartilage
(E) hyoid bone

117. Your patient requires an intravenous infusion and you have determined that the veins of the arms and hands are no longer suitable for this purpose. You observe a large neck vein that appears to be crossing perpendicularly the superficial surface of the sternocleidomastoid muscle and decide to cannulate it. This is the

(A) retromandibular vein
(B) anterior jugular vein
(C) posterior auricular vein
(D) external jugular vein
(E) internal jugular vein

118. Which of the following structures is located within the prevertebral layer of cervical fascia?

(A) vagus nerve
(B) common carotid artery
(C) internal jugular vein
(D) esophagus
(E) middle scalene muscle

119. As an endocrine gland, the thyroid gland has a rich blood supply, receiving vessels derived directly or indirectly from the subclavian artery, the external carotid artery, and occasionally from the brachiocephalic trunk or the arch of the aorta. The superior thyroid artery is usually the first branch of the

(A) thyrocervical trunk
(B) internal carotid artery
(C) external carotid artery
(D) facial artery
(E) brachiocephalic trunk

120. Your patient is in respiratory distress and cannot be intubated. As you prepare to create an artificial airway in the midline, you are concerned about damaging the isthmus of the highly vascular thyroid gland. You move with confidence as you recall that in the midline the isthmus of the thyroid gland covers the

(A) cricoid cartilage
(B) second, third, and fourth tracheal rings
(C) jugular notch
(D) thyroid cartilage
(E) hyoid bone

Questions 121 and 122

Your patient presented in your office complaining of hoarseness. During your examination you find that one vocal fold has deviated toward the midline and does not abduct during deep inspiration or vocalization. You also observe that touch sensation in the vestibule of the larynx appears to be intact.

121. Which laryngeal muscle is most important in abduction of the vocal folds?

(A) cricothyroid muscle
(B) posterior cricoarytenoid muscle
(C) thyroarytenoid muscle
(D) transverse arytenoid muscle
(E) lateral cricoarytenoid muscle

122. You suspect that a nerve has been damaged, but which nerve is most likely involved?

(A) superior laryngeal nerve
(B) inferior laryngeal nerve
(C) external laryngeal nerve
(D) internal laryngeal nerve
(E) glossopharyngeal nerve

123. Which of the following arteries commonly passes between the two roots of the auriculotemporal nerve?

(A) inferior alveolar artery
(B) middle meningeal artery
(C) infraorbital artery
(D) masseteric artery
(E) sphenopalatine artery

Questions 124 through 126

Your patient reports that several days earlier he "threw his back out" when he bent from the waist and picked up a very heavy package. The pain was immediate and extended from his hip, down the back of the thigh, and into his leg and foot. As he lies on the examining table, you raise his leg by the foot keeping the knee extended and elicit intense pain over the distribution of the sciatic nerve. A magnetic resonance imaging (MRI) scan confirms your conclusion that your patient has a herniated intervertebral disc between the fourth and fifth lumbar vertebrae.

124. Intervertebral discs may protrude or rupture in any direction, but they most commonly protrude in which direction?

(A) anteriorly
(B) posteriorly
(C) anterolaterally
(D) posterolaterally
(E) laterally

125. Herniation of the intervertebral disc between the fourth and fifth lumbar vertebrae would most likely impinge on the roots of which spinal nerve?

(A) L3
(B) L4
(C) L5
(D) S1
(E) S2

126. In examining this patient you also make note of a mild lateral curvature of the spine. Which of the following is commonly associated with a lateral curvature of the vertebral column?

(A) kyphosis
(B) ruptured disc
(C) scoliosis
(D) lordosis
(E) "gorilla" rib

127. Which of the following structures crosses the posterior surfaces of the obturator internus, the gemelli, and the quadratus femoris muscles?

(A) femoral artery
(B) common iliac veins
(C) obturator nerve
(D) sciatic nerve
(E) superior gluteal nerve and artery

128. Your young female patient has a large bulge on the anterior thigh below the inguinal ligament. You suspect an abdominal hernia that has passed through the femoral ring into the femoral sheath and then through the saphenous hiatus into the subcutaneous layer of the upper thigh. In addition to the hernial sac, you would expect the femoral canal to contain the

(A) femoral artery
(B) femoral vein
(C) femoral nerve
(D) connective tissue and lymph nodes
(E) great saphenous vein

129. The most anterior structure passing under the flexor retinaculum of the foot is the

(A) tendon of the peroneus longus muscle
(B) tendon of the tibialis posterior muscle
(C) tendon of the flexor digitorum longus muscle
(D) tendon of the flexor hallucis longus muscle
(E) tibial nerve

130. Careful study of this posteroanterior radiograph of the thorax (Figure 1–11) revealed two interesting contours marked with arrows A and B. Both were determined to be normal, but what is the feature marked A?

(A) ascending aorta
(B) descending aorta
(C) arch of the aorta
(D) pulmonary trunk
(E) superior vena cava

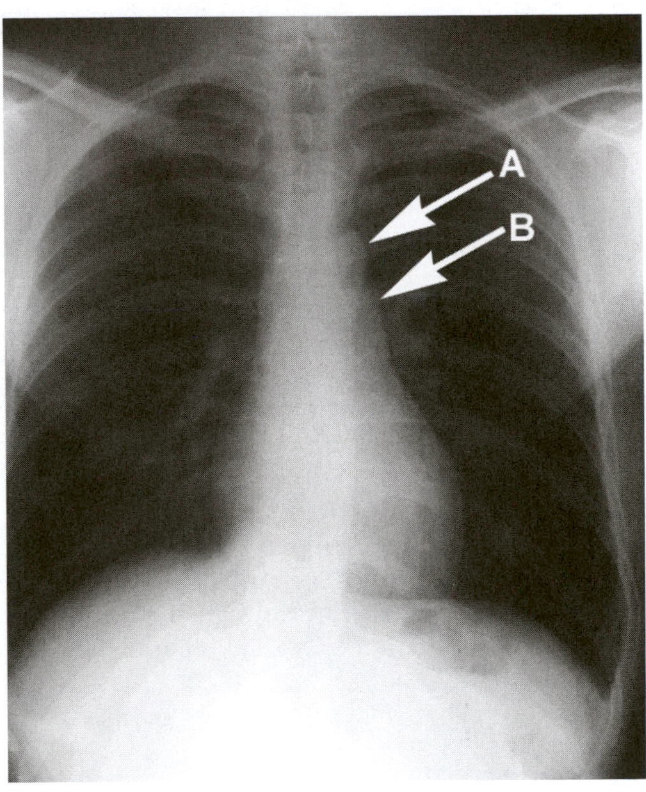

Figure 1–11

131. In examining radiographs of your patient's chest you notice that the contents of the middle mediastinum appear to be deviated to the right side. Which of the following structures is located within the middle mediastinum?

(A) trachea
(B) heart
(C) thymus
(D) aortic arch
(E) esophagus

132. You are concerned that your patient may have compromised function of the mitral valve. The sound of the mitral valve is best heard

(A) in the fifth intercostal space to the right of the sternum
(B) at the apex in the left fifth intercostal space in the midclavicular line
(C) in the second intercostal space to the left of the sternum
(D) at the xiphisternal junction
(E) in the second intercostal space to the left of the sternum

133. While performing surgery, you mobilize the duodenum and the head of the pancreas reflecting them to the left. Which of the following would you normally expect to find passing behind the first part of the duodenum?

(A) splenic artery
(B) common hepatic artery
(C) common hepatic duct
(D) superior mesenteric artery
(E) portal vein

134. Which of the following structures is located in the posterior interventricular sulcus?

(A) middle cardiac vein
(B) small cardiac vein
(C) coronary sinus
(D) oblique vein of the left atrium
(E) great cardiac vein

135. Cutaneous branches of the maxillary division of the trigeminal nerve include the

(A) supratrochlear
(B) infraorbital
(C) mental
(D) lacrimal
(E) supraorbital

136. Secretion of pulmonary surfactant is a function of

(A) alveolar dust cells
(B) endothelial cells of capillaries in the alveolar septum
(C) small granule cells
(D) type I pneumocytes (squamous alveolar cells)
(E) type II pneumocytes (greater alveolar cells)

137. Which blood cell differentiates in a site other than the bone marrow?

(A) B lymphocyte
(B) T lymphocyte
(C) neutrophil
(D) basophil
(E) eosinophil

138. The cytoplasm of a typical acinar secretory cell in the pancreas contains

(A) numerous lipid droplets
(B) abundant smooth endoplasmic reticulum (sER)
(C) mitochondria with tubular cristae
(D) abundant secretory granules at the cell apex
(E) a poorly developed Golgi complex

139. Which of the following is a mixed cranial nerve that includes axons with special visceral efferent, general visceral efferent, general visceral afferent, special visceral afferent, and general somatic afferent functions?

(A) oculomotor
(B) trigeminal
(C) abducens
(D) vagus
(E) hypoglossal

140. Which step in gamete development has a duration of about three weeks in spermatogenesis and many years in oogenesis?

(A) migration of primordial germ cells from yolk sac to gonad
(B) mitotic division of oogonia or spermatogonia
(C) final S phase preceding meiosis
(D) first meiotic division (including prophase)
(E) second meiotic division (including all its phases)

141. In routine H&E staining of tissue sections, the hematoxylin component of the stain mixture binds most avidly to

(A) Golgi complexes
(B) smooth endoplasmic reticulum
(C) ribosomes
(D) elastic fibers
(E) collagenous fibers

142. The presence in the plasmalemma of numerous receptors for the Fc portion of immunoglobulin E molecules is characteristic of

(A) neutrophils
(B) basophils and mast cells
(C) monocytes and macrophages
(D) B lymphocytes
(E) platelets

143. Some fertility problems can be aided by procedures that require mixing of spermatozoa and ova in vitro in order to achieve fertilization. Strategies to optimize success in retrieving mature oocytes from the ovaries of a woman include the daily administration of both gonadotropins and gonadotropin-releasing hormone (GnRH) during the first half of the menstrual cycle. The daily doses of GnRH would be expected to

(A) promote an LH (luteinizing hormone) surge
(B) directly stimulate development of ovarian follicles
(C) shut down the normal secretory activity of pituitary gonadotropic cells
(D) induce the second meiotic division by secondary oocytes
(E) directly stimulate the proliferative phase of the endometrium

144. General visceral efferent (autonomic) axons from cell bodies in the thoracic spinal cord terminate on

(A) smooth muscle cells in the wall of the stomach
(B) parasympathetic ganglion neurons in the wall of the stomach
(C) secretory cells in the submandibular salivary gland
(D) neurons in dorsal root ganglia
(E) neurons in sympathetic ganglia of the sympathetic trunk

145. The root of a tooth is anchored in its bony socket by

(A) odontoblast processes
(B) dentinal tubules
(C) the stellate reticulum
(D) fibers of the periodontal ligament
(E) the subodontoblastic plexus of Rashkow

146. Lymph nodes are populated by lymphocytes that exit the vascular compartment to gain access to the parenchyma of the node by passing through the walls of

(A) arterioles
(B) afferent lymphatic vessels
(C) efferent lymphatic vessels
(D) medullary sinuses
(E) high endothelial postcapillary venules

147. Myelination of large-caliber axons in peripheral nerves is a function of

(A) oligodendroglial cells (oligodendrocytes)
(B) Schwann cells
(C) fibroblasts
(D) perineurial cells
(E) astrocytes

148. In Figure 1–12, which labeled bracket (A through E) spans a sarcomere?

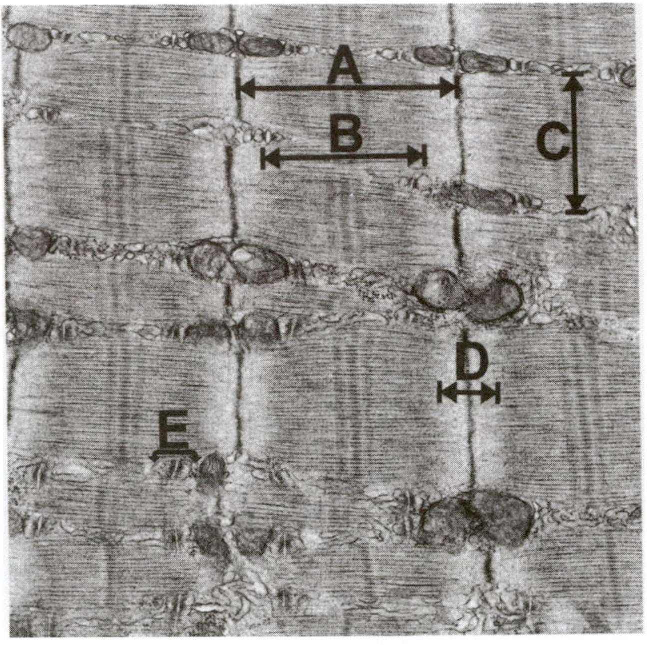

Figure 1–12

149. The vessel in the electron micrograph in Figure 1–13 is best classified as

(A) a continuous capillary
(B) a discontinuous capillary
(C) a fenestrated capillary
(D) a medium vein
(E) an arteriole

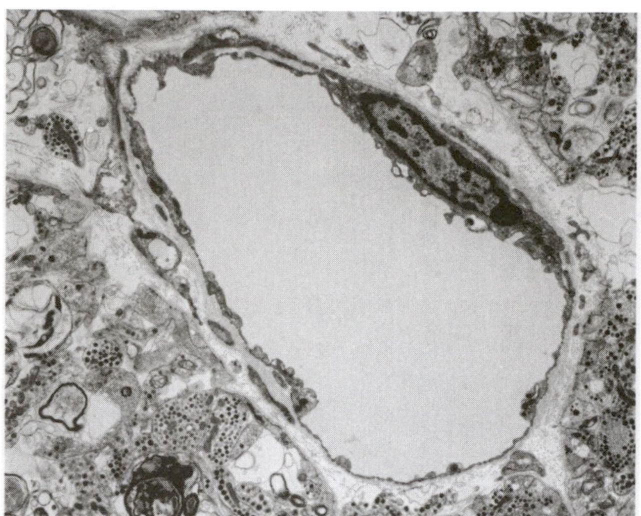

Figure 1–13

150. Which letter in the electron micrograph in Figure 1–14 indicates the structure that is seen as an intercalated disk in light microscopy?

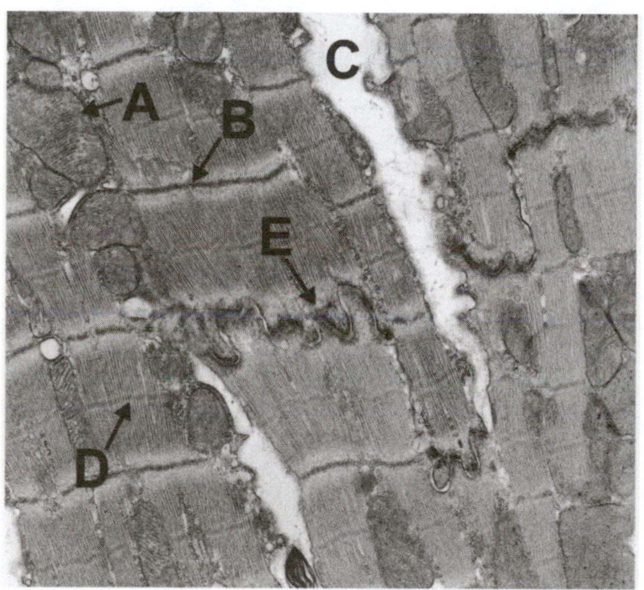

Figure 1–14

151. In the electron micrograph of a renal corpuscle in Figure 1–15, which letter (A through E) is located within the urinary space?

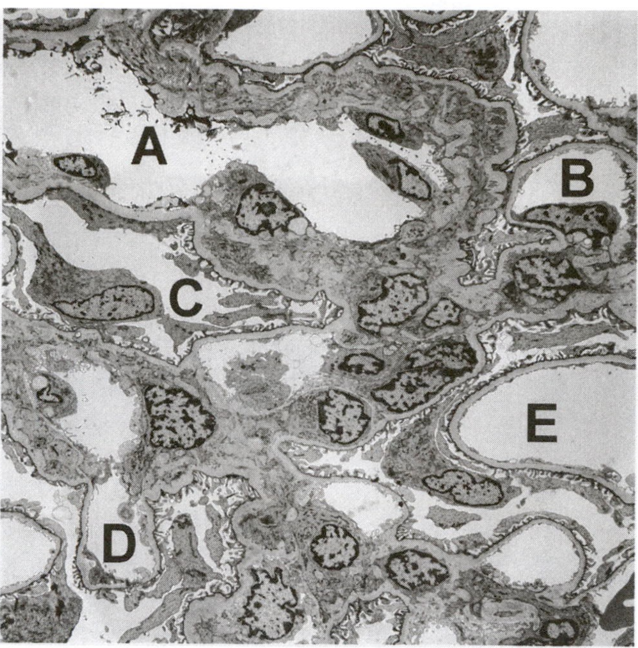

Figure 1–15

152. Which label in Figure 1–16 indicates profiles of smooth endoplasmic reticulum in this electron micrograph of an adrenal cortical cell?

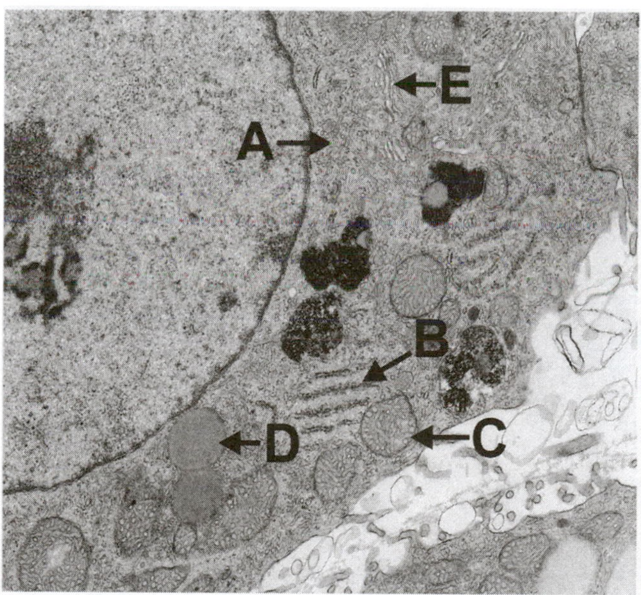

Figure 1–16

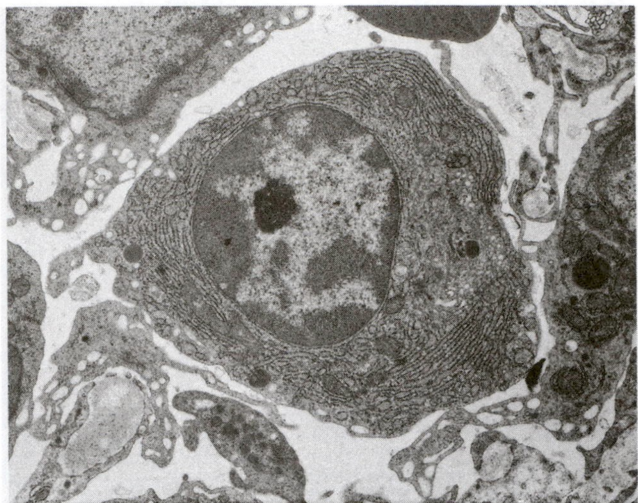

Figure 1–17

153. The electron micrograph in Figure 1–17 illustrates a

(A) lymphocyte
(B) plasma cell
(C) neutrophil
(D) basophil
(E) platelet

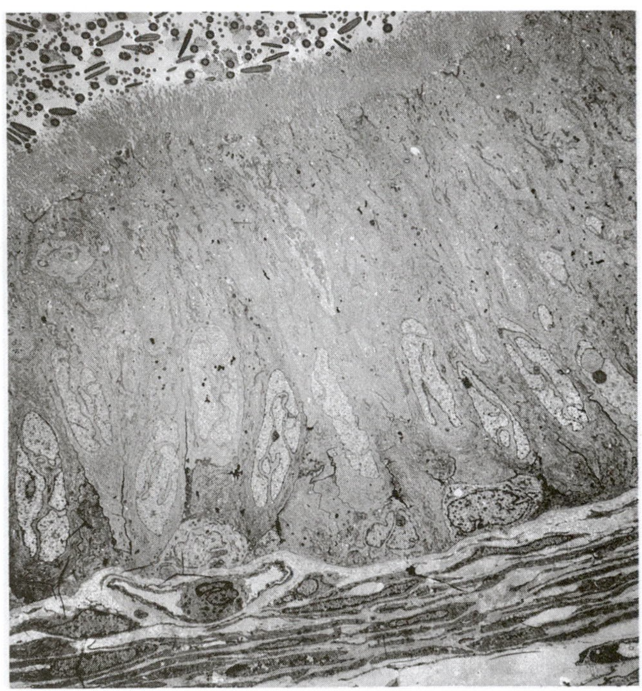

Figure 1–18

154. The epithelium in the electron micrograph in Figure 1–18 is characteristic of the lining of the

(A) esophagus
(B) small intestine
(C) trachea
(D) seminiferous tubule
(E) epididymal duct

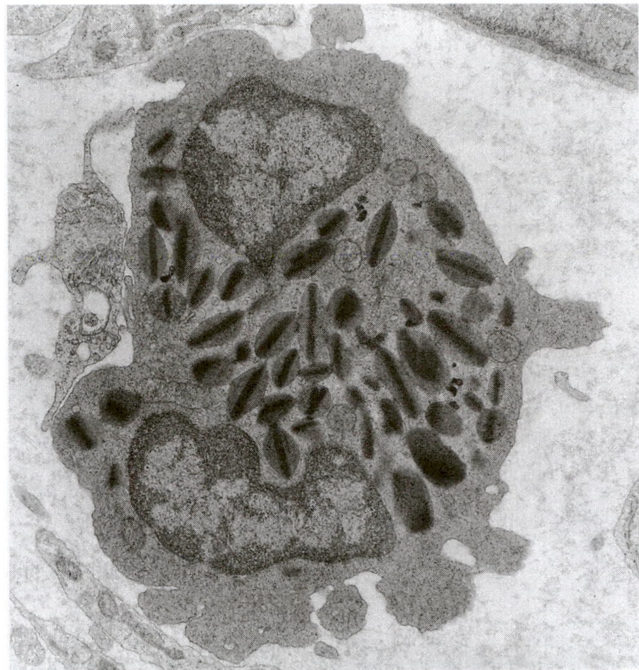

Figure 1–19

155. The leukocyte shown in the electron micrograph in Figure 1–19 is

(A) a lymphocyte
(B) a monocyte
(C) a neutrophil
(D) an eosinophil
(E) a basophil

Answers and Explanations

1. **(E)** All of the indicated brain regions or cell groups participate in smooth pursuit movements. The object to be tracked is first imaged on the fovea (choice A) and the signal is transmitted in sequence along the primary optic pathway from retina to dorsal lateral geniculate nucleus (choice B), to primary visual cortex (choice C). From the latter cortex, signals are eventually transmitted to the frontal eye field (choice D) and then sent downstream to the vestibulocerebellum.

2. **(A)** Traumatic lesions or compression of the left oculomotor nerve (choice A) will result in loss of parasympathetic innervation to the sphincter pupillae muscle and lead to mydriasis (dilation of pupil) along with lateral and downward deviation of the ipsilateral eye due to weakness in all ocular muscles innervated by the left third cranial nerve. Damage to the right trochlear nerve (choice B) would denervate the right superior oblique muscle and have no effect on the left eye. Compression of the left abducens nerve (choice C) would cause the left eye to be medially deviated and would not affect the sphincter pupillae muscle. Damage to the left trigeminal nerve (choice D) or the left facial nerve (choice E) would have no effect on ocular motility or the sphincter pupillae of the left eye.

3. **(C)** These are the classic signs of uncal herniation which involves compression of the third cranial nerve and the adjacent cerebral peduncle and its contingent of corticospinal fibers. This combination of symptoms is referred to as superior alternating hemiplegia and includes cranial nerve signs ipsilateral to the lesion and contralateral hemiplegia resulting from corticospinal tract involvement rostral to the pyramidal decussation. The combination of corticospinal tract involvement and damage to the VIth cranial nerve is classified as middle alternating hemiplegia (choice D), while inferior alternating hemiplegia combines hypoglossal nerve (XII) damage with corticospinal tract involvement. Wallenberg's syndrome (choice A) and syringomyelia (choice E) are primarily sensory disorders that involve a loss of pain sensation. Capsular hemiplegia (choice B) results in contralateral hemiplegia and corticobulbar signs (upper motor neuron cranial nerve signs) and is not associated with lower motor neuron signs of cranial nerve dysfunction.

4. **(B)** The lateral geniculate nucleus (LGN) of one side receives retinal input from both the ipsilateral and the contralateral eyes (choice B). It contains projection neurons whose axons synapse primarily in layer IV of the ipsilateral and not the contralateral (choice A) striate cortex. Projection neurons of the LGN can be either large (magnocellular) or small and are not entirely parvocellular (choice C). The axons of LGN projection neurons do not enter the optic tract (choice D) but rather course through the retrolenticular portion of the internal capsule to reach the striate cortex. The LGN does not receive parasympathetic innervation (choice E).

5. **(E)** Photons that pass through the lens eventually strike the photoreceptors after

passing through all of the intervening layers of the retina (choice A). In the absence of photic stimulation (darkness) the photoreceptors are depolarized as a result of dark current and are therefore continuously releasing neurotransmitter in the dark (choice B). The optic disc is located nasally with respect to the macula (choice C). Horizontal cells in the retina do form synapses with the synaptic portion (rod spherules or cone pedicles) of the photoreceptor cells (choice D).

6. **(A)** During early histogenesis in the cerebral hemisphere and elsewhere in the developing brain, germinal or matrix cells undergo cell division in the ventricular zone, the region that abuts the luminal space (future ventricular space) of the neural tube. Later, these cells lose their ability to divide and migrate laterally toward the perimeter of the neural tube where they accumulate as neuroblasts and form the mantle layer (choice B). As development proceeds, the sulcus limitans forms as a groove in the wall of the neural tube, and cells in the dorsal portion of the mantle layer give rise to the alar plate (choice C) and become associated with sensory functions. Cells ventral to this groove form the basal plate and eventually give rise to motor neurons. Cells that undergo mitosis are normally not found at the pial surface (choice D), nor are they evenly distributed throughout the thickness of the developing neural tube (choice E).

7. **(B)** Axons of Purkinje neurons use GABA as a neurotransmitter. Glutamate (choice A), acetylcholine (choice C), serotonin (choice D), and glycine (choice E) are neurotransmitters used by other types of neurons throughout the nervous system.

8. **(B)** Sensory fibers that arise from Golgi tendon organs synapse with interneurons which inhibit those motor neurons that innervate the muscle to which the tendon organ is related. Type Ib sensory fibers do play an important role in this reflex (choice C). Type Ia (choice A) and type II (choice E) sensory fibers originate from muscle spindles and are involved in the myotatic reflex but not the inverse myotatic reflex. An increase in the tension applied to the muscle tendon in which the tendon organ is located is the appropriate stimulus for this reflex. Stimulation of cutaneous pain endings (choice D) in the region of a Golgi tendon organ is not in itself sufficient to activate the reflex.

9. **(D)** The internal pyramidal layer is composed of large numbers of pyramidal neurons whose axons make up the bulk of those projections that extend to numerous subcortical locations including the spinal cord and basilar pontine gray. The external pyramidal layer (choice B) is also largely composed of pyramidal neurons, but most of their axons distribute intracortically. The axons of cells in the internal (choice C) and external granular (choice A) layers also distribute within the cortical gray matter, while the multiform layer (choice E) contains the bulk of neurons projecting to the thalamus.

10. **(A)** In middle alternating hemiplegia (choice B) the involved structures are the corticospinal tract and fibers of the abducens nerve, while superior alternating hemiplegia (choice C) involves corticospinal fibers and exiting fibers of the oculomotor nerve. Spina bifida (choice D) is a developmental defect involving failure of the neural tube to close. Syringomyelia (choice E) is due to the formation of a cyst-like cavity in the central portion of the spinal cord damaging the crossing pain fibers in the ventral white commissure, and resulting in a bilateral loss of pain and temperature sensation in the affected dermatomes.

11. **(A)** Compression of the surface of the cerebellum beginning with the pia would affect the layers of the cerebellar cortex in the following sequence: pia mater, molecular layer, Purkinje layer, and granular layer. The other choices (B–D) involve incorrect sequencing of the layers from the outer surface inward.

12. **(C)** Sensory neurons such as those found in the cochlear, spinal trigeminal, solitary, and vestibular nuclei arise from the alar plate. The hypoglossal nucleus (choice A), dorsal vagal

nucleus (choice B), and nucleus ambiguus (choice D) contain motor neurons that innervate either striated or smooth musculature, and such neurons arise from the basal plate.

13. **(D)** The posterior inferior cerebellar artery supplies the rostral, dorsolateral medulla. The posterior spinal (choice A) and anterior spinal (choice C) arteries supply dorsal and ventral portions respectively of the caudal medulla. The anterior inferior cerebellar (choice B) and superior cerebellar (choice E) arteries supply portions of the pons and mesencephalon.

14. **(A)** Pain and temperature receptors on the right side of the face send afferent signals to the right spinal trigeminal nucleus. Somatosensory information from the right face passes through the left ventral posterior medial (not VPL, choice B) nucleus of the thalamus. The right principal sensory (choice C) and mesencephalic (choice D) trigeminal nuclei receive proprioceptive and tactile sensory input from the right face, but not pain and temperature information. The right posterior limb (choice E) of the internal capsule carries pain and temperature signals from the left side of the face via the right thalamus.

15. **(E)** The characteristic feature of the lateral medullary syndrome is a loss of pain and temperature sensation that involves the ipsilateral face (the lesion side) and the contralateral side of the body. Pain and temperature sensation is lost in the ipsilateral and not the contralateral (choice A) face. The medullary pyramid (choice B) is typically not involved in this syndrome. Involvement of the ipsilateral upper and contralateral lower extremities (choice C) is not a feature of this syndrome. This syndrome is typically the result of a vascular lesion involving the posterior inferior (not anterior inferior) cerebellar artery (choice D).

16. **(D)** Patients with Weber's syndrome exhibit involvement of the ipsilateral oculomotor nerve. Interruption of this nerve on the right would eliminate parasympathetic outflow on that side, resulting in a dilated right pupil that does not react to light. Movements of the left eye (choice A) would not be affected. Involvement of corticospinal fibers in the right crus (choice C) would produce contralateral hemiplegia. Involvement of corticobulbar fibers coursing in the right crus cerebri might cause the protruded tongue to deviate to the left (not right, choice B), and cause paralysis of the facial expression musculature in the lower left portion (not complete paralysis on one side, choice E).

17. **(A)** This syndrome results from degeneration of neurons in the substantia nigra pars compacta, cells that normally release dopamine at their synaptic terminals in the neostriatum. The nigrostriatal projection degenerates as a result of the loss of neurons in the substantia nigra, but this utilizes dopamine at its terminals, not norepinephrine (choice B). Patients with this syndrome also exhibit bradykinesia (not tachykinesia, choice C), a generalized slowing of movement. This syndrome is treated with a variety of compounds (including carbidopa, choice D) that attempt to increase real, or effective, dopamine levels in the striatum, but the efficacy of most of these substances is minimal because they do not readily cross the blood–brain barrier. Parkinson's disease is characterized by a resting tremor (not an intention tremor, choice E) that usually involves the fingers and hands.

18. **(C)** Failure of the right eye to adduct on attempted lateral gaze to the left, accompanied by normal abduction of the left eye, suggests a lesion involving the right medial longitudinal fasciculus. Interruption of the right trochlear nerve (choice A) or the right (choice B) or left (choice D) abducens nerve alone would not result in defective conjugate horizontal eye movements, but would unilaterally affect eye movements in the eye innervated by the injured nerve. Damage to the left medial longitudinal fasciculus (choice E) would prevent adduction of the left eye on attempted right lateral gaze.

19. **(C)** A vascular lesion affecting the left caudal medulla would involve the left medial

lemniscus, left hypoglossal nerve fibers, and the left medullary pyramid. Involvement of the left medial lemniscus would produce somatosensory deficits involving the right side of the body. Damage to the left hypoglossal nerve would result in deviation of the protruded tongue to the left (and other lower motoneuron signs), while damage to the left pyramid would result in right hemiplegia (choices A and B involve incorrect combinations) along with other upper motoneuron signs. Choices D and E are incorrect because they fail to combine involvement of the tongue and contralateral hemiplegia.

20. **(B)** Since the left hemisphere is dominant in more than 95% of individuals, large left frontal lobe lesions typically produce a motor or expressive aphasia known as Broca's aphasia (not conduction, choice C, or Wernicke's, choices A and D). Broca's motor speech area in the left frontal operculum is near the primary motor cortex controlling the right upper extremity (not the left, choice E), and consequently patients with Broca's aphasia frequently exhibit motor deficits involving the right hand. Wernicke's aphasia (sensory or receptive aphasia) and conduction aphasia commonly result from parietal lobe lesions and consequently are not commonly seen in association with motor deficits in the hand.

21. **(C)** Lesions (usually vascular in nature) that involve the dorsolateral medulla produce the classic signs of the lateral medullary syndrome (Wallenberg's syndrome), which include a loss of pain and temperature sensibility over the face ipsilateral to the lesion and the contralateral side of the body. Since the left side of the face exhibits a loss of pain sensation, choice A is not correct. Syringomyelia (choice B) is a spinal cord lesion that typically does not affect the face. Unilateral lesions that involve somatosensory pathways coursing through the posterior limb of the internal capsule will give rise to a loss of all or some somatosensation over the contralateral face (not choice D) and the contralateral body surface. Weber's syndrome (choice E) does not typically produce somatosensory deficits.

22. **(D)** The opening of potassium channels in the apical membrane of auditory hair cells allows potassium ions to flow into the cell (not out of the cell, choice A or B) and depolarize (not hyperpolarize, choice C) it. The apical surface of these cells is exposed to endolymph containing a higher concentration of potassium ions than is found inside the cell. A potential difference of 160 mV (outside positive) exists across the apical membrane, resulting in a net movement of potassium ions into the cell when the stereocilia bundle is deflected and ion transduction channels are opened (not choice E).

23. **(C)** The appearance of right beating horizontal nystagmus with warm caloric stimulation of the right ear, coupled with the absence of nystagmus following warm caloric stimulation of the left ear, suggests that the left labyrinth (and not the right, choice D) or the left VIIIth cranial nerve has been damaged. The absence of left beating nystagmus under these conditions does not indicate that only the left lateral vestibulospinal tract (choice B) has been affected. The presence of right beating nystagmus indicates that receptors in the right ear (choice A) have not been damaged. The absence of nystagmus upon warm water irrigation of the left ear suggests that there is a lesion (not choice E) in the vestibular system.

24. **(E)** Each of the four areas listed (choices A–D) gives rise to some corticospinal axons. The largest number arises from the primary motor area, followed by the premotor, supplementary motor, and primary somatosensory regions.

25. **(B)** The effect of activity in the indirect pathway is to inhibit the output of thalamocortical projections, whereas activation of the direct pathway leads to an increase (not decrease, choice C) in motor activity produced by activation of thalamocortical projections. The degeneration of nigrostriatal projections affects both (not choice A) the indirect and direct pathways. Loss of function in the indirect (not direct, choice D) pathway leads to the production of involuntary movements.

The tremor of Parkinson's disease is best described as a resting tremor (not intention tremor, choice E) and is most obvious when the affected body part is at rest.

26. **(E)** The hypothalamus and amygdaloid complex contain the so-called "upper motoneurons" (not choice C) that control "lower motoneurons" found in the brainstem reticular formation (not the amygdala, choice D). The hypothalamus regulates autonomic function on a moment-to-moment (reflexive) basis (not long-term, choice A), whereas the amygdaloid complex provides more long-term regulation (not short-term, choice B).

27. **(B)** The wide-based stance and staggering gait are two of the characteristic features of cerebellar disease. Basal ganglia dysfunction, not cerebellar pathology, produces a resting-type tremor (choice A). Spasticity (choice C) and hyperreflexia (choice E) are prominent signs of upper motoneuron dysfunction. Somatosensory deficits such as the loss of pain and temperature sensation (choice D) are not typically seen with cerebellar disease.

28. **(A)** Interruption of the oculomotor nerve causes the affected eye to be directed down and out (not up and out, choice D) due to the pull of intact muscles innervated by cranial nerves IV and VI. The loss of parasympathetic fibers in the third nerve results in the impairment of the pupillary light reflex (choice B) and lens accomodation (choice C). In addition, third nerve involvement causes the ipsilateral eyelid (not contralateral, choice E) to droop (ptosis) due to denervation of the levator palpebrae superioris.

29. **(E)** The intrinsic muscles of the hand are derived mostly from the T1 myotome and to a lesser degree from the C8 myotome and, consequently, derive their innervation from the corresponding segmental spinal nerves. The segmental innervation to the intrinsic muscles of the hand is overwhelmingly from the T1 segmental nerve with some input from the C8 nerve. The supraspinatus muscle (choice A) is supplied by the suprascapular nerve which is derived from the upper trunk of the brachial plexus. Consequently, it receives innervation from the C5 and C6 spinal nerves, as do the other intrinsic muscles of the shoulder. The deltoid muscle (choice B) is an intrinsic muscle of the shoulder supplied by the axillary nerve. While the posterior cord of the brachial plexus which gives rise to the axillary nerve contains fibers from the C5 to T1 spinal nerves, the axillary nerve largely consists of C5 and C6 fibers which supply the deltoid and teres minor muscles. The biceps brachii muscle (choice C) is innervated by the musculocutaneous nerve derived from the lateral cord of the brachial plexus. While the lateral cord and musculocutaneous nerve contain fibers derived from the C5, C6, and C7 spinal nerves, the biceps muscle is mostly supplied by the C5 and C6 spinal nerves. The pronator teres muscle (choice D) is supplied by the median nerve. While the median nerve contains fibers derived from the C5 to T1 spinal nerves, the pronator teres muscle is mostly supplied by the C5 and C6 spinal nerves.

30. **(C)** Injury to the lower trunk of the brachial plexus would affect the C8 and T1 dermatomes. The C8 dermatome covers the little finger and the adjacent side of the ring finger and the medial side of the hand, wrist, and lower forearm. The T1 dermatome extends up the medial side of the forearm across the elbow onto the medial side of the arm. The web between the thumb and index finger (choice A) is covered by the C6 dermatome. The lateral side of the forearm (choice B) is divided between the C5 and C6 dermatomes. The deltoid muscle just above its insertion (choice D) is covered by the C5 dermatome. The dorsum of the wrist and the anatomical snuffbox (choice E) are covered by the C6 dermatome.

31. **(A)** Injury to the lower roots may occur when the arm is forcibly pulled upward above the head. The resulting injury is known as Klumpke's paralysis. Horner's syndrome (choice B) results from interruption of the sympathetic innervation to the head. Preganglionic sympathetic fibers arising from the T1 and T2 spinal cord segments ascend in

the sympathetic trunk to reach the cervical ganglia. These fibers may be damaged in injuries involving the lower roots of the brachial plexus. Waiter's tip hand (choice C) describes the position of the extremity in Erb–Duchenne palsy, resulting from injury to the upper roots of the brachial plexus. Erb–Duchenne palsy (choice D) involves injury to the C5 and C6 roots of the brachial plexus. It occurs when the shoulder is pushed downward and the head and neck are forced to the opposite side. Wrist drop (choice E) results from injury to the radial nerve and is caused by paralysis of the extensors of the wrist and fingers.

32. **(E)** The serratus anterior muscle draws the scapula forward against the thoracic wall when reaching forward and/or when pushing. Denervation of the serratus anterior muscle results in a characteristic "winged scapula" when attempting these movements. The serratus anterior muscle is innervated by the long thoracic nerve which has no cutaneous distribution. Damage to the upper roots of the brachial plexus (choice A) will affect the serratus anterior muscle and long thoracic nerve (C5, C6, and C7) but would also result in a sensory deficit over the corresponding dermatomes. Damage to the posterior cord of the brachial plexus (choice B) will have no effect on the serratus anterior muscle as it does not give rise to the long thoracic nerve. The accessory nerve (choice C) innervates the trapezius muscle and not the serratus anterior muscle. Damage to the accessory nerve produces a "drooping shoulder" resulting from an inbility to elevate the point of the shoulder. The suprascapular nerve (choice D) innervates the supraspinatus and infraspinatus muscles, two of the "rotator cuff" group. The supraspinatus muscle is an abductor at the shoulder joint and the infraspinatus is a lateral rotator.

33. **(D)** Figure 1–3 reflects the distribution of the superficial branch of the radial nerve over the dorsum of the hand. This nerve is entirely cutaneous and supplies no muscles. Damage to the ulnar nerve at the elbow (choice A) will produce a sensory deficit over the dorsal and ventral surfaces of the medial one-third of the hand, all of the little finger, and the medial half of the ring finger. Damage to the dorsal cutaneous branch of the ulnar nerve (choice B) will produce a sensory deficit over the dorsal surface of the medial one-third of the hand, little finger, and medial half of the ring finger. Damage to the radial nerve in the cubital fossa (choice C) will produce the same cutaneous deficit as injury to the superficial radial nerve (the correct answer) but will also affect the motor innervation to the muscles of the posterior compartment of the forearm. The posterior antebrachial cutaneous nerve (choice E) is a branch of the radial nerve in the posterior arm, and is distributed down the posterior forearm extending onto the dorsum of the wrist with distribution onto the hand.

34. **(B)** The blackened area in Figure 1–3 represents the C6 and C7 dermatomes. The C5 and C6 dermatomes (choice A) extend in a strip along the lateral surface of the upper extremity from the shoulder to the hand. The C6 dermatome extends onto the hand but the C5 dermatome does not. The C7 and C8 dermatomes (choice C) extend in a strip along the posterior and medial surfaces of the upper extremity from the shoulder to the hand. The C7 dermatome supplies the area indicated but the C8 dermatome covers the medial side of the hand rather than the lateral side. The C8 and T1 dermatomes (choice D) cover the little finger and the adjacent side of the ring finger and the medial side of the hand, wrist, and lower forearm (C8), and extend up the medial side of the forearm across the elbow onto the medial side of the arm (T1). The T1 dermatome (choice E) extends up the medial side of the forearm across the elbow onto the medial side of the arm. It has no representation on the hand.

35. **(C)** The trapezius muscle has an extensive attachment to the occipital bone, the ligamentum nuchae, the spinous processes and supraspinous ligaments down to T12, the spine of the scapula, the acromion, and the lateral third of the clavicle. Such a fan-shaped muscle has many actions. The upper and middle fibers, which attach to the clavicle

and acromion, lift the point of the shoulder. The trapezius is innervated by the accessory nerve, and the ability to shrug the shoulder is often used to test the function of the accessory nerve. The suprascapular nerve (choice A) innervates the supraspinatus and infraspinatus muscles. Damage to this nerve would affect the ability to raise the arm from the side (the supraspinatus muscle) and to laterally rotate the shoulder (infraspinatus muscle). The dorsal scapular nerve (choice B) innervates the rhomboideus major and minor muscles. Together they stabilize the scapula, and with the levator scapulae muscle they rotate the scapula so that the glenoid cavity points inferiorly. Damage to the thoracodorsal nerve (choice D) would affect the latissimus dorsi muscle which adducts, extends, and medially rotates the arm at the shoulder. Damage to the long thoracic nerve (choice E) affects the serratus anterior muscle. The serratus anterior muscle draws the scapula forward against the thoracic wall when reaching forward and/or when pushing.

36. (B) The axillary nerve, with the posterior humeral circumflex artery, passes through the quadrangular space and crosses the surgical neck of the humerus where it is susceptible to injury in fracture and in dislocation of the shoulder joint. The radial nerve (choice A) is most susceptible to injury as it lies in the spiral groove along the posterior aspect of the shaft of the humerus. The scapular circumflex artery (choice C) leaves the axilla through the triangular space at the lateral border of the scapula. It is separated from the quadrangular space by the long head of the triceps brachii muscle. The profunda brachii artery (choice D) is most susceptible to injury as it lies with the radial nerve in the spiral groove along the posterior aspect of the shaft of the humerus. The brachial artery (choice E) lies in a superficial position as it descends through the arm and therefore is not particularly vulnerable in fractures of the humerus.

37. (C) The axillary nerve arises from the posterior cord of the brachial plexus and supplies the deltoid and teres minor muscles. The serratus anterior muscle (choice A) is supplied by the long thoracic nerve which is derived from the roots of C5, C6, and C7. The median nerve is derived from the medial and lateral cords and supplies the pronator teres muscle (choice B). The biceps brachii muscle (choice D) is supplied by the musculocutaneous nerve which arises from the lateral cord. The suprascapular nerve from the upper trunk of the brachial plexus supplies the infraspinatus muscle (choice E).

38. (E) The posterior humeral circumflex artery arises from the third part of the axillary artery but has no anastomotic connections with branches of the subclavian artery. The suprascapular artery (choice A) is a branch of the thyrocervical trunk from the subclavian artery. As it descends in the infraspinous fossa deep to the infraspinatus muscle, it makes anastomotic connections with the scapular circumflex artery. The subscapular artery (choice B) is a branch from the third part of the axillary artery and gives rise to the scapular circumflex artery. Through this branch, it makes anastomotic connections with the suprascapular artery in the infraspinous fossa. The dorsal scapular artery (choice C) arises from the subclavian artery and descends along the vertebral border of the scapula. It anastomoses deep to the infraspinatus muscle with branches of the scapular circumflex branch of the subscapular artery, from the third part of the axillary artery. The scapular circumflex artery (choice D) anastomoses around the scapula with the suprascapular artery, a branch of the thyrocervical trunk, and the dorsal scapular artery, a branch of the subclavian artery.

39. (C) The radial notch of the ulna and the annular ligament form a ring in which the head of the radius rotates at its articulation with the capitulum of the humerus. The annular ligament narrows over the neck, cupping the head of the radius, and preventing downward dislocation. In a child the head of the radius is not fully developed and may slip from under the annular ligament with a twisting pull on the forearm. Separation of the ulna from its articulation with the trochlea (choice A) is not a common injury due to the strength and stability of the joint, but may occur when severe force is applied to it. Separation of the head of the radius from its articulation with the trochlea of the humerus (choice B) does not occur because the radius does not articulate with the trochlea. Stretching of the radial nerve as it passes around the medial epicondyle of the humerus (choice D) is not possible because the radial nerve enters the forearm in front of the lateral epicondyle. The ulnar nerve can be stretched as it passes behind the medial epicondyle. Compression of the median nerve as it penetrates the supinator muscle (choice E) is not possible because the median nerve passes through the pronator teres muscle, not the supinator. The radial nerve penetrates the supinator muscle, where it can be compressed.

40. (C) The thoracic duct ascends in the posterior mediastinum between the azygous vein and the descending aorta. The recurrent laryngeal nerves (choice A) have differing courses on the right and left sides. The left recurrent laryngeal nerve arises in the superior mediastinum adjacent to the aortic arch, and the right recurrent laryngeal nerve arises in the root of the neck, passing around the right subclavian artery to re-enter the neck. The tracheal bifurcation (choice B) lies at the level of the sternal angle and lies largely in the middle mediastinum. The phrenic nerves (choice D) descend through the superior and middle mediastina. The left atrium (choice E) lies completely within the middle mediastinum as does all of the heart.

41. (A) The circumflex branch of the left coronary artery circles to the posterior surface of the heart in the coronary sulcus (atrioventricular groove). It sends branches to the left atrium and left ventricle before anastomosing with the posterior interventricular branch of the right coronary artery. The right atrium and right ventricle (choice B) are largely supplied by the right coronary artery as it descends in the coronary sulcus between them. The apex of the heart (choice C) is supplied by the anterior interventricular branch of the left coronary artery as it descends in the anterior interventricular sulcus, and the posterior interventricular branch of the right coronary artery as it descends in the posterior interventricular sulcus. The right and left ventricles (choice D) are supplied by both the right and left coronary arteries, but the circumflex branch of the left coronary artery has little if any contribution to the right ventricle. The right ventricle and the interventricular septum (choice E) are supplied by both the right and left coronary arteries, but the circumflex branch of the left coronary artery has little if any contribution to the interventricular septum.

42. (E) The anterior abdominal wall is divided by two transverse and two vertical planes into nine regions used to locate the signs and symptoms of abdominal disease. From superior to inferior, the midline regions are the epigastric, umbilical, and the hypogastric regions, and the lateral regions are the hypochondriac, lateral, and inguinal regions. The splenic artery arises from the celiac trunk in the epigastric region and passes to the spleen located in the left hypochondrium. The superior epigastric artery (choice A) lies on the anterior abdominal wall descending into the umbilical region where it anastomoses with the inferior epigastric artery ascending from the hypogastric region. The superior mesenteric artery (choice B) supplies the coils of small intestine and the transverse colon lying in the umbilical region, the cecum and appendix lying in the right inguinal region, and the ascending colon lying in the right lateral region. The inferior mesenteric artery (choice C) arises from the abdominal aorta in the umbilical region and descends to the left to supply the descending colon in the left lateral region and the sigmoid colon in the left inguinal region. The renal arteries (choice D) and the hilum of the kidneys lie approximately along the transpyloric plane, with the kidneys located in both the hypochondrium and lateral regions.

43. (B) The greater peritoneal sac communicates with the lesser sac, or omental bursa, through the epiploic foramen (of Winslow). The superior boundary is the caudate lobe of the liver. The first part of the duodenum (choice A) is the inferior boundary of the epiploic foramen. The head of the pancreas (choice C) is separated from the epiploic foramen by the first part of the duodenum and does not form one of the boundaries of the opening. The common bile duct (choice D) lies in the free edge of the lesser omentum (the hepatoduodenal ligament) that forms the anterior boundary of the epiploic foramen. The hepatic veins (choice E) pass directly from the liver to join the inferior vena cava as it passes through the respiratory diaphragm. It is not related to the epiploic foramen.

44. (C) The lymphatic drainage of an organ is closely related to its blood supply. Lymphatic drainage from the testis travels along the testicular artery to reach lymph nodes along the aorta. The superficial inguinal nodes (choice A) receive lymph from the superficial tissues of the thigh and leg, the buttock, the lower abdominal wall, and the external genitalia, but not from the testis. The deep inguinal nodes (choice B) lie alongside the femoral vein and drain the deep tissue of the thigh and leg. The internal iliac nodes (choice D) generally drain the structures supplied by branches of the internal iliac artery including the pelvic organs (but not the ovaries), the gluteal region, and the deep structures of the perineum. The common iliac nodes (choice E) receive lymph from the inguinal, external iliac, and internal iliac nodes, none of which drain the testis.

45. (C) The artery to the hindgut and its derivatives is the inferior mesenteric artery. The celiac artery (choice A) supplies structures derived from the caudal foregut. The superior mesenteric artery (choice B) supplies the structures derived from the midgut. In the fetus the ductus arteriosus (choice D) shunts blood from the pulmonary trunk to the aorta to bypass the lungs. In the fetus the umbilical artery (choice E) delivers blood to the placental circulation.

46. (A) Urine may leak from the umbilicus when the lumen of the allantois remains patent (a urachal fistula) allowing the urinary bladder to communicate with the umbilicus. A persistent and patent vitelline duct (choice B) may allow feces or mucus to leak from the umbilicus due to the communication between the terminal ileum and the umbilicus. An omphalocele (choice C) is a congenital hernia through the anterior abdominal wall at the umbilicus that is covered only by the amnion. Gastroschisis (choice D) is a congenital defect in the anterior abdominal wall, not located at the umbilicus, that is accompanied by a herniation of the small intestine and part of the large intestine. An umbilical hernia (choice E) is a protrusion of the small intestine through the anterior abdominal wall at the umbilicus that is covered by peritoneum and skin.

47. (C) The long head of the biceps brachii muscle arises from the supraglenoid tubercle on the scapula. The radial tuberosity (choice B) marks the insertion of the tendon of the biceps brachii on the radius. The coracoid process of the scapula (choice A) provides attachment for the short head of the biceps brachii, coracobrachialis, and pectoralis minor muscles. The bicipital aponeurosis (choice D) is an aponeurotic sheet that extends from the biceps tendon to the deep fascia of the forearm, thus providing a secondary insertion into the ulna. The lesser tubercle of the humerus (choice E) provides attachment for the subscapularis muscle.

48. (C) A "claw hand" is best associated with injury to the ulnar nerve at the wrist affecting the interosseus, lumbrical, and hypothenar muscles of the hand. It is characterized by a wasted palm and hypothenar eminence, hyperextended metacarpophalangeal joints, and flexed interphalangeal joints. Injury to the median nerve (choice A) interferes with pronation of the forearm and with flexion of the phalanges of the thumb and digits two and three. In addition, the thenar muscles waste with an accompanying inability to oppose the thumb and fingers. Injury to the radial nerve (choice B) may affect the extensor muscles of the arm and forearm depending on the point of injury. It is associated with "wrist drop" due to loss of the extensors of the wrist and fingers. Injury to the axillary nerve (choice D) affects the deltoid and teres minor muscles. The deltoid muscle is primarily an abductor of the upper limb, and the teres minor muscle is a lateral rotator of the shoulder. Injury to the musculocutaneous nerve (choice E) primarily involves the flexors of the arm and forearm.

49. **(A)** The scaphoid bone lies in the floor of the anatomical snuffbox and acute tenderness over this area is indicative of a fracture of the scaphoid, even in the absence of radiographic verification. Approximately 70% of carpal fractures involve the scaphoid only. A fracture through its narrow middle part may deprive the scaphoid of its blood supply, causing its proximal part to undergo avascular necrosis. The pisiform bone (choice B) is a sesamoid bone in the tendon of the flexor carpi ulnaris on the lateral wrist. It is not related to the anatomical snuffbox. The hamate bone (choice C) lies in the distal row of carpal bones on the medial side of the wrist. It is not related to the anatomical snuffbox. The capitate bone (choice D) is the largest of the carpal bones occupying a central position in the distal row of carpal bones. It is not related to the anatomical snuffbox. The lunate bone (choice E) lies adjacent to the scaphoid in the proximal row of carpals and with the scaphoid articulates with the radius at the radiocarpal or wrist joint. It is not related to the anatomical snuffbox.

50. **(C)** Lesions of the radial nerve in the arm may paralyze all of the extensor muscles of the forearm, producing a "wrist drop" (flexion of the hand by gravity when the forearm is horizontal), as well as inability to extend the digits at the metacarpophalangeal joints. Injury to the axillary nerve (choice A) affects the deltoid and teres minor muscles. The deltoid muscle is primarily an abductor of the upper limb and the teres minor muscle is a lateral rotator of the shoulder. Injury to the musculocutaneous nerve (choice B) primarily involves the flexors of the arm and forearm. Injury to the median nerve (choice D) in the arm interferes with pronation of the forearm and with flexion of the phalanges of the thumb and digits two and three. In addition, the thenar muscles waste with an accompanying inability to oppose the thumb and fingers. Injury to the ulnar nerve (choice E) in the arm affects the flexor digitorum profundus to the ring and little fingers and the interosseus, lumbrical, and hypothenar muscles of the hand. It is characterized by a wasted palm and hypothenar eminence, hyperextended metacarpophalangeal joints, and flexed interphalangeal joints.

51. **(B)** The funnel-shaped infundibulum, or conus arteriosus, leads into the pulmonary trunk through the pulmonary orifice. The crista terminalis (choice A) partially divides the interior of the right atrium into two main parts: the posteriorly located, smooth-walled sinus venarum that is derived from the embryonic sinus venosus, and the anteriorly located, rough-walled remnant of the embryonic right atrium. The crista supraventricularis (choice C) divides the interior of the right ventricle into two portions, the upper one being the infundibulum that leads into the pulmonary trunk. The limbus fossa ovalis (choice D) forms a prominent margin for the fossa ovalis on the interatrial wall of the right atrium. The ostium of the coronary sinus (choice E) lies in the right atrium medial to the opening of the inferior vena cava.

52. **(C)** The musculocutaneous nerve passes through the coracobrachialis muscle and continues distally between the biceps brachii and brachialis muscles. It supplies all three muscles. Injury to the nerve will affect flexion at the shoulder (coracobrachialis and biceps brachii), flexion at the elbow (brachialis and biceps brachii), and supination of the forearm (biceps brachii). Weakened extension at the elbow (choice A) would result from injury to the radial nerve affecting the triceps brachii muscle. Weakened abduction at the shoulder (choice B) would result from injury to the axillary nerve affecting the deltoid muscle or injury to the suprascapular nerve affecting the supraspinatus muscle. Diminished cutaneous sensation over the medial forearm (choice D) would result from injury to the C8 or T1 spinal nerves, the medial cord of the brachial plexus, or the medial antebrachial cutaneous nerve arising from it. Diminished cutaneous sensation over the medial palm (choice E) would result from injury to the C8 spinal nerve, the ulnar nerve, or the palmar cutaneous branch of the ulnar nerve.

53. (A) The transpyloric plane is a hypothetical horizontal plane passing through the lower part of the body of the first lumbar vertebra. The liver, pancreas, kidneys, duodenum, and spleen all lie at this level. The bifurcation of the abdominal aorta (choice B) occurs over the body of the L4 vertebra. The celiac trunk (choice C) arises from the abdominal aorta over the body of the 12th thoracic vertebra. The transverse colon (choice D) lies in the umbilical region below the level of the transpyloric plane. The esophagus (choice E) ends and is continuous with the stomach as it passes through the respiratory diaphragm at the level of the tenth thoracic vertebra.

54. (D) Nucleus D belongs to a primary spermatocyte. This is one of a cohort of synchronized cells that have entered Prophase I of meiosis as indicated by their migration away from the basal compartment and into the adluminal compartment. These cells exemplify the longest subdivision of Prophase I, pachytene. At this stage, the nucleolus and nuclear envelope are intact, but the chromatin has condensed to give the appearance of thick ribbons formed by the pairing (synapsis) of homologous chromosomes. Two different cohorts (choices A and B) of spermatids can be identified in the micrograph. The group illustrated by A has nearly completed morphogenesis (spermiogenesis) as indicated by their dense, flattened nuclei. Cell B is an undifferentiated spermatid formed recently as a result of completion of the second (equational) meiotic division by secondary spermatocytes. The composition of this segment of seminiferous epithelium indicates that it is in Stage I of the six-stage, 16-day epithelial cycle. The cohort of nearly mature spermatids is 16 days further along in spermatogenesis than the cohort of undifferentiated spermatids which, in turn, is 16 days more advanced than the cohort of pachytene primary spermatocytes. Because the second (equational) meiotic division is completed rapidly, secondary spermatocytes are rarely seen in sections of testis, occurring only during Stage IV, the briefest of the six stages of the epithelial cycle. The Sertoli (sustentacular) cell (choice C) is a somatic cell that supports spermatogenesis by a wide variety of functions. Its distinguishing features are the large, elongated nucleus oriented perpendicular to the basement membrane and the large, often diamond-shaped, nucleolus. The cytoplasm of Sertoli cells spans the entire thickness of the epithelium, and junctions between neighboring Sertoli cells form the blood–testis barrier between the basal and adluminal compartments. The spermatogonium (choice E) has an interphase nucleus with the long axis parallel to the adjacent basement membrane. Spermatogonia comprise a heterogeneous population that includes the true stem cells of the male germ cell line.

55. (C) The letter C indicates the tectorial membrane. On the left, this flap-like structure of gelatinous extracellular material is anchored to the spiral limbus which contains a row of interdentate cells which secrete the tectorial membrane. The free edge of the tectorial membrane (the kink in this photomicrograph is a typical artifact) rests on the tallest stereocilia at the apical surfaces of the inner and outer hair cells, the sensory transducers of mechanical energy to electrical signals. Sound waves passing through the labyrinth create shear at the interface between the tectorial membrane and the stereocilia of the hair cells. The vestibular (Reissner's) membrane (choice A) separates the scala vestibuli, a perilymph-filled space above, from the scala media (cochlear duct), an endolymph-filled space below. The stria vascularis (choice B) is an epithelium that lines the outer wall of the scala media. This epithelium is thought to maintain the peculiar, high-potassium composition of the endolymph, and its name derives from the unusual feature of capillaries coursing within the epithelium. The apical surfaces of outer hair cells (cuticular plates) and outer phalangeal cells are indicated by D (choice D). Underneath, the upper row of nuclei belong to the hair cells and the lower row to the phalangeal cells. The organ of Corti rests on the basilar membrane (choice E). This separates the scala media above from the scala tympani below. The width of the basilar membrane is greatest at the apex of the cochlea, thus tuning this end of the organ of Corti to low-frequency sounds.

56. (D) Retinal separation typically occurs at the interface between the retinal pigment epithelium and the outer limit of the sensory (neural) retina. The weakness of this plane is attributed to the manner in which the retina develops, a process that involves obliteration of the space between two of the layers of the optic cup—an inner layer from which the sensory retina arises, and an outer layer from which the retinal pigment epithelium arises. Other retinal layers are bridged by neuronal processes, and Müller cells, the retina's glial cells, span the entire thickness of the neural retina. Plane A (choice A) marks the boundary between the nerve fiber layer above and the ganglion cell layer below. The nerve fiber layer is composed of axons of the retinal ganglion cells. Plane B (choice B) is within the inner plexiform layer, the site of synaptic contacts between bipolar neurons, retinal ganglion cells, and amacrine cells. Plane C (choice C) is within the outer plexiform layer, the site of synapses between bipolar cells, rods and cones, and horizontal cells. The boundary between the choroid (of the middle vascular tunic or uvea) and the sclera (of the external, fibrous tunic) is marked by plane E (choice E).

57. (C) Virus-infected cells are the main natural targets of cytotoxic T (CD8) cells. This class of lymphocyte recognizes antigens only when presented on the plasmalemmas of host (self) cells in association with Class I MHC. Typically, these would be viral antigens expressed by infected cells. Cytotoxic cells are also activated by allogenic tissue grafts (choice A) via recognition of non–self-MHC molecules; however, this phenomenon (which is a result of the polymorphic nature of Class I MHC genes) does not represent the typical natural function of these cells. Although regulatory T lymphocytes are important in defense against bacterial toxins (choice B), bacteria (choice D), and protozoan parasites (choice E), the direct destruction of these agents is brought about by other effector mechanisms, such as the complement system, macrophages, and granulocytic leukocytes, that are triggered by immunoglobulins, which are produced by B lymphocytes.

58. (A) The neuroectoderm of the optic cup gives rise to the neural retina, pigmented retinal epithelium, ciliary epithelium, posterior iridial epithelium, and anterior iridial epithelium. The lens epithelium (choice B) is derived from the lens placode, specialization of the surface ectoderm overlying the optic cup. The other structures (choices C, D, and E) are all mesenchymal derivatives. The ciliary muscle (choice C) and choriocapillaris layer (choice D) are derived from the uvea (choroidal or vascular coat). The extraocular muscles, including the lateral rectus (choice E) are derived from mesenchyme, although there is some uncertainty about their precise origin.

59. (D) At day 8 of the cycle, a dominant follicle has been selected, but its oocyte, although greatly enlarged, is still a primary oocyte. Oogonia (choice A) are absent by the time the female fetus reaches the fifth month of gestation because they have completed their mitotic divisions to produce primary oocytes. When a female individual is born, all germ cells in the ovaries are primary oocytes that are arrested in prophase of the first meiotic division. After the onset of the menstrual cycle (menarche), normally only one oocyte will resume meiosis during each cycle. This occurs in the dominant follicle following the midcycle LH (luteinizing hormone) surge and a few hours preceding ovulation. When this cell completes the first meiotic division at about day 14 of the cycle, the products will be a single secondary oocyte and the first polar body (choice B). Polar bodies are products of the completion of the first and second meiotic divisions. Thus, association of a primary oocyte with a polar body (choice C) does not occur. Conversely, a secondary oocyte will not normally occur without a first polar body as its companion (choice E).

60. **(A)** Antimitotic drugs disrupt microtubule assembly in the formation of the mitotic spindle. In addition to killing rapidly dividing tumor cells, this can deplete intestinal epithelial cells, blood cells, and other populations of normal cells that have a high rate of replacement. Because lens epithelial cells (choice B), neurons (choices C and D), and cardiac muscle cells (choice E) are all terminally differentiated, non-dividing cells, they are not susceptible to spindle poisons.

61. **(B)** The space between plasmalemmas of adjacent epithelial cells is obliterated at the tight junction (zonula occludens) which forms by fusion of the membranes along narrow anastomosing bands. The tight junction is the apical-most part of the junctional complex which is typical of epithelia lining tubular and hollow organs. The zonula adherens and desmosome (choice A) also contribute to the junctional complex, but they hold adjacent cells together. The hemidesmosome (choice C) is a specialization for adhesion of a cell to its basement membrane. The gap junction (choice D) functions to electrically and chemically couple adjacent cells. It consists of direct channels (connexons) between cells, but there is a significant space (about 2 nm) separating the membranes between the channels. The terminal bar (choice E) is not a type of junction, but rather a manifestation of the junctional complex seen with the light microscope.

62. **(B)** Action potentials (APs) are initiated at the myoneural junction on the surface of a muscle fiber. T tubules are narrow invaginations of the sarcolemma that channel the APs to the vicinity of the sarcoplasmic reticulum organized around myofibrils. The Z line (choice A) is a component of the sarcomere that serves as an anchor for actin filaments. Muscle spindles (choice C) are complex sensory structures that monitor changes in muscle length. The sarcoplasmic reticulum (choice D) does not conduct APs; rather it responds to APs by releasing calcium. The endomysium (choice E) is the thin connective tissue layer surrounding each muscle fiber.

63. **(E)** The macula densa is a modified segment of the distal tubule at the site of its passage adjacent to the vascular pole of the renal corpuscle. The name arises from the close spacing of nuclei of the epithelial cells forming this part of the distal tubule. These cells are thought to sense the chloride content in the passing filtrate and generate signals that regulate the caliber of the afferent arteriole. Mesangial cells (choice A) are incompletely understood cells found in the glomerulus and in the juxtaglomerular apparatus. The afferent arteriole (choice B) feeds blood to the glomerulus. As part of the juxtaglomerular apparatus, it is closely apposed to the macula densa. Bowman's capsule (choice C) encompasses the capillaries of the glomerulus in two layers of epithelium. The inner, closely applied, visceral layer of podocytes is continuous at the vascular pole with the outer, parietal layer of squamous cells. Between the two layers is the urinary space, which is continuous with the lumen of the proximal convoluted tubule (choice D), which is not a component of the juxtaglomerular apparatus.

64. **(D)** Among the constituents of the pars nervosa are axons of neurosecretory neurons, a rich vascular bed of fenestrated capillaries, and a large number of glial cells called pituicytes. Thus, most of the cell nuclei seen in the pars nervosa belong to pituicytes. The axonal processes and terminals of oxytocin-secreting and antidiuretic hormone (ADH)–secreting neurons (choice A) form much of the bulk of the pars nervosa, but the cell bodies of these cells are located in the hypothalamus (supraoptic and paraventricular nuclei), so their nuclei are not seen in the neurohypophysis. Basophils (choice B) and chromophobes (choice C) reside in the adenohypophysis, and Schwann cells (choice E) are peripheral nerve constituents.

65. (B) Oxytocin is synthesized by neurons that have their cell bodies in the hypothalamus. These cells project their axons to the pars nervosa, so this is where the hormone is secreted, not within the hypothalamus (choice A). Basophils (choice C) of the adenohypophysis secrete corticotropin, thyrotropin, or gonadotropic hormones. Acidophils (choice D) secrete either growth hormone or prolactin. Pituicytes (choice E) are not hormone-secreting cells, but are glial cells located in the pars nervosa.

66. (C) The thymus provides for development of new T lymphocytes in an environment shielded from foreign antigens. Like bone marrow, the thymus is a primary lymphoid organ, and not a site of reactions to foreign antigens. Lymphoid follicles are sites of B lymphocyte proliferation in response to antigen stimulation. These occur in the white pulp of the spleen (choice A), lymph nodes (choice B), Peyer's patches (choice D), and tonsils (choice E).

67. (A) Hair follicles and their associated sebaceous glands are restricted in distribution to thin skin. Both thin (hairy) and thick (glabrous) skin have sweat glands (choice B) and dermal papillae (choice C). The epidermis of thick skin is generally thicker than that of thin skin, but both have basal (choice D), spinous (choice E), granular, and cornified layers in the epidermis. The epidermis of thick skin has a thicker stratum corneum and an additional layer, the stratum lucidum.

68. (C) The normal laboratory values can be used to calculate the upper limit of the normal range of absolute counts/mm^3 for each leukocyte (maximum normal total leukocyte count times the maximum normal percentage for the cell type). The patient's differential percentages can each be multiplied by 24,000/mm^3 to obtain total counts per mm^3 for each leukocyte type. The following table shows the results of these calculations. Asterisks (*) indicate values that are elevated.

Leukocyte	Normal upper limit (per mm^3)	Patient's count (per mm^3)
Segmented neutrophils	6820	17,040*
Band form neutrophils	550	3840*
Eosinophils	330	960*
Basophils	82	48
Lymphocytes	3630	720
Monocytes	770	1440*

69. (B) Although numbers of eosinophils and monocytes are somewhat elevated, the most prominent change in circulating leukocyte numbers is a greatly elevated neutrophil count, with a "shift to the left" (increased numbers of immature forms). This is indicative of a bacterial infection. Parasitic infections (choice A) and severe allergic reactions (choice C) are more likely to result specifically in an eosinophilia. Chronic lymphocytic leukemia (choice D) would result in lymphocytosis. Fragile, abnormally shaped erythrocytes are produced in sickle cell disease (choice E) resulting in chronic hemolytic anemia.

70. (C) The space of Disse separates hepatocytes from the endothelial cells that form the hepatic sinusoids. Thus, it is bordered partly by endothelium on one side and by microvilli of the hepatocytes on the other side (choice A). The endothelium of the sinusoids allows free passage of plasma, but not cells (choice B), into the space of Disse. The initial channel for flow of bile (choice D) is the bile canaliculus formed by junctions between adjacent hepatocytes. The portal triad (choice E) comprises an arteriolar branch of the hepatic artery, a venule conducting blood from the hepatic portal vein, and a bile duct. These are accompanied by one or more lymphatic vessels.

71. (C) Generation of specific granules occurs during the myelocyte stage. Development of all three types of granulocytes follows a similar sequence of stages. Buildup of the protein synthesis machinery occurs during the myeloblast (choice A) and promyelocyte (choice B) stages. The promyelocyte stage is also characterized by production of primary (non-specific) granules. After the myelocyte stage, further condensation and reshaping of the nucleus occurs during the metamyelocyte stage (choice D). The granulocyte-colony–forming unit (choice E) is an undifferentiated progenitor cell of the granulocyte line.

72. **(E)** The term *acidophilic* describes the staining behavior of cellular components (e.g., proteins with a high content of basic amino acids) that attract acid dyes such as eosin. Concentrations of mitochondria, such as occur in parietal cells, confer cytoplasmic acidophilia. Parietal cells secrete hydrochloric acid (choice A), but they do not store it. Moreover, an acidic substance would attract basic dyes such as hematoxylin. Parietal cells are also the source of intrinsic factor (choice B), but they do not contain readily evident secretory granules. Chief cells, not parietal cells, synthesize pepsinogen (choice C) and store it in secretory granules. Rough endoplasmic reticulum (choice D), which occurs in only a small degree in parietal cells, is basophilic due to its high RNA content.

73. **(C)** Endothelial cells of the capillaries that form the renal glomerulus have fenestrations which, incidentally, are not bridged by the diaphragms typical of fenestrated capillaries elsewhere such as in endocrine glands. Continuous capillaries are typical of central nervous system tissue (choice A), skeletal muscle (choice B), and most connective tissue. The predominant capillary in the red pulp of the spleen (choice D) is the sinusoidal capillary, which allows free passage of formed elements between the pulp cord tissue and the vascular compartment. The epidermis (choice E) is not penetrated by blood vessels.

74. **(A)** The syncytiotrophoblast forms the surface layer of the chorionic villi and is bathed by maternal blood flowing through the intervillus space. The syncytiotrophoblast is a product of division and fusion of cells in the underlying cytotrophoblast (choice B). Fetal capillaries (choice C) course through the fetal connective tissue (choice D) that forms the core of all orders of villi and thus have no contact with maternal blood when placental structure is intact. As the syncytiotrophoblast is a derivative of the embryonic trophoblast layer, it is incorrect to state that maternal blood has no contact with fetally derived cells (choice E).

75. **(C)** The parotid gland is the only major salivary gland containing almost exclusively serous secretory cells. The submandibular (choice A) and sublingual glands (choice B) are mixed glands, with differing proportions of serous and mucous cells. Esophageal (choice D) and intestinal glands (choice E) are small mucus-secreting glands.

76. **(C)** The source of intrinsic factor in humans is parietal cells of gastric glands. Intrinsic factor is required for absorption of vitamin B_{12}. Pepsinogen (choice A) and lipase (choice B) are secreted by chief cells of gastric fundic glands, but pepsin and lipase are digestive enzymes unrelated to vitamin B_{12} absorption. Gastrin is a hormone that stimulates acid secretion by parietal cells. It is secreted by one type of enteroendocrine cell (choice D), type G, in the pyloric glands. Lysozyme is an enzyme found in Paneth cells (choice E) of the small intestine as well as in neutrophils. It hydrolyzes glycosides of the cell wall of some gram-positive bacteria, and may be involved in regulation of the intestinal flora.

77. **(B)** The spinal cord and its meninges do not entirely fill the vertebral canal. The space between the walls of this canal and the outer menix of the cord, the dura mater, is the epidural space, which is filled with fat, connective tissue, and a plexus of veins. This is the internal vertebral venous plexus which consists of anterior and posterior internal vertebral venous plexuses. The external venous plexuses (choice A), which communicate with the internal venous plexus, are located anterior to the vertebral bodies and posterior to the vertebral arches. The anterior spinal artery (choice C), posterior spinal arteries (choice D), and middle cerebral artery (choice E) are all located deep to the arachnoid mater.

78. (D) The glossopharyngeal nerve provides parasympathetic innervation for the parotid gland. The facial nerve provides the parasympathetic innervation of the lacrimal (choice A), submandibular (choice B), sublingual (choice C), and nasal glands (choice E).

79. (E) Respiratory (ciliated pseudostratified columnar) epithelium is characterized by a mixture of tall and short cell types, all of which contact the basement membrane. It is readily recognizable on the basis of the multiple layers of nuclei, the prominent cilia, and the thick basement membrane (the amorphous band at the base of the epithelium). Goblet cells are also characteristic. The esophagus (choice A) is lined by a non-keratinized stratified squamous epithelium. The colon (choice B) is also lined by a columnar epithelium which has goblet cells, but the nuclei form a single row and the apical surfaces bear microvilli, not cilia. The aorta (choice C), like all blood vessels, is lined by endothelium. With few exceptions, endothelium is a thin, simple squamous epithelium. Transitional epithelium lines the urinary bladder (choice D). This is a stratified epithelium adapted for stretching. A distinctive feature of transitional epithelium is the surface layer of large pillow-shaped cells.

80. (D) The distinctive feature of enteroendocrine cells is the presence of small granules located predominantly in the cytoplasm on the basal side of the cell nucleus. Other terms applied to enteroendocrine cells are DNES (diffuse neuroendocrine system) cells and, because they stain with silver salts, argentaffin cells. This diverse family of cells secretes signal molecules (polypeptides and biogenic amines) that act on neighboring (paracrine) or distant (endocrine) cells. The cell shown here extends to the apical surface of the epithelium, and thus would be designated an open type of enteroendocrine cell. The other listed cell types are all residents of intestinal crypts of the small intestine. Goblet cells (choice A) contain large, generally washed-out mucous granules in the apical cytoplasm and a narrow cell base. An example of a goblet cell can be seen in the micrograph above the arrow. Paneth cells (choice B) have large granules filling the apical cytoplasm, but these are intensely acidophilic. Paneth cells are limited in distribution to the small intestine, specifically localized to the basal ends of the crypts. Several such cells can be seen in the micrograph. Absorptive cells (choice C) are the majority cell type of the intestinal epithelium. With the light microscope, they appear as relatively nondescript columnar cells with a brush border of microvilli, but no secretory granules. Stem cells (choice E) are relatively undifferentiated, and accordingly lack distinguishing morphological features. Stem cells divide mitotically to produce cells that differentiate to replace goblet, absorptive, and Paneth cells.

81. (A) Sensory ganglia are characterized histologically by the presence of clusters or columns of spherical neuronal cell bodies (somas or perikarya) interposed between bundles of nerve fibers. The micrograph illustrates some other features typical of somas of primary sensory (pseudounipolar) neurons: (a) centrally located nucleus, (b) a distinct covering of satellite cells (note the layer of small nuclei around each soma), and (c) a wide range of sizes. The superior cervical ganglion (choice B) and pterygopalatine ganglion (choice C) are autonomic ganglia, which are sites of synaptic contact between preganglionic nerve fibers and the multipolar postsynaptic neurons that project directly to effector organs. Like sensory ganglia, autonomic ganglia are composed of nerve fibers and neuronal cell bodies, but there are distinguishing features: (a) somas are scattered homogeneously among the nerve fibers rather than clustered, (b) somas have a narrow range of sizes, (c) nuclei tend to have an eccentric location within the soma, and (d) the satellite cells encompassing each soma are less prominent. A peripheral nerve (choice D) is a bundle of nerve fibers; no cell bodies would be seen. The cerebellar cortex (choice E) is composed of both cell bodies and nerve fibers, but these are organized in distinct layers. Moreover, the cell bodies (principally Purkinje cells and granule cells) have distinctive sizes and shapes.

82. **(C)** The black areas in this section of dried, compact bone are empty spaces normally occupied by cells and soft tissues. The arrows indicate lacunae interspersed among lamellae of osteons (haversian systems). In life, these are occupied by osteocytes. The fine lines radiating from the lacunae are canaliculi which contained processes of the osteocytes. Osteoclasts (choice A) are large, multinucleated cells found at surfaces of bone at sites that are undergoing absorption. Osteoblasts (choice B) are restricted to surfaces of bone at sites of bone apposition. When osteoblasts become entrapped in lacunae as a result of their synthetic activity, they become osteocytes. Blood vessels (choice D) of compact bone course through Volkmann's canals (not shown) and haversian canals (seen here at the center of each osteon). Hematopoietic cells (choice E) occur in red marrow located within medullary canals of long bones and the cavities of cancellous bone.

83. **(C)** The buccinator is a muscle of facial expression and is therefore innervated by the facial nerve. The lateral pterygoid (choice A), masseter (choice B), anterior belly of the digastric (choice D), and temporalis (choice E) are all muscles of mastication and are therefore innervated by the mandibular division of the trigeminal nerve.

84. **(D)** The ciliary, sphincter pupillae, and medial rectus muscles participate in the near response. Signals originating in the right eye are directed to both the right and left pretectal region, not only the right side (choice A). Neurons in the left Edinger–Westphal nucleus receive input from both eyes, not only the the right eye (choice B). Dilation of the pupil is mediated via postganglionic neurons in the superior cervical ganglion, not the ciliary ganglion (choice C). The blink reflex involves the trigeminal (sensory limb) and facial (motor limb) nerves but not the oculomotor nerve (choice E).

85. **(A)** The cells of the first-order neurons that contribute to the ascending somatosensory pathways are located in dorsal root ganglia. Some dorsal horn neurons (choice B) contribute to ascending somatosensory pathways, but these signals do not reach the thalamus and cortex for conscious awareness. The dorsal primary rami (choice C) are nerve trunks and do not contain neuronal cell bodies. Nucleus gracilis and cuneatus (choice D), the dorsal column nuclei, contain second-order neurons in the ascending pathways. The nucleus dorsalis (choice E) contains second-order neurons in the pathway for ascending somatosensory signals that are directed to the cerebellum.

86. **(C)** The sensations of discriminative touch and vibration are transmitted through the medial lemniscus. The nucleus gracilis (choice A) contains neurons that process sensory signals from the lower extremity. Pain and temperature pathways decussate in the ventral white commisssure (choice B). The second-order fibers carrying discriminative touch and vibration from the upper limb originate from neurons in the nucleus cuneatus (choice D).

87. **(B)** The principal somatosensory pathways course through the posterior limb of the internal capsule and terminate in the postcentral gyrus, not the precentral gyrus (choice A). The somatosensory pathways decussate in the spinal cord or brainstem, not in the thalamus (choice C). The somatosensory pathways typically involve a three-neuron chain, not a two-neuron sequence (choice D). The ventral posterior nucleus of the thalamus is the principal processing station for somatosensation, not the ventral lateral nucleus (choice E).

88. **(D)** The ascending MLF provides input to the oculomotor and abducens nuclei. The lateral vestibulospinal tract originates from the lateral vestibular nucleus, not the medial vestibular nucleus (choice A). The medial vestibulospinal tract extends to cervical or upper thoracic levels but not to the lumbar spinal cord (choice B). The vestibulospinal tracts primarily influence extensor musculature, not flexors (choice C). The descending portion of the MLF courses into the spinal cord and has no influence over extraocular muscles (choice E).

89. (A) A patient with extensive damage in the lower brainstem is likely to have some involvement of the vestibular nuclei or their connections, and this will preclude nystagmus from being induced. In contrast, nystagmus can be induced (not choice B) with appropriate stimulation in a patient who has no involvement of the vestibular nuclei or their connections. The direction of nystagmus is defined as the direction of the fast component (not choice C) of the movement. When observed following the appropriate stimulation in a patient, the presence of nystagmus indicates that there is no damage to the vestibular system (not choice D). Nystagmus is not limited to horizontal (choice E) eye movements.

90. (A) Deflection of the stereocilia toward the kinocilium (toward the utricle) has a depolarizing influence on the hair cell. Deflection away from the kinocilium (away from the utricle) is hyperpolarizing, not depolarizing (choice B). Only movement of the stereocilia toward the kinocilium is depolarizing, not movement in any direction (choice C). If the stereocilia remain upright or vertical (choice D), the hair cell is not depolarized. If the stereocilia are detached from the kinocilium (choice E), the hair cell no longer functions normally.

91. (E) The near response, but not the pupillary light reflex, involves the visual cortex. The near response includes disconjugate, not conjugate (choice A) eye movements. The near response includes bilateral activation of the medial rectus muscles, not the lateral rectus muscles (choice B). The near response involves both the optic nerve (choice C) and the oculomotor nerve (choice D).

92. (E) The internal laryngeal nerve supplies the laryngeal mucosa above the level of the vocal fold as well as the mucosa of the piriform recess and the epiglottic valleculae. The external laryngeal nerve (choice A) is motor to the cricothyroid muscle and the lowest part of the inferior pharyngeal constrictor muscle. The inferior laryngeal nerve (choice B) is motor to the intrinsic muscles of the larynx except the cricothyroid muscle, and is sensory to the mucosa of the larynx below the level of the vocal fold. The glossopharyngeal nerve (choice C) carries afferent fibers from the mucosa of the middle ear, auditory tube, pharynx, palatine tonsils, and posterior one-third of the tongue, but does not supply the laryngeal mucosa. The pharyngeal plexus (choice D) supplies most of the innervation to the pharynx, including general visceral afferent fibers from the pharyngeal mucosa that are carried in the glossopharyngeal nerve.

93. (A) All four extremities can be moved in a coordinated manner through the actions of intrinsic spinal cord circuits. Type Ia sensory fibers (choice B) from muscle spindles primarily form synapses with alpha motoneurons, whereas type Ib sensory fibers (choice C) from Golgi tendon organs primarily form synapses with inhibitory interneurons. Type C pain fibers (choice D) form numerous synaptic contacts with spinal cord interneurons. The activation of a Golgi tendon organ (choice E) inhibits the muscle to which it is structurally related.

94. (B) A motor unit is composed of one alpha motoneuron and all the muscle fibers it innervates. A motor unit does not include alpha and gamma motoneurons (choice A), nor does it include sensory and motor fibers (choice C). The smallest motor units (choice D) contain alpha motoneurons with the smallest somal diameter, whereas large motor units are composed of motoneurons with the largest somal diameter. The motor units associated with extraocular muscles (choice E) are among the smallest, since a relatively small number of muscle fibers (10 to 15) are innervated by a single alpha motoneuron.

95. (A) A striosome or patch is one of the many relatively small acetylcholinesterase-poor regions which collectively form a mosaic distribution within the caudate nucleus and the putamen. Pyramidal neurons (choice B) are found in the cerebral cortex and hippocampus. Glomeruli (choice C) are complex synaptic structures found in several regions of the brain, including the thalamus, olfactory bulbs, and cerebellar cortex. Renshaw cells (choice D) are inhibitory neurons found in the spinal cord gray matter, while callosal neurons (choice E) are located in the cerebral cortex.

96. (A) Compression of cranial nerve III, in combination with descending corticospinal and corticobulbar fibers occurs as part of superior alternating hemiplegia. Middle alternating hemiplegia (choice B) and inferior alternating hemiplegia (choice C) involve cranial nerves VI and XII, respectively, in combination with corticospinal fibers. Patients with Broca's aphasia (choice D) typically do not exhibit involvement of the pupillary light reflexes. Wallenberg's syndrome (lateral medullary syndrome) (choice E) typically does not include damage to the corticospinal tract.

97. (C) The skin in the affected area is red and dry (not moist as in choice B) due to diminished sympathetic activity. The pupil on the affected side is constricted (myosis) (not dilated as in choice A) due to unopposed activity of the sphincter pupillae muscle. Motor deficits such as atrophy of tongue musculature (choice D) or paralysis of facial expression muscles (choice E) are typically not part of Horner's syndrome.

98. (A) The primary sensory neurons of the cranial nerve and dorsal root ganglia are derived from neural crest cells. The cerebellum (choice B) arises from the rhombic lip portion of the developing neural tube whereas the retina (choice C) is a derivative of the forebrain neural tube. The vestibular and cochlear nuclei (choice D) arise from the alar plate of the hindbrain neural tube, while ventral horn motoneurons (choice E) derive from the basal plate of the spinal cord neural tube.

99. (A) A lesion in the dominant hemisphere involving the ventrolateral parietal lobe is likely to include Wernicke's area. Damage to this cortical region produces a receptive (sensory) aphasia known as Wernicke's aphasia. Broca's (motor) aphasia (choice B) is the result of damage to the frontal operculum in the dominant hemisphere. Contralateral hemineglect (choice C) is typically caused by lesions in the non-dominant parietal lobe, whereas motor aprosodia (choice D), the inability to impart proper emotional tone to speech, is due to damage to the frontal operculum in the non-dominant hemisphere. Prosopagnosia (choice E), the inability to recognize familiar faces, most frequently results from bilateral damage to the ventral portion of the temporo-occipital association cortex.

100. (C) Neurons in the internal segment of the globus pallidus contribute axons to the ansa lenticularis. Degeneration of neurons in the pars compacta of the substantia nigra gives rise to resting tremor, not an intention tremor (choice A). The thalamic fasciculus (choice B) includes axons arising from cells in the globus pallidus and cerebellar nuclei. Most neurons in the pars reticulata of the substantia nigra utilize GABA (gamma-aminobutyric acid) as a neurotransmitter, not dopamine (choice D). The term *lenticular nucleus* (choice E) refers to the combination of the putamen and globus pallidus.

101. (D) Capsular lesions of the corticobulbar system produce the "central seven" symptoms. Loss of the descending cortical fibers to the contralateral facial nucleus (cranial nerve VII) primarily affects the muscles of facial expression in the lower portion of the face, particularly those around the angle of the mouth and the nasolabial fold. Spastic hemiplegia (choice A), deviation of the protruded tongue (choice B), and hypertonia/hyperreflexia (choice C) are symptoms that result from a capsular lesion, but they would be seen contralateral to the affected capsule, and in this case would involve the left side of the body. Paraplegia (choice E) is not typically seen following a unilateral capsular lesion.

102. (A) The cytoarchitectural subdivisions of the SI cortex are numbered from anterior to posterior as 3a, 3b, 1, and 2. All four subdivisions of the SI cortex (not just 3b as in choice B) contain a complete representation of the entire body surface. The somatotopic representation of the body surface in the primary somatosensory cortex is arranged in a "tongue to tail" (not the reverse as indicated in choice C) sequence from ventrolateral to dorsomedial. Areas 3a and 2 (choice D) receive input from muscle spindle afferents and Golgi tendon organs, whereas areas 3b and 1 (choice E) receive mostly cutaneous inputs.

103. (A) The entry of calcium into the axon terminal initiates the sequence of events leading to release of neurotransmitter. Docking proteins (choice B) attach synaptic vesicles to the presynaptic membrane. Fusion of vesicles with the presynaptic membrane (choice C) results in the release of one quantum of the transmitter agent. There are no actin bridges (choice D) that join the pre- and postsynaptic membranes. Following vesicular release, the neurotransmitter agent binds to receptors on the postsynaptic membrane, not the presynaptic membrane (choice E).

104. (C) The type Ia sensory fibers from a spindle form direct excitatory synapses with alpha motoneurons. Each muscle spindle contains a mixture of both nuclear bag and nuclear chain intrafusal fibers, not just one type as indicated in choice A. Each intrafusal muscle fiber (choice B) is innervated by only one gamma motoneuron. Activation of type Ia sensory fibers (choice D) leads to excitation of the muscle in which that spindle is located. Alpha motoneurons (choice E) synapse with extrafusal muscle fibers, whereas gamma motoneurons synapse with intrafusal muscle fibers.

105. (B) The Babinski sign, dorsiflexion of the great toe in response to stroking the plantar aspect of the foot, is a characteristic sign of pyramidal tract involvement. Signs and symptoms of corticospinal tract injury that are nearly always apparent to some degree include spastic paralysis, hypertonia, loss of deep tendon reflexes, and hyperactive abdominal and cremasteric reflexes. Flaccid paralysis and hypotonia (choice A) are commonly seen following lower motoneuron injury, as is loss of deep tendon reflexes (choice C). Muscle degeneration and atrophy (choice D) are not characteristic symptoms of corticospinal tract damage. The presence of an intention tremor (choice E) is a sign of cerebellar damage and is not seen with corticospinal tract lesions.

106. (D) Spastic muscles exhibit an increase in the resistance to passive manipulation by the examiner. The muscles typically affected by spasticity are physiological limb extensors and not postural muscles as indicated in choice A. Muscles that exhibit spastic paralysis are hypertonic, not hypotonic (choice B). Muscles that exhibit fibrillations (choice C) or decreased deep tendon reflexes (choice E) are demonstrating signs of lower motoneuron damage, not involvement of upper motoneurons that form the corticospinal tract.

107. (D) Basal ganglia lesions typically produce involuntary movements such as athetosis or choreiform movements. Basal ganglia disease does not usually result in muscle paralysis limited to antigravity muscles (choice A) or loss of tendon reflexes (choice B), symptoms that are more commonly associated with upper or lower motoneuron lesions. Ataxia and scanning speech (choice C) are symptoms associated with cerebellar lesions. Horizontal nystagmus (choice E) is typically seen following damage to the vestibular sensory apparatus, cranial nerve VIII, or central vestibular connections. In addition, cerebellar lesions may also cause nystagmus.

108. (C) The nucleus raphe magnus receives input from the periaqueductal gray and gives rise to descending serotonergic fibers of the raphespinal projection. The latter fibers activate enkephalinergic spinal cord interneurons that presynaptically inhibit incoming pain fibers at their initial synapse in the spinal cord dorsal horn. The ventral lateral nucleus of the thalamus (choice A) is primarily involved with motor function and does not contribute to descending pathways that influence pain transmission. The medial longitudinal fasciculus (choice B) is an ascending fiber system in the brainstem that is primarily involved in the control of eye movements. The rubrospinal system (choice

D) is a descending fiber tract involved with the control of limb musculature. The neurotransmitter dopamine (choice E) has not been shown to be involved in the descending systems that modulate pain transmission.

109. **(A)** Each taste receptor responds best to a specific type of stimulus quality, but may respond with less vigor to the other stimuli. The taste receptors are arranged in a rostrocaudal pattern (not medial to lateral as indicated in choice B), such that the most anterior respond best to sweet and salty stimuli, whereas sour and bitter sensations are represented posteriorly. Taste receptors generally have a relatively short life span of 7 to 10 days (not three months as indicated in choice C). Taste receptors are stimulated when a solid or fluid substance diffuses through its apical pore and depolarizes the cell. The only receptors that hyperpolarize (choice D) in response to their preferred stimulus are retinal photoreceptors. Taste receptors are not typically found on the lateral surfaces (choice E) of the tongue.

110. **(A)** The muscles that dorsiflex the ankle joint are located in the anterior compartment of the leg and are innervated by the deep peroneal nerve. The evertors of the foot occupy the lateral compartment of the leg and are supplied by the superficial peroneal nerve. Thus, the common peroneal nerve innervates both the dorsiflexors and evertors of the foot. The superficial peroneal nerve (choice B) supplies the evertors of the foot located in the lateral compartment of the leg, but not the dorsiflexors of the foot located in the anterior compartment. The deep peroneal nerve (choice C) supplies the dorsiflexors of the foot located in the anterior compartment of the leg, but not the evertors of the foot located in the lateral compartment. The tibial nerve (choice D) supplies the muscles of the posterior leg which are plantar flexors and invertors of the foot. The obturator nerve (choice E) supplies the adductor muscle group of the medial thigh.

111. **(C)** The common fibular nerve leaves the popliteal fossa to wind forward around the lateral surface of the neck of the fibula and is vulnerable at this point. It ends in the lateral compartment of the leg by dividing into the superficial and deep fibular nerves. The sural nerve (choice A) is a cutaneous nerve with distribution down the posterolateral side of the leg onto the lateral heel and foot. It is not vulnerable in a fracture of the neck of the fibula. The tibial nerve (choice B) is not commonly injured in a fracture of the leg because it does not lie adjacent to either the tibia or fibula in its course. The deep fibular nerve (choice D) arises from the common fibular nerve in the lateral compartment of the leg and enters the anterior compartment. It does not lie adjacent to the neck of the fibula and is unlikely to be injured by a fracture at that point. The femoral nerve (choice E) is the motor and cutaneous nerve of the anterior thigh and is not related to the neck of the fibula.

112. **(E)** The posterior cruciate ligament prevents backward sliding of the tibia on the femur. Abnormal anteroposterior movement when the knee is flexed is a "drawer" sign. The tibial collateral ligament (choice A) extends from the medial femoral condyle to the medial tibial condyle, blending with and reinforcing the medial part of the fibrous capsule. It does not significantly restrict anterior or posterior sliding movements between the tibia and femur. The oblique popliteal ligament (choice C) is an upward and lateral extension of the semimembranosus tendon which reinforces the capsule of the knee joint posteriorly. It helps to resist hyperextension of the knee, but does not significantly restrict anterior or posterior sliding movements between the tibia and femur. The anterior cruciate ligament (choice D) prevents forward sliding of the tibia on the femur, but not backward movement. The fibular collateral ligament (choice B) extends from the lateral femoral epicondyle to the head of the fibula. It does not significantly restrict anterior or posterior sliding movements between the tibia and femur.

113. **(C)** Transposition of the great vessels occurs when the truncoconal ridges fail to spiral as they divide the outflow tract into two

channels. This produces two totally independent circulatory loops with the right ventricle feeding into the aorta and the left ventricle feeding into the pulmonary artery. Persistent truncus arteriosus (choice A) results from a total failure of the truncoconal ridges to develop and partition the outflow tract of the developing heart. Tetralogy of Fallot (choice B) is a related group of defects with the primary malformation being an unequal division of the outflow tract resulting in pulmonary stenosis. The other features of tetralogy are an interventricular septal defect, an overriding aorta, and right ventricular hypertrophy. Survival of the infant depends on the maintenance of a patent ductus arteriosus. Persistent atrioventricular canal (choice D) results from a failure of the endocardial cushions to fuse and partition the atrioventricular canal into a right and left component. It is accompanied by defects of the atrial and ventricular septa. Common atrium (choice E) results from a complete failure of the septum primum and septum secundum to form.

114. (C) The oblique fissure separates the superior lobe from the inferior lobe. The horizontal fissure makes a further subdivision of the superior lobe of the right lung. The horizontal fissure and the inferior part of the oblique fissure form the boundaries of the middle lobe of the right lung. The apex of the left lung (choice A) is the part of the upper lobe that projects above the first rib into the neck. It is not bounded by a fissure. The lingula of the left lung (choice B) is part of the upper lobe and is separated from the lower lobe by the oblique fissure. The left lung has no horizontal fissure. The horizontal fissure and the superior part of the oblique fissure delineate the upper lobe of the right lung (choice D). The lower lobe of the left lung (choice E) is separated from the upper lobe by the oblique fissure.

115. (A) The pea-sized bulbourethral glands of the male lie on either side of the membranous urethra and are embedded in the fibers of the sphincter urethrae and deep transverse perineal muscles. The ischiocavernosus muscles (choice B) cover the crura of the penis (corpora cavernosa). The superficial transverse perineal muscles (choice C) are small muscles that arise from the ischial tuberosity and insert into the perineal body. The bulbospongiosus muscles (choice D) arise from the perineal body and the median raphe of the bulb and invest the bulb of the penis or the bulb of the vestibule. The corpora cavernosa (choice E) are the paired erectile bodies that together with the single corpus spongiosum form the body of the penis.

116. (E) The digastric muscle is a two-bellied muscle that attaches by an intermediate tendon to the hyoid bone. With the border of the mandible for a base, the digastric muscle completes the definition of the submandibular triangle, the apex of which is directed inferiorly. The sixth cervical vertebra (choice A) is not related to the digastric muscle or its intermediate tendon. The mandible (choice B) is one side of the submandibular triangle, the other two being the anterior and posterior bellies of the digastric muscle. The anterior belly of the digastric muscle inserts at the digastric fossa of the mandible. The mastoid process (choice C) provides attachment for the posterior belly of the digastric muscle (at the mastoid notch), but not for the intermediate tendon. The cricoid cartilage (choice D) is not related to the digastric muscle or its intermediate tendon.

117. (D) The external jugular vein passes perpendicularly across the superficial surface of the sternocleidomastoid muscle directly under the platysma muscle. The retromandibular vein (choice A) forms in the parotid gland by union of the superficial temporal and maxillary veins, and ends behind the mandible by dividing into branches that join the internal and external jugular veins. The anterior jugular vein (choice B) descends on the front of the neck near the midline. The posterior auricular vein (choice C) joins the retromandibular vein to form the external jugular vein posterior to the mandible. The internal jugular vein (choice E) runs in the carotid sheath deep to the sternocleidomastoid muscle.

118. (E) The prevertebral fascia crosses the midline anterior to the prevertebral muscles and continues laterally, covering the scalene muscles and forming the floor of the posterior triangle. The vagus nerve (choice A) lies within the carotid sheath. The common carotid artery (choice B) lies within the carotid sheath. The internal jugular vein (choice C) lies within the carotid sheath. The esophagus (choice D) is surrounded by the pretracheal (visceral) fascia.

119. (C) The superior thyroid artery is usually the first branch of the external carotid artery. The thyrocervical trunk (choice A) arises from the subclavian artery and gives rise to the inferior thyroid artery. The internal carotid artery (choice B) gives off no major branches in the neck. The facial artery (choice D) and the lingual artery arise as independent branches of the external carotid artery. The brachiocephalic artery (choice E) gives rise to the right subclavian artery, the right common carotid artery, and occasionally a single thyroidea ima (lowest thyroid) artery.

120. (B) The isthmus of the thyroid gland unites the two lateral lobes across tracheal rings two, three, and four. The cricoid cartilage (choice A) lies superior to the isthmus of the thyroid gland. The jugular notch (choice C) is the superior border of the manubrium. It lies at the level of the third thoracic vertebra, well below the isthmus of the thyroid gland. The thyroid cartilage (choice D) lies superior to the isthmus of the thyroid gland. The hyoid bone (choice E) lies superior to the thyroid cartilage and far above the isthmus of the thyroid gland.

121. (B) The vocal folds are abducted and the rima glottidis is widened by the posterior cricoarytenoid muscles that rotate the arytenoid cartilages laterally. The cricothyroid muscles (choice A) tense and lengthen the vocal ligament by tilting the thyroid cartilage forward. The thyroarytenoid muscles (choice C) decrease the tension and length of the vocal ligaments by tilting the thyroid cartilages posteriorly. The transverse arytenoid muscle (choice D) adducts the vocal folds by pulling the arytenoid cartilages together. The lateral cricoarytenoid muscles (choice E) adduct the vocal folds by medially rotating the arytenoid cartilages.

122. (B) The inferior laryngeal nerve is motor to the intrinsic muscles of the larynx except the cricothyroid muscle, and is sensory to the larynx below the level of the vocal fold. The superior laryngeal nerve (choice A) is sensory to the laryngeal mucosa above the vocal fold and also includes motor fibers to the cricothyroid muscle. The external laryngeal nerve (choice C) is the branch of the superior laryngeal nerve that contains the motor fibers to the cricothyroid muscle and to the cricopharyngeus muscle. The internal laryngeal nerve (choice D) is the branch of the superior laryngeal nerve that contains the sensory fibers to the laryngeal mucosa above the vocal fold. The glossopharyngeal nerve (choice E) does not supply either motor or sensory fibers to the larynx.

123. (B) The middle meningeal artery, a branch of the maxillary artery, is the principal artery of the cranial dura mater. It passes upward, superficial to the sphenomandibular ligament and between the two roots of the auriculotemporal nerve, and enters the middle cranial fossa via the foramen spinosum. The inferior alveolar artery (choice A) arises from the maxillary artery in the infratemporal fossa and passes with the inferior alveolar nerve into the mandibular foramen to supply the teeth of the lower jaw. The infraorbital artery (choice C) arises from the maxillary artery within the pterygopalatine fossa and passes forward through the inferior orbital fissure to reach the infraorbital canal. The masseteric artery (choice D) arises from the maxillary artery in the infratemporal fossa and passes through the mandibular notch with the masseteric branch of the mandibular nerve to reach the masseter muscle. The sphenopalatine artery (choice E) arises from the maxillary artery within the pterygopalatine fossa and reaches the nasal cavity through the sphenopalatine foramen.

124. (D) Intervertebral discs may protrude or rupture in any direction but do so most commonly in a posterolateral direction, just lateral to the strong central portion of the posterior longitudinal ligament. This is usually the weakest part of the disc, since the annulus is thinner here and is not supported by other ligaments. Anteriorly (choice A) the intervertebral discs are supported by the broad and strong anterior ligament. Herniation is less common in this direction. Posteriorly (choice B) the intervertebral discs are supported by the posterior longitudinal ligament. Herniation is less common in this direction. Anterolaterally (choice C) the intervertebral disc is supported by the broad anterior longitudinal ligament. The nucleus pulposus is also situated posteriorly in the disc, making herniation here less likely. Herniation of the intervertebral disc laterally (choice E) is not particularly common.

125. (C) A bulging or protruded disc typically affects the traversing nerve root; that is, the nerve affected is one number greater than the number of the disc. The L3 spinal nerve (choice A) would be affected by protrusion of the L2 intervertebral disc. The L4 spinal nerve (choice B) would be affected by protrusion of the L3 intervertebral disc. The S1 spinal nerve (choice D) would be affected by protrusion of the L5 intervertebral disc. The S2 spinal nerve (choice E) exits through the foramina of the fused sacrum and therefore is not subject to compression by herniated intervertebral discs.

126. (C) Abnormal lateral deviation of the spine is known as scoliosis. Kyphosis (choice A) is an increased posterior convexity of the vertebral column (hunchback). A ruptured disc (choice B) may produce irritation and spasm of the intrinsic back muscles but is not associated with lateral curvature of the vertebral column. Lordosis (choice D) is an increased anterior convexity of the vertebral column (swayback). Gorilla rib (choice E) is an abnormal rib associated with the first lumbar vertebra. It is not associated with abnormal lateral curvature of the spine.

127. (D) The sciatic nerve is the largest nerve in the body. It emerges below the piriformis and descends through the gluteal region crossing the posterior surfaces of the obturator internus, the gemelli, and the quadratus femoris muscles. The femoral artery (choice A) is a continuation of the external iliac artery below the inguinal ligament. It passes anterior to the hip joint. The common iliac veins (choice B) form in the major pelvis and ascend on the posterior abdominal wall to join and form the inferior vena cava. The obturator nerve (choice C) forms in the pelvis and enters the medial thigh through the obturator canal. The superior gluteal nerve and artery (choice E) enter the gluteal region above the piriformis muscle. The artery gives branches to the gluteus maximus muscle and then runs forward with the nerve to supply the gluteus medius, gluteus minimus, and tensor fasciae latae muscles.

128. (D) The femoral canal, the medial compartment of the femoral sheath, contains only a slight amount of loose connective tissue and one or two lymphatic vessels and nodes. The femoral artery (choice A) is found in the lateral compartment of the femoral sheath with the genital branch of the genitofemoral nerve. The femoral vein (choice B) occupies the intermediate compartment of the femoral sheath. The femoral nerve (choice C) is the most lateral structure in the femoral triangle, but it does not lie within the femoral sheath. The saphenous vein (choice E) is a superficial vein that passes through the saphenous hiatus to end in the femoral vein. It does not lie within the femoral canal.

129. (B) The flexor retinaculum of the foot runs between the medial malleolus and the calcaneus. The tendon of the tibialis posterior muscle passes under the flexor retinaculum immediately posterior to the medial malleolus. The tendon of the peroneus longus muscle (choice A) and the tendon of the peroneus brevis muscle pass beneath the superior and inferior peroneal retinacula on the lateral side of the foot. The tendon of the flexor digitorum longus muscle (choice C) passes beneath the flexor retinaculum immediately posterior to the tendon of the tibialis posterior. The tendon of the flexor hallucis longus muscle (choice D) passes beneath the flexor retinaculum posterior to the tendons of the tibialis posterior and flexor digitorum longus muscles. The tibial nerve (choice E) and the posterior tibial vessels pass beneath the flexor retinaculum between the tendons of the flexor digitorum longus and the flexor hallucis longus muscles.

130. (C) Considerable information concerning the size, shape, and function of the heart can be obtained from examining a simple posteroanterior projection of the heart. The arch of the aorta is seen as the prominence (the aortic bulb or knuckle) that lies most superiorly on the left margin of the heart shadow. The shadow of the ascending aorta (choice A) lies in the center of the heart shadow and cannot be seen along the margin. The shadow of the descending aorta (choice B) can be seen posterior to the heart shadow but does not lie along the margin of the shadow. The pulmonary trunk (choice D) is indicated by arrow B. Its shadow lies along the upper left margin between the shadows of the aortic arch above and the left auricle below. The shadow of the superior vena cava (choice E) lies along the upper right margin of the heart shadow opposite the shadows of the aortic arch and pulmonary trunk.

131. (B) The pericardial sac, the heart, and the roots of the great vessels occupy the middle mediastinum. The trachea (choice A) descends from the neck through the superior mediastinum and divides into the primary bronchi at the level of the sternal angle. The thymus (choice C) or its remnant lies in the superior mediastinum and the anterior mediastinum. The aortic arch (choice D) lies completely in the superior mediastinum, beginning and ending at the level of the sternal angle. The esophagus (choice E), vagus nerves, descending thoracic aorta, azygos veins, and thoracic duct are all located in the posterior mediastinum.

132. (B) There is only one point of the heart that can be directly identified on the precordium: the apex. A cardiac impulse may be visible at the apex, and palpation over it will confirm the presence of the apex beat. The apex is located in the left fifth intercostal space just medial to the midclavicular line, and is the point where the mitral valve is best heard. The tricuspid valve is best heard in the fifth intercostal space to the right of the sternum (choice A). The pulmonary valve is best heard in the second intercostal space to the left of the sternum (choice C). None of the heart sounds are best heard at the xiphisternal junction (choice D). The aortic valve is best heard in the second intercostal space to the left of the sternum (choice E).

133. (E) The portal vein forms posterior to the neck of the pancreas and ascends behind the first part of the duodenum to pass to the liver through the hepatoduodenal ligament. The splenic artery (choice A) arises from the celiac trunk in the bed of the stomach and passes to the left along the upper border of the pancreas. The common hepatic artery (choice B) arises from the celiac trunk in the bed of the stomach and passes to the right to enter the hepatoduodenal ligament. It passes above, not behind, the first part of the duodenum. The common hepatic duct (choice C) forms from the right and left hepatic ducts in the porta hepatis and becomes the common bile duct when it is joined by the cystic duct. The common bile duct descends behind the first part of the duodenum to join the main pancreatic duct. The superior mesenteric artery (choice D) arises from the abdominal aorta and enters the root of the mesentery where it passes anterior to the third part of the duodenum.

134. (A) The middle cardiac vein runs in the posterior interventricular sulcus with the posterior interventricular artery. The small cardiac vein (choice B) runs along the acute margin of the right ventricle to end in the right end of the coronary sinus. The coronary sinus (choice C) lies in the coronary sulcus between the left atrium and the right and left ventricles. The oblique vein of the left atrium runs downward on the left atrium to end in the coronary sinus (choice D). The great cardiac vein (choice E) lies in the anterior interventricular sulcus with the anterior interventricular artery.

135. **(B)** The cutaneous branches of the maxillary division of the trigeminal nerve include the infraorbital, inferior palpebral, external nasal, zygomaticofacial, and the zygomaticotemporal. The mental nerve (choice C) is a cutaneous branch of the mandibular division. The cutaneous branches of the ophthalmic division of the trigeminal nerve include the supratrochlear (choice A), lacrimal (choice D), supraorbital (choice E), infratrochlear, and external nasal branches.

136. **(E)** All the listed cell types are components of the respiratory system. Type II pneumocytes are the source of pulmonary surfactant. Alveolar dust cells (choice A) are macrophages. Endothelial cells (choice B) and type I pneumocytes (choice D) are components of the blood–air barrier. Small granule cells (choice C), which are members of the diffuse neuroendocrine system, function in paracrine and endocrine signaling.

137. **(B)** Although it is likely that T lymphocyte progenitor cells arise in bone marrow, differentiation and programming of new T lymphocytes occurs in the thymus. Bone marrow provides the environment for development of stem and precursor cells into B lymphocytes (choice A), granulocytes (choices C, D, and E), erythrocytes, platelets, and monocytes.

138. **(D)** Cells that secrete proteinaceous substances in response to endocrine signals characteristically store these products (or their precursors) in membrane delimited granules in the apical (toward the lumen of the acinus) region of the cytoplasm. Steroid hormones have several stereotypical ultrastructural features related to their function. Lipid precursor molecules are stored in lipid droplets (choice A), but there is no storage of the end product in secretory granules. Synthesis of steroid hormones is a cooperative activity of the well developed sER (choice B) and mitochondria with specializations that include tubular rather than shelf-like cristae (choice C). None of these features typify protein-secreting cells. Although a Golgi complex is a ubiquitous feature of metabolically active cells, it is particularly well developed in cells that synthesize and package proteins for secretion (choice E).

139. **(D)** The vagus nerve is a mixed nerve with functions including special visceral efferent (innervation of laryngeal muscles), general visceral efferent (parasympathetic innervation of thoracic and abdominal viscera), general visceral afferent (sensory innervation of thoracic and abdominal viscera), special visceral afferent (sensory innervation of pharyngeal taste buds), and general somatic afferent (cutaneous innervation of a portion of the external ear), but not general somatic efferent. The oculomotor nerve (choice A) contains nerve fibers that serve either a somatic efferent (motor innervation of extraocular muscles) or general visceral efferent (parasympathetic innervation of pupillary constrictor and ciliary body) function. The trigeminal nerve (choice B) consists of axons that are either general somatic afferent (sensory innervation of face and anterior oral and nasal cavities or special visceral efferent (motor innervation of mastication muscles). The abducens nerve (choice C) provides motor innervation of the lateral rectus extraocular muscle, and the hypoglossal nerve (choice E) provides motor innervation of the intrinsic and extrinsic skeletal muscles of the tongue. Thus, both nerves are classified as having somatic efferent as their sole functional component.

140. **(D)** The first meiotic division is protracted in both sexes. After completing DNA synthesis, primary spermatocytes enter prophase of the first meiotic division, but spend nearly three weeks in the pachytene stage of prophase before rapidly completing the remaining steps of the first meiotic division to produce secondary spermatocytes. At the time a female is born, all gametes are primary oocytes arrested in Prophase I of meiosis. Even the small number of oocytes that resume meiosis will remain arrested for approximately 12 to 50 years before doing so. Migration of primordial germ cells from the yolk sac wall to the developing gonad (choice A) occurs during part (weeks 4 to 6) of the embryonic period, and the two genders are morphologically indistinguishable at this time. Spermatogonia and oogonia undergo mitotic division (choice B) to produce the cells that begin meiosis (primary spermatocytes and primary oocytes). A given mitotic event has a duration of hours or days. In females, all oogonia have produced a lifetime supply of primary oocytes by the sixth month of gestation. In males, spermatogonia persist thoughout adult life as stem cells that give rise to new primary spermatocytes continuously. Prior to the initiation of meiosis, primary spermatocytes and primary oocytes in interphase undergo a round of DNA replication (choice C), a process that requires a few hours. No DNA synthesis occurs during the remaining stages of spermatogenesis. In spermatogenesis, the second meiotic division (choice E) is a very rapid event, requiring less than one day. A few hours prior to ovulation, the primary oocyte in the mature follicle completes the first meiotic division to produce a primary polar body and a secondary oocyte. The secondary oocyte (ovum) begins the second meiotic division but becomes arrested in metaphase. The division is completed only if fertilization occurs. Otherwise, the secondary oocyte degenerates within about a day without completing meiosis.

141. (C) Hematoxylin is a cationic dye that, although complex in its interactions with cellular and extracellular constituents, tends to bind to basophilic (i.e., acidic) substances. These include ribosomes because of their content of ribonucleic acid. The other dye of the H&E stain is eosin, an anionic dye that tends to bind to acidophilic (i.e., basic) substances. Golgi complexes (choice A) are not strongly stained by hematoxylin or eosin. Generally, the cytoplasm occupied by Golgi complexes is unstained. For example, the prominent Golgi complex of a plasma cell is seen adjacent to the nucleus as a poorly stained region of the otherwise intensely basophilic cytoplasm. Smooth endoplasmic reticulum (sER, choice B) lacks ribosomes or other nucleic acid–rich components, and the cytoplasm of cells rich in sER does not stain strongly with hematoxylin. Elastic fibers (choice D) and collagenous fibers (choice E) are stained by eosin, but not hematoxylin, in routine histological sections.

142. (B) The source of IgE molecules is a subpopulation of antigen-stimulated B lymphocytes (choice D) and their immunoglobulin-secreting plasma cell progeny. The IgE that is secreted by plasma cells into tissue fluid and blood is sequestered by the IgE receptors of mast cells and basophils. Mast cells and basophils are triggered to degranulate when antigen (typically allergens) binds to the IgE molecules that occupy their IgE receptors. This is the basis of allergic reactions. Neutrophils (choice A) and macrophages (choice C) have Fc receptors for immunoglobulins of the IgG class. Binding of IgG molecules to bacteria promotes their phagocytosis and destruction by neutrophils and macrophages. Platelets (choice E), which function primarily in hemostasis, are not directly involved in immune responses.

143. (C) Gonadotropin-releasing hormone normally acts on pituitary gonadotropic cells, those cells in the pars distalis that secrete FSH (follicle stimulating hormone) and LH. In order for the gonadotropes to function normally, hypothalamic neurons must intermittently secrete GnRH into the hypothalamohypophyseal portal system in brief pulses at an interval of about 90 minutes. Paradoxically, if the gonadotropic cells are exposed to a prolonged high level of GnRH signal, as when a pharmacologic dose of an agonist is administered, gonadotropic cells cease secretion of FSH and LH (choice A) and become desensitized; that is, they no longer respond to the normal estrogens and progestins in the normal feedback mechanisms. When the objective is to retrieve oocytes in a mature (fertilizable) condition, it is important to know the exact timing of the LH surge. This is a necessary event because it brings about the final maturation of the oocyte; however, ovulation occurs about 40 hours after the LH surge and the oocytes can be harvested effectively only before they are released from the ovary. Thus, the reason for disabling the normal hormonal signaling by gonadotropic cells is to avoid a natural LH surge and substitute a controlled surge by administering an LH analog when numerous large follicles have emerged as a result of the gonadotropic hormone therapy. The midcycle LH surge is normally brought about by the response of gonadotropes to elevated levels of estrogens (mainly estradiol) secreted by the ovarian follicle that has established dominance. The primary extra-ovarian signals that regulate development of ovarian follicles are FSH and LH. GnRH (choice B) is only indirectly involved. Immediately before ovulation, the primary oocyte of the (usually single) dominant follicle resumes meiosis, completing the first division to produce a polar body and a secondary oocyte which begins the second division (choice D), but becomes arrested in metaphase. This is one of many preovulatory changes that are brought about by the LH surge. The proliferative phase of the endometrium (choice E) is induced by estrogens released by developing ovarian follicles.

144. (E) The autonomic neurons of the thoracic and lumbar spinal cord are sympathetic preganglionic neurons with their cell bodies (somas) in the intermediolateral cell column. These cells project to postganglionic neurons located in the sympathetic paravertebral chain ganglia and in prevertebral ganglia. Axons of postganglionic, not preganglionic, neurons (choice A) project to the effector cells of the gut, including smooth muscle of the stomach. Parasympathetic ganglion cells in the stomach wall (choice B) receive termination and signals from axons of the vagus nerve. The submandibular salivary gland does receive both parasympathetic and sympathetic innervation (choice C); however, the direct source of the sympathetic innervation is the superior cervical ganglion. The dorsal root ganglia (choice D), which contain somas of sensory pseudounipolar neurons, are not targets of preganglionic sympathetic projections.

145. (D) Collagenous fibers of the periodontal ligament function to form a resilient suspension system for the tooth. These fibers are attached to the cementum covering of the root and to the alveolar bone of the tooth socket. Dentinal tubules (choice B) are minute canals that extend through the thickness of the dentin in both the crown and root. Each dentinal tubule contains processes of an odontoblast (choice A). Odontoblasts are the cells that produce dentin. The stellate reticulum (choice C) is a component of the enamel organ, a temporary epithelial structure that produces the enamel of the crown before the tooth erupts. The subodontoblastic plexus of Rashkow (choice E) is a network of nerve fibers in the dental pulp.

146. (E) High endothelial venules (HEV), located primarily in the deep cortex, are specialized to recruit circulating lymphocytes from the blood. Lymphocytes in the circulating blood adhere to the lining endothelial cells of HEV by way of an integrin-based recognition. Lymphocytes then gain access to the lymph node tissue by actively migrating (a process called diapedesis) between or through endothelial cells. Arterioles (choice A) are a component of the circulation of the lymph node, but they are not permeable to cell traffic. Afferent lymphatic vessels (choice B) conduct lymph, not blood, into the lymph node. The source of the lymph is either upstream lymph nodes or tissue fluid from the region supplied by the node. This component of the system serves as a filter and as a mechanism for antigen-presenting cells to enter the node. Efferent lymphatic vessels (choice C) conduct lymph and cells from the lymph node to either the blood circulation or to downstream lymph nodes. Lymph in efferent lymphatic vessels conveys immunoglobulins and recirculating lymphocytes to the bloodstream. Medullary sinuses (choice D) are part of a system of passages that filter lymph and direct it from the afferent lymphatic vessels to the efferent lymphatic vessels. Medullary sinuses occupy spaces between medullary cords, which are occupied by large numbers of plasma cells, the cells that secrete immunoglobulins.

147. (B) Schwann cells are neural crest derivatives that form the myelin sheaths of large axons in peripheral nerves. The myelin is composed of multiple, tightly packed layers of Schwann cell membrane. Oligodendrocytes (choice A) also form myelin, but they are restricted to the central nervous system. Fibroblasts (choice C) contribute to the formation of the perineurium, which is a sleeve covering bundles (fascicles) of nerve fibers, and to formation of the epineurium, a connective tissue sleeve that covers the entire nerve. Cells of the perineurium (choice D) are flattened, epithelium-like cells that contribute to the blood–nerve barrier. Astrocytes (choice E) are restricted to the central nervous system where they have multiple functions in support of neurons. These functions include mechanical support, scavenging of neurotransmitters, metabolic support, and contributions to the isolation of brain tissue from blood and cerebrospinal fluid.

148. (A) An individual sarcomere, the unit of contraction in striated muscle, spans the interval between successive Z-lines. Each sarcomere encompasses an A-band (choice B) and half of each of two I-bands (choice D). Each myofibril (choice B) of a striated muscle fiber is composed of a tandem series of sarcomeres. Coupling of excitation and contraction is a critical function of the triad (choice E), which is composed of a T-tubule interposed between two cisternae of the sarcoplasmic reticulum.

149. (C) The cytoplasm of the endothelial cell that lines this small blood vessel has a beaded appearance because it is interrupted by fenestrae that are bridged by diaphragms. Such capillaries are typical of the kidney, intestinal mucosa, and endocrine glands. This capillary in the neurohypophysis is surrounded by axon terminals filled with secretory granules. There are no breaks in the endothelial lining of continuous capillaries (choice A), a more widespread capillary found, for example, in muscle and nervous tissue. Discontinuous capillaries (choice B), such as the sinusoids of the liver and spleen, have large gaps within and between endothelial cells which allows traffic of cells through their walls. The walls of both medium veins (choice D) and arterioles (choice E) have smooth muscle and connective tissue components in addition to the endothelium.

150. (E) The intercalated disk is formed by junctional complexes between adjacent cardiac muscle cells. Note that the transverse component of the junctional complex (indicated by the arrow) is located at the position of the Z-line (hemi-Z band) of an adjacent terminal sarcomere of each of the two muscle cells. Mitochondria (choice A) are abundant in cardiac muscle. Like skeletal muscle, cardiac muscle contains myofibrils of tandemly arranged sarcomeres which are delimited by Z-bands (choice B). The sarcomeres exhibit the same components as in skeletal muscle, incuding the M-line (choice D). Choice C is the extracellular space between the lateral surfaces of two adjacent cardiac muscle cells.

151. (C) The urinary space is lined by podocytes. These can be identified by their interdigitating secondary processes (pedicles or foot processes), which are separated from glomerular endothelial cells by a thick basal lamina. The cell body of a podocyte with some of its processes can be seen in the urinary space labeled C. The other labels (choices A, B, D, and E) are located in the lumens of fenestrated glomerular capillaries.

152. (A) Cells of the adrenal cortex have abundant smooth endoplasmic reticulum (sER) consistent with the central role of the sER in synthesis of steroid hormones such as glucocorticoids, mineralocorticoids, and androgenic hormones. In electron micrographs, the sER appears as profiles of membranous tubules (choice A). In contrast to sER, rough endoplasmic reticulum (choice B) is composed of flattened membranous cisternae that are studded with ribosomes. Steroid hormone synthesis requires collaboration between the sER and mitochondria (choice C). As seen in the micrograph, cells that synthesize steroid hormones have mitochondria with tubular, rather than shelf-like, cristae. An additional feature common to cells that secrete steroid hormones is the presence in the cytoplasm of lipid droplets (choice D). These are not sites of hormone storage; rather, they contain precursors such as cholesterol. Another organelle that is composed of membranous cisternae is the Golgi complex (choice E). The distinguishing feature is the arrangement of the flattened cisternae in a short stack. The Golgi complex is the major site of post-translational modification of newly synthesized proteins, and packaging of the proteins so they are directed to appropriate destinations, for example, the plasmalemma or lysosomes.

153. **(B)** Each plasma cell synthesizes and secretes large quantities of a single immunoglobulin (antibody) molecule. The ultrastructural features of these cells are dictated by their function. The cytoplasm is packed with rough endoplasmic reticulum (rER) consistent with an elevated level of protein synthesis for export. A prominent Golgi complex (not clearly evident here) performs in glycosylation and packaging of the immunoglobulin molecule for secretion. Secretory granules are not conspicuous in plasma cells because the immunoglobulin is not stored, but secreted as rapidly as it is synthesized. Also consistent with active protein synthesis is the presence of a prominent nucleolus, the source of ribosomal RNA. The peripheral distribution of heterochromatin in the nucleus is characteristic of plasma cells. Lymphocytes (choice A) are the immediate precursors of plasma cells. The scant cytoplasm of a resting lymphocyte contains only a modest amount of rER and other organelles. Neutrophils (choice C) and basophils (choice D) are distinguished by the numerous specific and non-specific granules in the cytoplasm. These cells have little rER. Platelets (choice E) are complex fragments of cells (megakaryocytes) that have granules of several types, but no nucleus or protein synthesis machinery. An example of a platelet can be seen adjacent to the plasma cell in the electron micrograph.

154. **(E)** The epithelial lining of the epididymal duct is a pseudostratified columnar epithelium. As illustrated in the micrograph, both tall columnar cells and rounded basal cells compose the epithelium. A prominent apical specialization of the columnar cells is the thick array of extremely long microvilli (stereocilia). The presence of spermatozoa in the lumen is a strong clue that this specimen is a component of the male reproductive system. The other choices are structures lined by different classes of epithelia. The esophagus (choice A) is lined by a stratified squamous epithelium. The small intestine (choice B) is lined by a simple columnar epithelium with microvilli that form a short brush border. Like the epididymal duct, the trachea (choice C) is lined by a pseudostratified columnar epithelium, but the apical specialization consists of cilia rather than microvilli. Spermatozoa may be evident in the lumen of seminiferous epithelium (choice D), but the construction of the epithelium is a complex arrangement of Sertoli cells and spermatogenic cells in several different stages of development.

155. **(D)** Like the other granulocytes, eosinophils are characterized by the content in the cytoplasm of specific granules. The distinctive ultrastructural feature of eosinophil granules is the presence of an electron dense (dark) rod-shaped crystalline core. In addition, the nucleus of an eosinophil is usually bi-lobed, as is evident in the illustration. Lymphocytes (choice A) have a round or oval nucleus, a relatively small amount of cytoplasm, and an absence of specific granules. Compared to a lymphocyte, a monocyte (choice B) usually has a larger, more irregularly shaped nucleus and more abundant cytoplasm, but like the lymphocyte it does not have specific cytoplasmic granules. Neutrophils (choice C) have multi-lobed nuclei and specific cytoplasmic granules; however, neutrophilic granules are much smaller than eosinophilic granules and they contain no crystalline cores. The granules of basophils (choice E) are large, but they are more homogeneously electron dense, lacking crystalline cores.

REFERENCES

Hall-Craggs ECB. *Anatomy as a Basis for Clinical Medicine,* 3rd edition. Baltimore: Williams & Wilkins, 1995

Moore KL. *Clinically Oriented Anatomy,* 3rd edition. Baltimore: Williams & Wilkins, 1992

Rosse C, Gaddum-Rosse P. *Hollinshead's Textbook of Anatomy,* 5th edition. Philadelphia: Lippincott Raven Publishers, 1997

Woodburne RT, Burckel WE. *Essentials of Human Anatomy,* 9th edition. New York: Oxford University Press, 1994

Subspecialty List: Anatomy

Question Number and Subspecialty

1. Nervous system
2. Nervous system
3. Nervous system
4. Nervous system
5. Eye
6. Nervous system
7. Nervous system
8. Nervous system
9. Nervous system
10. Nervous system
11. Nervous system
12. Nervous system
13. Nervous system
14. Nervous system
15. Nervous system
16. Nervous system
17. Nervous system
18. Nervous system
19. Nervous system
20. Nervous system
21. Nervous system
22. Auditory system
23. Vestibular system
24. Nervous system
25. Nervous system
26. Nervous system
27. Nervous system
28. Nervous system
29. Trunk and upper extremity
30. Trunk and upper extremity
31. Trunk and upper extremity
32. Trunk and upper extremity
33. Trunk and upper extremity
34. Trunk and upper extremity
35. Trunk and upper extremity
36. Trunk and upper extremity
37. Trunk and upper extremity
38. Trunk and upper extremity
39. Trunk and upper extremity
40. Thorax
41. Heart
42. Abdomen
43. Abdomen
44. Reproductive system
45. Vascular system
46. Abdomen
47. Trunk and upper extremity
48. Trunk and upper extremity
49. Trunk and upper extremity
50. Trunk and upper extremity
51. Thorax
52. Trunk and upper extremity
53. Abdomen
54. Reproductive system
55. Auditory system
56. Eye
57. Hematopoietic system
58. Eye
59. Reproductive system
60. Cellular biology
61. Cellular biology
62. Muscular system
63. Urinary system
64. Nervous system
65. Endocrine system
66. Lymphoid system
67. Skin
68. Hematopoietic system
69. Hematopoietic system
70. Liver
71. Hematopoietic system
72. Digestive system
73. Urinary system
74. Placenta

75. Digestive system
76. Digestive system
77. Nervous system
78. Nervous system
79. Respiratory system
80. Digestive system
81. Nervous system
82. Skeletal system
83. Nervous system
84. Eye
85. Nervous system
86. Nervous system
87. Nervous system
88. Nervous system
89. Eye
90. Vestibular system
91. Eye
92. Larynx
93. Nervous system
94. Nervous system
95. Nervous system
96. Nervous system
97. Nervous system
98. Nervous system
99. Nervous system
100. Nervous system
101. Nervous system
102. Nervous system
103. Cellular biology
104. Muscular system
105. Nervous system
106. Nervous system
107. Nervous system
108. Nervous system
109. Taste
110. Lower extremity
111. Lower extremity
112. Lower extremity
113. Heart
114. Respiratory system
115. Reproductive system
116. Muscular system
117. Head and neck
118. Head and neck
119. Thyroid
120. Head and neck
121. Larynx
122. Larynx
123. Head and neck
124. Spine
125. Spine
126. Spine
127. Lower extremity
128. Lower extremity
129. Lower extremity
130. Thorax
131. Thorax
132. Heart
133. Abdomen
134. Heart
135. Nervous system
136. Respiratory system
137. Hematopoietic system
138. Digestive system
139. Nervous system
140. Reproductive system
141. Cellular biology
142. Hematopoietic system
143. Endocrine system
144. Nervous system
145. Head and neck
146. Lymphoid system
147. Nervous system
148. Muscular system
149. Vascular system
150. Heart
151. Urinary system
152. Endocrine system
153. Lymphoid system
154. Reproductive system
155. Hematopoietic system

CHAPTER 2

Physiology
Questions

Andreas Carl, MD, PhD

DIRECTIONS (Questions 156 through 282): Each of the numbered items or incomplete statements in this section is followed by answers or by completions of the statement. Select the ONE lettered answer or completion that is BEST in each case.

156. A 17-year-old primigravida asks you what to expect during her pregnancy. You tell her that normally during pregnancy

(A) blood volume increases
(B) hematocrit increases
(C) respiratory tidal volume decreases
(D) pulmonary functional residual capacity increases
(E) gastrointestinal muscle tone and motility increase

157. Tremor that is caused by a cerebellar lesion is most readily differentiated from that caused by loss of the dopaminergic nigrostriatal tracts in that

(A) it is present at rest
(B) it is decreased during activity
(C) it only occurs during voluntary movements
(D) its frequency is very regular
(E) its amplitude remains constant during voluntary movements

158. You are called for consultation on a patient with diabetes insipidus. Although vasopressin (ADH) significantly contributes to fluid and electrolyte balance, it does not appear to closely regulate blood volume in the long run. Blood volume is maintained at near normal levels in this patient because

(A) the peripheral renin–angiotensin system is stimulated
(B) water intake is appropriately adjusted
(C) plasma oncotic pressure increases
(D) sympathetic reflexes decrease glomerular filtration
(E) renal blood flow decreases

159. Elderly patients often lose control over their bladder function. Which of the following statements about micturition is correct?

(A) Sympathetic fibers originating in L1 and L2 provide continuous tone to the external sphincter, thereby preventing micturition unless desired.
(B) Patients with damage to the lumbar spinal cord lose their micturition reflex (atonic bladder).
(C) Patients with damage to the sacral spinal cord have an intact micturition reflex but lose almost all voluntary control over micturition (automatic bladder).
(D) Higher centers in the brainstem primarily serve to enhance the micturition reflex.
(E) Urination will occur if inhibition of the external sphincter through spinal reflex pathways is stronger than the voluntary constrictor signals to the external sphincter from the brain.

Questions 160 and 161

Figure 2–1 illustrates histological changes in the endometrium during the menstrual cycle.

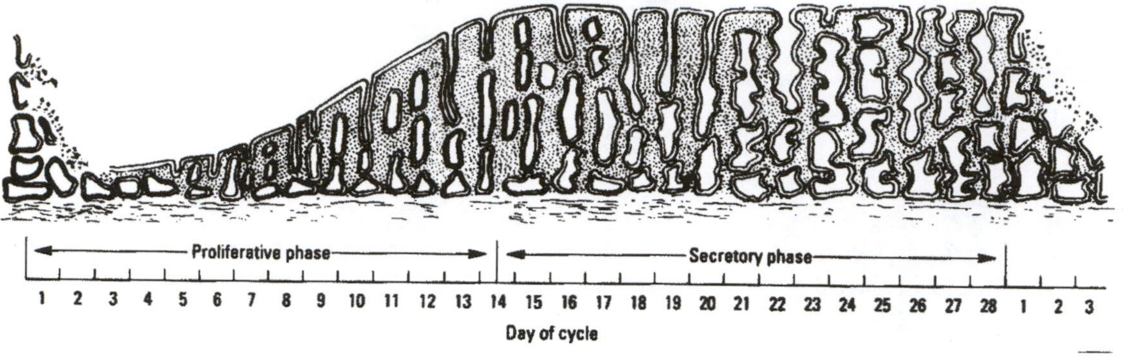

Figure 2–1. *(Reprinted with permission from Ganong, WF.* Review of Medical Physiology. *17th ed. Appleton & Lange, 1995.)*

160. Progesterone levels are highest around

(A) day 7
(B) day 12
(C) day 14
(D) day 21
(E) day 28

161. Estrogen levels are highest around

(A) day 7
(B) day 12
(C) day 14
(D) day 21
(E) day 28

162. Pupil size is an important indicator of brainstem function. Which of the following statements about pupil diameter is correct?

(A) General increase in sympathetic tone during emotional excitement results in pupil constriction.
(B) Increase in sympathetic activity in fibers innervating the inner eye muscles during darkness results in pupil constriction.
(C) Decrease in parasympathetic activity in fibers innervating the inner eye muscles during darkness results in pupil constriction.
(D) Phentolamine causes pupil constriction.
(E) Atropine causes pupil constriction.

163. The introduction of cold water into one ear may cause giddiness and nausea. The primary cause of this effect of temperature is

(A) temporary immobilization of otoliths
(B) decreased movement of ampullar cristae
(C) increased discharge rate in vestibular afferents
(D) decreased discharge rate in vestibular afferents
(E) convection currents in endolymph

164. A 17-year-old female with iron deficiency anemia remains anemic despite treatment with an oral iron preparation. Which of the following statements about iron metabolism is correct?

(A) Iron is more efficiently absorbed in the ferrous state (Fe^{2+}) than in the ferric state (Fe^{3+}).
(B) The gastrointestinal rate of iron absorption is extremely high.
(C) Most iron in the body is stored as hemosiderin.
(D) Hemosiderin is a product of hemoglobin degradation.
(E) Ferritin is a plasma protein that transports iron in the blood.

165. Which of the following physiologic responses occurs as the pitch of a sound is increased?

(A) The amplitude of maximal basilar membrane displacement increases.
(B) The location of maximal basilar membrane displacement moves toward the base of the cochlea.
(C) A greater number of hair cells become activated.
(D) The frequency of action potentials in auditory nerve fibers increases.
(E) Units in the auditory nerve become responsive to a wider range of sound frequencies.

166. You are called for consultation on a patient with a history of progressive muscle weakness. Which of the following diagnostic signs or procedures would support a diagnosis of myasthenia gravis?

(A) Response of skeletal muscles to direct electrical stimulation is weakened.
(B) Response of skeletal muscle to nerve stimulation is weakened.
(C) A small dose of physostigmine is likely to worsen the symptoms.
(D) A large dose of physostigmine is likely to improve the symptoms.
(E) The patient should be given alpha-bungarotoxin to determine the number of acetylcholine binding sites at the post-junctional membrane.

167. Which of the following statements about blood coagulation is correct?

(A) Absence of Ca^{2+} promotes blood coagulation.
(B) Patients with hemophilia A usually have a normal bleeding time.
(C) Von Willebrand factor suppresses platelet adhesion.
(D) Von Willebrand factor suppresses blood coagulation.
(E) Disseminated intravascular coagulation (DIC) results in depletion of fibrin split products.

168. The stimulation of nerve endings in the Golgi tendon organs leads directly to

(A) contraction of extrafusal muscle fibers
(B) contraction of intrafusal muscle fibers
(C) reflex inhibition of motor neurons
(D) increased gamma-efferent discharge
(E) increased activity in group II afferent fibers

169. Typical findings in patients with idiopathic hyperfunction of the juxtaglomerular apparatus (Bartter's syndrome) are

(A) very high blood pressure
(B) low renin levels
(C) low angiotensin levels
(D) low aldosterone levels
(E) decreased sensitivity of blood vessels to angiotensin

170. Colonoscopy of a 34-year-old patient with long-standing ulcerative colitis revealed multiple foci of high-grade dysplasia. The entire colon of this patient had to be removed to prevent colon carcinoma. Which of the following statements about patients with total colectomy and ileostomy is correct?

(A) Long-term survival is not possible, since the colon is a vital organ.
(B) Long-term survival is possible, but parenteral nutrition is required to maintain fluid and electrolyte balance.
(C) These patients are at increased risk of anemia due to malabsorption of iron.
(D) These patients are at increased risk of anemia due to malabsorption of vitamin B_{12}.
(E) Following total colectomy and ileostomy, the volume and water content of ileal discharge decreases over time.

171. Soldiers exposed to nerve gas (organophosphate) usually die of respiratory and cardiovascular failure. The expected effect of organophosphate poisoning on the heart would be to

(A) decrease the rate of rhythmicity of the sinoatrial (SA) node by inducing hyperpolarization
(B) depolarize cells of the SA node by closing potassium channels under the control of the muscarinic acetylcholine receptor
(C) increase the rate of rhythmicity of the SA node by increasing the upward drift in membrane potential caused by sodium leakage
(D) increase conductivity at the atrioventricular (AV) junction by inducing depolarization
(E) decrease the force of myocardial contractions by potentiating the vagal tone to the ventricular muscle

172. A karate fighter who received a direct stroke to his left carotid sinus during a tournament immediately fainted. Which of the following occurred during this event?

(A) decreased pressure at the carotid sinus baroreceptors
(B) decreased firing rate of the carotid sinus fibers
(C) decreased firing rate of cardiac sympathetic fibers
(D) decreased firing rate of the vagus nerve efferents
(E) increased heart rate

173. You are about to attend your first delivery of a baby. Which of the following circulatory changes normally take place in the newborn within five minutes after birth?

(A) decrease in systemic artery resistance
(B) increase in pulmonary artery resistance
(C) closure of the foramen ovale
(D) closure of the ductus arteriosus
(E) closure of the ductus venosus

174. Glucagon is secreted by the α-cells of the pancreatic islets. Which of the following is most likely to induce glucagon secretion?

(A) low serum concentrations of amino acids
(B) low serum concentrations of glucose
(C) high serum concentrations of glucose
(D) secretion of somatostatin by the pancreatic δ-cells
(E) parasympathetic stimulation

Questions 175 through 177

A 52-year-old male has a history of anginal pain that until recently was responsive to nitrates. He is now evaluated for possible angioplasty.

175. The graph in Figure 2–2 shows the ECG of this patient. Blood flow across the mitral valve is largest around

(A) point A
(B) point B
(C) point C
(D) point D
(E) point E

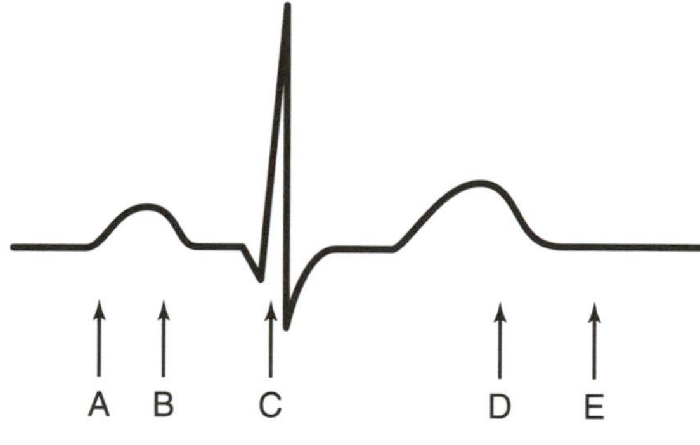

Figure 2–2

176. The graph in Figure 2–3 shows the pressure–volume curve of the left ventricle of this patient (shaded area). The pressure–volume curve of a normal subject is shown for comparison (broken lines).

Compared to normal this patient most likely has

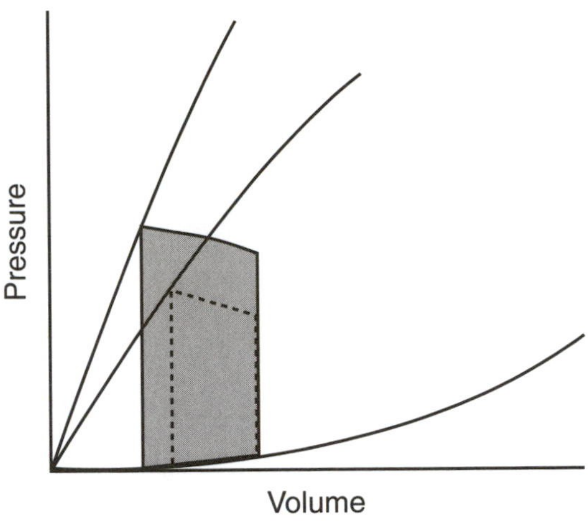

Figure 2–3

(A) an increased force of contraction
(B) an increased preload
(C) a decreased preload
(D) a decreased afterload
(E) a decreased stroke volume

177. The graph in Figure 2–4 shows the jugular vein pressure curve of this patient. Which part of the curve represents the atrial contraction?

(A) peak A
(B) peak B
(C) peak C
(D) peak D
(E) peak E

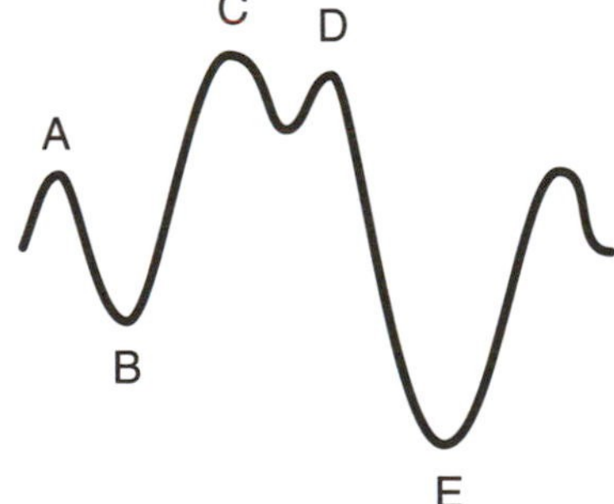

Figure 2–4

178. A neuronal soma has a resting membrane potential of –60 mV. Opening chloride channels in the neuronal membrane will most likely cause

(A) depolarization to about –30 mV
(B) depolarization to about +30 mV
(C) hyperpolarization to about –70 mV
(D) no change in membrane potential
(E) initiation of an action potential

179. A 24-year-old male with essential hypertension has a blood renin level of 5 ng/mL/h (normal 1 to 2.5 ng/mL/h). Which of the following could be a major stimulus for the release of renin from the juxtaglomerular apparatus in this patient?

(A) overhydration
(B) hypertension
(C) dilatation of renal arteries
(D) increased delivery of sodium to the distal tubules
(E) increased sympathetic activity via renal nerves

180. Which of the following statements most accurately describes the response of a cell to a decrease in the conductance of the cell membrane to chloride ions?

(A) The cell will hyperpolarize if its membrane potential is positive with respect to the equilibrium potential for chloride ions.
(B) The cell will depolarize if its membrane potential is positive with respect to the equilibrium potential for chloride ions.
(C) The cell will hyperpolarize if the external chloride concentration is greater than the internal chloride concentration.
(D) The cell will hyperpolarize if the external chloride concentration is less than the internal chloride concentration.
(E) No change in membrane potential will occur if the external and internal chloride ion concentrations are equal.

181. Which of the following statements is true for hypertensive patients with secondary hyperaldosteronism? Aldosterone release occurs primarily in response to

(A) hypokalemia
(B) hypernatremia
(C) high volume states (fluid overload)
(D) angiotensin II
(E) atrial natriuretic peptide

182. Miniature end-plate potentials that can be recorded from a muscle fiber are believed to represent

(A) the postsynaptic action of a single neurotransmitter molecule released from the presynaptic terminal
(B) the opening of a single receptor–ion channel in the muscle membrane
(C) the opening of multiple ion channels in the muscle membrane caused by spontaneous release of a small amount of neurotransmitter
(D) the spontaneous opening of ion channels in the muscle membrane in the absence of presynaptically released transmitter
(E) the opening of multiple ion channels in the postsynaptic membrane in response to a single presynaptic action potential

183. Which of the following statements correctly describes effects of autonomic nerve activity on the cardiovascular system in a healthy subject?

(A) Stimulation of parasympathetic nerves decreases the strength of cardiac ventricular contractions.
(B) Stimulation of sympathetic nerves decreases the strength of cardiac ventricular contractions.
(C) Inhibition of parasympathetic nerves increases heart rate.
(D) Inhibition of parasympathetic nerves increases total peripheral resistance.
(E) Inhibition of parasympathetic nerves decrease total peripheral resistance.

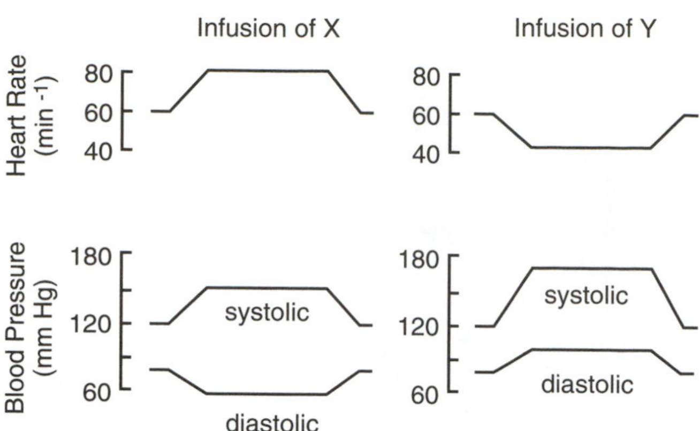

Figure 2–5. *(Reprinted with permission from Ganong, WF.* Review of Medical Physiology. *17th ed. Appleton & Lange, 1995.)*

184. Figure 2–5 shows the effects of infusion of a catecholamine X and a catecholamine Y on heart rate and systolic and diastolic blood pressure. Which of the following statements correctly describes the actions of these drugs?

(A) the decrease in heart rate following infusion of Y is due to the effect of this drug on cardiac α-adrenergic receptors
(B) the decrease in heart rate following infusion of Y is due to the effect of this drug on cardiac β-adrenergic receptors
(C) the decrease in heart rate following infusion of Y is due to the effect of acetylcholine on cardiac muscarinic receptors
(D) the decrease in diastolic blood pressure following infusion of X is due to the effect of this drug on vascular smooth muscle α-adrenergic receptors
(E) catecholamine X is norepinephrine and catecholamine Y is epinephrine

185. A patient with acute glomerulonephritis has a total plasma [Ca^{2+}] = 2.5 mM/L and a glomerular filtration rate of 160 L/day. What is the estimated daily filtered load of calcium?

(A) 64 mM/day
(B) 120 mM/day
(C) 240 mM/day
(D) 400 mM/day
(E) 800 mM/day

186. If a person suffered a stab injury and air entered the intrapleural space (pneumothorax), the most likely response would be for the

(A) lung to expand outward and the chest wall to spring inward
(B) lung to expand outward and the chest wall to spring outward
(C) lung to collapse inward and the chest wall to collapse inward
(D) lung to collapse inward and the chest wall to spring outward
(E) lung volume to be unaffected and chest wall to spring outward

187. Normally, O_2 transfer is perfusion limited; that is, the amount of O_2 taken up is a function of pulmonary blood flow. Which of the following conditions would favor a diffusion limitation of O_2 transfer from alveolar to pulmonary capillary blood?

(A) chronic obstructive lung disease
(B) lung edema
(C) breathing hyperbaric gas mixture
(D) increased ventilatory rate
(E) mild exercise

188. A 48-year-old man died of immediate respiratory failure due to a self-inflicted gunshot wound injuring his brainstem. Which of the following statements accurately describes the interaction of respiratory centers in the brainstem and their effect on respiration?

(A) The medullary rhythmicity center is a discrete group of neurons whose rhythmicity is abolished when the brain is transected above and below this area.
(B) Sectioning the brainstem above the pons, near the inferior colliculus of the midbrain results in immediate respiratory arrest.
(C) Transection above the apneustic center results in prolonged expiration and very short inspiration.
(D) Transection of the afferent fibers of the vagus and glossopharyngeal nerves results in prolonged inspiration and shortened expiration.
(E) The apneustic and pneumotaxic centers of the pons are essential for maintenance of the basic rhythm of respiration.

Questions 189 and 190

Figure 2–6 shows a pair of action potentials.

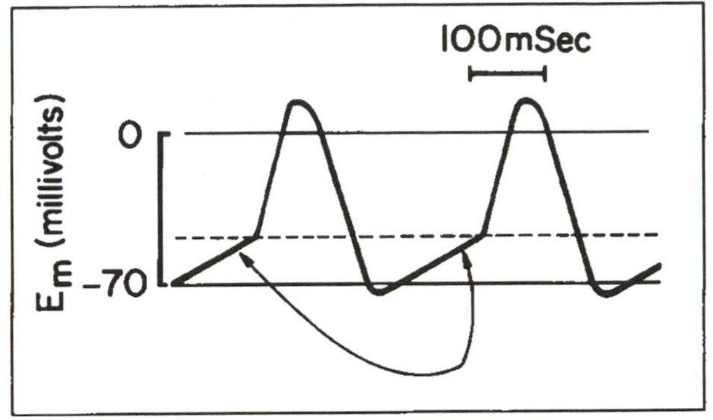

Figure 2–6

189. The action potentials shown represent those of

(A) myelinated motor axons
(B) skeletal muscle fibers
(C) vascular smooth muscle cells
(D) cardiac nodal cells
(E) ventricular Purkinje cells

190. The gradual depolarization between action potentials (see arrows) is mainly the result of

(A) a gradual increase in inward Na^+ current through fast Na^+ channels (I_{Na})
(B) an increase in the "delayed rectifier" current due to outward movement of K^+ (I_K)
(C) a combination of gradual inactivation of outward I_K along with the presence of an inward "funny" current (I_f) due to the opening of channels permeable to both Na^+ and K^+ ions
(D) changes in permeability of cells to the principal extracellular anions, Cl^- and HCO_3^-
(E) a gradual change in the ratio of extracellular to intracellular ion concentrations across the cell membrane

191. When measuring the tension that a skeletal muscle develops during an isometric contraction, it is observed that

(A) active tension increases monotonically with the length of the fiber
(B) active tension first increases then decreases with the length of the fiber
(C) passive tension first increases then decreases with the length of the fiber
(D) total tension is inversely proportional to the length of the fiber
(E) total tension increases monotonically with the length of the fiber

Questions 192 and 193

A middle-aged male with smaller-than-normal-sized kidneys on ultrasound and a history of chronic glomerulonephritis has the following laboratory values:

Arterial blood	Urine
pH = 7.33	pH = 6.0
Pao_2 = 95 mm Hg	protein = positive
$Paco_2$ = 35 mm Hg	glucose = negative
HCO_3^- = 18 mEq/L	

192. This patient most likely has

(A) respiratory acidosis with some renal compensation
(B) respiratory acidosis without renal compensation
(C) metabolic acidosis with some respiratory compensation
(D) metabolic acidosis without respiratory compensation
(E) diabetic ketoacidosis

193. The most likely cause of his acid–base imbalance is

(A) hypoventilation
(B) hyperventilation
(C) decreased ability to produce adequate urinary NH_4^+ excretion
(D) excess beta-hydroxybutyric and acetoacetic acids in his blood
(E) decreased catabolism of sulfur-containing amino acids (e.g., methionine, cysteine)

194. A 15-year-old girl had a past episode of minimal change glomerulonephritis. On follow-up examination, her urinary protein normalized and now is negative. There is very little protein in her glomerular filtrate because

(A) all serum proteins are too large to fit through the glomerular pores
(B) positive charges line the pores, which repel serum proteins
(C) a combination of pore size and negative charges lining the pores
(D) active reabsorption of filtered protein by the glomerular epithelial cells
(E) metabolism of filtered proteins by the urinary flora

195. Patients recovering from myocardial infarction are advised to avoid vigorous physical exercise because in contrast to skeletal muscle fibers, the heart is unable to function anaerobically even for short periods of time. The extra energy required by skeletal muscle fibers for a burst of vigorous physical activity lasting between 20 and 100 seconds comes from

(A) the breakdown of glycogen to lactic acid
(B) the breakdown of adenosine triphosphate (ATP) in muscle cells
(C) the breakdown of creatine phosphate
(D) gluconeogenesis
(E) oxidative reactions

196. During a routine preschool examination a 5-year-old boy is found to have difficulty focusing on distant objects. Which of the following is true during far accommodation of the eyes?

(A) the ciliary muscles are relaxed
(B) the zonula fibers are relaxed
(C) the lens is rounded
(D) the focal length of the lens is short
(E) the pupils are constricted (accommodation response)

197. A patient with ventricular fibrillation is resuscitated and now shows shortened, irregular QT intervals on his ECG. Which of the following ion channels is responsible for the plateau phase of the cardiac action potential that is reflected by the QT interval?

(A) K^+ channels
(B) Na^+ channels
(C) L-type Ca^{2+} channels
(D) T-type Ca^{2+} channels
(E) Cl^- channels

198. A 47-year-old female presents for elective cholecystectomy. Shortly after induction of anesthesia with halothane, the patient develops circulatory instability, tachypnea, and a sharp rise in body temperature (malignant hyperthermia). What is the cause of fever in this patient?

(A) increased heat production by skeletal muscle
(B) increased hypothalamic temperature set point
(C) increased blood levels of interleukin-1
(D) decreased convectional heat loss
(E) increased sweat production

199. A 65-year-old woman complains about chronic fatigue. Her hematocrit is 30%, erythrocytes are $4 \cdot 10^6/\mu L$, and her hemoglobin level is 8 g/dL. In order to determine the likely cause of her anemia, red blood cell indices are calculated by the Coulter counter. Which of the following is correct?

(A) MCHC = hemoglobin concentration · 10/erythrocyte number
(B) MCHC = hemoglobin concentration/hematocrit
(C) MCV = hematocrit · 1000/hemoglobin
(D) MCV = hemoglobin concentration · 10/erythrocyte number
(E) MCV = hemoglobin concentration/hematocrit

200. A patient with difficulty breathing is sent for diagnostic spirometry. Figure 2–7 shows the expiratory and inspiratory flow-volume curves of this patient (solid lines) and a healthy person (broken lines) for comparison. Which of the following disease states best explains this finding?

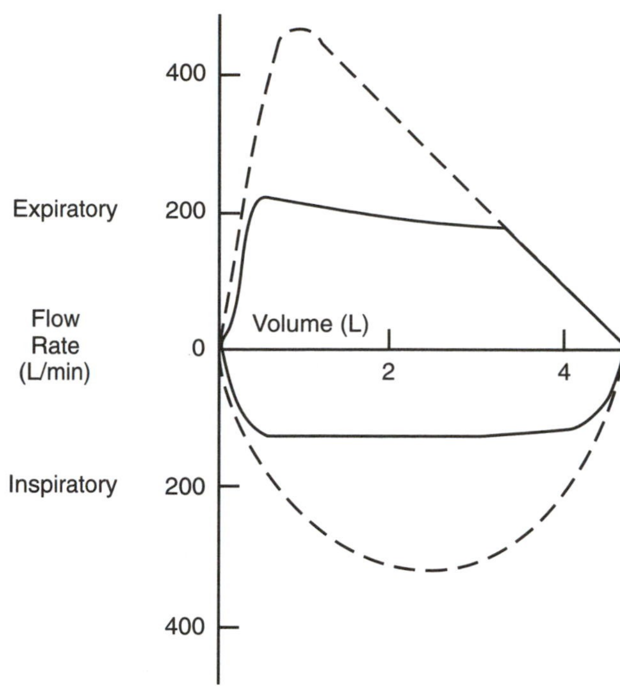

Figure 2–7. *(Reprinted with permission from West, JB.* Pulmonary Pathophysiology—The Essentials. *4th ed. Williams & Wilkins, 1992.)*

(A) severe epiglottitis
(B) panacinar emphysema
(C) centrilobular emphysema
(D) chronic obstructive lung disease
(E) chronic restrictive lung disease

201. A patient with chronic renal insufficiency due to renal vascular disease has a net functional loss of nephrons. If we assume that production of urea and creatinine is constant and that the patient is in a steady state, a 50% decrease in the normal glomerular filtration rate (GFR) will

(A) not affect plasma creatinine
(B) decrease plasma urea concentration
(C) greatly increase plasma Na^+
(D) increase the percent of filtered Na^+ excreted
(E) significantly decrease plasma K^+

202. Which of the following events typically occurs during REM sleep?

(A) somnambulism
(B) enuresis
(C) night terrors
(D) sleep spindles
(E) penile erections

203. A patient with multiple trauma in the ICU is on artificial respiration. If alveolar ventilation is halved (and if CO_2 production remains unchanged), then

(A) alveolar CO_2 pressure (P_{ACO_2}) will be halved
(B) arterial O_2 pressure (P_{aO_2}) will double
(C) arterial CO_2 pressure (P_{aCO_2}) will double
(D) arterial O_2 pressure (P_{aO_2}) will not change
(E) alveolar O_2 pressure (P_{AO_2}) will double

204. You see a patient with damage to the left cervical sympathetic chain ganglia as a result of a neck tumor. Which of the following physical signs would be expected?

(A) ptosis (hanging of the upper eye lid) on the left
(B) pupil dilation of the left eye
(C) pale skin on the left side of the face
(D) increased sweat secretion on the left side of the face
(E) lateral deviation of the left eye

205. A patient at rest has a systolic/diastolic blood pressure of 130/70 mm Hg and a cardiac output of 5 L/min. What is his total peripheral resistance?

(A) 18 mm Hg · min/L
(B) 20 mm Hg · min/L
(C) 22 mm Hg · min/L
(D) 0.05 L/min · mm Hg
(E) 20 L/min · mm Hg

206. A patient is admitted to the hospital with respiratory acidosis. The patient's renal excretion of potassium would be expected to

(A) rise, since acid and potassium excretion are coupled
(B) rise, since acidosis is a stimulus to renin secretion by the juxtaglomerular apparatus
(C) rise, since acidosis increases the affinity of the aldosterone receptor for aldosterone
(D) fall, since the filtered load of potassium to the tubules falls in acidosis
(E) fall, since tubular secretion of potassium is inversely coupled to acid secretion

207. A patient is given 100% O_2 to breathe, arterial blood gases are determined and a P_{aO_2} of 125 mm Hg is measured. This result is associated with

(A) diffusion abnormality
(B) ventilation/perfusion inequality
(C) anatomic right-to-left shunting
(D) profound hypoventilation
(E) the normal response

208. Which of the following statements concerning the action of β-receptors is correct? Stimulation of β-receptors

(A) promotes glycogen synthesis in liver cells
(B) promotes glycogen synthesis in muscle cells
(C) promotes lipolysis
(D) decreases insulin secretion by pancreatic β-cells
(E) decreases glucagon secretion by pancreatic β-cells

209. A routine ECG on a patient reveals a prolonged PQ interval. Which of the following cardiac pathways is most likely damaged and responsible for this patient's prolonged PQ interval?

(A) between the sinoatrial (SA) and the atrioventricular (AV) nodes
(B) the AV node
(C) the bundle of His
(D) the Purkinje fibers
(E) the ventricular muscle

210. Which of the following statements is true for a patient with hyperopia?

(A) This patient is nearsighted.
(B) The lens of this patient has unusually large refractive power.
(C) Hyperopia can be corrected with convex glasses.
(D) The eyeball of this patient is too long.
(E) The lens of this patient has reduced elasticity.

211. A patient with low arterial oxygen saturation is evaluated for anatomic and physiologic lung dead space. The anatomic dead space in this patient with a tidal volume of 500 mL is 125 mL when determined by plotting nitrogen concentration versus expired volume after a single inspiration of 100% O_2 (Fowler's method). If the patient's lungs are healthy and the Pa_{CO_2} is 40 mm Hg, the mixed expired CO_2 tension (P_{ECO_2}) should be about

(A) 0 mm Hg
(B) 10 mm Hg
(C) 20 mm Hg
(D) 30 mm Hg
(E) 40 mm Hg

Questions 212 and 213

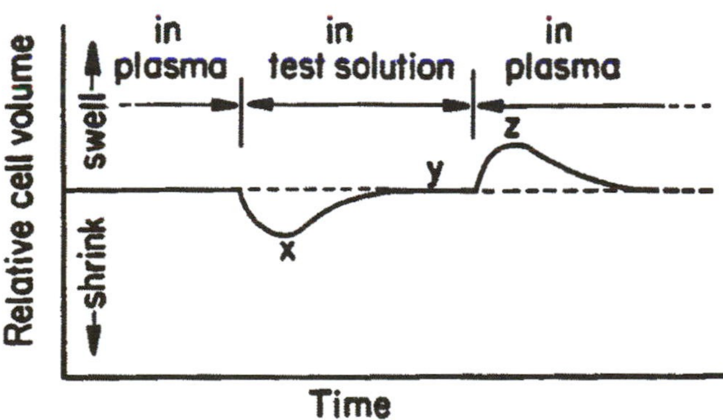

Figure 2–8

Figure 2–8 represents a continuous record of the relative cell volume of a red blood cell as it is changed from being immersed in a large volume of normal plasma, to being immersed in a large volume of a test solution, and then returned to the plasma. Changes in cell volume are passive (not due to cell volume regulation).

212. The change in cell volume that has peaked at point x on the diagram resulted from

(A) net exit of water from cell
(B) net extracellular water entry into cell
(C) net solute entry into cell
(D) no net water movement
(E) increased rate of solute entry into cell

213. The cell volume change that has peaked at point z is a result of

(A) net exit of water from cell
(B) no net water movement
(C) net entry of water into cell caused by prior net entry of solute
(D) neither net solute nor water movement
(E) net solute exit that occurred during prior exposure to test solution

214. In a normal kidney, a large increase in glomerular filtration rate (GFR) would be expected to occur following

(A) vasoconstriction of glomerular afferent arterioles
(B) vasoconstriction of glomerular efferent arterioles
(C) substantial increases in renal blood flow (RBF)
(D) an increase in mean arterial pressure from 90 mm Hg to 140 mm Hg
(E) strong, acute sympathetic stimulation to kidney

215. Head injuries can lead to a syndrome in which the hormone vasopressin (ADH) is secreted at abnormally high levels. Patients manifesting a syndrome of inappropriate ADH secretion (SIADH) would be expected to have

(A) low serum sodium due to the dilutional effect of ADH-induced water retention in the collecting tubules
(B) low serum sodium due to a direct inhibitory effect of ADH on distal tubular sodium resorption
(C) no change in serum sodium, since the dilutional effect of ADH-induced water retention is balanced by a direct stimulatory effect of ADH on distal tubular sodium resorption
(D) high serum sodium due to the direct stimulatory effect of ADH on distal tubular sodium resorption
(E) high serum sodium due to the concentrating effect of ADH-induced water excretion in the collecting tubules

216. A patient with asbestosis due to work-related exposure comes for evaluation of his lung function. In order to calculate inspiratory reserve volume, the following must be known

(A) tidal volume and vital capacity
(B) tidal volume and expiratory reserve volume
(C) tidal volume and residual volume
(D) tidal volume, vital capacity, and expiratory reserve volume
(E) tidal volume, vital capacity, and residual volume

217. A 33-year-old female with congenital aortic stenosis is in her second month of pregnancy. In order to evaluate the potential risk this pregnancy poses to her, she is admitted for cardiac function testing. O_2 consumption (measured by analysis of mixed expired gas) in this patient is 300 mL/min, arterial O_2 content is 20 mL/100 mL blood, pulmonary arterial O_2 content is 15 mL/100 mL blood, and her heart rate is 60/min. Her cardiac stroke volume is

(A) 1 mL
(B) 10 mL
(C) 60 mL
(D) 100 mL
(E) 200 mL

218. Which of the following statements regarding fetal circulation is correct?

(A) The liver and heart of the fetus receive blood with very high O_2 saturation.
(B) Po_2 of fetal blood leaving the placenta is slightly greater than maternal mixed venous Po_2.
(C) The presence of fetal hemoglobin shifts the oxyhemoglobin dissociation to the right.
(D) The foramen ovale closes during the third trimester unless the fetus has an atrial septal defect.
(E) The major portion of right ventricular output passes through the lungs.

219. The resistance to blood flow in the cerebral circulation of humans will increase when

(A) Pao_2 decreases to < 50 mm Hg
(B) an individual inhales a gas mixture enriched with CO_2
(C) an individual's hematocrit is decreased to < 0.30 by isovolemic exchange transfusion
(D) systemic arterial pressure increases from 100 to 130 mm Hg
(E) an individual suffers an epileptic seizure

Questions 220 through 222

A 68-year-old coal miner with decades of work-related exposure to dust is examined for pulmonary fibrosis. His FEV_1 is 75% (normal > 65%) and his arterial oxygen saturation is 92%. His alveolar ventilation is 6000 mL/min at a tidal volume of 600 mL and a breathing rate of 12 breaths/min. Pathologic changes in lung compliance and residual volume are also documented in this patient.

220. Which of the following describes this patient's lung compliance measured under static conditions?

(A) change in lung volume divided by change in distending pressure ($P_{alv} - P_{pl}$)
(B) change in distending pressure ($P_{alv} - P_{pl}$) divided by change in lung volume
(C) change in distending pressure ($P_{alv} - P_{pl}$) minus the change in lung volume
(D) lung volume divided by recoil pressure ($P_{alv} - P_{pl}$)
(E) change in elastic recoil pressure ($P_{alv} - P_{pl}$)

221. This patient's residual volume

(A) is part of vital capacity
(B) is part of the expiratory reserve volume
(C) cannot be measured directly with a spirometer
(D) represents the resting volume of the lungs
(E) is the volume at which the lungs tend to recoil outward

222. What is this patient's anatomic dead space?

(A) 100 mL
(B) 120 mL
(C) 150 mL
(D) 200 mL
(E) 250 mL

223. A patient's arterial blood analysis shows a pH of 7.56, bicarbonate 21 mEq/L, PO_2 = 50 mm Hg, and PCO_2 = 25 mm Hg. This patient probably

(A) has severe chronic lung disease
(B) is an emergency room patient with severely depressed respiration as a result of a heroin overdose
(C) is a subject in a clinical research experiment who has been breathing a gas mixture of 10% oxygen and 90% nitrogen for a few minutes
(D) is a lowlander who has been vacationing at high altitude for two weeks
(E) is an adult psychiatric patient who swallowed an overdose of aspirin

224. A patient with newly diagnosed schizophrenia is given chlorpromazine. Which of the following is an expected side effect of this medication?

(A) increased gastrointestinal motility
(B) decreased gastrointestinal sphincter tone
(C) emptying of urinary bladder and rectum
(D) dry mouth
(E) bradycardia

225. Which of the following conditions is associated with a decrease in skeletal muscle tone?

(A) upper motor neuron lesions
(B) lower motor neuron lesions
(C) activation of γ-fibers
(D) Parkinson's disease
(E) anxiety

226. If the cabin of an airplane is pressurized to an equivalent altitude of 10,000 ft (barometric pressure of 523 mm Hg), the P_{AO_2} in a healthy person compared with his or her predicted P_{AO_2} at sea level will

(A) decrease to < 100 mm Hg because the fraction of inspired air that is O_2 (F_{IO_2}) will be < 0.2
(B) decrease to < 100 mm Hg even though the F_{IO_2} is still around 0.2
(C) not change because water vapor pressure is low at high altitude
(D) not change because P_{aCO_2} will decrease because of hyperventilation
(E) not change because the cabin is pressurized

227. On routine examination a patient has an arterial oxygen (P_{aO_2}) slightly below the alveolar oxygen (P_{AO_2}). This finding

(A) is normal and due to shunted blood
(B) is due to significant diffusion gradients
(C) is due to reaction time of O_2 with hemoglobin
(D) is due to unloading of CO_2
(E) is the result of a major cardiac right-to-left shunt (ventricular septal defect)

228. Which of the following statements about cystic fibrosis is correct?

(A) Sweat of cystic fibrosis patients has elevated Na^+ and low Cl^- content.
(B) The gene that is abnormal in cystic fibrosis encodes a cAMP regulated Cl^- channel.
(C) Cystic fibrosis is more common in African-Americans than in Caucasians.
(D) The gene that is abnormal in cystic fibrosis is located on the X chromosome.
(E) Cystic fibrosis is caused by a defective Na^+ transporter across airway epithelial cells, resulting in thick airway mucus.

229. Cutting sympathetic nerve fibers that supply blood vessels in the arms or legs usually results in acute vasodilatation due to

(A) parasympathetic fibers dilating blood vessels
(B) loss of sympathetic tone
(C) development of hypersensitivity to circulating catecholamines
(D) compensatory increase of epinephrine release from the adrenal medulla
(E) compensatory increase of norepinephrine release from the adrenal medulla

230. Figure 2–9 shows an EEG recording of a 12-year-old child with suspected attention deficit hyperactivity disorder. Which of the following events most likely causes the change at the time marked by the arrow?

(A) patient closes eyes
(B) patient opens eyes
(C) patient's mind "wandering off"
(D) patient falling asleep
(E) petit mal attack

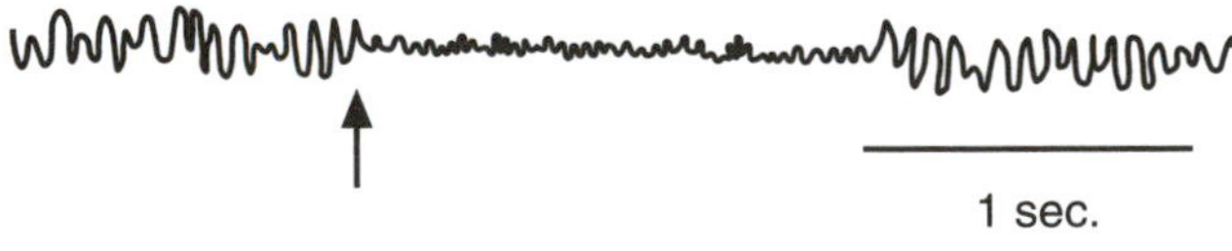

Figure 2–9

231. Prostaglandins are important mediators of inflammation. Which of the following statements about the role of prostaglandins during inflammatory processes is correct?

(A) Thromboxane A_2 inhibits platelet aggregation.
(B) $PGF_{2\alpha}$ relaxes bronchial smooth muscle.
(C) PGE_2 contracts bronchial smooth muscle.
(D) $PGF_{2\alpha}$ and PGE_2 relax uterine smooth muscle.
(E) PGE_2 sensitizes nociceptive nerve endings, causing pain.

232. One year after suffering a myocardial infarction a 49-year-old male is admitted for evaluation of his cardiac function. The left ventricular pressure–volume loop of this patient is shown in Figure 2–10.

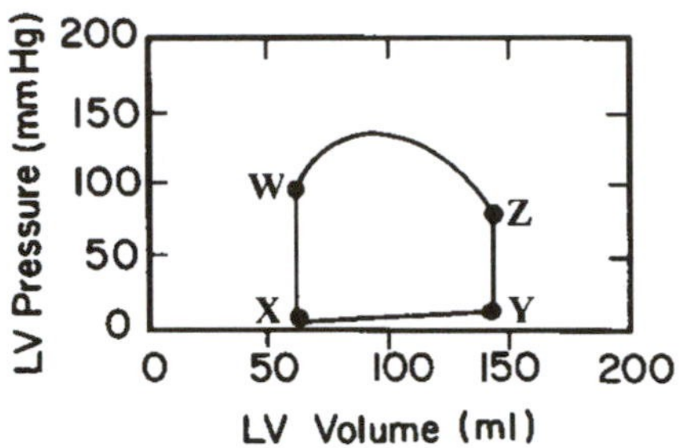

Figure 2–10

The part of the cardiac cycle described as isovolumetric relaxation is between points

(A) W and X
(B) X and Y
(C) Y and Z
(D) Z and W

233. You are called for consultation on a patient with asthma. To determine residual volume the following measurements were made (helium method):

- Spirometer volume 6 L
- Initial helium fraction in spirometer 10%
- Helium fraction after 20 deep breaths 9%

Residual volume of this patient is

(A) 1.0 L
(B) 0.666 L
(C) 0.6 L
(D) 0.54 L
(E) 0.5 L

234. A 28-year-old woman with chronic fatigue is admitted to the sleep laboratory for 24-hour monitoring of her sleep and breathing patterns. Her sleep latency is 90 minutes (normal 20 to 30 minutes). An hour later she appears asleep but her EEG pattern reverts to beta waves. Most likely, this patient

(A) has just entered light sleep (stage 1)
(B) has just entered deep sleep (stage 4)
(C) has entered REM sleep
(D) just woke up
(E) suffers from central sleep apnea

235. A patient with acute myocardial infarction is treated with streptokinase to reduce a blood clot in his left coronary artery. Which of the following statements about fibrinolysis is correct? Fibrinolysis in this patient

(A) is due to hydrolysis of fibrin by plasmin
(B) is due to hydrolysis of fibrin by streptokinase
(C) is inhibited by plasmin
(D) is inhibited by streptokinase
(E) is due to activation of tissue plasminogen activator by streptokinase

Questions 236 and 237

236. The graph in Figure 2–11 shows the static expiratory pressure–volume curve of a patient's lung and thorax (solid line). The broken line indicates the pressure–volume curve of a normal person for comparison.

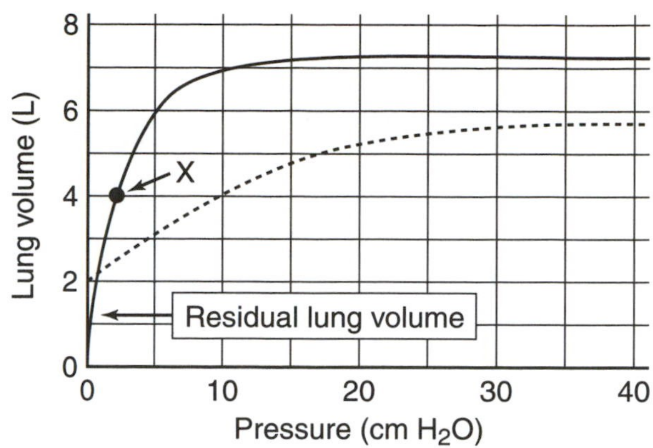

Figure 2–11

The lung compliance (at point x) of this patient is approximately

(A) 4 L/cm H_2O
(B) 2 L/cm H_2O
(C) 1 L/cm H_2O
(D) 1 cm H_2O/L
(E) 0.5 cm H_2O/L

237. This patient most likely suffers from

(A) tuberculosis
(B) sarcoidosis
(C) asbestosis
(D) acute obstruction of the glottis
(E) alpha-1-antitrypsin deficiency

238. You are called for consultation on a patient with aortic stenosis. The following measurements are made: oxygen uptake 200 mL/min, oxygen concentration in peripheral vein 7 vol% (7 mL oxygen/100 mL blood), oxygen concentration in pulmonary artery 10 vol% (10 mL oxygen/100 mL blood), oxygen concentration in aorta 15 vol% (15 mL oxygen/100 mL blood). The cardiac output of this patient equals:

(A) 1333 mL/min
(B) 2000 mL/min
(C) 2500 mL/min
(D) 3000 mL/min
(E) 4000 mL/min

239. A newlywed 23-year-old female and her 28-year-old husband are evaluated for infertility. They have been unable to conceive a child despite regular intercourse for the past 12 months. The first step of this couple's infertility workup is to determine whether ovulation occurs regularly. Which of the following hormones is primarily responsible for ovulation?

(A) estradiol
(B) estriol
(C) luteinizing hormone (LH)
(D) follicle-stimulating hormone (FSH)
(E) inhibin

240. Neuronal function is critically dependent on oxygen supply. Blood flow through the brain is most increased by

(A) intensive thinking
(B) barbiturates
(C) increased arterial pressure to 160/90 mm Hg
(D) decreased arterial oxygen to 75 mm Hg
(E) increased arterial carbon dioxide to 45 mm Hg

241. The solid line in Figure 2–12 represents a normal hemoglobin oxygen-binding curve.

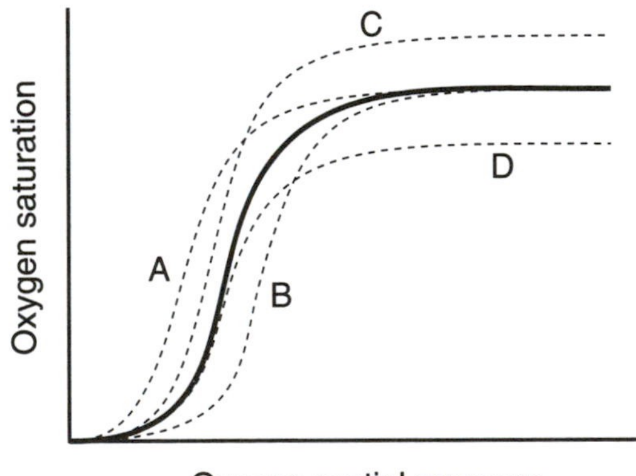

Figure 2–12

Strenuous physical exercise will shift this oxygen binding curve to

(A) line A
(B) line B
(C) line C
(D) line D

242. A 75-year-old male with a 40-plus–year history of smoking one to two packs per day is evaluated for lung transplantation. Figure 2–13 shows a Davenport diagram plotting arterial plasma bicarbonate against arterial blood pH. Dashed lines are different levels of arterial P_{CO_2} (isobars). Which of the points labeled A through I most likely describes the acid–base state of this patient?

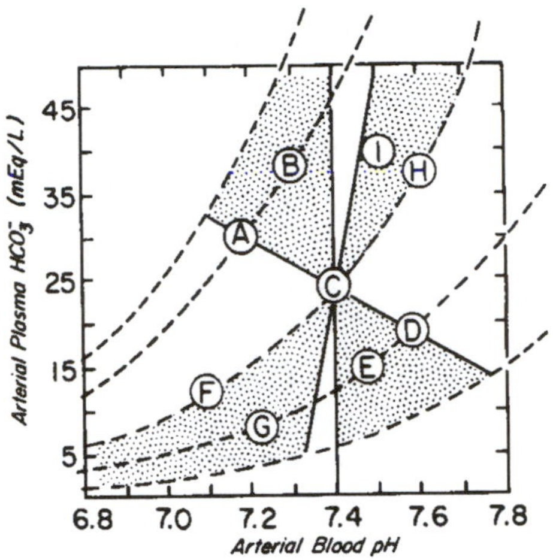

Figure 2–13

(A) point A
(B) point B
(C) point C
(D) point D
(E) point E
(F) point F
(G) point G
(H) point H
(I) point I

243. Which of the following is a major secretory product of gastric chief cells?

(A) mucus
(B) pepsinogen
(C) gastrin
(D) hydrogen
(E) intrinsic factor

244. During a marathon attempt a runner collapses and is admitted with severe acute dehydration. This patient most likely has

(A) decreased plasma osmolarity
(B) decreased baroreceptor firing rate
(C) low plasma ADH levels
(D) low water permeability of collecting duct tubular cells
(E) high renal water excretion

245. Figure 2–14 illustrates simultaneous changes in left ventricular (LV) pressure and LV volume over time. There are nine lettered points on the LV pressure curve (points A through I). At which of these points does LV pressure equal diastolic aortic blood pressure?

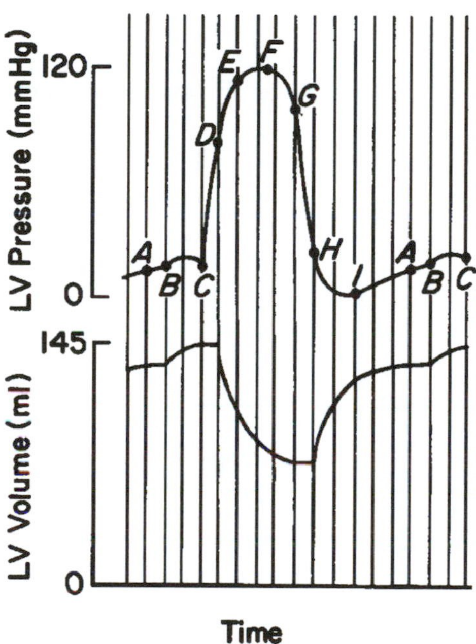

Figure 2–14

(A) point A
(B) point B
(C) point C
(D) point D
(E) point E
(F) point F
(G) point G
(H) point H
(I) point I

246. A patient on intensive care is ventilated with a frequency of 12 per minute and a tidal volume of 0.6 liters. His arterial pH increases to > 7.6. In order to correct this respiratory alkalosis, you should

(A) increase oxygen fraction
(B) increase minute ventilation
(C) decrease dead space
(D) decrease tidal volume
(E) use positive end expiratory pressure (PEEP)

247. Figure 2–15 illustrates the extracellular and intracellular volume–osmolarity status of a patient (broken lines) and that of a normal subject (solid lines) for comparison.

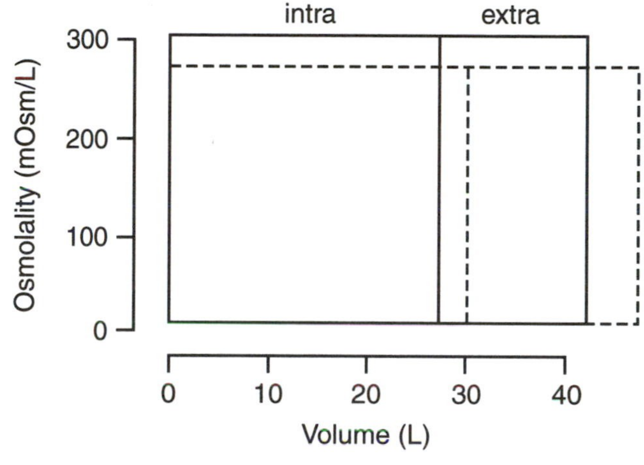

Figure 2–15

This patient most likely suffers from

(A) chronic vomiting
(B) adrenal insufficiency
(C) SIADH
(D) iatrogenic fluid overload with 0.9% NaCl
(E) iatrogenic fluid overload with hypertonic solution

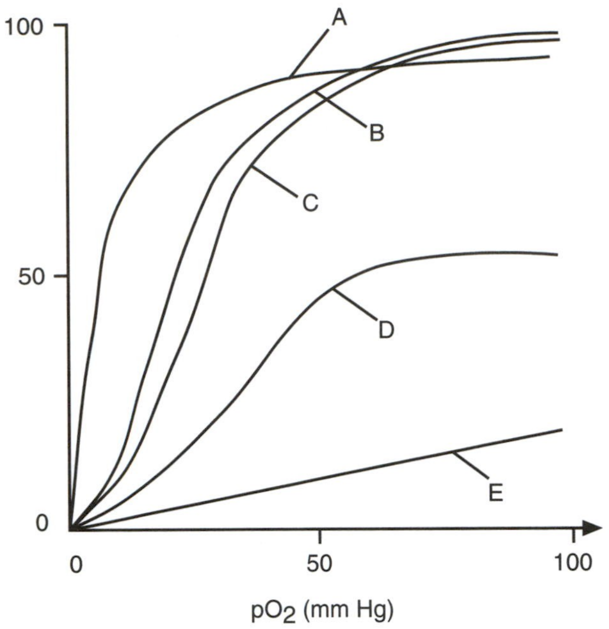

Figure 2–16

248. A series of oxygen-binding curves is shown in Figure 2–16. Which of these curves represents the binding of oxygen to myoglobin?

(A) curve A
(B) curve B
(C) curve C
(D) curve D
(E) curve E

249. The "dark current" of retinal photoreceptors is generated by

(A) Cl^- channels
(B) nonselective cation channels
(C) nonselective anion channels
(D) the ryanodine receptor
(E) the Na^+/K^+ pump

250. Creatinine clearance is often used to evaluate glomerular function. Which of the graphs in Figure 2–17 best represents the relationship between plasma creatinine concentration and creatinine clearance in a normal healthy person?

(A) curve A
(B) curve B
(C) curve C
(D) curve D
(E) curve E

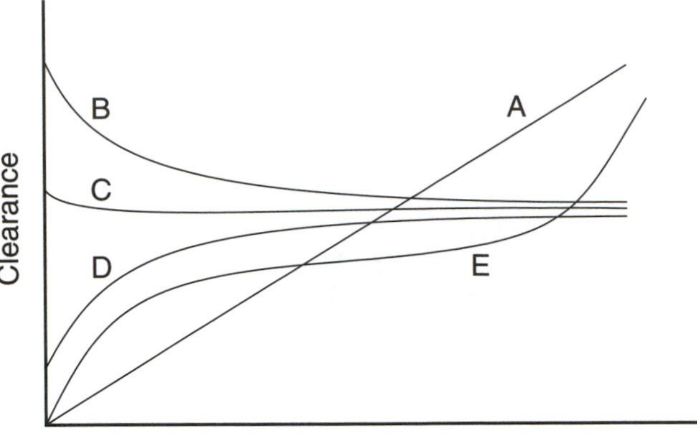

Figure 2–17

251. Which of the following cytokines is produced by T cells and induces MHC-II (major histocompatibility) proteins?

(A) α-interferon
(B) β-interferon
(C) γ-interferon
(D) interleukin-1
(E) tumor necrosis factor

252. Under resting conditions athletes (compared to untrained persons) have a higher

(A) cardiac output
(B) cardiac stroke volume
(C) heart frequency
(D) oxygen consumption
(E) respiratory frequency

253. A 56-year-old male presents with headache, nausea, left-sided ocular pain, and blurred vision. On examination his cornea appears cloudy and the pupils are fixed in a mid-dilated position. Ocular pressure is 48 mm Hg (normally < 20 mm Hg). Which of the following statements about intraocular pressure is correct?

(A) Intraocular pressure varies by as much as 50% from day to day.

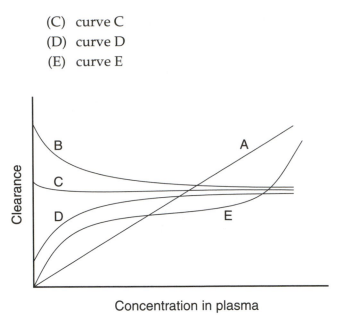

(B) Intraocular pressure is mainly determined by the rate of production of the aqueous humor.
(C) Decreased pupil size reduces flow out of ocular chamber.
(D) Anti-inflammatory corticosteroids are the drug of choice for this patient.
(E) Glaucoma is a rare cause of blindness in the U.S.

254. Which of the following hormones is produced in the duodenum and stimulates the pancreas to produce an enzyme-rich secretion?

(A) secretin
(B) gastrin
(C) cholecystokinin (CCK)
(D) gastric inhibitory peptide (GIP)
(E) vasointestinal inhibitory peptide (VIP)

255. Chronic non-erosive gastritis is often associated with decreased gastric acid secretion. Which of the following best describes the main ion transport at the apical membrane of gastric parietal cells?

(A) active secretion of H^+ in exchange for K^+
(B) active H^+ and Cl^- cotransport
(C) Na^+/K^+ pump
(D) Cl^-/HCO_3^- exchange
(E) passive diffusion of H^+

256. Plasma renin levels are decreased in patients with

(A) primary aldosteronism
(B) salt restriction
(C) upright posture
(D) heart failure
(E) renal artery stenosis

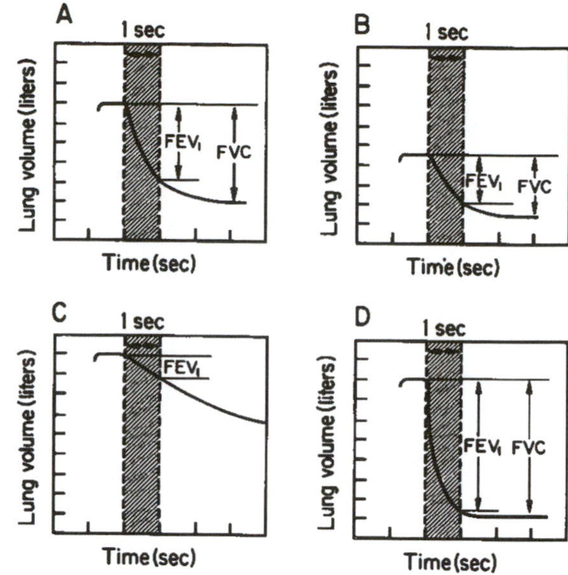

Figure 2–18

257. A 19-year-old patient has a 5-year history of moderate to severe asthma and comes in for his yearly pulmonary function test. Illustrated in Figure 2–18 are four different patterns of forced expiratory volume in one second (FEV_1) and forced vital capacity (FVC). Which of these patterns do you expect to see in this patient?

(A) curve A
(B) curve B
(C) curve C
(D) curve D

258. A patient asks you for advice about travel to the Himalayas. You recommend acetazolamide (a carbonic anhydrase inhibitor) for prevention of mountain sickness. Which of the following statements about the action of acetazolamide is correct? Acetazolamide

(A) causes metabolic alkalosis
(B) directly suppresses the respiratory drive
(C) directly increases the respiratory drive
(D) increases bicarbonate concentration in the urine
(E) increases hydrogen concentration in the urine

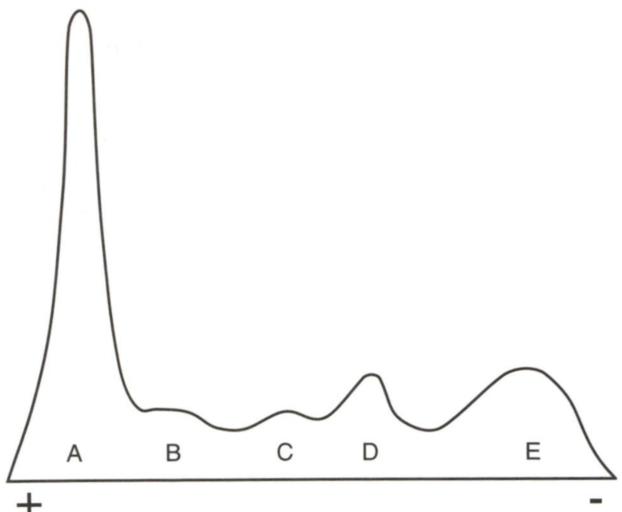

Figure 2–19

259. Figure 2–19 illustrates a plot of a blood protein electrophoresis from a 6-month-old boy with a suspected congenital immunodeficiency syndrome. Proteins in which of the electrophoretic fraction are responsible for humoral immunity?

(A) fraction A
(B) fraction B
(C) fraction C
(D) fraction D
(E) fraction E

260. A 56-year-old female presents with microcytic anemia, low ferritin serum level, and low transferrin saturation. Which of the following statements correctly describes intestinal iron absorption in this patient?

(A) Intestinal iron absorption depends on intrinsic factor.
(B) Iron is mainly absorbed in the distal ileum.
(C) Free iron is more readily absorbed than iron bound to organic molecules.
(D) Iron is more readily absorbed in the ferric state (Fe^{3+}) than in the ferrous state (Fe^{2+}).
(E) Dietary iron is more readily absorbed in this patient due to low ferritin stores of the intestinal epithelium.

261. ADH secretion is most increased by

(A) increased plasma osmolarity
(B) decreased plasma osmolarity
(C) increased plasma volume
(D) decreased plasma volume
(E) hypothalamic releasing factor

262. One of your diabetic patients has a blood glucose level of 200 mg/dL. Surprisingly, a dipstick test is negative for urinary glucose. How could this finding be explained?

(A) Patient has significantly reduced glomerular filtration rate.
(B) Patient has diabetes insipidus.
(C) Patient is in a state of antidiuresis.
(D) Patient has defective tubular glucose transporters.
(E) Dipstick tests are more sensitive for reducing sugars other than glucose.

263. A 79-year-old patient with congestive heart failure and peripheral edema is given a diuretic. Which of the following diuretics promotes diuresis by opposing the action of aldosterone?

(A) mannitol
(B) thiazide
(C) loop diuretic
(D) carbonic anhydrase inhibitor
(E) potassium-sparing diuretic

264. Liver glycogen content is affected by several hormones. Which of the following shows the correct effects of hormones on liver glycogen content?

	Catecholamines	Glucocorticoids	Glucagon
(A)	decreased	decreased	decreased
(B)	decreased	decreased	decreased
(C)	decreased	increased	decreased
(D)	increased	decreased	increased
(E)	increased	increased	decreased

265. A 37-year-old female presents with a plasma TSH 12.5 mU/L (normal < 5 mU/L) and a T3 resin uptake of 19% (normal 25 to 35%). Which of the following clinical symptoms and signs would you expect in this patient?

(A) tachycardia
(B) periorbital swelling and lethargy
(C) increased body temperature
(D) palpitations
(E) anxiety

266. Following an automobile accident a patient suffers a pelvic fracture and significant internal blood loss resulting in hemorrhagic shock. Which of the following organs has the largest specific blood flow (blood flow per gram of tissue) under resting conditions and is especially vulnerable during the shock phase?

(A) brain
(B) skin
(C) kidneys
(D) heart muscle
(E) skeletal muscle

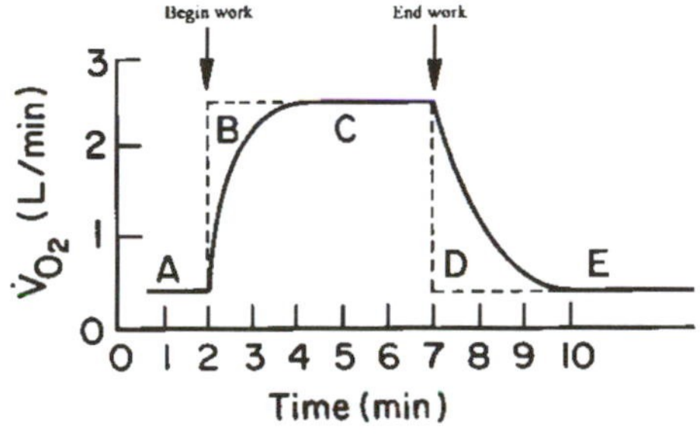

Figure 2–20

267. During training for a 1000 meter run the oxygen consumption ($\dot{V}O_2$) of an athlete is monitored before, during, and after the run. His energy requirements are indicated by dashed lines in Figure 2–20. Several different periods are marked by letters A through E. O_2 delivery to exercising muscles is less than that required for aerobic metabolism during

(A) period A
(B) period B
(C) period C
(D) period D
(E) period E

268. Following an acute stroke a patient denies the presence of paralysis of his left upper and lower extremities. The most likely cortical lesion in this patient is localized in the

(A) right posterior parietal cortex
(B) right precentral gyrus
(C) right postcentral gyrus
(D) posterior inferior gyrus of left frontal lobe
(E) posterior superior gyrus of left temporal lobe

269. Which of the following is the primary site for salt and water reabsorption in the kidneys?

(A) glomerulus
(B) proximal tubule
(C) juxtaglomerular apparatus
(D) thick ascending limb of Henle's loop
(E) collecting duct

270. Which of the following renal sites is characterized by low water permeability under all circumstances?

(A) glomerulus
(B) proximal tubule
(C) juxtaglomerular apparatus
(D) thick ascending limb of Henle's loop
(E) collecting duct

Questions 271 and 272

271. A 58-year-old male visits your office and complains about impotence. Upon questioning you learn that he is capable of erections, but they don't last as long and are of lesser strength than previously. Which of the following neurotransmitters is primarily responsible for dilation of the penile artery during erections?

(A) epinephrine
(B) norepinephrine
(C) acetylcholine
(D) nitric oxide
(E) GABA

272. Nitric oxide causes penile artery dilation by

(A) increasing cellular cAMP
(B) decreasing cellular cAMP
(C) increasing cellular cGMP
(D) decreasing cellular cGMP
(E) increasing cellular inositol-tris-phosphate

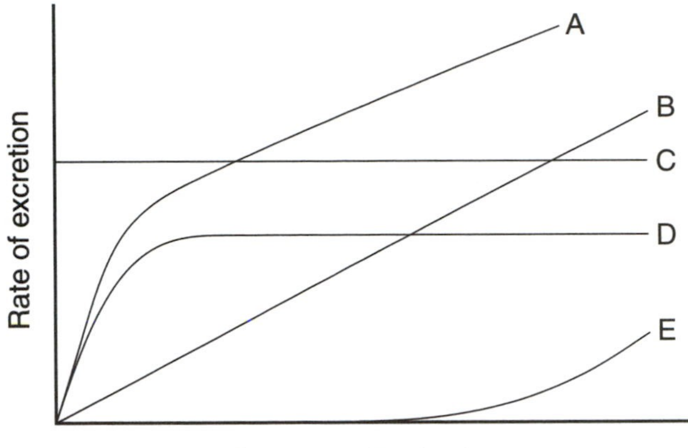

Figure 2–21

273. Creatinine clearance is used to estimate glomerular filtration rate in patients with chronic renal diseases. Which of the graphs in Figure 2–21 shows the correct relationships between renal rate of excretion and plasma concentration of creatinine?

(A) curve A
(B) curve B
(C) curve C
(D) curve D
(E) curve E

274. One of your obstetric patients is 5 months pregnant with her second child. Pregnancy and delivery of her first child were unremarkable. Which of the following combinations poses a significant risk of hemolytic anemia for her second child?

	Mother	First Child	Second Child
(A)	Rh-negative	Rh-negative	Rh-positive
(B)	Rh-negative	Rh-positive	Rh-positive
(C)	Rh-positive	Rh-positive	Rh-negative
(D)	Rh-positive	Rh-negative	Rh-positive
(E)	Rh-positive	Rh-positive	Rh-positive

275. Which of the following statements about human chorionic gonadotropin (hCG) is correct?

(A) hCG is often negative in patients with ectopic pregnancy.
(B) hCG is usually negative in patients with choriocarcinoma.
(C) hCG can be detected in the urine prior to the first missed period.
(D) hCG levels are highest at the end of pregnancy.
(E) hCG directly suppresses fetal production of steroids.

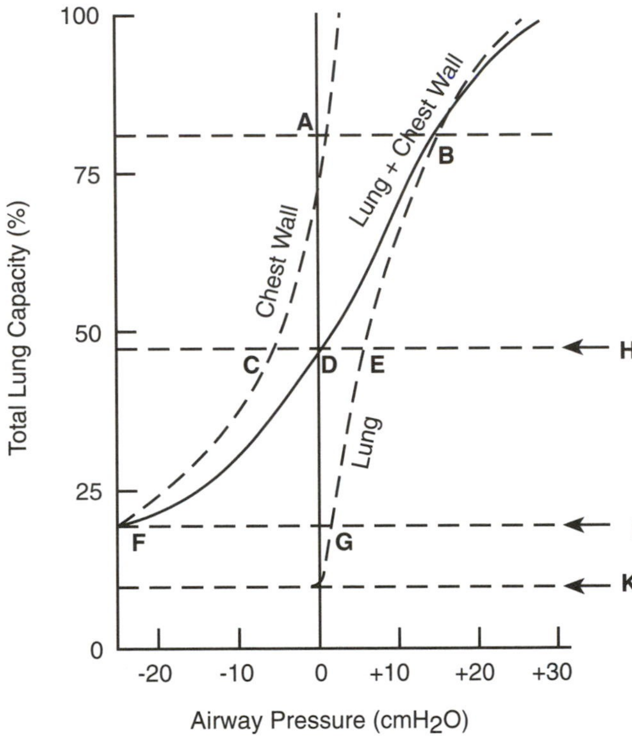

Figure 2–22. *(Reprinted with permission from Rahn, H.* American Journal of Physiology *146.)*

276. The graph in Figure 2–22 shows a passive relaxation pressure–volume curve of the lung and the chest wall. The residual volume of the lung is indicated by

(A) point A
(B) point B
(C) point C
(D) point D
(E) point E

(F) point F
(G) point G
(H) point B to point E
(I) level H
(J) level I
(K) level K

277. Which of the following transmembrane proteins is mainly responsible for the resting membrane potential of vascular smooth muscle cells?

(A) K^+ channels
(B) Na^+/K^+ pump
(C) Na^+ channels
(D) Cl^- channels
(E) nonselective cation channels

Questions 278 and 279

Normal values (female):
Hemoglobin: 12–16 g/dL
Mean corpuscular volume (MCV): 80–100 fL
Mean corpuscular hemoglobin concentration (MCHC): 31–37 g/dL

A female patient presents with an RBC count of 3.0 million/μL, a hematocrit of 27%, and a hemoglobin of 11 g/dL. Laboratory examination of a blood sample reveals increased osmotic fragility of this patient's erythrocytes.

278. This patient's erythrocytes have

(A) normal MCV
(B) decreased MCV
(C) normal MCHC
(D) decreased MCHC
(E) increased cell diameter

279. Which of the following is a likely cause of this patient's findings?

(A) iron deficiency anemia
(B) sickle cell anemia
(C) thalassemia
(D) spherocytosis
(E) liver disease

Questions 280 to 282

A 79-year-old male patient with chronic renal failure and a glomerular filtration rate of 25 mL/min (normal 120 mL/min) is admitted to the hospital because of a spontaneous fracture of the left humerus. X-ray shows numerous subperiosteal erosions with low bone density.

280. The most likely cause of this patient's fracture is

(A) osteoporosis due to old age
(B) osteoporosis due to lack of sex steroids
(C) osteomalacia due to primary hyperparathyroidism
(D) osteomalacia due to secondary hyperparathyroidism
(E) rickets due to lack of dietary vitamin D

281. Which of the following statements about renal handling of phosphate is correct? In this patient

(A) the filtration rate of phosphate is lower than normal, resulting in phosphate accumulation
(B) the tubular secretion rate is higher than normal, resulting in phosphate loss
(C) the tubular reabsorption rate is higher than normal, resulting in phosphate accumulation
(D) increased urinary phosphate binds urinary calcium, resulting in a loss of both phosphate and calcium
(E) most of the filtered phosphate is excreted

282. Which of the following statements is correct? Phosphate reabsorption in the proximal tubule

(A) is due to active cotransport with calcium ions
(B) is due to active cotransport with chloride ions
(C) is due to passive diffusion down its electrochemical gradient
(D) is inhibited by calcitonin
(E) is inhibited by parathormone

Answers and Explanations

156. (A) During pregnancy many physiological changes take place in the mother's body. Maternal blood volume increases up to 40% due to elevated aldosterone and estrogen levels. Bone marrow production of erythrocytes also increases, but does not keep up with the plasma volume expansion, resulting in a decrease in hematocrit ("physiological anemia of pregnancy") (choice B). Respiratory minute volume increases by about 50% because of the increased basal metabolic rate and oxygen consumption. This increase is largely due to an increase in tidal volume without increase in respiratory rate (choice C). Both residual volume and expiratory reserve volume decrease (choice D). Gastrointestinal tone and motility decrease because of the inhibitory effect of progesterone on these smooth muscles (choice E).

157. (C) The cerebellum is generally considered to play an important role in the coordination and smoothing out of voluntary movements. Intention tremor, which may be observed in cerebellar disease, is absent at rest (choice A) but appears at the onset of voluntary movements (choice B). This aspect of the tremor readily differentiates it from tremor observed with degeneration of the nigrostriatal dopaminergic tracts in Parkinson's disease, which produces tremor that is present at rest. Frequency of tremor is a less reliable means to distinguish these types of tremor (choice D), and the amplitude of oscillations is not generally constant throughout a voluntary movement (choice E).

158. (B) In diabetes insipidus, appropriate water intake from thirst will adequately compensate for the potential excess volume loss. Only if access to appropriate intake is prevented will a large volume loss occur. All of the other changes listed would tend to maintain blood volume, but all are either short-term effects (choices A and C) or the result of extreme stimuli, such as hemorrhage or intense sympathetic activity (choices D and E).

159. (E) Urination occurs whenever the bladder pressure exceeds the sphincter tone. The external sphincter is a skeletal muscle innervated by motor neurons from the pudendal nerve, not by sympathetic fibers (choice A). As the bladder fills, sensory signals from bladder stretch receptors elicit a micturition reflex via parasympathetic fibers originating in the sacral spinal cord. These transient contractions elicit an urge to urinate, but normally urination does not occur unless the external sphincter relaxes. If the lumbar spinal cord is damaged (choice B) while the sacral segments are intact, micturition reflexes will occur, resulting in spontaneous and uncontrolled bladder emptying (automatic bladder). If the sacral spinal cord is damaged (choice C), micturition reflexes are lost and the bladder fills to capacity resulting in overflow incontinence (atonic bladder). Higher centers in the brainstem keep the micturition reflex inhibited except when micturition is desired (choice D).

160. (D) Figure 2–1 shows the endometrial changes expected during a textbook menstrual cycle of 28 days' length. Ovulation occurs on day 14, counting as day 1 the first day of the last menstrual period. Progesterone produced by the corpus luteum reaches its peak around day 21. In the absence of fertilization, the corpus luteum then degenerates and progesterone levels begin to drop.

161. **(B)** In contrast to progesterone, which is detectable in significant amounts only during the secretory phase, estrogen levels show a biphasic time course. Peak levels are secreted by the growing follicle about 36 hours prior to ovulation (which occurs on day 14), inducing the LH surge. A second but smaller increase of estrogen occurs during the luteal phase of the cycle.

162. **(D)** Pupil diameter is determined by the balance between sympathetic tone to the radial fibers of the iris and parasympathetic tone to the pupillary sphincter muscle. Phentolamine is a blocker of α-adrenergic receptors which causes pupil constriction. Pupil dilation occurs during increased sympathetic activity, e.g., emotional excitement (choice A), decreased parasympathetic activity during darkness (choices B and C), or block of muscarinic receptors by atropine (choice E).

163. **(E)** Water that is either higher or lower than body temperature when introduced into the external auditory meatus may set up convection currents within the endolymph of the inner ear. These currents may result in the stimulation of the semicircular canals by causing movements of the ampullar cristae. Conflicting information from the right and left sides may in turn result in vertigo and nausea. Decreased movement or immobilization of the otoliths (choice A) or the ampullar cristae (choice B) is not caused by such changes in temperature. Furthermore, changes in the discharge rate of vestibular afferents (choices C and D), which must occur with caloric stimulation, are most likely to be caused by the changes in the activity of the receptors, rather than being a direct response of the afferents to changes in temperature.

164. **(A)** The absorption of non-heme iron in any food is strongly affected by the composition of the meals. Iron is more efficiently absorbed in the ferrous state (Fe^{2+}) than in the ferric state (Fe^{3+}), and commercial iron preparations often contain vitamin C to prevent oxidation of Fe^{2+} to Fe^{3+}. Still, only 3 to 6% of the ingested daily iron is actually absorbed in the upper gastrointestinal tract (choice B). Seventy percent of the total body iron is used for hemoglobin and myoglobin; the remainder is stored as readily exchangeable ferritin, and some is stored in less easily mobilized hemosiderin (choice C). When old red blood cells are destroyed by the tissue macrophage system, heme is separated from globin and degraded to biliverdin (choice D). Iron in the plasma is bound to the iron-transporting protein transferrin (choice E). Transferrin level (total iron binding capacity) and saturation are clinically important indicators of iron deficiency anemia.

165. **(B)** The primary change in the cochlea due to an increase in the frequency of a sound wave is a change in the position of maximal displacement of the basilar membrane. A sound of low pitch produces the greatest displacement toward the apex of the cochlea and produces the greatest activation of hair cells at that location. As the pitch is increased, the position of greatest displacement moves closer to the base of the cochlea. Increased amplitude of basilar membrane displacement (choice A), and increases in the number of hair cells that are activated (choice C) and in the frequency of discharge of units in the auditory nerve fibers (choice D), together with an increase in range of frequencies to which such units respond (choice E), are all more likely to be observed in response to increases in the intensity of a sound stimulus rather than to increases in pitch. In the auditory cortex, sound frequencies are organized topographically so that a change in pitch may be represented by a change in the location of activated cortical units.

166. **(B)** Myasthenia gravis is an autoimmune disease characterized by progressive muscle weakness due to formation of antibodies against the nicotinic ACh receptor of the motor end-plate. Impairment of neuromuscular transmission results in a weakened response of the muscle to nerve stimulation, but a normal response to direct electrical stimulation (choice A). Improvement of muscle weakness by small doses of acetylcholinesterase inhibitors physostigmine or edrophonium are diagnostic for this disease (choice C). A large dose of physostigmine worsens muscle weakness because of desensitization of the end-plate to persistent ACh (choice D). Radiolabeled snake venom α-bungarotoxin is a useful investigative tool to quantify the number of ACh receptors at the motor endplate and should be performed in vitro on a muscle biopsy specimen (choice E).

167. **(B)** Prolonged bleeding time is characteristic of platelet disorders, e.g., thrombocytopenia. Patients with hemophilia A or B (i.e., absence of factor VIII or IX, respectively) have a prolonged partial thromboplastin time (PPT), but do not have a prolonged bleeding time. Ca^{2+} is a necessary cofactor for blood coagulation, and chelation of Ca^{2+} ions by citrate inhibits coagulation (choice A). Von Willebrand factor is part of the factor VIII complex and also promotes platelet adherence to the vascular subendothelium (choice C). Patients who lack this factor (von Willebrand's disease) have both a prolonged PPT and a prolonged bleeding time (choice D). Disseminated intravascular coagulation results in depletion of coagulation factors and accumulation of fibrin split products (choice E).

168. **(C)** The stimulation of receptors in the Golgi tendon organs leads to the inverse stretch reflex. This reflex is responsible for the relaxation that is observed when a muscle is subjected to a strong stretch. Impulses from the organs travel in type Ib fibers to the spinal cord, where they activate inhibitory interneurons. These in turn suppress the activity of motor neurons and therefore lead to relaxation of the extrafusal muscle fibers (choice A) attached to the tendons. The state of contraction of intrafusal fibers (choice B), the gamma-efferent discharge rate (choice D), and the activity in group II afferent fibers (choice E) control the stretch reflex, which is distinct from the inverse stretch reflex mediated by the Golgi tendon organs.

169. **(E)** Blood vessels of patients with Bartter's syndrome adapt to the increased angiotensin levels by down-regulating their angiotensin II receptors. This explains why these patients usually have normal blood pressure (choice A). Patients with Bartter's syndrome have primary elevated renin (choice B) due to idiopathic hyperfunction of the juxtaglomerular apparatus. Consequently, these patients have elevated levels of angiotensin II (choice C) and aldosterone (choice D).

170. **(E)** Following total colectomy and ileostomy, the volume and water content of ileal discharge decreases over time, and most patients can lead an essentially normal life. (choices A and B). Iron absorption occurs in the upper GI tract, not the colon (choice C) and the vitamin B_{12}–intrinsic factor complex is absorbed in the ileum (choice D). As long as the ileum remains intact, deficiency of these factors essential for erythropoiesis is not expected.

171. **(A)** The toxic effects of nerve gas derive from its ability to inhibit the enzyme cholinesterase. The inhibition of this naturally occurring degradative enzyme engenders a massive accumulation of acetylcholine, evoking an overstimulation of the acetylcholine receptors throughout the body. In the heart, specifically, acetylcholine released by the vagal nerve stimulates muscarinic receptors in the cells of the SA node. This results in the opening of potassium channels and hyperpolarization of the SA node (choice B). It therefore takes longer for sodium leakage to cause the membrane potentials of these cells to reach the threshold required for an action potential (choice C). The rate of rhythmicity is thus decreased. A similar hyperpolarization of the fibers at the AV junction decreases conduction velocity of atrial impulses to the ventricle (choice D). The force of ventricular contractions is not affected by the vagus nerve (choice E).

172. (C) Cardiac sympathetic nerves show decreased action potential frequency as a result of carotid sinus pressure or massage. The increased pressure at the sinus baroreceptors (choice A) causes an increase in the firing rate of the afferent carotid sinus nerve (choice B) that inhibits the medullary vasomotor center. Consequently, both a decrease in sympathetic tone and an increase in efferent vagal discharge (choice D) contribute to the fall in heart rate (choice E) and arterial blood pressure following massage or a stroke to the carotid sinus. When performing this maneuver on your patients or peers, be prepared for cardiac sinus arrest and avoid vigorous massage, which might dislodge an embolus and cause permanent neurological damage.

173. (C) With the first breath of life, pulmonary arterial resistance drops dramatically. This is due to the oxygenation of the lungs causing vasodilatation of the pulmonary vessels. Clamping of the umbilical cord doubles peripheral resistance and causes an increase in arterial blood pressure. As soon as right atrial pressure drops below left atrial pressure, the foramen ovale will close (valve-like mechanism), establishing the adult-type blood circulation. The rising systemic (choice A) and falling pulmonary artery pressure (choice B) cause a flow reversal through the ductus arteriosus from right to left to left to right within minutes of birth. Complete closure of the ductus arteriosus appears to be due to a decline of local prostacyclin levels and usually occurs within 24 to 48 hours after birth (choice D). The ductus venosus (choice E) closes even later.

174. (B) Hypoglycemia is the most potent stimulus for glucagon secretion. High serum levels of amino acids (especially alanine and arginine) will also induce glucagon release (choice A). Hyperglycemia (choice C) is a potent stimulus for insulin release from pancreatic beta cells. Somatostatin inhibits glucagon secretion (choice D). While parasympathetic stimulation to the pancreas stimulates acinar secretion, it does not stimulate α-cells to secrete glucagon (choice E).

175. (E) The most rapid filling of the ventricles occurs in early diastole, immediately after opening of the atrioventricular valves. This happens after the repolarization phase (T wave) and resulting relaxation of the cardiac ventricular muscle. Excitation of the atria (choice A) also results in increased blood flow into the ventricles, occurring around choice B. However, the flow at that time is less than during early diastole. Ventricular contraction begins with the QRS complex (choice C) and lasts until the end of the T wave (choice D). During this time, the mitral and tricuspid valves are closed.

176. (A) Note that the end-diastolic volume of this patient is the same as that of a normal subject. Since the patient's stroke volume is larger than that of a normal subject, the force of contraction must also be larger. This could be due to increased sympathetic tone or to the fact that the patient took inotropic medications. The volume remaining after the ventricular contraction is correspondingly smaller compared to normal. Preload (choices B and C) equals end-diastolic volume and is the same in patient and normal subject. Afterload (choice D) is equal to arterial pressure. Both afterload and stroke volume (choice E) are larger in this patient compared to normal.

177. (C) Figure 2–23 shows the jugular vein pressure curve. Pressure in the jugular vein reflects atrial pressure and is highest during the atrial contraction (a-wave). The v-wave (choice A) represents the rise in atrial pressure before the tricuspid valve opens during diastole. The y-notch (choice B) is due to fall

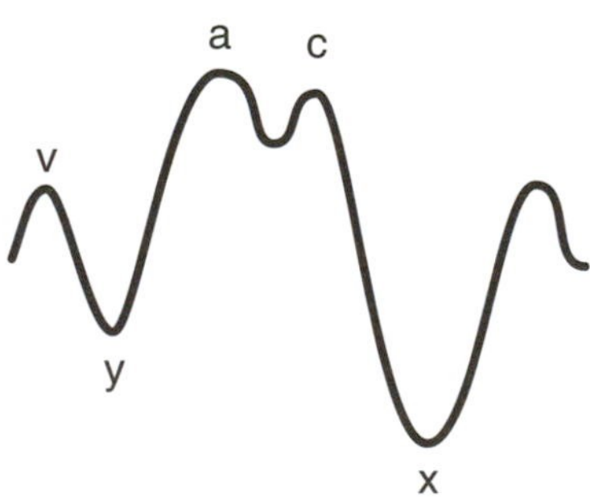

Figure 2–23

of atrial pressure during the ventricular filling phase. The c-wave (choice D) is due to the rise in atrial pressure produced by the bulging of the mitral valve during isometric contraction of the left ventricle. The x-notch (choice E) coincides with the ventricular ejection phase.

178. (C) Increasing the membrane's conductance to chloride will result in chloride influx and the membrane potential approaching the value dictated by the chloride equilibrium potential (calculated from the Nernst equation), which is about –70 mV for neurons. Minus thirty mV (choice A) is near the Nernst potential for Cl^- ions in smooth muscle cells, but not in neurons. Plus thirty mV (choice B) is near the Nernst potential for Na^+ ions. The membrane potential would remain unchanged (choice D) only if the cell resting membrane potential is already at the Nernst potential of the ion channels that were opened. Action potentials occur if the cell membrane is depolarized above threshold (choice E).

179. (E) Renin secretion is enhanced by sympathetic activity via renal nerves. Fifteen percent of patients with essential hypertension have elevated plasma renin levels, while 85% of patients with essential hypertension have normal or decreased plasma renin levels. Reasons for this difference are not well understood. Generally speaking, conditions of decreased extracellular fluid volume or decreased blood pressure stimulate renin secretion from juxtaglomerular cells located in the media of the afferent arterioles, while overhydration (choice A) and hypertension (choice B) tend to suppress renin secretion. There are two major mechanisms that stimulate renin release: (1) decreased pressure in the afferent arterioles, and (2) decreased delivery of Na^+ and Cl^- to the distal tubules at the level of macula densa cells. Dilation of renal arterioles (i.e., increased pressure) (choice C) and increased delivery of Na^+ and Cl^- to the distal tubules (choice D) both decrease renin secretion.

180. (B) Although electrogenic pumps may contribute to the membrane potential of certain cells, the major determinants of membrane potential are the external and internal concentrations of permeant ions and their relative permeabilities in the membrane. Decreasing the conductance causes the membrane potential to move away from the equilibrium potential for that ion. Thus, a decrease in the conductance of a membrane to chloride ions causes the cells to depolarize—that is, become more positive—if the membrane potential is positive with respect to the chloride equilibrium potential. Conversely, increasing the conductance for an ion causes the membrane potential to approach the equilibrium potential for that ion (choice A). External and internal ion chloride concentrations are needed to calculate the Nernst potential for this ion, but a simple comparison of these two values does not allow predictions about the change in membrane potential (choices C, D, and E).

181. (D) Secondary aldosteronism in hypertensive states either is secondary to a primary overproduction of renin by the kidneys or is caused by an overproduction of renin secondary to a decrease in renal blood flow or perfusion pressure (e.g., malignant hypertension). Principal stimuli for aldosterone release are circulating ACTH from the pituitary gland, angiotensin II, and high plasma K^+ levels. In addition, low plasma Na^+ may also have a direct stimulatory effect on the adrenal cortex. Hypokalemia (choice A) and hypernatremia (choice B) reduce aldosterone secretion. Volume depletion, e.g., hemorrhage, increases aldosterone release through activation of the renin–angiotensin system. Overhydration (choice C) has the opposite effect. Atrial natriuretic peptide (choice E) is secreted from atrial myocytes under conditions of expanded extracellular volume and acts on renal mesangial cells and ductal epithelium to decrease Na^+ reabsorption.

182. (C) Acetylcholine, the transmitter at the muscle end-plate, may be released spontaneously in small packets or quanta, without the presynaptic terminal being depolarized by an action potential. These quanta are believed to represent the contents of single vesicles containing about 10,000 molecules of ACh (choice A). Release of acetylcholine activates many ion channels in the muscle to produce a miniature end-plate potential (choice B). Current through single ion channels can only be observed with special methods (patch clamping), but not with microelectrodes used to measure membrane potentials. While ion channels do open spontaneously even in the absence of neurotransmitter (choice D), the amplitude of these currents is much smaller than the amplitude of miniature end-plate potentials occurring during spontaneous release of vesicles from the nerve terminal. The opening of multiple ion channels in the postsynaptic membrane in response to a single presynaptic action potential (choice E) would produce a large end-plate potential of much greater amplitude than miniature end-plate potentials possess.

183. **(C)** Heart rate will increase whenever sympathetic firing rate increases or parasympathetic firing rate decreases, since the cardiac atria receive tonic input from both sympathetic and parasympathetic nerves. In humans, the ventricles are not innervated by parasympathetic nerves (choice A), and the strength of contraction increases with increasing preload (Frank–Starling mechanism), increasing sympathetic firing rate (choice B). With few exceptions, blood vessels are not innervated by parasympathetic nerves, and there is little effect of changes in parasympathetic tone on total peripheral resistance (choices D and E).

184. **(C)** Figure 2–5 shows the effects of epinephrine (X) and norepinephrine (Y) on heart rate and blood pressure. Epinephrine is more potent to β-receptors than α-receptors, while norepinephrine reacts predominantly with α-receptors and β_1-receptors. Both catecholamines increase heart rate (choices A and B) and cardiac output of the isolated heart preparation identically. Because of its β-adrenergic effect (choice D), epinephrine dilates blood vessels and lowers overall peripheral resistance; norepinephrine, due to its potent action on α-receptors, causes a steep increase in peripheral resistance. This increase in peripheral resistance is reflected in an immediate increase in diastolic and mean arterial blood pressure, causing a reflex bradycardia due to activation of the baroreceptor reflex. Therefore, it is acetylcholine from vagal nerve fibers that is responsible for the decrease in heart rate seen after norepinephrine infusion. Catecholamine X is epinephrine and catecholamine Y is norepinephrine (choice E).

185. **(C)** About 40% of total plasma Ca^{2+} is bound to proteins and not filtered at the glomerular basement membrane. Therefore, the estimated daily filtered load is 1.5 mM/L · 160 L/d = 240 mM/d. The exact amount of free versus total Ca^{2+} depends on the blood pH: free Ca^{2+} increases during acidosis and decreases during alkalosis.

186. **(D)** The response to a stab wound that punctures the lung demonstrates the elasticity of the lung and chest wall. The tendency of the lung to collapse is normally balanced by the tendency of the chest wall to spring out. Thus intrapleural pressures are subatmospheric. Introduction of air in this space allows the lung to collapse and not to expand outward (choices A and B). At the same time the chest wall will spring outward, not inward (choice C). Lung collapse obviously results in very low lung volume (choice E).

187. **(B)** Normally, O_2 is transferred from air spaces to blood via a perfusion-limited process. Thus, O_2 moves across the alveolar–capillary membrane by a process of simple diffusion, and the amount of gas taken up depends entirely on the amount of blood flow. Processes that impair diffusion of O_2 transform the normal relationship to a diffusion-limited process. Thus, if O_2 must move a greater distance because of a thickened barrier, as would occur with increased extravascular lung water (pulmonary edema) or cell components (interstitial fibrosis or asbestosis), the diffusion process is limited. Chronic obstructive lung diseases have little effect on pulmonary diffusion capacity (choice A). Breathing a hyperbaric gas mixture (choice C) would increase the driving force and may overcome diffusion limitation in patients with mild fibrosis or interstitial edema. Increasing the ventilatory rate (choice D) will not have this effect and will only serve to maintain a high gradient of O_2 from air to blood. Strenuous, but not mild exercise (choice E), decreases passage time and may also favor diffusion limitation.

188. **(D)** Afferent fibers from pulmonary mechanoreceptors are carried with the vagal and glossopharyngeal nerves to the brainstem and serve to limit inspiration. The respiratory center of the CNS consists of a diffuse group of neurons whose inherent activity is not abolished (choice A) even after all known afferent stimuli have been eliminated. Although sectioning the brain and observing respiratory changes is a useful approach to locating important areas of respiratory regulation, this approach interferes with many complex pathways which may interact. Nonetheless, transection of the brain above the pons has little effect (choice B)—an apneustic center may be located in the pons. Transection above the center results in prolonged inspiration, but not prolonged expiration (choice C). Apparently, a pneumotaxic center in the upper pons together with vagal afferents limit inspiration. The medullary center is capable of initiating and maintaining respiration even if separated from the pons (choice E).

189. **(D)** The action potentials illustrated must be those of cardiac nodal cells (SA node or AV node). The duration of these action potentials is too long for either motor axons (2 msec) (choice A) or skeletal muscle fibers (5 msec) (choice B). Also, the configuration is different. They cannot represent vascular smooth muscle cells, which have no appreciable action potential at all (choice C). They cannot be ventricular Purkinje action potentials (choice E) as these have a more negative diastolic component that does not gradually depolarize, a longer duration (200 msec), and a plateau region.

190. **(C)** One of the principal distinguishing features of nodal cell action potentials is the gradual diastolic depolarization, the so-called pacemaker potential. When the pacemaker potential reaches threshold (dashed line in illustration), an action potential is generated and propagated along conducting pathways to other cardiac fibers (the basis of autorhythmicity of cardiac pacemaker cells). During the diastolic period the outward I_K (or delayed rectifier current mainly responsible for repolarization) is slowly deactivated. At the same time there is activation of poorly selective channels (permeable to both Na^+ and K^+), which gives rise to a slow "funny" inward current due mainly to Na^+. Fast Na^+ channels (choice A) are responsible for action potentials in nerve cells and skeletal muscle fibers. An increase in delayed rectifier K^+ current (choice B) would counteract any cell membrane depolarization. Changes in anion permeability (choice D) do not contribute significantly to the pacemaker potential, but may play a role in the repolarization phase of the ventricular action potential. The ratio of intracellular to extracellular ion concentration shows no measurable change during action potentials (choice E). Due to the small membrane capacitance, movement of a very small number of ions across the cell membrane is sufficient to create the membrane potential.

191. **(B)** The total tension that is developed on stimulating a muscle isometrically is the sum of the passive tension of the unstimulated muscle and the active tension exerted by stimulation. The passive tension, but not the active tension, increases monotonically with the length of the fiber (choices A and C). Active tension, however, increases up to the resting length of the fiber and then declines as the length is increased further. The total tension therefore also shows first an increase and then a decrease as a fiber is lengthened (choices D and E).

192. **(C)** With arterial blood pH of 7.33, the patient clearly has an acidosis. The first question you should ask yourself is, "Is it respiratory or non-respiratory (metabolic)?" If it were respiratory (choices A and B), the $Pa{CO_2}$ would have been above normal. Since it is lower than normal, this indicates the acidosis is metabolic with some respiratory compensation in response to the acidemia. Uncompensated metabolic acidosis (choice D) would show normal Pa_{CO_2}. It is unlikely that the metabolic acidosis is due to diabetic ketoacidosis (choice E); if this were the case, you would expect glucose to be present in the urine.

193. (C) In healthy subjects on a normal diet, about 70 mEq of hydrogen ion is produced each day (largely from oxidation of sulfur-containing amino acids). This would produce a progressive metabolic acidosis if the H^+ were not excreted in the urine as NH_4^+ and $H_2PO_4^-$. Both are decreased in the later stages of renal failure (e.g., from chronic glomerulonephritis). Since NH_4^+ excretion plays the major role in disposing of daily H^+, a deficiency in ammonium excretion explains the metabolic acidosis (probably simply a reflection of the diminished number of functioning nephrons). Hypoventilation (choice A) or hyperventilation (choice B) are not the cause of this patient's acidosis. Excess beta-hydroxybutyric and acetoacetic acids (i.e., ketoacidosis) (choice D) is unlikely in this patient. Decreased catabolism of methionine and cysteine (choice E) also could not account for the metabolic acidosis.

194. (C) Glomerular pores have a diameter of approximately 8 nm. Albumin, the smallest serum protein (with a molecular weight of 69,000) has a diameter of approximately 6 nm and therefore pore size alone (choice A) cannot explain the virtual absence of albumin in the urine. However, albumin is prevented from passing through the pores by electrostatic repulsion, since the pores are lined by negative charges (choice B), and albumin, like most serum proteins, is itself negatively charged. Filtered amino acids and some very low weight proteins (choice D) are reabsorbed in the renal tubuli, but this does not explain the virtual absence of protein in the urine of this patient. Urine is usually sterile and filtered proteins are not metabolized (choice E).

195. (A) Energy can be derived from either aerobic or anaerobic sources. Although aerobic oxidative processes can provide a significant amount of energy, these processes are too slow to provide all of the energy required. Although stores of ATP (choice B) and creatine phosphate (choice C) are present in muscle, they provide sufficient energy for only very brief periods of exercise (a few seconds). Deaminated proteins may undergo gluconeogenesis (choice D), in which they are converted to glucose or glycogen, but this pathway is not normally used for strenuous exercise. The breakdown of glycogen to lactic acid provides sufficient energy rapidly enough to support brief periods of strenuous exercise (many seconds to a few minutes). The depletion of glycogen and production of lactic acid contribute to an energy debt, which is repaid via oxidative metabolism (choice E) in the period after exercise.

196. (A) This patient probably suffers from myopia (nearsightedness). Myopia is either due to eyeballs that are too long or a lens that is too strong. In order to focus a distant object onto the retina (far accommodation) the lens has to decrease its refractive power, i.e., increase its focal length. This is accomplished through relaxation of the ciliary muscles that oppose the pull of the sclera, resulting in a tightening of the zonula fibers and a flattening of the lens. Relaxation of the zonular fibers (choice B), rounding of the lens (choice C), and shortening of the focal length (choice D), all occur during near accommodation. The pupils also constrict during near accommodation (choice E), perhaps to increase depth of field.

197. (C) The cardiac myocyte action potential is characterized by a rapid depolarization due to opening of fast Na^+ channels and a more slowly developing plateau phase lasting about 200 msec. The plateau is due to opening of slowly inactivating high-threshold dihydropyridine-sensitive L-type Ca^{2+} channels. This action potential spreads rapidly across the myocardium since cardiac myocytes are electrically coupled via gap junctions. A subclass of K^+ channels (namely inwardly rectifying K^+ channels) (choice A) determine the cardiac resting membrane potential. Opening of Na^+ channels (choice B) causes the rapid upstroke of the action potential. Fast inactivating low-threshold dihydropyridine-insensitive T-type Ca^{2+} channels (choice D) are activated at thresholds intermediate between I_{NA} and $I_{CA\text{-}L}$, and contribute to the inward current of late stage phase 4 depolarization in sinus node and His/Purkinje cells. Cl^- channel activity (choice E) is increased by adrenergic stimulation and contributes to repolarization of the action potential.

198. **(A)** Malignant hyperthermia is due to a genetic variation of the skeletal muscle ryanodine receptors (sarcoplasmic Ca^{2+} release channels). Halothane and several other drugs may trigger excessive Ca^{2+} release, leading to muscle contractures, increased muscle metabolism, and an enormous increase in heat production. This condition is fatal if not treated promptly with a ryanodine receptor antagonist such as dantrolene. An increased hypothalamic temperature set point (choice B) occurs during febrile episodes of infectious diseases. Such change of set point is due to increased blood levels of interleukin-1 (choice C). Convectional heat loss (e.g., lack of appropriate clothing during winter) (choice D) would result in cooling of the body temperature. Increased sweat production (choice E) is a consequence, but not the cause, of malignant hyperthermia.

199. **(B)** Mean corpuscular hemoglobin concentration (MCHC) is calculated simply by dividing the hemoglobin concentration (8 g/dL) by the hematocrit (0.3). Normal range is 31 to 36 g/dL and this patient has a hypochromic anemia (MCHC = 8/0.3 = 26.7 g/dL). Dividing hemoglobin concentration · 10 by erythrocyte number (choice A) yields mean corpuscular hemoglobin (MCH). Normal range is 25.4 to 34.6 pg/cell and this patient has significantly reduced cellular hemoglobin content (MCH = 8 · 10/4 = 20 pg/cell). Mean corpuscular volume (MCV) (choices C, D, and E) is calculated by dividing hematocrit · 1000 by erythrocyte number ($4 \cdot 10^6/\mu L$). Normal range is 80 to 100 fL and this patient has a microcytic anemia (MCV = 0.3 · 1000/4 = 75 fL). Microcytic, hypochromic anemia is characteristic for iron deficiency.

200. **(A)** The diagram shows an expiratory and inspiratory flow–volume curve of a patient with an upper airway obstruction, e.g., severe epiglottitis or tracheal narrowing due to a compressing tumor. Upper airway obstructions limit the maximal flow rate of both inspiration and expiration. Patients with panacinar (choice B) or centrilobular (choice C) emphysema or COPD (choice D) typically have an increased residual volume and a normal to increased total lung volume. Patients with restrictive lung diseases (choice E) typically have decreased residual volume and decreased total lung volume.

201. **(D)** Both Na^+ and K^+ excretion are tightly regulated. Thus, as GFR decreases in disease, the percentage of filtered Na^+ or K^+ that is excreted increases in order to maintain a normal amount of Na^+ or K^+ excretion (assuming Na^+ and K^+ intake remain the same). Substances like creatinine (choice A) (almost exclusively excreted by glomerular filtration) and urea (choice B) (some reabsorption) have no adaptive mechanisms to regulate plasma levels. Thus, a significant decrease in GFR results in significant increases in plasma creatinine and urea (assuming production of both substances remains constant). This is because the amount of substance x that is excreted ($U_x \cdot V$) equals the amount produced. Furthermore, $U_x \cdot V$ equals GFR · P_x. If GFR decreases, P_x increases. Because of the increase in percent filtered Na^+ and K^+ that is excreted, an increase in plasma Na^+ (choice C) or a decrease in plasma K^+ (choice E) would not be expected with a GFR that is 50% of normal. U_x: urine concentration of x, P_x: plasma concentration of x, V: urine volume.

202. **(E)** Normal sleep occurs in alternating cycles between slow-wave sleep (non-REM sleep) and rapid eye movement (REM) sleep, the latter characterized by high metabolic brain activity and desynchronization of the EEG. Somnambulism (sleep walking) (choice A), enuresis (bedwetting) (choice B), and night terrors (choice C) occur during slow-wave sleep or arousal from slow-wave sleep. During REM sleep there is hypotonia of all major muscle groups except the ocular muscles, due to a generalized spinal inhibition that prevents acting out of dreams. Dreams, nightmares, and penile erections in the male all occur during REM sleep. Sleep spindles (choice D) in the EEG are characteristic for the early sleep stages.

203. **(C)** The relationship between alveolar ventilation ($\dot{V}_A$) and alveolar CO_2 pressure (P_{ACO_2}) is represented as

$$\dot{V}_A = (\dot{V}_{CO_2}/P_{ACO_2}) \cdot K$$

where K is a constant such that $P_{ACO_2} = F_{ACO_2} \cdot K$. ($F_{ACO_2}$ is the fraction of alveolar CO_2). Since $\dot{V}_{CO_2}$ is constant if CO_2 production remains unchanged, P_{ACO_2} will double if $\dot{V}_A$ is halved. In normal persons, alveolar CO_2 pressure (P_{ACO_2}) is virtually identical to arterial CO_2 pressure (Pa_{CO_2}). Therefore, Pa_{CO_2} will also double if $\dot{V}_A$ is halved. On the other hand, alveolar CO_2 pressures (P_{ACO_2}) (choice A) would decrease if ventilation were increased. Unless inspired air is enriched with O_2, arterial O_2 pressure (Pa_{O_2}) (choices B and D) and alveolar O_2 pressure (P_{AO_2}) (choice E) will decrease.

204. **(A)** The patient in question has Horner's syndrome. Unilateral loss of sympathetic innervation of the face results in ptosis and pupil constriction, not dilation (choice B). Vasodilation of the skin vessels and loss of sweating results in dry and red skin, not pale (choice C) or sweaty skin (choice D). Lateral deviation of the eye (choice E) would suggest damage to the third cranial nerve.

205. **(A)** Flow = pressure difference/resistance. If central venous pressure is negligibly small compared to mean arterial pressure, we can calculate the peripheral resistance from the data given. The key in obtaining a correct answer is being able to determine mean arterial pressure from systolic pressure P_S and diastolic blood pressure P_D. Because of the particular shape of the pressure curve, this is not simply the arithmetic mean, but rather

$$\text{mean arterial pressure} = P_D + 1/3\,(P_S - P_D), \text{ i.e., } 70 + 20 = 90 \text{ mm Hg}$$

Therefore, resistance = 90 mm Hg/5 L/min = 18 mm Hg · min/L.

206. **(E)** Secretion of acid and potassium by the renal tubule are inversely related. Thus, increased excretion of H^+ during renal compensation for respiratory acidosis will result in decreased secretion (or increased retention) of potassium ions, with the result that the body's potassium store rises. An increase in K^+ excretion (choices A, B, and C) would be associated with renal compensation for respiratory alkalosis. The filtered load of K^+ (choice D) depends only on K^+ plasma concentration and glomerular filtration rate, not on plasma pH.

207. **(C)** Breathing 100% O_2 should increase the Pa_{O_2} to almost 670 mm Hg in healthy persons (same as alveolar P_{AO_2}). Diffusion abnormalities (choice A) and ventilation/perfusion inequality (choice B) are also common causes of hypoxemia. Breathing 100% O_2 will greatly relieve the hypoxemia in these cases, but not if the patient has an anatomic right-to-left shunt (for example, a ventricular septal defect). One hundred percent O_2 also greatly increases the Pa_{O_2} in profound hypoventilation (choice D). The Pa_{O_2} will greatly increase in the normal individual as well (choice E). In abnormalities of diffusion (e.g., alveolar wall thickening) the Pa_{O_2} will be below 670 mm Hg, but not as low as 125 mm Hg. In ventilation/perfusion abnormalities, P_{AO_2} will be quite high in all communicating air spaces after 100% O_2, and both alveolar and arterial P_{O_2} will be quite high. Only in true right-to-left shunting would breathing 100% O_2 not substantially elevate the Pa_{O_2}, which could be as low as 125 mm Hg. The small rise over normal Pa_{O_2} comes mainly from a small amount of additional dissolved O_2 in blood passing through ventilated areas.

208. (C) Norepinephrine is the neurotransmitter at autonomic nerve terminals, whereas the main catecholamine released by the adrenal medulla under conditions of acute stress is epinephrine. These circulating catecholamines have numerous effects on metabolism, mostly mediated by β-receptors. Epinephrine has a direct lipolytic effect on fat cells because it activates the hormone-sensitive lipase, releasing free fatty acids into the circulation. Epinephrine has a potent effect on liver cells causing glycogenolysis, releasing large quantities of glucose within minutes into the bloodstream. It inhibits glycogen synthesis (choice A). This action is mediated by β-receptors linked to adenylate cyclase. By the same mechanism, epinephrine also inhibits glycogen synthesis in skeletal muscle cells (choice B) and promotes muscle glycogenolysis. However, the freed glucose is directly utilized by the muscle and not released into the bloodstream. Under some conditions stimulation of sympathetic nerves can increase insulin (choice D) and glucagon (choice E) secretion, however it is doubtful that these effects are of physiological significance. The main factor controlling both insulin and glucagon secretion is the blood glucose level. Increased blood glucose levels increase insulin secretion and suppress glucagon secretion, while low blood glucose levels increase glucagon secretion and inhibit insulin secretion.

209. (B) Under normal circumstances, depolarization is initiated in the SA node and then propagates to the AV node. From there, action potentials are propagated through the bundle of His and through the Purkinje system to the ventricular muscle. Conduction in the AV node is slower than conduction from the SA node to the AV node (choice A), from the AV node to ventricular muscle (choices C and D), or conduction within the ventricular muscle (choice E). The AV nodal delay is typically on the order of 100 msec.

210. (C) Hyperopia, or farsightedness, is due either to an insufficient refractive power of the lens or too short an eyeball. This condition can be corrected using glasses with convex lenses. Myopia, or nearsightedness (choice A), is either due to unusually large refractive power of the lens (choice B) or too long an eyeball (choice D). This condition can be corrected using glasses with concave lenses. Presbyopia is a condition of decreased accommodation range of the lens due to a decline of lens elasticity with age (choice E). Like hyperopia, this condition can also be corrected with convex glasses (reading glasses).

211. (D) Bohr's equation states that

$$\dot{V}_D/\dot{V}_T = (P_{ACO_2} - P_{ECO_2})/P_{ACO_2}$$

where P_{ECO_2} is mixed expired CO_2. In a normal person, Pa_{CO_2} is virtually identical to P_{ACO_2}. Thus

$$\dot{V}_D/\dot{V}_T = (Pa_{CO_2} - P_{ECO_2})/Pa_{CO_2}$$

Since by Fowler's method, $\dot{V}_D/\dot{V}_T = 0.25$ in the patient described in the question, the $(Pa_{CO_2} - P_{ECO_2})/Pa_{CO_2} = (40 - P_{ECO_2})/40 = 0.25$. Therefore $P_{ECO_2} = 30$ mm Hg. If considerable inequality of blood flow and ventilation were present, P_{ECO_2} could be much less than 30 mm Hg, and the patient's physiologic dead space would exceed the anatomic dead space.

212. (A) The test solution was isotonic but hyperosmotic. When the red cell was removed from normal isotonic plasma and placed in the test solution, two things happened: (1) the cell shrank, and (2) it then gradually returned to normal size. This would happen if the test solution had two components: (1) a concentration of impermeant solutes giving the same osmolality as plasma, plus (2) an additional amount of permeant solute capable of gradually penetrating the red cell membrane (at a slower rate than water). Examples of such permeant solutes are urea and NH_4^+. When the cell was placed in the test solution, it initially shrank, as if the test solution were hypertonic due to its higher osmolality. However, as the permeant solute became equilibrated (with the same concentration inside the cell as outside), the cell volume returned to normal. That is, although the test solution initially acted as if it were hypertonic due to its total solute concentration, this effect was only transient because of the penetration of the permeant particles. Net water entry (choice B) results in an increase in cell volume. Net solute entry (choice C) increases intracellular osmotic pressure and leads to net water entry. In this case the net solute entry resulted in a return of cell volume to the initial level (y). Changes in cell volume are always accompanied by changes in net water movement across the cell membrane (choice D), and the rate of entry merely determines the speed with which a new equilibrium is established (choice E).

213. **(C)** When the cell, with its accumulated gain of permeant solute (from prior exposure to test solution), was placed back into plasma, it had by then a total solute osmolality higher than plasma, so there was a period of net entry of water into the cell, causing it to swell, reaching a peak at point z. However, as the accumulated solute diffused out of the cell, the cell eventually lost all of this permeant solute and therefore ultimately returned to normal volume. Net water exit (choice A) would cause cell shrinkage, and lack of net water movement (choices B and D) would not cause any change in cell volume. If the solute had exited the cell during the exposure to test solution (choice E), the cell volume would have shrunk when returned to plasma.

214. **(C)** An increase in the rate of blood flow through the kidney (RBF) greatly increases the glomerular filtration rate (GFR). The filtrate formed is derived by ultrafiltration of plasma in the glomerular capillaries. The more plasma available (from increased RBF), the more filtrate is formed. Vasoconstriction of glomerular afferent arterioles (choice A) would not increase GFR but decrease it, because of a decrease in both RBF and capillary ultrafiltration pressure. Vasoconstriction of efferent arterioles (choice B) could produce a slight increase in GFR, but not much because of offsetting effects on RBF (decrease) and glomerular colloid osmotic pressure (increase). Indeed, because of a very substantial decrease in RBF with moderate to severe increases in efferent arteriolar resistance, there is actually a decrease in GFR despite increased capillary pressure. Because of the autoregulatory ability of the kidneys, an increase in mean arterial pressure (choice D) from 90 mm Hg to 140 mm Hg would not have much of an effect on either RBF or GFR. Autoregulation acts to maintain a constant blood flow and capillary pressure by its influence on afferent arteriolar resistance. A strong, acute stimulation of sympathetic activity to the kidneys (choice E) results in decreased RBF, decreased GFR, and may produce renal shutdown with zero urinary output.

215. **(A)** ADH acts on the collecting tubules of the kidney to induce water retention. Inappropriately high levels of ADH, as are achieved in SIADH, result in the renal retention of free water, which consequently exerts a dilutional effect on serum ion concentrations. Thus, serum sodium can fall dramatically in SIADH. While ADH also increases Na^+ reabsorption in the papillary collecting ducts, this effect is not enough to overcome the dilution of plasma caused by the increased renal water reabsorption in the presence of ADH (choices B, C, and D). High sodium levels (choices D and E) might be expected with decreased ADH levels, decreased renal responsiveness to ADH, or in patients dehydrated from any other cause.

216. **(D)** Vital capacity is the sum of inspiratory reserve volume, tidal volume, and expiratory reserve volume. Therefore, in order to calculate inspiratory reserve volume, the tidal volume and expiratory volume have to be subtracted from the vital capacity. All of these values can be measured by spirometry. The other choices (choices A, B, C, and E) are not sufficient to calculate inspiratory reserve volume. Residual volume (choices C and E) cannot be measured by spirometry.

217. **(D)** The Fick principle is derived by applying the law of conservation of mass ("what comes in must go out"):

$$\dot{V}O_2 = \dot{Q} \cdot (CaO_2 - CvO_2)$$

where $\dot{V}O_2$ equals O_2 consumption ("what comes in"), $\dot{Q}$ is cardiac output, and CaO_2 and CvO_2 are arterial and mixed venous O_2 content, respectively. First, we calculate cardiac output:

$$300 \text{ mL } O_2/\text{min} = \dot{Q} \cdot (20\text{–}15) \text{ mL } O_2/100 \text{ mL blood}$$
$$300 \text{ mL } O_2/\text{min} = \dot{Q} \cdot 5 \text{ mL } O_2/100 \text{ mL blood}$$
$$\dot{Q} = 6000 \text{ mL blood/min}$$

Next, we calculate stroke volume using the formula:

$$\text{stroke volume} = \text{cardiac output} \div \text{heart rate}$$

plugging in our value of 6,000 mL/min for cardiac output and 60/min for heart rate yields

$$\text{stroke volume} = 6{,}000 \text{ mL/min} \div 60 \text{ /min}$$
$$\text{stroke volume} = 100 \text{ mL}$$

218. **(A)** Since the liver is supplied by umbilical venous blood from the placenta, and the heart and head receive blood before it has mixed with significant amounts of desaturated blood, these important organs receive blood that is relatively high in saturated oxyhemoglobin. The high rate of blood flow at the placenta and the significant resistance of the placenta to diffusion of O_2 result in blood in the umbilical vein that has a lower PO_2 (30 mm Hg) than maternal mixed venous blood (choice B). However, the left shift in fetal oxyhemoglobin concentration (choice C) and the Bohr effect both act to increase the transport of O_2 to fetal tissues. A number of significant differences in circulating patterns are present in the fetus. The foramen ovale (choice D) remains open until after birth and a significant portion of inferior vena cava flow is shunted through it to the left. The major portion of right ventricular output is shunted through the ductus arteriosus to the aorta, not the lungs (choice E). The net effect of these shunts in the presence of high fetal pulmonary vascular resistance is very low fetal pulmonary blood flow. At birth, these patterns normally are quickly changed to ex utero patterns with high pulmonary perfusion.

219. **(D)** The brain autoregulates, and consequently an increase in blood pressure is offset by an increase in local vascular resistance to maintain constant cerebral blood flow. Cerebral blood flow will increase when PaO_2 is decreased to < 50 mm Hg or when $PaCO_2$ increases above normal. A decrease in arterial oxygen (choice A) or an increase in arterial CO_2 (choice B) would therefore cause vasodilation and decreased resistance to cerebral blood flow. A decrease in viscosity (choice C) would also increase blood flow. Cerebral blood flow is closely linked to brain parenchymal metabolism, and intense activity during a seizure (choice E) results in large, widespread increases in blood flow.

220. **(A)** P_{alv} is ambient atmospheric pressure, or zero reference pressure, and P_{pl} is a negative intrapleural pressure that becomes even more negative during inspiration. The lungs will expand to a higher volume during inhalation as a result of an increase in the transpulmonary pressure, or distending pressure ($P_{alv} - P_{pl}$). Static compliance is measured under conditions of no airflow (stepwise changes in volume with no airflow during measurement of distending pressure). With each increase in distending pressure there is a corresponding increase in lung volume. Compliance is $\Delta V/\Delta P$. Distending pressure divided by change in lung volume (choice B) gives the lung elasticity. The lung volume divided by recoil pressure ($P_{alv} - P_{pl}$) (choice D) equals compliance only during the first linear part of the lung distention/pressure relationship. Generally speaking, V/P does not equal $\Delta V/\Delta P$. Change in elastic recoil pressure (choice E) is only part of the compliance calculation.

221. (C) The volume of air remaining in the lungs after a maximal effort to exhale all the air possible is the residual volume. Therefore, this volume is not part of the vital capacity (choice A) and cannot be measured directly by a spirometer, which measures only changes in volume. Since you cannot voluntarily change your lung volume below the residual volume, the spirometer cannot measure it. Other methods (e.g., body plethysmography, inert gas dilution) must be used to measure residual volume. Expiratory reserve volume (choice B) is vital capacity minus inspiratory capacity, and the resting volume of the lungs (choice D) is the sum of residual volume and expiratory reserve volume. Lungs will recoil inward (choice E) until the recoil pressure ($P_{alv} - P_{pl}$) equals zero, a volume significantly below the residual volume.

222. (A) The product of tidal volume (volume moved in or out with each breath) times the frequency or breathing rate (number of breaths/min) is the total ventilation per minute (also called minute ventilation). In this case, the total ventilation is 600 mL times 12 breaths/min = 7200 mL/min. As stated in the problem, the alveolar ventilation (air ventilating the respiratory zone for gas exchange each minute) is 6000 mL/min. The difference is that part of the total ventilation going only to non-exchanging conducting airways = 1200 mL/min, or 100 mL per breath at 12 breaths/min. This 100 mL is the dead space volume.

223. (C) Breathing a low-oxygen gas mixture is similar to being at high altitude, but if this is done for only a few minutes, there will be no time for renal compensation. The hypoxia stimulates hyperventilation, which lowers the P_{CO_2}. The slightly lowered bicarbonate is due to buffering by nonbicarbonate buffers. Decreased P_{CO_2} results in decreased H_2CO_3. Decreased H_2CO_3 results in the following reaction being pulled to the right:

$$HCO_3^- + H^+ \rightarrow H_2CO_3 \rightarrow H_2O + CO_2$$

thus lowering the plasma bicarbonate HCO_3^- to slightly below normal. Had there been time for renal compensation, the bicarbonate would have been much lower. Severe chronic lung disease (choice A) or an overdose of heroin (choice B) would have caused respiratory acidosis due to abnormally high arterial P_{CO_2} (not low P_{CO_2}, which this subject has). A lowlander at high altitude for two weeks (choice D) would have had both low P_{O_2} and low P_{CO_2} like this subject, but would have had an abnormally low plasma bicarbonate and a more nearly normal pH, due to renal compensation in the form of bicarbonate excretion. Acute aspirin overdose (choice E) in adults usually presents first with a respiratory alkalosis, which includes a low P_{CO_2}, but not a low P_{O_2}.

224. (D) Chlorpromazine is an antipsychotic drug and has significant anticholinergic action, i.e., it inhibits the effects of parasympathetic stimulation. Functions of the parasympathetic nervous system include increasing gastrointestinal motility, decreasing gastrointestinal sphincter tone, and emptying of the rectum and urinary bladder. Therefore, patients on chlorpromazine often complain about constipation and urinary retention. Increased motility (choice A), decreased sphincter tone (choice B), or bladder emptying (choice C) are not expected. Parasympathetic fibers slow the heart rate and anticholinergic drugs cause tachycardia rather than bradycardia (choice E).

225. (B) Muscle tone is determined by the basal firing rate of the α-motor neurons and damage to these so-called lower motor neurons will result in flaccid paralysis. In contrast, damage to the corticospinal tract (i.e., upper motor neuron lesions) (choice A) will result in spastic paralysis because of hyperactive stretch reflexes. Activation of γ-efferent fibers (choice C) to muscle spindles also increases muscle tone due to reflex activation of the α-motor neurons (stretch reflex). Pathologically increased γ-efferent discharge results in muscle clonus. Parkinson's disease (choice D) is characterized by muscle rigidity and tremors.

Anxiety (choice E) is also associated with increased muscle tension.

226. **(B)** Even though the cabin of the airplane described in the question is pressurized, the barometric pressure decreased to 523 mm Hg. Thus, the FIO_2 (choice A) remains the same (0.2), but inspired PO_2 decreases, since it is the product of FIO_2 and barometric pressure. Water vapor pressure (choice C) remains at 47 mm Hg as long as body temperature is normal, and thus PO_2 of humidified alveolar air must be less than that at sea level. Although a decrease in $PACO_2$ due to some hyperventilation (choice D) may slightly enhance PAO_2, this is not sufficient to prevent the decrease in PAO_2 due to the drop in barometric pressure. Since cabin pressure (choice E) is less than at sea level, alveolar O_2 will also be lower.

227. **(A)** Shunted blood is blood that bypasses ventilated parts of the lung and directly enters the arterial circulation. In normal persons, this is largely due to mixing of arterial blood with bronchial venous and some myocardial venous blood, which drains into the left heart. Diffusion limitation (choice B), although finite, is usually immeasurably small, as is reaction velocity with hemoglobin (choice C). Unloading of CO_2 (choice D) may affect alveolar oxygen partial pressure, but would have no effect on the difference between alveolar and arterial PO_2. A large ventricular septal defect (choice E) would result in a significantly lower arterial O_2 compared to alveolar O_2.

228. **(B)** The gene that is abnormal in cystic fibrosis encodes a cAMP-regulated Cl^- channel (CFTR). Since Cl^- flux via this channel plays different roles in different epithelia, it is not surprising that the symptoms of cystic fibrosis are quite diverse. The volume-absorbing airway epithelium in CF patients shows increased Na^+ reabsorption, probably because lack of CFTR increases the transepithelial potential difference. This results in a thick, dehydrated mucus predisposing to airway infections. This is in contrast to sweat glands, where CF patients secrete nearly normal volumes of sweat into the acinus, but are unable to absorb NaCl from sweat as it moves through the sweat duct. Therefore, the Na^+ and Cl^- content of sweat are both elevated in CF patients (choice A). Lack of Cl^- and water secretion in gastrointestinal epithelia can lead to severe constipation and obstruction of the small and large bowels. Impairment of the Cl^-/HCO_3^- exchange in pancreatic ductal epithelium results in water and enzyme retention and may eventually destroy the pancreas. Cystic fibrosis is more common in Caucasians than in African-Americans (choice C), and is one of the most common genetic disorders, occurring in 1 of 2,000 Caucasian births. The abnormal gene is not located on the X chromosome (choice D), but on chromosome 7 (autosomal recessive). Sodium channels (choice E) are not defective in cystic fibrosis.

229. **(B)** With few exceptions, blood vessels are not innervated by parasympathetic nerves (choice A), and there is little effect of parasympathetic tone on total peripheral resistance. In contrast, sympathetic nerve activity contributes to the basal vascular smooth muscle tone, and cutting these nerve fibers results in immediate vasodilation of the affected extremity. While hypersensitivity to circulating catecholamines (choice C) will develop over time, this does not contribute to the vasodilation. Epinephrine and norepinephrine release from the adrenal medulla (choices D and E) is regulated by its direct sympathetic innervation (preganglionic cholinergic fibers from the splanchnic nerve), and not affected by sympathetic fibers to the extremities or circulating catecholamines.

230. **(B)** The initial segment of this EEG recording shows normal alpha brain wave activity. Alpha waves are indicative of a relaxed state, with eyes closed and the mind wandering freely. At the point marked by the arrow, the EEG becomes desynchronized (beta brain waves). Beta waves are seen when the patient performs specific mental tasks such as calculations or when he or she observes objects after opening the eyes. Closing one's eyes (choice A) would show the opposite pattern

(EEG becomes synchronized). The EEG cannot discriminate thought content such as the mind "wandering off" (choice C). Falling asleep (choice D) is associated with sleep spindles and increased synchronization of brain waves. Petit mal (absence seizures) (choice E) is characterized by a unique 3-per-second "spike and dome" pattern.

231. (E) Local inflammatory processes are often painful. This is due to sensitization of nociceptive nerve endings by PGE_2. Nonsteroidal anti-inflammatory drugs (NSAIDs) inhibit prostaglandin synthesis and help to alleviate the pain. Thromboxane A_2 (choice A) and prostacyclin (PGI_2) are both derived from PGH_2, but have opposite effects on platelets and blood vessels. Thromboxane A_2, released from platelets, promotes vasoconstriction and platelet aggregation while PGI_2, released from endothelial cells, is a potent vasodilator and inhibits platelet aggregation. Most prostaglandins have a large range of actions, and they may contract or relax smooth muscle cells depending on tissue source and species. In humans $PGF_{2\alpha}$ (choice B) constricts bronchial smooth muscle and PGE_2 (choice C) relaxes it. An increase in prostaglandin production by fetal membranes is believed to be a major factor for onset of uterine contractions and labor in humans (choice D).

232. (A) The pressure–volume relationship of this patient is essentially normal. Isovolumetric relaxation involves a drop in left ventricular pressure, with no change in left ventricular volume (hence the term "isovolumetric"). This occurs between points W (point at which the aortic valve closes) and X (point at which the mitral valve opens and ends the isovolumetric period). X to Y (choice B) is the filling phase of the ventricle and point Y denotes the end-diastolic volume (pre-load). Y to Z (choice C) is the isometric contraction before opening of the aortic valve, while Z to W (choice D) is the ejection phase of the systole.

233. (B) In order to measure the residual lung volume, the patient is connected to the spirometer after maximal expiration. After about 20 deep breaths the helium will be equally distributed between the spirometer and the residual volume. In this case:

$$6\ \text{L} \cdot 10\% = (6\ \text{L} + \text{RSV}) \cdot 9\%$$
$$6.666\ \text{L} = 6\ \text{L} + \text{RSV}$$
$$\text{RSV} = 0.666\ \text{L}$$

234. (C) Alert wakefulness and REM sleep are both characterized by beta waves, which indicate a high degree of brain activity. In the first stage of slow-wave sleep, which is associated with very light sleep (choice A), the EEG pattern shows very-low-voltage waves punctuated by occasional bursts of alpha activity, called sleep spindles. As sleep progresses, frequency of the EEG waveform decreases until it is approximately 2 to 3 cycles per second. This pattern, called delta waves, is characteristic of the deep sleep (choice B) of slow-wave stage 4. Quiet wakefulness is associated with alpha waves. If the patient woke up (choice D) her EEG would also show beta waves, but it's unlikely that she would still appear asleep. Central sleep apnea (choice E) is characterized by a sudden cessation of respiratory activity and drop of arterial oxygen saturation.

235. (A) Plasmin lyses fibrin and fibrinogen and is the active component of the fibrinolytic system. Plasminogen is a protein made in the liver. Cleavage of a single arginine–valine bond converts plasminogen to active plasmin. Streptokinase (choice B) has no direct effect on fibrin. Its action is due to formation of plasmin from its inactive precursor plasminogen. Neither plasmin (choice C) nor streptokinase (choice D) inhibit fibrinolysis. ε-aminocaproic acid inhibits fibrinolysis by inhibiting the conversion of plasminogen to plasmin. Streptokinase does not act on tissue plasminogen activator TPA (choice E). Streptokinase, urokinase, and recombinant human TPA all activate plasminogen and are used clinically in early treatment of myocardial infarction.

236. (C) Compliance (stretchability) of the lung is the change in lung volume divided by the change in airway pressure (δV/δP) and is usually measured at the steepest portion of the pressure–volume curve. This patient's lungs have a compliance of 5L/5 cm H_2O = 1 L/cm H_2O (Fig. 2–24). Lung elasticity (choice D) equals 1 divided by compliance, and this patient's lungs have an elasticity of 1 cm H_2O/L.

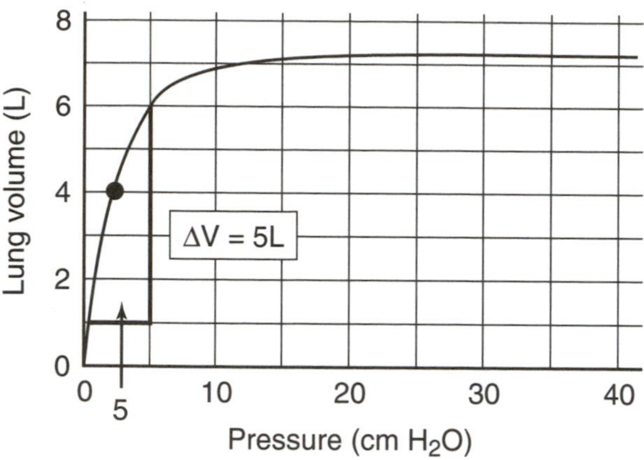

Figure 2–24

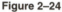

237. **(E)** Normal lung compliance is about 0.2 L/cm H_2O and this patient's lung compliance is significantly higher than normal. This occurs in emphysema resulting from chronic obstructive lung diseases or alpha-1-antitrypsin deficiency. Tuberculosis (choice A) and sarcoidosis (choice B) are chronic granulomatous lung diseases that have little effect on overall lung stretchability. Asbestosis (choice C) is a restrictive lung disease and would have a compliance less than normal (< 0.2 L/cm H_2O). Acute obstruction of the glottis (choice D) does not affect lung compliance, but would make this measurement difficult or impossible.

238. **(E)** Fick's principle states that the uptake of a substance by an organ equals the arteriovenous difference of the substance multiplied by the blood flowing through the organ. Measuring pulmonary arterial (i.e., mixed venous) oxygen content, aortic oxygen content, and oxygen uptake, the pulmonary blood flow can be calculated. Assuming there are no intracardiac shunts, pulmonary blood flow, systemic blood flow, and cardiac output are the same.

$$
\begin{aligned}
\text{Cardiac output} &= \text{oxygen uptake/(aortic} - \text{mixed venous oxygen content)} \\
&= 200\ \text{mL/min/}(15\ \text{mL}\ O_2/100\ \text{mL} - 10\ \text{mL}\ O_2/100\ \text{mL}) \\
&= 200\ \text{mL/min/}(5\ \text{mL}\ O_2/100\ \text{mL}) \\
&= 200\ \text{mL/min/}0.05 \\
&= 4000\ \text{mL/min}
\end{aligned}
$$

The cardiac output of this patient is significantly below normal (~6000 mL/min). If your calculation was 1333 mL/min (choice A) or 2000 mL/min (choice B) you probably forgot to subtract oxygen concentrations. When measuring cardiac output by Fick's method, it is important to use pulmonary arterial oxygen content rather than peripheral vein oxygen content (choice C), since different organs vary widely in their oxygen extraction.

239. **(C)** Although the early maturation of an ovarian follicle is dependent on the presence of FSH, ovulation is induced by a surge of LH. Although estrogens (choices A and B) usually have a negative feedback effect on LH and FSH secretion, the LH surge seems to be a response to elevated estrogen levels. In concert with FSH, LH induces rapid follicular swelling. LH also acts directly on the granulosa cells to cause them to decrease estrogen production, as well as to initiate production of small amounts of progesterone. These changes lead to ovulation. FSH (choice D) causes follicle maturation, and is also required for Sertoli cells to mediate the development of spermatids into mature sperm cells. Inhibin (choice E) is a polypeptide secreted by the testes and ovaries that inhibits FSH secretion.

240. **(E)** The brain depends on continuous blood flow and consciousness is lost after as little as 8 to 10 seconds of flow interruption. Dilation of cerebral blood vessels occurs during hypoxia, acidosis, and hypercapnia. Of these, hypercapnia (increased CO_2) is the main effector. Regional blood flow can increase by as much as 50% in response to metabolic demands of cortical neurons and may be visualized by PET scan. However, these local increases of flow have little effect on overall cerebral blood flow (choice A). Barbiturates reduce neuronal oxygen demand (choice B). Blood flow through the brain is largely autoregulated, and increased systemic blood pressure has little effect on cerebral blood flow (choice C). Decreased arterial oxygen content will also dilate cerebral vessels and increase cerebral flow, however a decrease of arterial O_2 to 75 mm Hg (choice D) is less effective than an increase of arterial CO_2 to 45 mm Hg.

241. (B) During strenuous physical exercise lactate is produced from anaerobic metabolism of skeletal muscle cells. This results in acidification of the blood (lactate acidosis). A right shift in oxygen binding occurs during acidosis, increased PCO_2, increased 2,3-DPG concentration inside erythrocytes, and increased temperature. A right shift in oxygen binding also enhances release of oxygen from hemoglobin in peripheral tissues. A left shift in oxygen binding (choice A) occurs during alkalosis, decreased PCO_2, decreased 2,3-DPG concentration inside erythrocytes, and decreased temperature. The oxygen carrying capacity of the blood depends on hematocrit and erythrocyte hemoglobin concentration; however, oxygen saturation (choices C and D) expressed in percent is not affected by changes in oxygen-carrying capacity.

242. (B) A normal, healthy individual in acid–base balance is represented by point C (pH 7.4, bicarbonate 24 mEq/L, and $Paco_2$ 40 mm Hg). Changes in $Paco_2$ cause changes in pH along the line A-C-D, which is a CO_2 titration curve. Moving either upward or downward along this titration curve represents these changes in pH with changes in $Paco_2$ (to higher or lower CO_2 isobars). There are small secondary changes in bicarbonate due to buffer reactions with nonbicarbonate buffers. These are not compensatory changes in bicarbonate concentration. At point A no compensation in the form of increased renal production of bicarbonate has yet occurred. A patient with end-stage lung disease most likely is in a state of respiratory acidosis with some renal compensation in the form of increased production of bicarbonate. This partially returns the pH toward normal. (Point A): uncompensated respiratory acidosis. (Point B): partially compensated respiratory acidosis. (Point C): normal state. (Point D): uncompensated respiratory alkalosis. (Point E): partially compensated respiratory alkalosis. (Point F) represents a simple uncompensated metabolic acidosis (a rare circumstance). But as the pH falls, alveolar ventilation is stimulated (e.g., Kussmaul breathing in ketoacidosis of diabetes), producing a lower $Paco_2$. Lowering the $Paco_2$ (point G) moves the pH back toward normal along a lower CO_2 isobar. (Point H): uncompensated metabolic alkalosis. (Point I): partially compensated metabolic alkalosis.

243. (B) Gastric chief cells secrete pepsinogen, the precursor of the pepsin in gastric juice. Mucus (choice A) is secreted by the neck and surface mucous cells in the body and fundus. Gastrin (choice C) is produced by G cells in the antral portion of the gastric mucosa in response to stomach dilation and peptides or amino acids in the gastric lumen. Hydrogen ions (choice D) and intrinsic factor (choice E) are secretory products of parietal (oxyntic) cells.

244. (B) Acute dehydration results in decreased plasma volume and increased plasma osmolarity (choice A), since more water than salt is lost in sweat. The decrease in plasma volume leads to an inhibition of the baroreceptors and a lower firing rate. The increase in plasma osmolarity leads to increased ADH secretion (choice C) and high plasma ADH levels, which increases water permeability of collecting duct cells (choice D). Therefore more water is reabsorbed by the kidneys and renal water excretion is low (choice E).

245. (D) The aortic blood pressure oscillates between a peak (called the systolic blood pressure) and a nadir (called the diastolic blood pressure). This nadir is reached just after the beginning of systole, when the rising left ventricular pressure equals, or just exceeds, the aortic blood pressure and forces the left ventricular blood to be ejected through the aortic valve. At this time (the end of the isovolumetric contraction and the beginning of ejection), the left ventricular pressure essentially equals aortic diastolic blood pressure at point D. (Points A and B): filling phase of the ventricle. (Point C): closure of mitral valve, beginning of isometric contraction. (Points D, E, F, G, and H): ejection phase. Note decreasing LV volume. (Point F): The T wave of the electrocardiogram represents ventricular repolarization (which leads to relaxation). By the peak of the T wave, enough ventricular muscle has begun to relax that the ventricular pressure starts to fall. Thus, the peak of the T wave and the peak of the ventricular pressure (point F in the illustration) are simultaneous. (Point H): opening of mitral valve. During ventricular systole, the blood returning to the heart from the pulmonary circulation causes a gradual rise in left atrial volume and pressure. When ventricular isovolumetric relaxation ends, blood suddenly exits from the left atrium into the left ventricle (beginning of ventricular rapid filling). It is the opening of the mitral valve that brings an end to the decreasing LV volume. (Point I): end of rapid filling phase.

246. (D) Respiratory alkalosis is due to hyperventilation, which lowers CO_2. Decreasing tidal volume will reduce alveolar ventilation and correct the respiratory alkalosis. Assuming a dead space of 150 mL, alveolar ventilation in this patient is 450 mL · 12/min = 5400 mL/min. If the tidal volume were decreased from 600 to 300 mL and the frequency increased from 12 to 24 per minute, then the alveolar ventilation would decrease to 150 · 12/min = 1800 mL/min even though the minute ventilation (12 · 600 mL/min = 24 · 300 mL/min) remained unchanged. The fraction of O_2 (choice A) in the respiratory air does not affect respiratory volumes or frequencies in a mechanically ventilated patient. Increasing minute ventilation (choice B) or decreasing dead space (choice C) would increase alveolar ventilation and worsen respiratory alkalosis. PEEP (choice E) is positive pressure applied during the expiratory phase to prevent the collapse of alveoli and to increase functional residual capacity of the lungs. It is used primarily to improve arterial oxygenation in severely hypoxic patients.

247. (C) This patient has increased extra- and intracellular volumes and a decreased osmolarity. SIADH (syndrome of inappropriate ADH secretion) results in inappropriately low water permeability of the renal collecting duct tubular cells and inappropriate water retention. As a result, patients with SIADH often present with hypotonic overhydration. Chronic vomiting (choice A) and adrenal insufficiency, i.e., lack of aldosterone (choice B), lead to dehydration. Fluid overload with isotonic NaCl (choice D) results in volume expansion without change in osmolarity. Fluid overload with hypertonic solution (choice E) results in volume expansion with increased osmolarity.

248. (A) Myoglobins and hemoglobins are oxygen-carrying proteins that differ in their O_2 affinity. These differences reflect their functional adaptation. HbA, which accounts for 95% of normal adult hemoglobin, consists of 2 alpha chains and 2 beta chains, each carrying one molecule of heme. Initial binding of oxygen to hemoglobin facilitates further binding of additional oxygen, resulting in a characteristic sigmoidal binding curve (curve C). Fetal hemoglobin HbF consists of 2 alpha chains and 2 gamma chains and differs from HbA in two important respects: (1) it doesn't bind organic phosphates including 2,3-DPG as effectively as HbA, and (2) its oxygen-binding curve is shifted to the left (curve B). Therefore, the oxygen content of umbilical vein blood is higher than that of placental vein blood, even though the PO_2 of umbilical blood is slightly lower than that of the placental veins. Myoglobin resembles hemoglobins but binds only 1 molecule O_2 rather than 4 molecules. Its oxygen-binding curve therefore is not sigmoidal but has a higher affinity compared to hemoglobins, resulting in a transfer of oxygen from arterial blood to skeletal muscle fibers. Percent saturation should always top at 100% since it is a normalized measure and not at 50% (curve D).

Physically dissolved O_2 in plasma shows a linear relationship (curve E).

249. (B) The photoreceptor cell membrane is relatively depolarized in darkness due to Na^+ entry through nonselective cation channels. Openings of these channels are maintained by the high intracellular cGMP levels in photoreceptors during darkness, and the Na^+ inward current through these channels is usually called "dark current." Illumination by light causes a conformational change in the photosensitive pigment rhodopsin, which is linked via a G protein to a cGMP specific phosphodiesterase. Activation of phosphodiesterase lowers cGMP levels and, since cGMP is required to maintain openings of the nonselective cation channels, results in membrane hyperpolarization with light exposure. Cl^- channels (choice A) or nonselective anion channels (choice C) do not contribute to the dark current of photoreceptors. Ryanodine receptors (choice D) are located on the sarcoplasmic reticulum (SR) and when opened release stored Ca^{2+} from the SR. These channels are locked into the open state by the plant alkaloid ryanodine (hence the name). Like in most other cells, the Na^+/K^+ pump (choice E) is responsible for the high intracellular K^+ concentration in photoreceptor cells.

250. (C) Creatinine clearance is independent of plasma creatinine concentration, otherwise creatinine would not be a useful measure of glomerular filtration rate. Clearance is defined as the amount of plasma that delivered the excreted substance, and for a substance that is neither actively secreted nor reabsorbed by the kidneys, its clearance equals the amount of plasma filtered through the glomerular membrane. All creatinine contained in that amount of plasma is excreted by the kidney, no matter what the concentration of creatinine in that plasma volume was. Since in the normal person a small amount of creatinine is secreted by the tubuli, clearance at low plasma concentrations is slightly higher than at elevated plasma concentration (slight initial upward bend of curve). Curve A describes the relationship between creatinine plasma concentration and renal excretion of creatinine. Note that excretion and clearance are not synonymous (also compare with question 273). Curves B and D describe the clearance of a substance that is secreted and filtered, or secreted and reabsorbed, respectively. At large plasma concentration the active transporters become saturated and the clearance of these substances approaches the creatinine clearance. Curve E depicts an improbable event with relatively increased clearance at both low and high concentrations of a substance, while there is an independent linear clearance at intermediate substance concentrations.

251. (C) Despite tremendous progress in understanding the role of cytokines in normal and pathological processes, the therapeutic and research potential of these substances has just begun to be explored. Interferons, by definition, elicit a nonspecific antiviral activity by inducing specific RNA synthesis and protein expression in neighboring cells. Common interferon inducers are viruses, double-stranded RNA, and microorganisms. INF-γ is produced mainly by CD4- and CD8-positive T cells, and to a lesser extent by B cells and natural killer cells. INF-γ has antiviral and antiparasitic activity and is synergistic with INF-α and INF-β, but its main biological activity appears to be immunomodulatory. Among its many functions are activation of macrophages and enhanced expression of MHC-II proteins (DP, DQ, and DR) on macrophages. The other two common human interferons are INF-α (choice A) and INF-β (choice B), derived from leukocytes and fibroblasts, respectively. INF-α is currently in clinical use against hairy cell leukemia, Kaposi's sarcoma, and venereal warts (condyloma acuminata). In addition to the common inducers, INF-β production by fibroblasts is also elicited by TNF and IL-1. In contrast to INF-α, INF-β is strictly species specific. INF-β appears to be useful for treatment of squamous sarcomas, viral encephalitis, and possibly multiple sclerosis. Macrophages produce IL-1 (choice D) and TNF (choice E). The effects of IL-1 and TNF are widespread and include activation of T cells, B cells, fever induction, and many others.

252. (B) Trained athletes have a larger heart volume (muscular hypertrophy) compared to untrained persons. This results in a significantly higher stroke volume at rest and an increased cardiac reserve (maximal cardiac output during exercise). Under resting conditions however, the cardiac output of trained and untrained persons is nearly the same (choice A), and this is due to a correspondingly lower resting heart frequency (choice C). It is not uncommon to find resting heart frequencies of 40 to 50 beats/min in trained athletes. Oxygen consumption (choice D) and respiratory frequency (choice E) at rest are little affected by athletic training.

253. (C) This patient suffers from an acute glaucoma attack. The aqueous humor leaves the eye in the anterior chamber, passes through a meshwork of trabeculae, and enters the canal of Schlemm which empties into extraocular veins. Pupil dilation tends to open the canal of Schlemm and enhance outflow because of the proximity of the pupillary dilator muscle insertion at the sclera to the canal and trabeculae. Normal ocular pressure is around 15 mm Hg, and remains constant in a normal eye throughout the day, usually within about ± 2 mm Hg (choice A). The production rate of aqueous humor is approximately 2 to 3 μL/min, and intraocular pressure is mainly determined by the balance of rate of production and outflow (choice B). Closure of the ocular angle (canal of Schlemm) leads to an acute glaucoma attack. Because of the high risk of permanent damage to the retina and optic nerve, this medical emergency should be treated with drugs that dilate the pupils. Drugs of choice are antimuscarinics (pilocarpine) or β-blockers (timolol). In addition, carbonic anhydrase inhibitors reduce the rate of production of aqueous humor during acute attacks, but are not useful for long-term treatment. Corticosteroids (choice D) play no role in the emergency management of acute glaucoma. Glaucoma is not a rare cause of blindness in the United States (choice E), but rather one of the most common causes of acquired blindness.

254. (C) Cholecystokinin is produced by the duodenum and reaches the pancreas via the bloodstream. It causes secretion of large quantities of digestive enzymes by the pancreatic acinar cells. Secretin (choice A) is produced by duodenal mucosa glands when highly acidic food enters the small intestine. This hormone stimulates secretion of a bicarbonate-rich solution from pancreatic ductal epithelium, but does not stimulate pancreatic enzyme secretion. Gastrin (choice B) is produced by G cells in the stomach antrum following vasovagal reflexes, stomach distention, or chemical stimuli, in particular amino acid and protein-rich food. Together with histamine and acetylcholine, gastrin stimulates acid secretion from parietal cells. GIP (choice D) is produced in the duodenum in response to sugars and fat. This peptide inhibits gastric secretion and motility, but its main effect appears to be stimulation of insulin production in pancreatic beta cells. VIP (choice E) stimulates water and electrolyte secretion by intestinal mucosa.

255. (A) Parietal cells secrete an essentially isotonic solution of pure HCl containing 150 mM Cl^- and 150 mM H^+ (pH < 1). Intracellular [H^+] of parietal cells is 10^{-4} mM/L (pH ≈ 7.0) and active transport is necessary to transport H^+ against this gradient. This is achieved by an H^+/K^+-ATPase in the apical membrane that exchanges H^+ for K^+. Cl^- (choice B) is extruded passively down its electrical gradient through Cl^- selective ion channels rather than transported actively. Na^+/K^+-ATPase (choice C) constitutes the major active transport process at the basolateral, but not the apical, membrane of parietal cells. The Cl^-/HCO_3^- exchange (choice D) also takes place at the basolateral membrane of the parietal cell. HCO_3^- comes from H_2CO_3 (the product of carbonic anhydrase enzyme), and is extruded from the cell in exchange for Cl^- to maintain electroneutrality. Passive diffusion (choice E) occurs always down an electrochemical gradient, never against a gradient.

256. (A) Most patients with primary aldosteronism (Conn's syndrome) have an adrenal adenoma. The increased plasma aldosterone concentration leads to increased renal Na^+ reabsorption, which results in plasma volume expansion. The increase in plasma volume suppresses renin release from the juxtaglomerular apparatus and these patients usually have low plasma renin levels. Salt restriction (choice B) and upright posture (choice C) decrease renal perfusion pressure and therefore increase renin release from the juxtaglomerular apparatus. Secondary aldosteronism is due to elevated renin levels and may be caused by heart failure (choice D) or renal artery stenosis (choice E).

257. **(C)** What is recorded in all of the examples is the forced expiratory volume in one second (FEV_1). The patient is connected to a spirometer, and after taking in as much air as possible (maximal inhalation), is asked to expire as forcefully as he or she can to exhale as much air as possible as rapidly as possible. The volume exhaled in the first second (shaded area of examples) is the FEV_1. The difference between the beginning total lung capacity (TLC) and the residual volume (RV) is the vital capacity. The forced vital capacity (FVC), shown in all but example C, is not always the same as in a less forced measurement. Curve C represents a patient with an obstructive disease that makes it difficult to force large volumes of air out at a high rate of flow. Thus, the slope is less steep than normal, and it takes a long time to reach the residual volume (it may take 20 or 30 seconds; this is why example C doesn't include FVC). Asthma, emphysema, and chronic bronchitis are common obstructive diseases. Both the TLC and the RV are higher than normal in such patients. At the bedside the same kind of information can be obtained by asking the patient to blow out a lighted match. Patients with obstructive disease have difficulty doing so. Curve A represents a normal, healthy adult. The flow rate is high at first (steep downward slope) near the beginning of TLC, but then becomes less and less steep as the lung volume decreases, until it plateaus (becomes flat) at residual volume and zero flow. Curve B represents the FEV_1 of a patient with restrictive lung disease (lungs are restricted in volume). Pulmonary fibrosis is a chronic condition that can follow pulmonary inflammation (pneumonitis) brought about by a number of conditions. Other examples of restrictive disease include problems with chest wall movement (Pickwickian syndrome, scoliosis, myasthenia gravis, etc.) and loss of lung compliance (e.g., lack of surfactant, pulmonary edema, fibrosis, etc.). Although flow rates are quite good at any given volume (comparable to that of a normal subject at that same lung volume), the TLC, VC, and RV are all below normal. Curve D (increased flow rates with normal or larger than normal lung volumes) is not realistic.

258. **(D)** Acetazolamide is an inhibitor of carbonic anhydrase, an enzyme found in large quantities in the brush border of the proximal tubule. This enzyme has two important functions: In the tubular lumen it promotes the dissociation of H_2CO_3 into H_2O and CO_2 and thereby helps to recover filtered bicarbonate. Inside the epithelial cells it promotes the formation of H_2CO_3. Inhibition of this enzyme therefore increases bicarbonate concentration in the urine, and results in a mild metabolic acidosis that counteracts the effect of respiratory alkalosis caused by hyperventilation in an oxygen-poor environment. Metabolic alkalosis (choice A) would worsen the symptoms of mountain sickness. Acetazolamide has no direct effect on respiratory drive (choices B and C). Hydrogen concentration in the urine (choice E) plays only a minor role in acid–base regulation by the kidneys. Most of the excess hydrogen is excreted in the form of non-titratable acid (NH_4^+).

259. **(E)** Plasma proteins consist of albumin, globulins, and fibrinogen. These can be separated by their rate of migration in an electrical field (electrophoresis). The fractions shown in the figure are (fraction A) albumin, (fraction B) α_1-globulins, (fraction C) α_2-globulins, (fraction D) β-globulins, and (fraction E) γ-globulins. The smallest of these proteins (albumins) are also the most numerous and are responsible for much of the oncotic pressure of plasma (about 25 mm Hg). Iron bound to transferrin and β-lipoproteins are transported in the β-globulin fraction, while bilirubin, fatty acids, and many drugs are transported adsorbed to albumin. Antibodies (immunoglobulins) constitute the bulk of γ-globulins.

260. **(E)** Only a small amount (5 to 15%) of dietary iron is absorbed by the body. Much of the iron entering the intestinal mucosa is not transferred to the plasma, but remains trapped as ferritin inside the epithelial cells and is lost when the cells are shed. Patients with chronic iron deficiency anemia have low ferritin stores and therefore a larger rate of intestinal iron absorption because of this mucosal regulatory mechanism. Intrinsic factor (choice A) is produced by parietal cells of the stomach. Its presence is crucial for intestinal absorption of vitamin B_{12}, but not iron. Its absence causes a macrocytic megaloblastic anemia. Iron is virtually exclusively absorbed in the duodenum and proximal jejunum and not the terminal ileum (choice B). Only iron kept soluble, either as hemoglobin or myoglobin, or bound to low weight organic molecules is absorbed by intestinal epithelial cells (choice C). Ferrous iron (Fe^{2+}) is better absorbed than ferric iron (Fe^{3+}) (choice D), and commercial iron preparations often contain an antioxidant like vitamin C to keep iron in the ferrous state.

261. **(A)** Increased plasma osmolarity is the most potent stimulus for ADH release. An increase in plasma osmolarity of only 1% is sufficient to increase ADH levels. Decreased plasma volume (choice D) also stimulates ADH release but is a less potent stimulus. Plasma ADH levels are not affected until blood volume is reduced by about 10%. Nevertheless the decreased blood volume and arterial pressure in patients with severe hemorrhage results in ADH secretion, causing increased water reabsorption by the kidneys that helps to restore blood pressure and volume. Hypothalamic releasing factors (choice E) control release of anterior pituitary hormones TSH, ACTH, FSH, LH, GH, and prolactin, but not the release of posterior pituitary hormones ADH and oxytocin.

262. **(A)** Glucose excretion by the kidneys depends on the glomerular filtration and tubular reabsorption rates. Glucose first appears in the urine when the capacity of the glucose transporters in the proximal tubuli cells is exceeded. This usually occurs at plasma glucose levels higher than 180 mg/dL. Patients with long-standing diabetes mellitus often have decreased renal function and reduced glomerular filtration rate. Under these circumstances the threshold (i.e., plasma level) for excretion of glucose will be higher than in a healthy person. Patients with diabetes insipidus (choice B) have a large urine output due to absence of ADH or defective renal ADH receptors, but should not have a plasma glucose level of 200 mg/dL. Antidiuresis (choice C) increases the concentration of solutes in the urine and increases the sensitivity to detect urine glucose. Reabsorption of filtered glucose occurs in the proximal tubule by active transport. A defect in glucose transporters (choice D) would result in glucosuria even at normal plasma glucose concentration. Urine dipsticks nowadays are both sensitive and specific for glucose, detecting as little as 100 mg/dL (choice E). Earlier dipstick tests were sensitive but not specific, i.e., they detected other reducing sugars in addition to glucose.

263. **(E)** Potassium-sparing diuretics act by either antagonizing the action of aldosterone (spironolactone) or by inhibiting Na^+ reabsorption in the distal tubules (amiloride). Mannitol (choice A) is freely filtered at the glomerulus, but in contrast to glucose is not reabsorbed and produces an osmotic diuresis. Clinically it is used to treat cerebral edema, and in prerenal azotemia to convert oliguric acute renal failure. Thiazides (choice B) inhibit Na^+ and K^+ reabsorption in the distal tubule, and loop diuretics (choice C) (e.g., furosemide, ethacrynic acid) inhibit the Na^+-K^+-2 Cl^- cotransporter in the thick ascending loop of Henle. Carbonic anhydrase inhibitors (choice D) reduce H^+ secretion and HCO_3^- reabsorption in the proximal tubules. Since these are coupled to Na^+ reabsorption through the Na^+/H^+ countertransport in the luminal membrane, a decrease in HCO_3^- reabsorption also reduces Na^+ reabsorption, causing these ions to remain in the tubular fluid and act as an osmotic diuretic.

264. (C) Glycogen synthesis and breakdown depend on the balance of glycogen synthase activity (glycogen synthesis) and glycogen phosphorylase activity (glycogen breakdown). These enzymes are under the control of cAMP-dependent protein kinases. Phosphorylation of glycogen phosphorylase activates this enzyme and promotes glycogen degradation. This phosphorylation is carried out by an enzyme called glycogen phosphorylase kinase, which itself is activated by a cAMP-dependent protein kinase. Therefore, hormones that increase liver cell cAMP promote glycogen breakdown, while hormones that decrease liver cell cAMP promote glycogen synthesis. Epinephrine and glucagon stimulate the mobilization of glycogen by triggering the cAMP cascade. Cortisol, the main glucocorticoid, regulates the metabolism of proteins, fats, and carbohydrates. On most organs cortisol acts catabolic, however on the liver it has anabolic effects, increasing glycogen synthesis and accumulation in the liver.

265. (B) An increased TSH combined with a low T3 resin uptake (and low free T4) are characteristic of hypothyroidism. Clinical signs and symptoms of hypothyroidism include dull facial expression, puffiness and periorbital swelling caused by infiltration with mucopolysaccharides, decreased adrenergic drive, lethargy, bradycardia, and cold intolerance. The periorbital swelling must be distinguished from exophthalmus due to increased retro-orbital tissue, which is a specific sign for hyperthyroidism caused by Graves' disease. Tachycardia (choice A), fever (choice C), palpitations (choice D), and anxiety (choice E) are all seen in hyperthyroidism. Additional clinical signs seen with hyperthyroidism may include heat intolerance, tremor, sweating, and sleeplessness.

266. (C) During resting conditions, approximately 15% of the cardiac output goes to the brain, 15% to the muscles, 30% to the GI tract, and 20% to the kidneys. However, when normalized by organ weight, the kidneys receive the largest specific blood flow (400 mL/min · 100 g) at rest and are particularly vulnerable during hemorrhagic shock. The brain (choice A) also receives relatively high specific blood flow (50 mL/min · 100 g). Blood flow through the skin (choice B) varies between 1 and 100 ml/min · 100 g and serves temperature regulation. Heart muscle (choice D) not surprisingly also has a relatively high resting specific blood flow (60 mL/min · 100 g), which may increase fivefold during exercise. Skeletal muscles (choice E) have low specific blood flow (2 to 3 mL/min · 100 g) at rest, which may increase up to 20-fold during strenuous exercise.

267. (B) This is the period of oxygen deficit during which part of the energy requirements are being met anaerobically by depletion of high energy phosphates (period B of illustration). The direct source of energy for muscle contraction comes from ATP hydrolysis. The most efficient means of generating new ATP to replace that used is through aerobic metabolism (mainly by the Krebs cycle). Aerobic metabolism depends on the supply of oxygen to muscle and cannot immediately rise to supply ATP as fast as it is used (period B illustration). This period is one of an "oxygen deficit." Time is required for sufficient increase in cardiac output and pulmonary ventilation to supply oxygen at the rate needed. During period A (before exercise) and period C (steady state exercise), $\dot{V}O_2$ matches the metabolic needs. Between the onset of exercise (at "Begin work" in illustration) and the highest level of oxygen supply and consumption (plateau in illustration), energy is mainly supplied by anaerobic depletion of high energy phosphate stores (ATP and CP) and anaerobic glycolysis. Resynthesis of these stores requires that $\dot{V}O_2$ remain above normal for a while after cessation of exercise (after "End work" in illustration) (period D). This period of time is described as repayment of an "oxygen debt." Period E (after exercise and repayment of debt): $\dot{V}O_2$ again matches the metabolic needs.

268. (A) Large injury to the nondominant parietal cortex may cause the patient to ignore the serious nature of his illness, and to neglect or even deny the presence of the paralysis affecting the side of the body opposite to the lesion. Occasionally this neglect may involve not only the patient's body but also the perception of the external world. Smaller injuries to the nondominant parietal cortex involving the precentral gyrus (primary motor cortex) (choice B), or postcentral gyrus (primary sensory cortex) (choice C), result in contralateral spastic paralysis or contralateral loss of tactile sensation, respectively. Injury to the dominant hemisphere involving the posterior inferior gyrus of the frontal lobe (choice D) (Broca's area) produces an expressive or motor aphasia in which the patient's comprehension of language is preserved, but his ability to form words is impaired. Injury to the dominant hemisphere involving the posterior superior gyrus of the temporal lobe (choice E) (Wernicke's area) produces a sensory aphasia in which words are spoken fluently but without meaning. The patient does not understand his own word salad, either.

269. (B) The proximal tubule reabsorbs the majority (about two-thirds) of filtered salt and water. This is done in an essentially iso-osmotic manner. Both the luminal salt concentration and the luminal osmolality remain constant (and equal to plasma values) along the entire length of the proximal tubule. Water and salt are reabsorbed proportionally because the water is dependent on and coupled with the active reabsorption of Na^+. The water permeability of the proximal tubule is high, and therefore a significant transepithelial osmotic gradient is not possible (a minute gradient of as little as 1 mosm/L may exist). Sodium is actively transported, mainly by basolateral sodium pumps, into the lateral intercellular spaces; water follows. The glomerulus (choice A) is where solutes are filtered from the plasma. The juxtaglomerular apparatus (choice C) produces renin. The thick ascending limb of Henle's loop (choice D) actively transports Na^+ and Cl^- from lumen to the peritubular space using a $Na^+/K^+/Cl^-$ cotransporter. About 30 to 35% of filtered salt is reabsorbed here. The collecting duct (choice E) reabsorbs only a small fraction of filtered Na^+.

270. (D) Both the thin and the thick ascending limbs of Henle's loop have very low permeability to water. Since there are no regulatory mechanisms to alter its permeability, it remains poorly permeable to water under all circumstances. Sodium and chloride are transported out of the luminal fluid into the surrounding interstitial spaces where they are reabsorbed. Since water must remain behind since it is not reabsorbed, the solute concentration becomes less and less (the luminal fluid becomes more dilute). This is one of the principal mechanisms (along with diminution of ADH secretion) for the production of a dilute, hypo-osmotic urine (water diuresis). The glomerulus (choice A) is completely permeable to water, acting as a filter. The proximal tubule (choice B) is characterized by high water permeability, preventing the establishment of an osmotic gradient across the proximal tubular epithelium, and reabsorption of any solute here is accompanied by reabsorption of water. The juxtaglomerular apparatus (choice C) produces renin. Water permeability of the collecting duct (choice E) is under control of ADH, allowing adjustment of the renal function according to the body's state of hydration.

271. (D) Nitric oxide has recently been discovered to have important neurotransmitter-like functions. Its short half-life due to spontaneous decay limits its range and action. Nitric oxide acts on smooth muscle cells in a generally inhibitory manner; it relaxes the gastrointestinal muscles and sphincters and dilates blood vessels. In blood vessels, nitric oxide is derived from endothelial cells and has been identified as the long-hypothesized EDRF (endothelium derived relaxing factor). Epinephrine (choice A) and norepinephrine (choice B) play a role during the ejaculation phase of the male sexual act, but do not contribute to penile artery dilation during the erectile phase. Acetylcholine (choice C) is the classic neurotransmitter of the parasympathetic nervous system. While activation of the pelvic parasympathetic nerves leads to erection, it is nitric oxide and not acetylcholine that relaxes penile artery smooth muscle cells. GABA (choice E) is an inhibitory neurotransmitter found in the central nervous system.

272. **(C)** Nitric oxide relaxes vascular smooth muscle by activating guanylate cyclase and increasing production of cGMP, which activates protein kinase G and possibly also protein kinase A. Viagra (sildenafil) inhibits type V guanylate phosphodiesterase, increases cGMP levels and thereby supports the vasodilatory effect of nitric oxide. Increased cAMP levels (choice A) also relax vascular smooth muscle. Epinephrine binds to vascular β-receptors, which stimulate adenylate cyclase via a G protein, increasing cellular cAMP. A decrease in cAMP (choice B) or cGMP (choice D) promotes contraction of vascular smooth muscle, rather than dilation. Inositol-tris-phosphate (IP_3) (choice E) is another important second messenger contributing to vascular smooth muscle contraction. For example, angiotensin II is a potent vasoconstrictor, whose action is mediated by AT_{1A} receptors coupled to phospholipase, leading to hydrolysis of PIP_2 to IP_3 and diacylglycerol (DAG).

273. **(B)** Measurement of glomerular filtration rate is a sensitive index of renal function. Clearance is defined as the amount of plasma that delivered the substance excreted. In the case of a substance like inulin or creatinine, which is filtered through the glomerular basement membrane, but neither reabsorbed nor secreted by renal tubular epithelial cells, this equals the amount of plasma filtered. Therefore the rate of excretion is a linear function of the substance's plasma concentration. Any deviation from linearity in the excretion versus plasma concentration relation indicates active transport processes. Since creatinine is also slightly secreted by the tubular cells, the actual line should be slightly above line B. Substances like PAH and penicillins that are both filtered and actively secreted show a steep excretion rate at low plasma concentrations (choice A). When the active transporters are saturated, this relationship becomes parallel to the curve for inulin. Line C is impossible, simply because renal excretion has to be 0 at a plasma concentration of 0. Substances which are actively secreted by tubular cells, but are too big to be filtered through the glomerular basement membrane, show initially steep excretion rates (choice D). When the transporters become saturated no further increase in excretion rate is possible. Glucose is readily filtered through the glomerular basement membrane, but almost completely reabsorbed by tubular cells (choice E). Renal excretion of glucose typically occurs at venous plasma concentrations above 180 mg/dL.

274. **(B)** The main difference between the ABO system of blood groups and the Rh system is the following: ABO antibodies are naturally occurring while a person missing an Rh antigen will not have antibodies against Rh in his serum unless sensitized. Sensitization of Rh-negative persons can occur through massive blood transfusions or through a prior pregnancy with an Rh-positive child. Having a first Rh-negative child does not pose a risk of sensitization for the mother (choice A). However the second Rh-positive child may still be at risk if the mother was sensitized by other means, for example previous transfusion with Rh-positive blood. Rh-positive mothers (choices C, D, and E) do not develop Rh antibodies and there is no risk of hemolytic transfusion reactions due to Rh incompatibility.

275. **(C)** New generation pregnancy tests using an immunoconcentration method (ICON) can detect urine hCG as early as 4 to 5 days before the first missed period. hCG is a glycoprotein produced by the syncytiotrophoblast. It is composed of an α and a β subunit, and the α subunit is identical to the α subunits of LH, FSH, and TSH. hCG is usually positive in patients with ectopic pregnancy (choice A) or a choriocarcinoma (choice B). hCG has its highest levels at the end of the first trimester, not the end of pregnancy (choice D). Levels of estradiol, estriol, and progesterone, however, continue to rise until term. The role of hCG is to maintain the corpus luteum in the ovary and it has no direct effect on fetal production of steroids (choice E).

276. (J) The relaxation pressure–volume diagram shows the interaction between lung elasticity and chest wall elasticity. Note that the combined pressure–volume curve (solid line) is simply the sum of lung and chest wall pressure curves. Point A: maximal passive chest wall expansion. Point B: lung expanded to point of maximal passive chest wall expansion. Point C: chest wall at resting level. Point D: resting level of lungs and chest wall combined. Point E: lungs at resting level. Point F: lungs and chest wall compressed to point of maximal expiration. Point G: lungs at point of maximal expiration (note that airway pressure is still positive: lungs will collapse further if allowed). At rest, when all respiratory muscles are relaxed, the corresponding lung volume (level H) is the functional reserve capacity (FRC). Below FRC, the combined lung and chest wall will spring outwards when the respiratory muscles are relaxed, thus generating a negative relaxation pressure. Residual volume (level I) is achieved after maximal expiration. The isolated lung would further collapse to its minimal volume (level K).

277. (A) The resting membrane potential of excitable cells is largely due to the selective permeability of the cell membrane to potassium ions. The Na^+/K^+ pump (choice B) generates the ion gradient across the cell membrane (i.e., high intracellular K^+, high extracellular Na^+), but it is the back diffusion of K^+ ions through K^+ channels that are open at rest which charges the cell membrane. If the cell membrane were a perfect K^+ electrode, the membrane potential would equal the equilibrium potential for K^+ as predicted by the Nernst equation. In reality, the resting membrane potential is more positive because of small contributions by Na^+ channels (choice C), Cl^- channels (choice D), and nonselective cation channels (choice E).

278. (A) Mean corpuscular volume is calculated from hematocrit and RBC count: MCV [fL] = hematocrit $\cdot$ 1000/RBC [$10^6/\mu L$] = 0.27 $\cdot$ 1000/3 = 90 fL, which is within the normal range. Mean corpuscular hemoglobin concentration (choices C and D) is calculated from blood hemoglobin and RBC count: MCHC [g/dL] = hemoglobin [g/dL]/hematocrit = 11/0.27 = 41 g/dL, and is higher than normal. Red blood cell diameter (choice E) cannot be calculated from the data given, but is likely less than normal in this patient.

279. (D) Spherocytes are small, round red blood cells with a decreased cell membrane surface area. They usually have a normal mean corpuscular volume but a smaller than normal diameter since they are rounded. This makes them more vulnerable to plasma or salt solutions with decreased osmotic pressure. Spherocytes are seen in hemolytic anemias and hereditary spherocytosis, an autosomal dominant disorder involving a molecular abnormality of the cytoskeleton (spectrin deficiency). The decreased cell surface area makes the red blood cells less flexible when traversing the spleen's microcirculation, resulting in anemia and sometimes jaundice. Iron deficiency anemia (choice A) is characterized by smaller-than-normal cells with a decreased mean corpuscular volume, and since membrane flexibility is not affected, these cells have normal or near normal osmotic fragility. Sickle cells (choice B) and target cells as seen in thalassemia (choice C) or chronic liver disease (choice E) have a decreased osmotic fragility (i.e., are less vulnerable to changes in osmolarity).

280. (D) Osteomalacia in chronic renal failure is caused by decreased production of vitamin D and phosphate retention by the kidneys. The rise in serum phosphate causes increased binding of calcium, resulting in a decrease in ionized calcium concentration, which stimulates PTH secretion by the parathyroid glands (secondary hyperparathyroidism). PTH stimulates release of calcium from the bones, leading to demineralization. Osteoporosis (choice A) is a reduction in bone mass, particularly a decrease in cortical thickness. In contrast to osteomalacia, the ratio of mineral to organic phase is normal in osteoporosis. Bone loss occurs with age in both males and females at a rate of about 0.5% per year. Osteoporosis predominantly involves the spine, hip, and distal radius. In postmenopausal women, an accelerated loss of bone mass is superimposed on the age-related loss due to declining estrogen levels. In men, bone modeling is less dependent on sex steroids (choice B). Osteomalacia occurs with both primary (choice C) and secondary hyperparathyroidism. In patients with chronic renal failure, hyperparathyroidism is secondary to reduced ionized calcium concentration in the serum. Lack of active vitamin D also contributes to osteomalacia in this patient. In chronic renal failure the conversion of 25-hydroxycholecalciferol to the active 1,25-dihydroxycholecalciferol by the kidneys is impaired. Lack of dietary vitamin D (choice E) is less likely in this patient.

281. **(A)** In the normal adult about 90% of the filtered phosphate is reabsorbed in the proximal tubule, and about 10% of filtered phosphate is excreted by the kidneys. Patients with chronic renal failure accumulate phosphate because of the low glomerular filtration rate. Phosphate is not secreted by renal tubular epithelium cells (choice B), but is actively reabsorbed. Since the phosphate load to the proximal tubule is low in patients with a reduced glomerular filtration rate, the rate of reabsorption (in percent of filtered phosphate) is indeed higher than normal (choice C), but this is not the cause for the phosphate accumulation. It is the decreased glomerular filtration, and not the increased reabsorption rate, that is primarily responsible for phosphate accumulation in patients with chronic renal disease. Increased serum phosphate binds ionized calcium in the serum, leading to low serum calcium levels. Binding of phosphate with calcium in the urine (choice D) does not result in increased serum phosphate. Depending on the activity of PTH, between 5 and 40% of filtered phosphate is excreted (choice E).

282. **(E)** Regulation of phosphate excretion is accomplished primarily by PTH, which inhibits phosphate reabsorption in the proximal tubule. At high PTH concentration, as much as 40% of filtered phosphate may be excreted. Reabsorption of phosphate by renal tubular cells occurs via a carrier cotransport of phosphate and sodium. This mechanism is similar to the reabsorption of glucose and amino acids and is driven by the Na^+ gradient built by the Na^+/K^+-ATPase at the basolateral membrane of the tubular epithelium. Cotransport with calcium (choice A) or chloride (choice B) does not occur. Reabsorption of phosphate occurs against its electrochemical gradient (choice C) and therefore cannot be passive. Calcitonin (choice D) has only minor effects on renal calcium and phosphate handling. It lowers serum calcium by suppressing bone osteoclasts, thus shifting the balance in favor of calcium deposition in the bone.

REFERENCES

Aidley DJ. *The Physiology of Excitable Cells,* 3rd edition. Cambridge University Press, 1991

Berne RM, Levy MN, eds. *Physiology,* 3rd edition. St. Louis: Mosby-Year Book, 1993

Davenport HW. *The ABC of Acid-Base Chemistry,* 7th edition. Chicago: University of Chicago Press, 1974

Ganong WF. *Review of Medical Physiology,* 17th edition. Los Altos, CA: Appleton & Lange, 1995

Guyton AC, Hall JE. *Textbook of Medical Physiology,* 9th edition. Philadelphia: WB Saunders, 1995

Isselbacher KJ, et al. *Harrison's Principles of Internal Medicine,* 13th edition. New York: McGraw-Hill, 1994

Kandel ER, Schwartz JH, Jessel TM. *Principles of Neural Science,* 3rd edition. New York: Elsevier, 1993

Ibelgaufts H. *Dictionary of Cytokines.* New York: VCH, 1994

McArdle WD, Katch FI, Katch VL. *Exercise Physiology,* 3rd edition. Philadelphia: Lea & Febiger, 1991

Mountcastle VB. *Medical Physiology,* 14th edition. St. Louis: CV Mosby Co, 1980

Rose DB. *Clinical Physiology of Acid-Base and Electrolyte Disorders,* 4th edition. New York: McGraw-Hill, 1994

Vander AJ. *Renal Physiology,* 5th edition. New York: McGraw-Hill, 1995

West JB, ed. *Best and Taylor's Physiological Basis of Medical Practice,* 12th edition. Baltimore: Williams & Wilkins, 1991

West JB. *Pulmonary Pathophysiology—The Essentials,* 4th edition. Baltimore: Williams & Wilkins, 1992

Subspecialty List: Physiology

Question Number and Subspecialty

156. Pregnancy
157. Nervous system
158. Circulation
159. Urogenital system
160. Endocrinology
161. Endocrinology
162. Nervous system
163. Sensory system
164. Gastrointestinal
165. Sensory system
166. Muscle
167. Blood
168. Muscle
169. Circulation
170. Gastrointestinal
171. Cardiac
172. Circulation
173. Circulation
174. Endocrinology
175. Cardiac
176. Cardiac
177. Cardiac
178. Cell physiology
179. Renal
180. Cell physiology
181. Endocrinology
182. Muscle
183. Circulation
184. Circulation
185. Renal
186. Respiratory
187. Respiratory
188. Respiratory
189. Cardiac
190. Cardiac
191. Muscle
192. Acid/Base
193. Acid/Base
194. Renal
195. Muscle
196. Sensory system
197. Cardiac
198. Thermoregulation
199. Blood
200. Respiratory
201. Renal
202. Sleep physiology
203. Respiratory
204. Nervous system
205. Circulation
206. Acid/Base
207. Respiratory
208. Cell physiology
209. Cardiac
210. Sensory system
211. Respiratory
212. Cell physiology
213. Cell physiology
214. Renal
215. Endocrinology
216. Respiratory
217. Circulation
218. Circulation
219. Circulation
220. Respiratory
221. Respiratory
222. Respiratory
223. Respiratory
224. Nervous system
225. Muscle
226. Respiratory
227. Respiratory
228. Cell physiology
229. Circulation

230. Nervous system
231. Inflammation
232. Cardiac
233. Respiratory
234. Sleep physiology
235. Blood
236. Respiratory
237. Respiratory
238. Circulation
239. Endocrinology
240. Circulation
241. Exercise physiology
242. Respiratory
243. Gastrointestinal
244. Circulation
245. Cardiac
246. Respiratory
247. Circulation
248. Cell physiology
249. Sensory system
250. Renal
251. Immunology
252. Exercise physiology
253. Sensory system
254. Gastrointestinal
255. Gastrointestinal
256. Renal
257. Respiratory
258. Acid/Base
259. Immunology
260. Blood
261. Endocrinology
262. Renal
263. Renal
264. Gastrointestinal
265. Endocrinology
266. Circulation
267. Exercise physiology
268. Nervous system
269. Renal
270. Renal
271. Cellular physiology
272. Cellular physiology
273. Renal
274. Blood
275. Endocrinology
276. Respiratory
277. Muscle
278. Blood
279. Blood
280. Bone
281. Renal
282. Renal

CHAPTER 3

Biochemistry

Questions

Michael W. King, PhD

DIRECTIONS: (Questions 283 through 409): Each of the numbered items or incomplete statements in this section is followed by answers or by completions of the statement. Select the ONE lettered answer or completion that is BEST in each case.

283. A 22-year-old black male was given the anti-malaria drug primaquine to take while on an expedition on the Amazon River. After taking the drug, he developed an acute anemia. The anemia was secondary to an intravascular hemolytic crisis. This crisis was reversed when he discontinued taking the primaquine. This drug-induced hemolytic anemia arises in persons who have a deficiency in which of the following enzymes?

(A) glyceraldehyde-3-phosphate dehydrogenase
(B) pyruvate dehydrogenase
(C) succinate dehydrogenase
(D) glucose-6-phosphate dehydrogenase
(E) glycerol-3-phosphate dehydrogenase

284. Competitive inhibitors

(A) increase the apparent K_m of the enzyme
(B) decrease the apparent K_m of the enzyme
(C) increase the apparent V_{max} of the reaction
(D) decrease the apparent V_{max} of the reaction
(E) do not affect the K_m or the V_{max}

285. Lactate that is released into the circulation from skeletal muscle is converted back to glucose primarily in

(A) liver
(B) heart muscle
(C) erythrocytes
(D) adipose tissue
(E) brain

286. A percentage of the population manifests the ABO blood group antigens in saliva and other mucous secretions and are thus referred to as "secretors," whereas those that do not are termed "nonsecretors." The difference between these two populations results from

(A) ABO antigens on circulating lipids
(B) mild hemolysis that releases cellular ABO antigens
(C) ABO antigens present on circulating proteins
(D) inappropriate activation of the ABO-specific glycosyltransferases in mucus-secreting tissues
(E) presence of a mutant glycosyl hydrolase which releases the ABO antigens from cell surfaces

287. A deficiency of vitamin D in adults can lead to

(A) osteomalacia
(B) xerophthalmia
(C) macrocytic anemia
(D) scurvy
(E) rickets

288. A deficiency in vitamin B_{12} can result from

(A) its being trapped in the form of N^5-methyltetrahydrofolate
(B) the lack of intrinsic factor
(C) lipid malabsorptive disorders
(D) the lack of transcobalamin II in the liver

289. The carbohydrate employed in the biosynthesis of nucleic acids is made in which of the following pathways?

(A) glycolysis
(B) gluconeogenesis
(C) urea cycle
(D) citric acid cycle
(E) pentose phosphate pathway

290. Decreased wound healing, osteoporosis, hemorrhaging, and muscle fatigue are all symptoms caused by the lack of vitamin

(A) E
(B) B_6
(C) K
(D) C
(E) D

291. The ATPase activity required for muscle contraction is associated with which protein?

(A) myosin
(B) troponin
(C) myosin light chain kinase
(D) tropomyosin
(E) actin

292. An adult male suffered from stable angina pectoris for 15 years, during which time there was progressive heart failure and repeated pulmonary thromboembolism. Upon his death at age 63, autopsy disclosed enormous cardiomyopathy (1100 g), cardiac storage of globotriaosylceramide (11 mg lipid/g wet weight) and restricted cardiocytes. The lipid storage disease indicated by these results would most likely be

(A) Gaucher's disease
(B) Niemann–Pick disease
(C) Tay–Sachs disease
(D) Fabry's disease
(E) Krabbe's disease

293. The rate-limiting step in glycolysis occurs at the step catalyzed by

(A) glyceraldehyde 3-phosphate dehydrogenase
(B) phosphofructokinase-1
(C) pyruvate kinase
(D) phosphoglycerate kinase
(E) phosphofructokinase-2

294. The primary positive control of gluconeogenesis is exerted by

(A) high acetyl-CoA levels
(B) high citrate levels
(C) low citrate levels
(D) low ATP levels
(E) high ATP levels

295. Regulation of gene expression in bacterial operons occurs exclusively at the level of transcriptional initiation. Certain proteins termed *repressors* inhibit transcriptional initiation by

(A) inducing methylation of DNA sequences, which prevents RNA polymerase binding
(B) binding to RNA polymerase, inhibiting its activity
(C) binding to sequences near the promoter, thereby interfering with RNA polymerase binding
(D) inducing inhibitory secondary structure in the DNA at the site of RNA polymerase binding
(E) inducing phosphorylation of RNA polymerase leading to its inactivation

296. Fluorouracil is a drug that is used in the chemotherapy of several solid tumors. The mechanism of action of fluorouracil is that it is an inhibitor of

(A) ribonucleotide reductase
(B) thymidylate synthase
(C) thymidine kinase

(D) de novo pyrimidine biosynthesis
(E) de novo purine biosynthesis

297. The activity of the malate–aspartate shuttle is reduced under conditions of high ATP concentrations primarily because

(A) the high ATP levels lead to high NADH levels in the mitochondria, which inhibits conversion of malate to oxaloacetate catalyzed by malate dehydrogenase
(B) the high ATP levels lead to high NADH levels in the cytoplasm, which inhibits conversion of malate to oxaloacetate catalyzed by malate dehydrogenase
(C) the high ATP levels lead to high NADH levels in the mitochondria, which inhibits conversion of oxaloacetate to malate catalyzed by malate dehydrogenase
(D) the high ATP levels lead to high NAD^+ levels in the mitochondria, which inhibits conversion of malate to oxaloacetate catalyzed by malate dehydrogenase
(E) the high ATP levels lead to high NADH levels in the cytoplasm, which favors conversion of malate to oxaloacetate catalyzed by malate dehydrogenase

298. Which of the following is the single most important force in stabilizing protein tertiary structure?

(A) peptide bonds
(B) disulfide bonds
(C) hydrogen bonds
(D) polar interactions
(E) hydrophobic interactions

299. Under conditions of anaerobic glycolysis, the NAD^+ required by glyceraldehyde 3-phosphate dehydrogenase is supplied by a reaction catalyzed by

(A) pyruvate dehydrogenase
(B) α-ketoglutarate dehydrogenase
(C) glycerol-3-phosphate dehydrogenase
(D) malate dehydrogenase
(E) lactate dehydrogenase

300. Pyruvate dehydrogenase activity is regulated by its state of phosphorylation. The activity of the kinase which catalyzes the phosphorylation of pyruvate dehydrogenase is increased by

(A) acetyl-CoA
(B) cAMP
(C) AMP
(D) NAD^+
(E) coenzyme-A

301. The eukaryotic translation initiation factor (designated Factor ? in Figure 3–1) required as a component of the eIF-2 cycle is

(A) eIF-1
(B) eIF-2B
(C) eIF-3
(D) eIF-4A
(E) eIF-4F

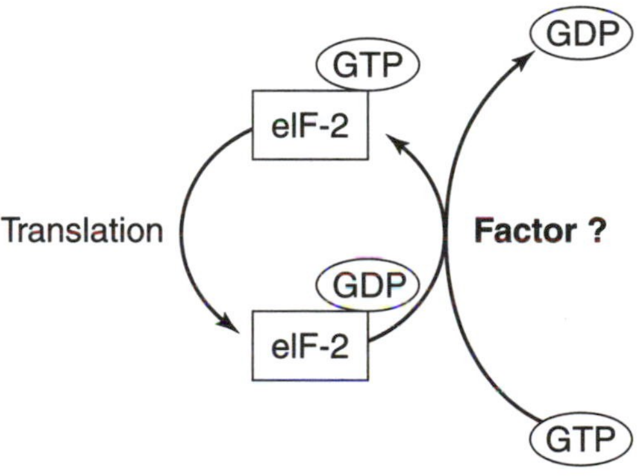

Figure 3–1

302. The key regulatory enzyme of fatty acid synthesis is

(A) enoyl reductase
(B) ATP citrate lyase
(C) acetyl-CoA carboxylase
(D) malonyl-CoA decarboxylase
(E) 3-ketoacyl reductase

303. Which of the following is a characteristic physiological consequence of type II diabetes?

(A) impaired glucagon-dependent inhibition of glycolysis
(B) elevated insulin secretion
(C) decreased glucagon secretion
(D) decreased insulin secretion
(E) impairment of insulin-dependent glucose uptake

304. The major site of regulation of cholesterol synthesis is

(A) cyclization of squalene to lanosterol
(B) 3-hydroxy-3-methylglutaryl-CoA synthase
(C) 3-hydroxy-3-methylglutaryl-CoA lyase
(D) 3-hydroxy-3-methylglutaryl-CoA reductase
(E) synthesis of squalene from isoprenoid isomers

305. Lack of which of the following hepatic enzymes leads to fructose intolerance?

(A) fructokinase
(B) fructose-1-phosphate aldolase
(C) phosphoglucomutase
(D) phosphohexose isomerase
(E) glucose-6 phosphatase

306. Synthesis of glycogen is inhibited in hepatocytes in response to glucagon stimulation primarily as a result of

(A) a decrease in the levels of phosphorylated phosphoprotein phosphatase inhibitor-1
(B) an increase in the level of the dephosphorylated form of glycogen synthase
(C) a decrease in the level of phosphorylated phosphorylase kinase
(D) an increase in the level of the phosphorylated form of glycogen synthase
(E) a decrease in the level of phosphoprotein phosphatase

307. Which of the following occurs in the lipidosis known as Tay–Sachs disease?

(A) synthesis of a specific ganglioside is excessive
(B) xanthomas due to cholesterol deposition are observed
(C) phosphoglycerides accumulate in the brain
(D) ganglioside GM_2 is not catabolized by lysosomal enzymes
(E) synthesis of a specific ganglioside is decreased

308. In diabetes, the increased production of ketone bodies is primarily a result of

(A) elevated acetyl-CoA levels in skeletal muscle
(B) a substantially increased rate of fatty acid oxidation by hepatocytes
(C) increased gluconeogenesis
(D) decreased cyclic AMP levels in adipocytes
(E) an increase in the rate of the citric acid cycle

309. Which of the following represents the primary function of the pentose phosphate pathway in erythrocytes?

(A) production of NADPH
(B) production of ribose-5-phosphate
(C) remodeling of dietary carbon atoms into 2,3-bisphosphoglycerate
(D) synthesis of ATP
(E) reduction of H_2O_2 to two moles of H_2O

310. Which of the following is considered the central molecule of gluconeogenesis?

(A) lactate
(B) malate
(C) phosphoenolpyruvate
(D) pyruvate
(E) oxaloacetate

311. Hepatocytes deliver ketone bodies to the circulation primarily because they lack

(A) the form of the β-ketothiolase necessary to hydrolyze acetoacetyl-CoA
(B) hydroxymethylglutaryl-CoA-lyase

(C) hydroxymethylglutaryl-CoA-synthetase
(D) succinyl-CoA-acetoacetate-CoA-transferase
(E) β-hydroxybutyrate dehydrogenase

312. An overdose of insulin in diabetic persons leads to

(A) hypoglycemia
(B) glucosuria
(C) ketonuria
(D) hyperglycemia
(E) ketonemia

313. Refsum's disease results from a greatly reduced capacity to carry out which of the following processes of lipid metabolism?

(A) β-oxidation of fatty acids
(B) activation of acetyl-CoA for cholesterol synthesis
(C) α-oxidation of fatty acids
(D) proper regulation of acetyl-CoA carboxylase
(E) lipoxygenase-catalyzed leukotriene synthesis

314. Consumption of raw eggs, which contain the protein avidin, could lead to a deficiency resulting in

(A) an inhibition of decarboxylation reactions
(B) an inability to form acetylcholine
(C) a decrease in CoA formation
(D) an increase in transaminations
(E) an inhibition of carboxylation reactions

315. Both glutamate transaminase and alanine transaminase require a prosthetic group derived from

(A) vitamin B_6 (pyridoxine)
(B) vitamin B_1 (thiamine)
(C) vitamin B_{12} (cobalamin)
(D) vitamin B_2 (riboflavin)
(E) biotin

316. Figure 3–2 represents the electron-transport chain of oxidative phosphorylation. Which component of the chain is the site for the inhibitory action of cyanide?

(A) Complex II
(B) Coenzyme Q
(C) Complex III
(D) Complex I
(E) Complex IV

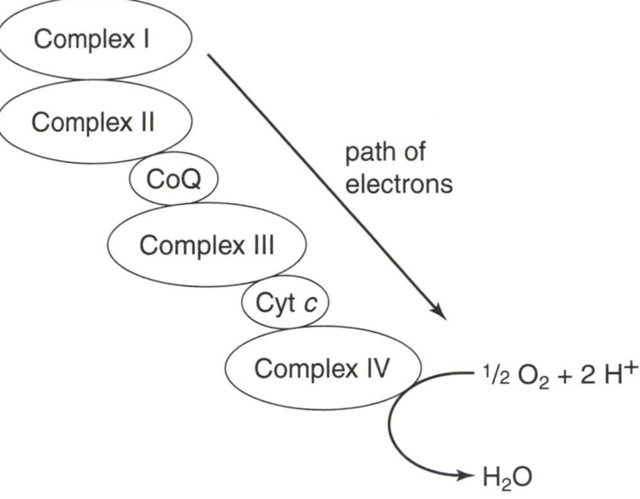

Figure 3–2

317. Which of the following is quantitatively the major contributor to routine clinical measurements of circulating plasma cholesterol concentrations?

(A) chylomicrons
(B) low-density lipoproteins (LDLs)
(C) high-density lipoproteins (HDLs)
(D) intermediate-density lipoproteins (IDLs)
(E) very-low-density lipoproteins (VLDLs)

318. Long-term treatment of hypercholesterolemia with the cholesterol synthesis inhibitor lovastatin (and related drugs) can lead to toxicity. This is most accurately explained by which of the following statements?

(A) Products of the cholesterol pathway are necessary for the synthesis of other compounds.
(B) A buildup of lovastatin in the liver leads to hepatic cell death.
(C) Lovastatin is lipid soluble and over long-term treatment enters the brain, leading to neuropathies.
(D) The loss of cholesterol biosynthesis leads to decreased bile acid production and a concomitant inability of the liver to excrete bilirubin, leading to jaundice.
(E) As cholesterol is required for normal membrane integrity, long-term inhibition of its synthesis ultimately leads to disruptions in normal membrane transport processes and cell death.

319. The process of activating a free fatty acid such that it can enter the β-oxidation pathway uses the equivalent of how many moles of ATP?

(A) 1
(B) 3
(C) 2
(D) 0
(E) 4

320. Activated core oligosaccharides that are transferred to the asparagine of proteins are carried by

(A) guanosine diphosphate (GDP)-mannose
(B) N-acetylglucosamine
(C) dolichol phosphate
(D) N-acetylgalactosamine
(E) UDP-glucose

321. Which of the following statements best characterizes ATP synthase?

(A) It couples ATP export from the mitochondrial matrix to ATP synthesis.
(B) Oligomycin binds to ATP synthase, directly preventing ATP export.
(C) Its catalytic function is to synthesize ATP in a reaction driven by a chemiosmotic potential.
(D) The low H^+ ion concentration outside the inner mitochondria membrane establishes an electrochemical gradient that drives ATP synthesis.
(E) It is a soluble protein found inside the mitochondrial matrix.

322. Which of the following is considered to be rate limiting in detoxification of ethanol in alcoholic individuals?

(A) the oxidized form of nicotinamide adenine dinucleotide (NAD^+)
(B) the oxidized form of flavin adenine dinucleotide (FAD)
(C) the oxidized form of nicotinamide adenine dinucleotide phosphate ($NADP^+$)
(D) alcohol dehydrogenase
(E) acetaldehyde dehydrogenase

For questions 323 and 324 use the following clinical case:

A 4-month-old male presents with painful progressive joint deformity (particularly the ankles, knees, elbows, and wrists), hoarse crying, and granulomatous lesions of the epiglottis and larynx leading to feeding and breathing difficulty. Biopsy of the liver indicates an accumulation of ceramides.

323. The observed symptoms and the results of the liver biopsy are indicative of which disease?

(A) metachromic leukodystrophy
(B) Farber's lipogranulomatosis
(C) Sandhoff–Jatzkewitz disease
(D) fucosidosis
(E) Gaucher's disease

324. Specific diagnosis of this disease requires assay of skin fibroblasts for a deficiency in which enzyme?

(A) hexosaminidase A
(B) sphingomyelinase

(C) acid ceramidase
(D) galactocerebrosidase
(E) arylsulfatase A

325. Which of the following reactions is the major oxidation reaction of energy metabolism in erythrocytes?

(A) NADPH ↔ $NADP^+$
(B) $FADH_2$ ↔ FAD
(C) dihydroxyacetone phosphate + NADH ↔ glycerol-3-phosphate + NAD^+
(D) pyruvate + NADH ↔ lactate + NAD^+
(E) acetaldehyde + NADH ↔ ethanol + NAD^+

326. The affinity of Hb for O_2 is increased by

(A) the formation of salt bridges in Hb
(B) the cross-linking of the β-chains of Hb
(C) lowering of pH
(D) decreases in 2,3-bisphosphoglycerate (BPG)
(E) increases in the partial pressure of CO_2

327. A 42-year-old male presents with hepatomegaly, jaundice, refractory ascites, and renal insufficiency, with peripheral leukocytes exhibiting only 20% of normal glucocerebrosidase activity. Which of the following would explain his symptoms?

(A) Fabry's disease
(B) Gaucher's disease
(C) Niemann–Pick disease
(D) Tay–Sachs disease
(E) Krabbe's disease

328. The increased intracellular concentrations of 5-phosphoribosyl-1-pyrophosphate (PRPP) and urate in the genetic hyperuricemia called the Lesch–Nyhan syndrome is most likely a consequence of

(A) allopurinol inhibition of xanthine formation
(B) increased purine synthesis
(C) elevated synthesis of hypoxanthine
(D) deficiency of hypoxanthine–guanine phosphoribosyltransferase (HGPRT)
(E) elevated PRPP synthetase activity

329. Which of the following amino acids are strictly ketogenic?

(A) lysine and leucine
(B) valine and isoleucine
(C) leucine and isoleucine
(D) lysine, leucine, and isoleucine
(E) tyrosine and tryptophan

330. Numerous related inherited disorders result from defects in the synthesis and/or processing of connective tissue proteins. Which of the following disorders results from a defect in the synthesis of fibrillin?

(A) osteogenesis imperfecta
(B) cutis laxa
(C) Marfan syndrome
(D) occipital horn syndrome
(E) Ehlers–Danlos syndrome

331. Which important metabolic pathway is depicted in Figure 3–3?

(A) non-oxidative cycle in pentose phosphate pathway
(B) purine nucleotide cycle
(C) urea cycle
(D) hypoxanthine–guanine phosphoribosyltransferase cycle
(E) adenosine deaminase cycle

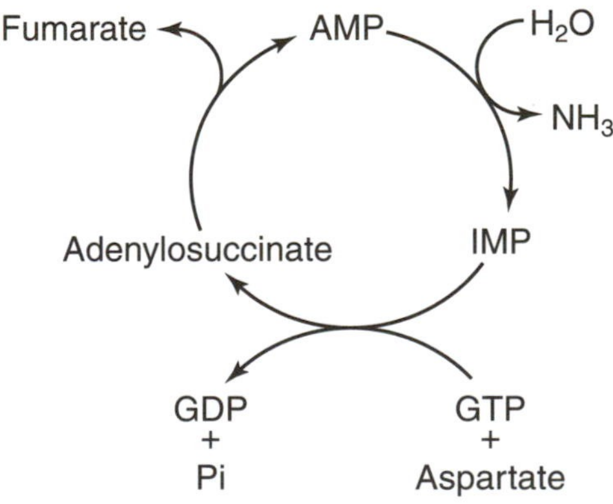

Figure 3–3

332. During the hydrolysis of which compound is sufficient free energy released that it can be coupled to the synthesis of ATP from ADP and P_i?

(A) glucose-1-phosphate
(B) 2,3-bisphosphoglycerate
(C) glycerol-3-phosphate
(D) phosphoenolpyruvate
(E) glucose-6-phosphate

333. Which of the following steps is common to both gluconeogenesis and glycolysis?

(A) fructose-6-phosphate to glucose-6-phosphate
(B) pyruvate to oxaloacetate
(C) glucose-6-phosphate to glucose
(D) fructose-1,6-bisphosphate to fructose-6-phosphate
(E) oxaloacetate to phosphoenolpyruvate

334. Patients with poorly controlled diabetes mellitus have elevated levels of blood glucose. This leads to an increase in the formation of glycosylated

(A) albumin
(B) hemoglobin
(C) cholesterol
(D) transferrin
(E) fatty acids

For Questions 335 and 336 refer to the clinical vignette below.

A child born and raised in Chicago planned to spend the summer on a relative's fruit farm and help with the harvest. The summer passed uneventfully, but several days after the harvest began the child became jaundiced and very sick. Upon admission to the hospital the following clinical findings were made: In addition to the expected hyperbilirubinemia, the patient was hypoglycemic, had a markedly elevated rise in blood fructose concentration, and was hyperlactic acidemic. Further history taking revealed that during the harvest it was customary for the family to indulge in fruit-filled meals and to snack freely on fruit while carrying out the harvest. The following conclusions were reached.

335. The elevated blood fructose was due to

(A) defective hepatic glucokinase
(B) defective hepatic fructokinase
(C) an allergic reaction to constituents in the fruit diet
(D) defective hepatic fructose-1,6-bisphosphate aldolase (aldolase A)
(E) defective hepatic fructose-1-phosphate aldolase (aldolase B)

336. The hyperlactic acidemia was attributed to

(A) an inability to carry out liver oxidative phosphorylation and gluconeogenesis, secondary to a severe deficiency of available inorganic phosphate in hepatocytes
(B) excess production of pyruvate from dietary fructose sources
(C) inability to metabolize pyruvate because of a dietary vitamin insufficiency, leading to inhibition of the pyruvate dehydrogenase complex
(D) an allergic reaction to a constituent in the fruit diet
(E) a diet-induced insufficiency of niacin, leading to low cell levels of available NAD^+ and NADH

337. Which of the following compounds would be used by a person on a carbohydrate-free diet as a source of carbon atoms for de novo glucose synthesis?

(A) palmitate
(B) β-hydroxybutyrate
(C) glycerol
(D) cholesterol
(E) acetoacetate

338. Which of the following symptoms can occur frequently in infants suffering from medium-chain acyl-CoA dehydrogenase (MCAD) deficiency if periods between meals are protracted?

(A) hyperuricemia and darkening of the urine

(B) metabolic alkalosis with decreased bicarbonate
(C) hyperammonemia with decreased ketones
(D) bone and joint pain and thrombocytopenia
(E) hypoglycemia and metabolic acidosis with normal levels of ketones

339. A decrease in the level of heme leads to a reduction in globin synthesis in reticulocytes. Which of the following best explains this phenomenon?

(A) RNA polymerase activity is decreased in reticulocytes by low heme.
(B) The initiation factor eIF-2 becomes phosphorylated, reducing its level of activity.
(C) Heme normally activates peptidyltransfersase in reticulocytes.
(D) A tRNA degrading enzyme is active in the absence of heme.
(E) A heme-controlled phosphatase dephosphorylates cap-binding factor, which prevents recognition of globin mRNA by the ribosomes.

340. Which of the following hormones functions to increase glycogen breakdown by binding to and activating a transmembrane receptor?

(A) epinephrine
(B) retinoic acid
(C) insulin
(D) parathyroid hormone
(E) thyrotropin

341. Which of the following lipoproteins plays a crucial role in the regulation at the cellular level of nonhepatic tissue cholesterol?

(A) LDLs
(B) VLDLs
(C) IDLs
(D) HDLs
(E) chylomicrons

342. A 28-year-old man has the following symptoms: diffuse grayish corneal opacities, anemia, proteinuria, and hyperlipemia. Renal function is normal and serum albumin level is only slightly elevated. Plasma triglycerides and unesterified cholesterol levels are elevated as are levels of phosphatidylcholine. These symptoms are indicative of which lipoprotein-associated disorder?

(A) familial hypercholesterolemia
(B) familial lecithin–cholesterol acyltransferase (LCAT) deficiency
(C) Wolman's disease
(D) Bassen–Kornzweig syndrome
(E) familial hypertriacylglycerolemia

343. Which of the following post-translationally modified amino acids is found in several proteins of the blood clotting cascade?

(A) hydroxyproline
(B) γ-carboxyglutamate
(C) phosphoserine
(D) N-acetylmethionine
(E) hydroxylysine

344. I-cell disease (also identified as mucolipidosis type II) is characterized by the presence of inclusion bodies in fibroblasts (hence the derivation of the term I-cell), severe psychomotor retardation, corneal clouding, and dystosis multiplex. These symptoms arise from a defect in the targeting of lysosomal enzymes due to an inability to

(A) remove mannose-6-phosphates from lysosomal enzymes prior to their transport to the lysosomes
(B) recycle the lysosomal receptor for mannose-6-phosphate present on lysosomal enzymes
(C) synthesize the mannose-6-phosphate receptor found in lysosomes
(D) transport mannose-6-phosphate receptors to lysosomes
(E) produce mannose-6-phosphate modifications in lysosomal enzymes

345. A 30-month-old child is presented with coarse facial features, corneal clouding, hepatosplenomegaly, and exhibiting disproportionate short-trunk dwarfism. Radiographic analysis indicates enlargement of the diaphyses of the long bones and irregular metaphyses, along with poorly developed epiphyseal centers. Other skeletal abnormalities typify the features comprising dystosis multiplex. The child's physical stature and the analysis of bone development indicate the child is suffering from

(A) Hurler's syndrome
(B) Sanfilippo's disease type A
(C) Hunter's syndrome
(D) Morquio's syndrome type B
(E) Maroteaux–Lamy syndrome

346. Which of the following amino acids is a major source of carbon for the one-carbon pool?

(A) serine
(B) asparagine
(C) glutamine
(D) glutamate
(E) aspartate

347. Which of the following polypeptides is derived by posttranslational processing of the pro-opiomelanocortin (POMC) gene product?

(A) oxytocin
(B) cholecystokinin
(C) atrial natriuretic factor
(D) β-endorphin
(E) bradykinin

348. A deficiency in the amino acid metabolizing enzyme α-keto acid decarboxylase results in neonatal vomiting, lethargy, and poor suckling behavior. Progressive neurological signs include decerebrate posturing. Which one of the following disorders corresponds to this defect?

(A) phenylketonuria
(B) alkaptonuria
(C) maple syrup urine disease
(D) isovaleric acidemia
(E) homocystinuria

349. Which of the following glycosaminoglycans exhibits antithrombic activity when released into the circulation?

(A) hyaluronate
(B) keratan sulfate
(C) dermatan sulfate
(D) heparin
(E) chondroitin sulfate

350. A 37-year-old male is presented with tophaceous deposits within the articular cartilage, synovium, tendons, tendon sheaths, pinnae, and the soft tissue on the extensor surface of the forearms. These clinical observations suggest the patient is suffering from

(A) gout
(B) Lesch–Nyhan syndrome
(C) von Gierke's disease
(D) purine nucleotide phosphorylase deficiency
(E) adenosine deaminase deficiency

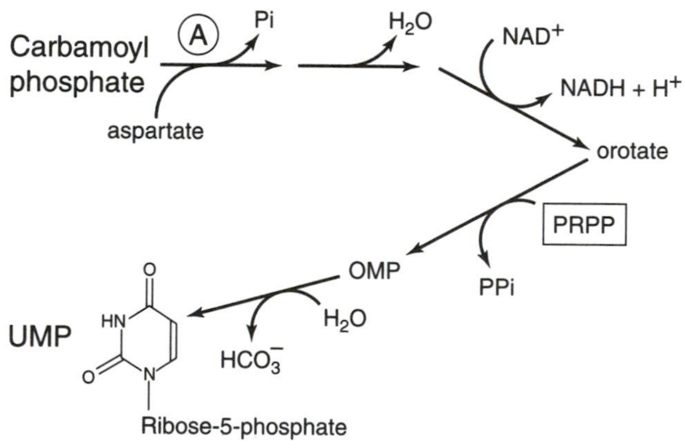

Figure 3–4

351. Figure 3–4 represents the de novo pathway of pyrimidine biosynthesis. The enzyme represented as "A" in the figure is

(A) phosphoribosylpyrophosphate (PRPP) synthetase

(B) PRPP amido transferase
(C) aspartate transcarbamoylase
(D) OMP decarboxylase
(E) ribonucleotide reductase

352. One important function of nitric oxide (NO) is the induction of vascular smooth muscle relaxation in response to acetylcholine. The production of NO requires which amino acid?

(A) lysine
(B) asparagine
(C) glutamine
(D) arginine
(E) cysteine

353. In renal insufficiency, calcium absorption is reduced and leads to increased bone resorption, a condition referred to as renal osteodystrophy. Treatment with which of the following can assist in the amelioration of the symptoms of this condition?

(A) calcitonin
(B) parathyroid hormone
(C) growth hormone
(D) antidiuretic hormone
(E) calcitriol

354. A 32-year-old female is diagnosed with hypertension, hypernatremia, hypokalemia, and alkalosis. Measurements of plasma glucocorticoid levels show them to be within the normal range, however, renin and angiotensin II levels are suppressed. Ultrasound indicates the possible existence of an adrenal cortical mass. These symptoms are likely due to excess production of

(A) androstenedione
(B) aldosterone
(C) estradiol
(D) dehydroepiandrosterone (DHEA)
(E) testosterone

355. The neurotransmitters epinephrine, norepinephrine and dopamine are all derived from which amino acid?

(A) phenylalanine
(B) tyrosine
(C) tryptophan
(D) arginine
(E) asparagine

356. A 17-year-old male who reports to his physician that he is incapable of obtaining an erection is also quite embarrassed by the apparent enlargement of his breast (gynecomastia). These symptoms when present in males are associated with an excessive production of

(A) growth hormone
(B) gonadotropin-releasing hormone
(C) prolactin
(D) corticotropin-releasing hormone
(E) melanocyte-stimulating hormone

357. Numerous inherited disorders are the result of the expansion of trinucleotide (triplet) repeats either within the coding regions of genes or the untranslated regions of the resultant RNAs. Which of the following diseases has been shown to be caused by triplet expansion?

(A) Huntington's disease
(B) cystic fibrosis
(C) Duchenne's muscular dystrophy
(D) Menkes' disease
(E) familial hypercholesterolemia

358. Figure 3–5 represents a portion of the glycolytic pathway. Which lettered step in this pathway represents the rate-limiting reaction of glycolysis?

(A) A
(B) B
(C) C
(D) D
(E) E

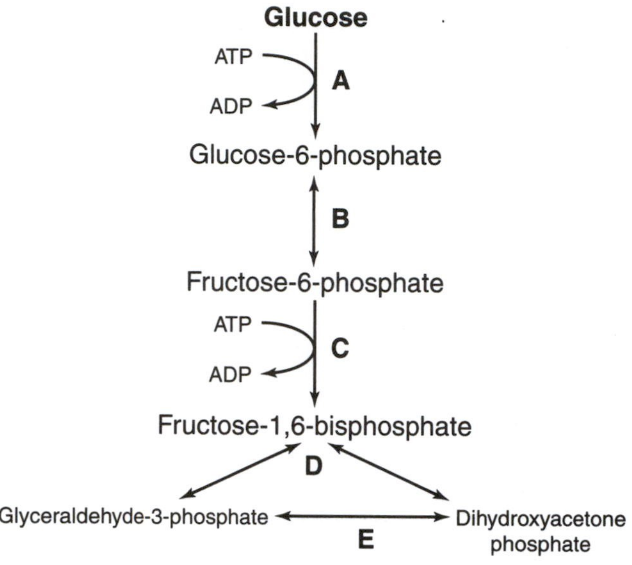

Figure 3–5

359. Severe combined immunodeficiency disease (SCID) is characterized by a complete lack of cell-mediated and humoral immunity. This disorder results from a deficiency in

(A) purine nucleoside phosphorylase
(B) orotic acid decarboxylase
(C) aspartate transcarbamoylase
(D) hypoxanthine–guanine phosphoribosyltransferase
(E) adenosine deaminase

360. The forensic analytical technique identified as DNA fingerprinting refers to

(A) the specific association of complimentary strands of DNA to one another
(B) the identification of sequences of DNA to which specific proteins bind, thereby rendering them resistant to digestion by DNA degrading nucleases
(C) the synthetic oligonucleotide-directed enzymatic amplification of specific sequences of DNA
(D) the use of repeat sequences to establish a unique pattern of fragments for any given individual
(E) the establishment of a complete collection of cloned fragments of DNA

361. Which of the following represents the rate-limiting step in the biosynthesis of heme?

(A) δ-aminolevulinic acid (ALA) dehydratase
(B) porphobilinogen (PBG) deaminase
(C) ferrochetalase
(D) δ-aminolevulinic acid (ALA) synthetase
(E) uroporphyrinogen decarboxylase

362. Polyamines are highly cationic molecules involved in the process of DNA replication. These molecules are synthesized from which amino acid?

(A) asparagine
(B) methionine
(C) arginine
(D) lysine
(E) glutamine

363. A 3-month-old infant exhibits profound neurological deficit in addition to being blind and deaf. Pathological examination indicates renal cysts, hepatomegaly, and facial dysmorphism. Biochemical analysis reveals plasma accumulations of very long chain fatty acids, abnormal intermediates of bile acid synthesis, and a marked deficiency of plasmalogens. These physical and biochemical features are characteristic of

(A) neonatal adrenoleukodystrophy
(B) infantile Refsum's disease
(C) Zellweger syndrome
(D) hyperpipecolic acidemia
(E) rhizomelic chondrodysplasia punctata (RCDP)

364. Which of the following apoproteins is found exclusively associated with chylomicrons?

(A) apo-B-48
(B) apo(a)
(C) apo-E
(D) apo-C-II
(E) apo-D

365. Which lettered reaction in Figure 3–6 (representing the non-oxidative portion of the pentose phosphate pathway) is catalyzed by transaldolase?

(A) A
(B) B
(C) C
(D) D
(E) E

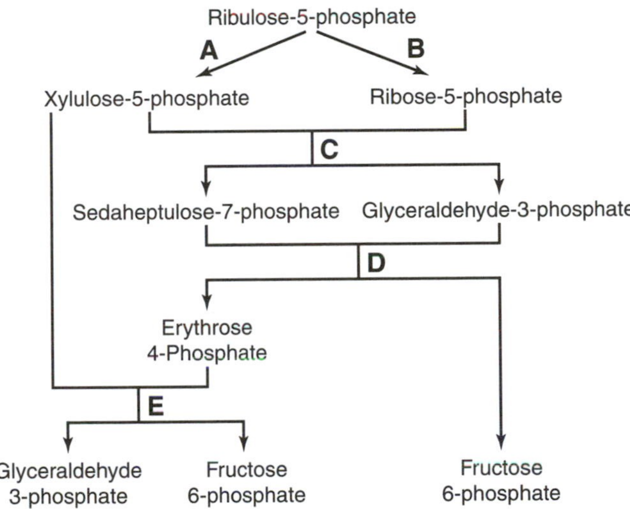

Figure 3–6

366. Acromegaly is characterized by protruding jaw, enlargement of the nose, hands, feet, and skull, and a thickening of the skin. This disorder is the result of excessive production of

(A) insulin-like growth factor II
(B) gonadotropin-releasing hormone
(C) growth hormone
(D) corticotropin-releasing hormone
(E) thyroid-stimulating hormone

367. The primary protein responsible for iron homeostasis is

(A) ceruloplasmin
(B) metallothionein
(C) transferrin
(D) ferritin
(E) haptoglobin

368. The primary site of action of the analgesic aspirin and other related non-steroidal anti-inflammatory drugs (NSAIDs) is at the level of which enzyme?

(A) phospholipase A_2
(B) HMG-CoA reductase
(C) lipoxygenase
(D) 15-hydroxyprostaglandin dehydrogenase
(E) cyclooxygenase

369. A 3-month-old infant, who otherwise appeared normal during the first two months of life except for a bout of hyperbilirubinemia, is now clearly exhibiting developmental delay. In addition, the infant's hair has become grayish and dull and there is a stubble of broken hairs over the occiput and temporal regions. The facial appearance has also changed such that the infant has very pudgy cheeks, abnormal eyebrows, and sagging jowls. The occurrence of frequent convulsions was the stimulus for the parents to bring their child to the emergency room. These rapidly deteriorating symptoms are indicative of

(A) Menkes' disease
(B) hemochromatosis
(C) Refsum's disease
(D) Gilbert syndrome
(E) Crigler–Najjar syndrome type I

370. Acute intermittent porphyria (AIP) is the major autosomal dominant acute hepatic porphyria. This disease is caused by a deficiency in porphobilinogen deaminase, an enzyme of heme biosynthesis. Patients afflicted with this disease would be expected to excrete excess amounts of

(A) coproporphyrinogen III
(B) δ-aminolevulinic acid
(C) hydroxymethylbilane
(D) type III uroporphyrinogen
(E) protoporphyrin IX

371. The phosphorylase kinase-associated regulatory protein identified by the letter A in Figure 3–7 is a calcium-binding protein. This subunit of phosphorylase kinase is

(A) glycogen synthase kinase-3
(B) phosphoprotein phosphatase
(C) fructose-2,6-bisphosphate
(D) phosphoprotein phosphatase inhibitor-1
(E) calmodulin

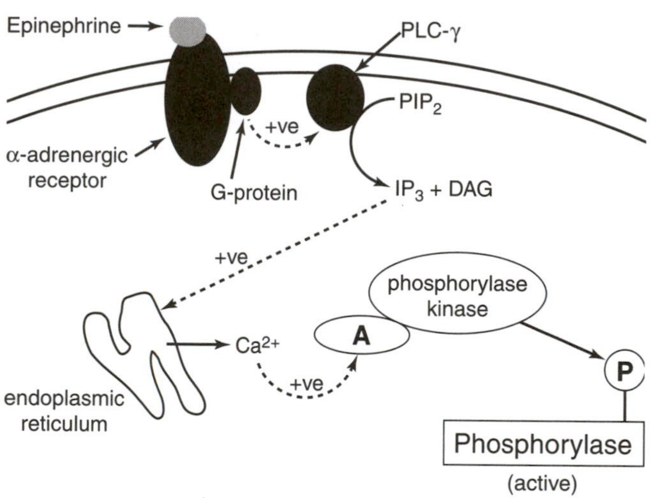

Figure 3–7

372. Which of the following enzymes of the urea cycle is found in the mitochondria?

(A) ornithine transcarbamoylase
(B) arginase
(C) argininosuccinase
(D) argininosuccinate synthetase

373. An 18-month-old boy was referred to the pediatrics clinic because of persistent anemia and associated failure to thrive. Laboratory analysis confirmed a microcytic anemia and revealed blood lead levels of 50 mg/dL (two times normal) and high levels of coproporphyrinogen III in the urine. The child was put on chelation therapy and recovered uneventfully. The cause of the child's difficulty was most likely due to the effects of lead inhibiting which of the following enzymes of heme biosynthesis?

(A) δ-aminolevulinic acid (ALA) dehydratase
(B) ferrochelatase
(C) porphobilinogen (PBG) deaminase
(D) uroporphyrinogen III cosynthase
(E) uroporphyrinogen decarboxylase

374. The terminal processing of the carbohydrate portion of glycoproteins occurs in the

(A) mitochondria
(B) Golgi complex
(C) plasma membrane
(D) endoplasmic reticulum
(E) lysosomes

375. Vitamin K is required for which of the following amino acid modifications?

(A) proline to hydroxyproline
(B) aspartate to β-carboxyaspartate
(C) lysine to β-methyllysine
(D) lysine to hydroxylysine
(E) glutamate to γ-carboxyglutamate

376. Steroid hormones interact with specific receptors within target cells. The steroid/receptor complexes then regulate the rate of

(A) replication of DNA
(B) post-transcriptional processing of specific mRNAs
(C) transcription of specific genes
(D) translation of specific mRNAs
(E) post-translational processing of specific proteins

377. Which of the following vitamins is required as a cofactor during both the synthesis and degradation of fatty acids?

(A) pantothenic acid
(B) thiamine
(C) biotin
(D) cobalamin
(E) riboflavin

378. Which of the following is an essential amino acid for humans?

(A) cysteine
(B) methionine
(C) serine
(D) glycine
(E) glutamate

379. Deficiencies in the enzyme glucose-6-phosphatase are likely to lead to which of the following?

(A) decreased glucagon production
(B) decreased skeletal muscle glycogen accumulation
(C) hyperglycemia
(D) increased hepatic glycogen accumulation
(E) increased accumulation of unbranched glycogen

380. Which of the following is a primary source of fuel for the brain during periods of prolonged starvation?

(A) fatty acids produced in adipose tissue
(B) glycogen stores of the liver
(C) amino acids from skeletal muscle
(D) glycogen stores of the brain
(E) ketone bodies produced in the liver

381. Acetyl-CoA enhances the rate of gluconeogenesis by acting as an allosteric activator of

(A) pyruvate carboxylase
(B) acetyl-CoA carboxylase
(C) pyruvate kinase
(D) phosphoenolpyruvate carboxykinase
(E) pyruvate dehydrogenase

382. A reaction important in oxygen transport is catalyzed by carbonic anhydrase. This reaction is

(A) ionization of carbonic acid
(B) production of CO_2 from carbonic acid
(C) protonation of hemoglobin
(D) carbamoylation of hemoglobin
(E) transport of chloride ion in exchange bicarbonate ion

383. The lack of which enzyme in skeletal muscle prevents its cells from delivering free glucose to the blood?

(A) phosphorylase kinase
(B) phosphohexose isomerase
(C) phosphoglucomutase
(D) glucose-6-phosphate dehydrogenase
(E) glucose-6-phosphatase

384. The accumulation of an oxygen debt during strenuous physical exercise may be accompanied by

(A) an increase in NAD^+ in muscle
(B) an increase in lactate in blood
(C) a decrease in pyruvate in blood
(D) an increase in citrate in muscle
(E) an increase in ATP in muscle

385. Dietary triacylglycerols are transported in the plasma as

(A) VLDLs
(B) HDLs
(C) chylomicrons
(D) LDLs
(E) albumin conjugates

386. Which of the following antibiotics is an inhibitor of transcription?

(A) streptomycin
(B) erythromycin
(C) tetracycline
(D) puromycin
(E) rifamycin

For question 387, refer to Figure 3–8.

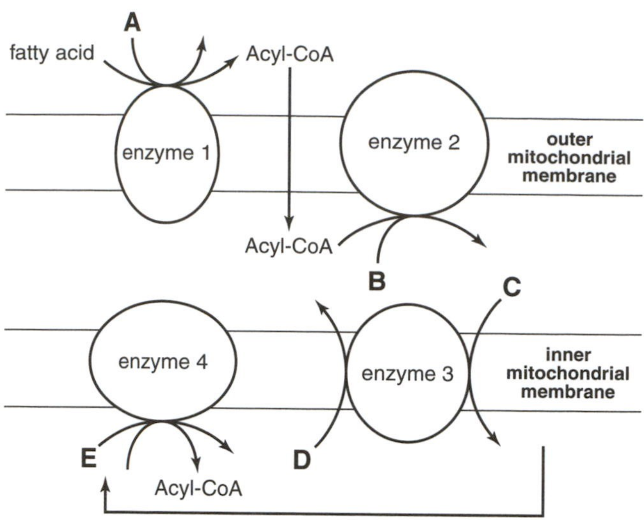

Figure 3–8

387. Carnitine, a zwitterionic compound derived from lysine, is involved in fatty acid metabolism and is required at which two points in the transport of fatty acids from the cytoplasm to the mitochondria?

(A) B and C
(B) E and D
(C) A and E
(D) B and D
(E) A and C

Questions 388 and 389 are based upon the following clinical case.

A male infant, delivered at 38 weeks' gestation, presents with severe bowing of long bones, blue sclera, and craniotabes at birth. Radiographs show severe generalized osteoporosis, broad and crumpled long bones, beading ribs, and poorly mineralized skull. Histological examination of the long bones revealed the trabecula of the calcified cartilage with an abnormally thin layer of osteoid, and the bony trabeculae are thin and basophilic.

388. The symptoms observed in the infant are characteristic of which disease?

(A) Marfan syndrome
(B) osteogenesis imperfecta
(C) Ehlers–Danlos syndrome
(D) scurvy
(E) occipital horn syndrome

389. The disease with the symptoms described results from the defective biosynthesis of

(A) α-collagen
(B) fibrillin
(C) cytokeratin
(D) vimentin
(E) desmin

390. The formula for the kinetic parameter identified as A in Figure 3–9 is

(A) $-1/K_m$
(B) v_1/V_{max}
(C) k_1/k_{-1}
(D) K_m/V_{max}
(E) $1/V_{max}$

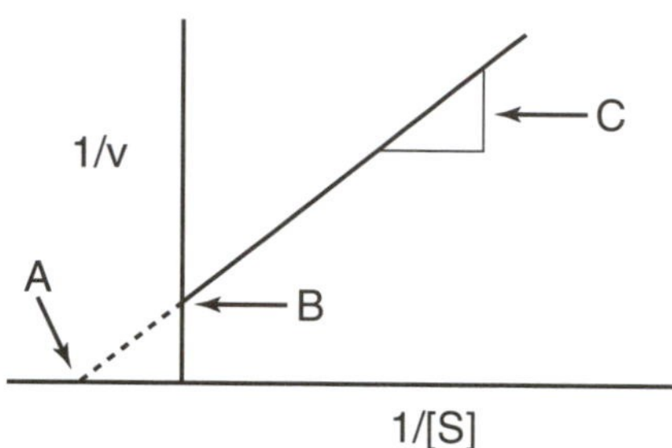

Figure 3–9

391. Which of the following enzyme abnormalities would be expected to lead to hyperuricemia?

(A) xanthine oxidase deficiency
(B) adenosine deaminase deficiency
(C) hypoxanthine–guanine phosphoribosyltransferase (HGPRT) deficiency (Lesch–Nyhan syndrome)
(D) purine nucleoside phosphorylase deficiency
(E) PRPP aminotransferase deficiency

392. Cockayne syndrome is a rare disorder that leads to sun sensitivity (without increased frequency of skin cancer), short stature, progressive neurological degeneration, mental retardation, and progressive deafness. This disease is the result of a deficiency in which process?

(A) transcription
(B) translation
(C) RNA processing
(D) DNA repair
(E) DNA replication

393. In the presence of arsenate, which of the following may or may not occur during glycolysis?

(A) 1,3-bisphosphoglycerate is formed
(B) NADH is formed
(C) P_i reacts with glyceraldehyde-3-phosphate
(D) 3-phosphoglycerate is not formed
(E) pyruvate is not formed

394. In analyzing a sample of double-stranded DNA, it has been determined that the molar ratio of adenosine is 20%. Given this information, what is the content of cytidine?

(A) 20
(B) 30
(C) 60
(D) 10
(E) 40

395. Measurement of the rate of creatinine clearance is used as a key determinant of renal function. In which of the following tissues is creatinine generated?

(A) liver
(B) kidney
(C) lung
(D) skeletal muscle
(E) adipose

396. Numerous cancers are caused by a genetic phenomenon termed "loss of heterozygosity." This phenomenon led to the identification of genes termed tumor suppressors, because it is the loss of their function that leads to cancer. Which of the following has been shown to result from defects in a tumor suppressor gene?

(A) Huntington's disease
(B) Crouzon's syndrome
(C) Creutzfeldt–Jakob disease
(D) Li–Fraumeni syndrome
(E) Prader–Willi syndrome

397. Following a relatively normal early developmental period, a 6-month-old male becomes pale and lethargic and begins to show signs of deteriorating motor skill. The infant has severe megaloblastic anemia; however, serum measurements of iron, folate, vitamins B_{12} and B_6 demonstrate they are within normal range. Urine samples were clear when fresh, but when left to stand for several hours showed an abundant white precipitate that was composed of fine needle-shaped crystals. Analysis of the crystals identified them as orotic acid. Significant improvement is observed in the infant following oral administration of a nucleoside. Which of the following is most likely the nucleoside used?

(A) thymidine
(B) cytidine
(C) uridine
(D) adenosine
(E) guanosine

398. Using the DNA shown as a template, what would be the sequence of the resultant mRNA following transcription?

5′-CATTCCATAGCATGT-3′

(A) 5′-CAUUCCAUAGCAUGU-3′
(B) 5′-ACAUGCUAUGGAAUG-3′
(C) 5′-UGUACGAUACCUUAC-3′
(D) 5′-GUAAGGUAUCGUACA-3′

399. Use the following table of codons to determine the sequence of the peptides translated from the mRNA generated in Question 398.

ACA	threonine	(T)	CAU	histidine	(H)
ACG	threonine	(T)	CUA	leucine	(L)
AUG	methionine	(M)	CGU	arginine	(R)
AAU	asparagine	(N)	CCU	proline	(P)
AGG	arginine	(R)	UGC	cysteine	(C)
AUA	isoleucine	(I)	UGU	cysteine	(C)
GGA	glycine	(G)	UAU	tyrosine	(Y)
GUA	valine	(V)	UAC	tyrosine	(Y)
GCA	alanine	(A)	UCC	serine	(S)
			UGG	tryptophan	(W)

(A) M-L-W-N
(B) H-S-I-A-C
(C) V-R-Y-R-T
(D) T-C-Y-G-M
(E) C-T-I-P-Y

400. Which of the following statements most correctly reflects the effect of epinephrine stimulation of adipocytes?

(A) increased synthesis and activation of lipoprotein lipase
(B) enzyme-dependent addition of fatty acids to glycerol-3-phosphate
(C) release of glycerol-3-phosphate for gluconeogenesis in the liver
(D) increased synthesis of HDL to transport fatty acids to peripheral tissues
(E) enzyme-dependent stepwise release of fatty acids from triglycerides

401. Which of the following familial cancers results from a defect in the tumor suppressor gene, p53?

(A) familial adenomatous polyposis
(B) Wilms' tumor
(C) Li–Fraumeni syndrome
(D) neurofibromatosis type 1
(E) retinoblastoma

402. Which of the following clotting factors forms an active complex with tissue factor (factor III) to initiate the extrinsic clotting cascade?

(A) I (fibrinogen)
(B) VIII
(C) protein S
(D) IX
(E) VII (proconvertin)

403. The liver is the only body organ that is capable of

(A) urea formation
(B) ganglioside synthesis
(C) nucleotide synthesis
(D) medium-chain fatty acid catabolism
(E) glycogen degradation

404. The cofactor not required for conversion of pyruvate to acetyl-CoA is

(A) NAD^+
(B) FAD
(C) thiamine
(D) biotin
(E) lipoic acid

405. The disease pellagra can be prevented by a dietary sufficiency of

(A) vitamin D
(B) riboflavin
(C) vitamin A
(D) thiamine
(E) niacin

406. Which of the following factors of blood coagulation is the major inhibitor of the extrinsic clotting cascade?

(A) antithrombin III
(B) lipoprotein-associated coagulation factor (LACI)
(C) protein C
(D) high molecular weight kininogen (HMWK)
(E) α_2-macroglobulin

407. Certain receptors function through the activation of phospholipase Cγ (PLCγ). Which of the following most accurately depicts the result of activated PLCγ?

(A) decreased release of inositol phospholipids from the plasma membrane
(B) activation of adenylate cyclase with increased production of cAMP
(C) increased release of diacylglycerol from plasma phospholipids
(D) activation of phosphodiesterase, thereby decreasing the concentration of cAMP
(E) increased cellular uptake of Ca^{2+} resulting in depolarization of the cell

408. When adipose tissue is stimulated to release fatty acids to the circulation, these fatty acids are transported in the plasma associated with

(A) VLDLs
(B) albumin
(C) β_2-microglobulin
(D) chylomicrons
(E) α_2-macroglobulin

409. Regulatory DNA sequences and repetitive genes such as those for rRNA account for roughly 10% of the DNA of the human genome. What approximate percentage of the human genome is accounted for by single copy mRNA genes?

(A) 0.5%
(B) 30%
(C) 90%
(D) 5%
(E) 50%

Answers and Explanations

283. (D) Erythrocytes are dependent upon the function of the pentose phosphate pathway to prevent permanent damage from the numerous reactive oxygen species that are present as a result of their role as oxygen transporters. The pentose phosphate pathway generates large quantities of NADPH through the actions of glucose-6-phosphate dehydrogenase and 6-phosphogluconate dehydrogenase. The need for NADPH stems from the fact that it is required for the action of glutathione reductase. Glutathione reductase converts oxidized glutathione (GSSG) to reduced glutathione (GSH). Red blood cells require GSH as a scavenger of reactive oxygen species to prevent oxidative damage. Deficiencies in glucose-6-phosphate dehydrogenase therefore lead to erythrocytes that are highly sensitive to oxidative damage with resultant hemolysis. The accelerated rate of hemolysis leads to anemia. Primaquine and related drugs are metabolized within erythrocytes to oxidative derivatives, which accelerate the rate of glutathione oxidation, as well as hydrogen transfer from NADPH and hemoglobin. Normally, under these conditions, the rate of flux through the pentose phosphate pathway is greatly accelerated providing increased amounts of NADPH. In persons with glucose-6-phosphate dehydrogenase deficiencies this acceleration is not possible and oxidative stress leads to hemolysis. None of the other enzymes (choices A, B, C, or E) generates NADPH as a byproduct of their respective reactions and can therefore have no influence on erythrocyte oxidative management.

284. (A) Compounds that can competitively inhibit enzyme catalyzed reactions are usually structurally similar to substrate. However, once bound, the enzyme cannot convert the inhibitor to product. Addition of increasing amounts of substrate leads to the displacement of the inhibitor and conversion of substrate to product. Since the inhibitor and substrate are competing for the substrate binding site, the K_m for substrate exhibits an apparent increase. No inhibitor will decrease the apparent K_m (choice B) or the apparent V_{max} (choice D) as these changes would not be inhibition, but an increase in enzyme activity. Non-competitive inhibitors increase the apparent V_{max} (choice C). A reaction with unaffected K_m and V_{max} (choice E) would not be inhibited in any way.

285. (A) Under anaerobic conditions (e.g., intense exercise), the production of pyruvate via glycolysis exceeds its oxidation by the citric acid cycle. This results in the synthesis of lactate by muscle. Lactate diffuses into the bloodstream and is taken up by the liver, where it is oxidized back to pyruvate. The latter is converted to glucose in the liver via gluconeogenesis. The only other tissue that performs the reactions of gluconeogenesis to any significant degree is the kidney cortex. Although the brain, skeletal muscle, and cardiac muscle (choices B and E) have the capacity to carry out gluconeogenesis, the rate is insignificant relative to the need for glucose production. Erythrocytes (choice C) and adipose tissue (choice D) do not carry out gluconeogenesis.

286. (C) The carbohydrates that constitute the ABO blood groups are covalently attached either to membrane sphingolipids or to circulating proteins. When present on the surface of cells, the ABO carbohydrates are linked to sphingolipid, and are therefore of the glycosphingolipid class (choice A). When the ABO carbohydrates are associated with protein in the form of glycoproteins, they are found in the serum and are referred to as the secreted forms. Some individuals produce the glycoprotein forms of the ABO antigens while others do not. This property distinguishes secretors from nonsecretors, a property that has forensic importance such as in cases of rape. Secretor/nonsecretor status is not due to any acute clinical situation (choice B) nor to defects in any gene function (choices D and E).

287. (A) Calcitriol (1,25-dihydroxy D_3) is the hormonally active form of vitamin D. The primary function of calcitriol is to regulate calcium and phosphorous homeostasis in cooperation with parathyroid hormone and calcitonin. Calcitriol activates the expression of a specific calcium binding protein in intestinal epithelial cells to facilitate absorption and delivery of dietary calcium. On bone, calcitriol functions with parathyroid hormone to stimulate resorption by stimulating osteoblast production and function. Deficiencies in vitamin D in children will lead to poorly mineralized osteoid matrix of the bone due to the severely reduced capacity to absorb calcium from the intestine. This leads to rickets (choice E). In adults, lack of vitamin D leads to demineralization of preexisting bone causing them to become soft. This condition is known as osteomalacia. The distinction between osteomalacia and osteoporosis is the presence of the osteoid matrix in the former and its absence in the latter. Deficiencies in vitamin A lead to progressive keratinization of the cornea referred to as xerophthalmia (choice B). Deficiencies in folate cause various anemias, and a defect in erythrocyte maturation leads to macrocytic anemia (choice C). Deficiency in vitamin C leads to scurvy (choice D).

288. (B) Vitamin B_{12} (cobalamin) is synthesized by microorganisms and stored in the liver of animals. Only two reactions in mammalian cells require cobalamin as a cofactor, these being conversion of homocysteine to methionine catalyzed by methionine synthase, and conversion of methylmalonyl-CoA to succinyl-CoA catalyzed by methylmalonyl-CoA mutase. The significance of a cobalamin deficiency relates to its indirect effects on thymidine nucleotide biosynthesis. The inability to convert homocysteine to methionine leads to entrapment of folate, in the form of tetrahydrofolate (required for thymidine nucleotide biosynthesis at the thymidylate synthase catalyzed step) as the N^5-methyltetrahydrofolate form (choice A). Absorption of vitamin B_{12} from the intestine is mediated by specific receptors that only recognize cobalamin bound to intrinsic factor. Therefore, the lack of gastric parietal cell–derived intrinsic factor prevents its absorption from intestine. As cobalamin is water soluble, lipid malabsorptive disorders have no effect on the uptake of the vitamin from the intestines (choice C). No known deficiencies in transcobalamin II production exist, therefore transport of cobalamin from the intestinal circulation to the liver is unaffected (choice D).

289. (E) The carbohydrate moieties in RNA and DNA are ribose and deoxyribose, respectively. A major product of the pentose phosphate pathway is ribose 5-phosphate. The latter is converted to 5-phosphoribosyl-1-pyrophosphate (PRPP), which serves as the donor of ribose in the biosynthesis of nucleotides. Ribose is made only by the pentose phosphate pathway, therefore each of the other pathways (choices A, B, C, and D) play no direct role in its production. Of course, the pentose phosphate pathway would not function were it not for the shunting (the pathway is also referred to as the hexose monophosphate shunt) of glucose from glycolysis into the pathway, but this does not confer a direct role for glycolysis in ribose production.

290. **(D)** Vitamin C is a reducing agent capable of reducing cytochromes a and c and molecular oxygen as well as other compounds, and may act as a general water soluble antioxidant. Vitamin C is also involved in the synthesis of bile acids and epinephrine and the degradation of tyrosine. Additionally, vitamin C is required as a cofactor for numerous hydroxylation reactions in the body, in particular the hydroxylation of lysine and proline residues in procollagen. In this capacity, the lack of vitamin C leads to the inability of procollagen to cross-link into normal collagen fibrils. The net result is an inability to maintain normal connective tissue and poor wound healing, since connective tissue is synthesized first in the healing process. Collagen is a necessary component in the organic portion of bone matrix and of the ground substance of capillary walls. Therefore, lack of properly processed collagen leads to impaired bone mineralization and weakened capillaries resulting in increased hemorrhaging. No major disease states have been associated with vitamin E deficiency (choice A) since it is amply supplied in the average American diet. Deficiencies of vitamin B_6 (choice B) are rare and usually related to an overall deficiency of all the B complex vitamins. Deficiency in vitamin K (choice C) is rare, but will lead to bleeding disorders if severe and chronic. Deficiency in vitamin D (choice E) leads to rickets (poorly formed bone) in children and osteomalacia (demineralization of preformed bone) in adults. As indicated in the answer to 287, the distinction between osteomalacia and osteoporosis is the presence of the osteoid matrix in the former and its absence in the latter.

291. **(A)** Myosin contains the ATPase activity that hydrolyzes ATP and allows contraction to proceed. The binding of actin to myosin enhances the ATPase activity of myosin. In fact, actin alternatively binds to myosin and is released from it as ATP is hydrolyzed. This reaction requires Mg^{2+} and is the driving force of contraction. Although troponin is not directly involved in the ATPase reaction, it binds calcium released by the sarcoplasmic reticulum, and in doing so allows conformational changes in tropomyosin and actin to occur, permitting contraction. Myokinase catalyzes the formation of ATP and AMP from two molecules of ADP. The proteins troponin (choice B), tropomyosin (choice D), and actin (choice E) are components of the thin filaments of muscle and perform structural functions without catalytic activity. The activity of myosin light chain kinase (choice C) is to phosphorylate the light chain of myosin, which then associates with actin and alters the conformation of the latter.

292. **(D)** Fabry's disease is an X-linked disorder that results from a deficiency in α-galactosidase A. This leads to the deposition of neutral glycosphingolipids with terminal α-galactosyl moieties in most tissues and fluids. Most affected tissues are heart, kidneys, and eyes. The predominant glycosphingolipid accumulated is globotriaosylceramide [galactosyl-(α1→4)-galactosyl-(β1→4)-glucosyl-(β1→1′)-ceramide]. With increasing age the major symptoms of the disease are due to increasing deposition of glycosphingolipid in the cardiovascular system. Indeed, cardiac disease occurs in most hemizygous males. Three types of Gaucher's disease (choice A) have been characterized and are caused by defects in lysosomal acid β-glucosidase (glucocerebrosidase). Defects in this enzyme lead to the accumulation of glucosylceramides (glucocerebrosides) which leads, primarily, to central nervous system dysfunction and also hepatosplenomegaly and skeletal lesions. Niemann–Pick disease, NPD, (choice B) comprises three types of lipid storage disorder, two of which (type A and B NPD) result from a defect in acid sphingomyelinase. Type A is a disorder that leads to infantile mortality. Type B is variable in phenotype and is diagnosed by the presence of hepatosplenomegaly in childhood and progressive pulmonary infiltration. Pathological characteristics of Niemann–Pick are the accumulation of histiocytic cells that result from sphingomyelin deposition in cells of the monocyte–macrophage system. Tay–Sachs disease (choice C) results from a defect in hexosaminidase A leading to the accumulation of GM_2 gangliosides, particularly in neuronal cells. This defect leads to severe mental retardation, progressive weakness, and hypotonia, which prevents normal motor development. Progression of the disease is rapid and death occurs within the second year. Krabbe's disease (choice E), also called globoid-cell leukodystrophy, results from a deficiency in galactosylceramidase (galactocerebroside β-galactosidase). This disease progresses rapidly and invariably leads to infantile mortality.

293. (B) There are three reactions of glycolysis that are thermodynamically irreversible. These are the hexokinase (glucokinase), phosphofructokinase-1 (PFK-1), and pyruvate kinase catalyzed reactions. Reactions that are essentially irreversible in most metabolic pathways are subject to complex regulatory controls and represent rate-limiting steps in the pathway. The primary site of regulation of glycolysis occurs at the level of the PFK-1 catalyzed step. Hence, this reaction is the rate-limiting step in glycolysis. PFK-1 is subject to allosteric control by numerous compounds. Citrate and ATP inhibit the activity of PFK-1 while AMP and fructose-2,6-bisphosphate (F-2,6-BP) activate the enzyme. The principal control of PFK-1 activity is exerted by alterations in the level of F-2,6-BP. This compound is synthesized from fructose-6-phosphate (F-6-P) by the bifunctional enzyme, phosphofructokinase-2 (PFK-2). PFK-2 (choice E) contains two catalytic domains, one a kinase and the other a phosphatase, the activities of which are affected by the state of phosphorylation. The phosphatase domain is active when the enzyme is phosphorylated and converts F-2,6-BP back to F-6-P, thereby reducing the levels of this powerful activator of PFK-1. Thus, although the activity of PFK-2 will determine the rate of activity of PFK-1, it is itself not the rate-limiting enzyme in glycolysis. Glyceraldehyde-3-phosphate dehydrogenase (choice A) and phosphoglycerate kinase (choice D) are not regulated enzymes of glycolysis. Pyruvate kinase (choice C) is regulated during glycolysis, but does not constitute a rate-limiting step.

294. (A) The first step in gluconeogenesis is the formation of oxaloacetate from pyruvate. The enzyme controlling this step is pyruvate carboxylase, an allosteric enzyme that does not function in the absence of its primary effector, acetyl-CoA, or closely related acyl-CoA. Thus, a high level of acetyl-CoA signals the need for more oxaloacetate. If there is a surplus of ATP, oxaloacetate will be used for gluconeogenesis. Under conditions of low ATP, oxaloacetate will be consumed in the citric acid cycle. Citrate is the primary negative effector of glycolysis, and the primary positive effector of fatty acid synthesis. High levels of citrate (choice B), but not low levels (choice C), do positively affect the activity of fructose-1,6-bisphosphatase, one of the bypass enzymes of gluconeogenesis, but this is not the primary site of control, since the carbon atoms must first go through the pyruvate carboxylase reaction. Low ATP levels (choice D) would be reflected in an elevation in ADP levels, and ADP negatively affects the activity of pyruvate carboxylase. High ATP levels (choice E) are necessary in order for gluconeogenesis to proceed, and will negatively affect glycolysis at the level of PFK-1, allowing for an increased net flow of carbon into glucose. However, increased levels of ATP do not directly regulate the enzymes of gluconeogenesis.

295. (C) Bacterial repressors function by binding to DNA sequences that overlap some of the same sequences bound by RNA polymerase. The repressor binding sequences are referred to as the *operator*. The sequences bound by RNA polymerase are termed the *promoter*. When repressor is bound to the operator sequences, RNA polymerase cannot interact with and bind to the promoter sequences. Repressors do not have catalytic activity, and therefore cannot induce the modification of DNA (choice A) or RNA polymerase (choice E), nor can they influence the overall structure of DNA (choice D). Repressors bind to DNA, not to the other transcriptional proteins such as RNA polymerase (choice B).

296. (B) Thymidylate (TMP) is synthesized by methylation of deoxyuridylate (dUMP) at the five-carbon in a reaction catalyzed by thymidylate synthase. TMP is the only precursor for DNA synthesis that is produced separately from the major biosynthetic pathways for purine and pyrimidine ribonucleotides. For this reason, reactions required for TMP biosynthesis are specific targets for drugs that will inhibit DNA synthesis. 5-Fluorouracil is a modified uracil that contains a fluorine attached to the five-carbon. It binds to thymidylate synthase because it is a structural analog of dUMP and forms a covalent complex with the enzyme. This results in complete inactivation of thymidylate synthase. Cells that are rapidly proliferating, such as tumor cells, carry out high levels of DNA synthesis. They therefore require larger amounts of TMP than normal cells and, for this reason, are more susceptible to the action of fluorouracil. Ribonucleotide reductase (choice A) is necessary for converting ribonucleotides to their corresponding deoxy forms and is not the target of uracil analogs. Thymidine kinase (choice C) is a nucleotide salvage enzyme, and the enzymes of de novo pyrimidine (choice D) and purine (choice E) are not targets for uracil analogs.

297. **(A)** The malate–aspartate shuttle is the major pathway by which electrons are transferred from cytoplasmic NADH to mitochondrial NADH for entry into the oxidative–phosphorylation process. When the energy charge of a cell is high (the level of ATP is high relative to that of ADP and AMP), the flux of electrons from the reduced electron carriers NADH and $FADH_2$ through the oxidative phosphorylation pathway is reduced. Therefore, concomitant with a rise in cellular ATP levels will be a rise in NADH levels both in the mitochondria and cytoplasm. Within the cytoplasmic portion of the malate–aspartate shuttle, the electrons of NADH are transferred to oxaloacetate, generating malate catalyzed by malate dehydrogenase. The malate is transported into the mitochondria, where the electrons are transferred to NAD^+ in a reversal of the reaction occurring in the cytoplasm. This mitochondrial reaction requires a steady supply of NAD^+ which is supplied as the electrons are transferred to the oxidative–phosphorylation pathway. However, as oxidative–phosphorylation slows down, the level of NAD^+ declines and NADH increases in the mitochondria leading to inhibition of the malate-to-oxaloacetate conversion. Each of the various combinations of ATP and NADH or NAD^+ in choices B, C, D, and E do not exert the effects on the malate–aspartate shuttle as outlined.

298. **(E)** Tertiary structure refers to the three-dimensional arrangement of amino acid residues in a protein. Studies of many proteins reveal that the nonpolar (hydrophobic) amino acid residues are buried in the interior of the protein structure, whereas the polar residues are on the outside in contact with the aqueous environment. The protein folds so as to shield its nonpolar groups from interaction with water molecules. These hydrophobic interactions are the driving force of protein folding. The tertiary structure is further stabilized by hydrogen bonding (choice C), polar interactions (choice D), and the formation of disulfide bonds (choice B). Peptide bonds (choice A) are only involved in formation of the primary structure of a protein.

299. **(E)** When glycolysis (a cytoplasmic pathway) is proceeding under anaerobic conditions, the electrons transferred to NAD^+ (generating NADH) during the glyceraldehyde-3-phosphate dehydrogenase (G3PDH) catalyzed step cannot be transferred to mitochondrial NADH nor $FADH_2$, which would regenerate cytoplasmic NAD^+ levels. This would lead to a deficiency in the NAD^+ required by G3PDH and an eventual cessation of glycolysis. Therefore, under anaerobic conditions, tissues such as skeletal muscle reduce pyruvate (the end product of anaerobic glycolysis) to lactate catalyzed by lactate dehydrogenase (LDH). This reaction requires electrons to be donated from NADH and thereby regenerate NAD^+ which can be used by G3PDH. If pyruvate dehydrogenase (choice A) were to utilize any NAD^+ in the oxidation of pyruvate to acetyl-CoA, there would be reduced levels available for G3PDH and glycolysis would cease, hence pyruvate is reduced by LDH. The citric acid cycle enzymes, α-ketoglutarate dehydrogenase (choice B) and malate dehydrogenase (choice D) require NAD^+, as well as being found in the mitochondria, and therefore would not be able to supply glycolysis with NAD^+. Although there is a cytoplasmic malate dehydrogenase and glycerol-3-phosphate dehydrogenase (choice C) is cytoplasmic, these enzymes are involved in the transfer of cytoplasmic electrons from NADH into the mitochondria, a process that is restricted by the lack of O_2 during anaerobic metabolism.

300. **(A)** Pyruvate dehydrogenase (PDH) activity is regulated both allosterically and by the state of phosphorylation. When phosphorylated the activity of PDH is reduced. The PDH kinase is associated with the PDH complex and is itself regulated by allosteric factors. High activity of PDH will be observed under conditions of reduced energy charge in order to supply the TCA cycle with acetyl-CoA. As the level of ATP rises, the rate of flux through the TCA cycle will begin to decline, leading to a buildup of acetyl-CoA. The increased acetyl-CoA in turn allosterically activates the PDH kinase, leading to an increased level of phosphorylation of PDH and a concomitant decline in its activity. Cyclic-AMP (choice B) and AMP (choice C) have no effect on the activity of PDH kinase. Both NAD^+ (choice D) and CoA (choice E) are negative regulators of the activity of PDH kinase.

301. **(B)** The eIF-2 cycle consists of the translation initiation factors, eIF-2A and eIF-2B (also called guanine nucleotide exchange factor, GEF). The cycle involves the binding of GTP by eIF-2A forming a complex that then interacts with the initiator methionyl-tRNA. When the initiator methionyl-tRNA is placed into the correct position of the 40S ribosomal subunit, the GTP is hydrolyzed to provide the energy necessary to correctly position the incoming mRNA such that the initiator AUG codon and the initiator methionyl-tRNA anticodon are aligned. In order to regenerate an active eIF-2A for subsequent translation initiation events, the GDP must be exchanged for GTP. The exchange reaction is catalyzed by eIF-2B (GEF). The initiation factor, eIF-1 (choice A) facilitates the correct positioning of the initiator methionyl-tRNA and the mRNA. eIF-3 (choice C) binds to the 40S ribosomal subunit and acts as a ribosome anti-association factor. This interaction is necessary to induce dissociation of the 40S and 60S subunits following completion of translation. Factor eIF-4A (choice D) binds to the mRNA and is required to "melt" any secondary structure that may exist at the 5′-end of the mRNA. Factor eIF-4F (choice E) binds to the cap structure that is added posttranscriptionally to all mRNAs.

302. **(C)** The formation of the three-carbon CoA thioester malonyl-CoA from acetyl-CoA is the regulatory step of fatty acid synthesis. Acetyl-CoA carboxylase (ACC) catalyzes this reaction.

$$\text{Acetyl-CoA} + HCO_3^- + \text{ATP} \rightarrow \text{malonyl-CoA} + \text{ADP} + P_i$$

Citrate, which serves as the means of transport of acetyl-CoA from the mitochondria to the cytosolic site of fatty acid synthesis, is the key allosteric regulator of acetyl-CoA carboxylase. It shifts the enzyme from an inactive protomer to an active filamentous polymer. The end product of the cytosolic fatty acid synthetase complex, palmitoyl-CoA, inhibits the carboxylase. Although acetyl-CoA carboxylase is the prime regulatory enzyme of fatty acid synthesis, it is not a part of the fatty acid synthetase complex, the site where most of the reactions of fatty acid synthesis take place. Enoyl reductase (choice A), malonyl-CoA decarboxylase (choice D), and 3-ketoacyl reductase (choice E) are all engaged in activities associated with fatty acid synthase which cannot function without first being activated by malonyl-CoA generated by the rate-limiting enzyme ACC. ATP citrate lyase (choice B) is involved in the transfer of acetyl-CoA from within the mitochondria to the cytoplasm, and as such its activity will have an effect on the rate of fatty acid synthesis. However, the acetyl-CoA that is transferred to the cytoplasm is not restricted to utilization in fatty acid synthesis, so the ATP citrate lyase reaction does not constitute a rate-limiting step for fatty acid synthesis.

303. (E) Type II diabetes is the non–insulin-dependent form of diabetes mellitus, and thus the disorder does not result from a lack of insulin production and secretion as in type I diabetes. The primary defect in type II diabetes is an impaired ability of cells to respond to insulin. There are several different factors leading to this impairment. Some patients exhibit reduced affinity of insulin receptors for insulin; others have receptors that bind insulin normally but have defects in post-receptor signaling processes. All of these defects lead to reduced insulin-dependent glucose uptake by all cells of afflicted individuals. Non–insulin-dependent diabetes patients have no defect in the action of glucagon (choice A) or in its secretion (choice C). Neither is the defect principally a result of altered insulin secretion (choices B and D), although in some patients, as the disease progresses a reduction in insulin levels can be detected.

304. (D) Cholesterol is obtained from the diet as well as by de novo synthesis. Although many cells can synthesize cholesterol, the liver is the major site of its production. The rate of cholesterol production is highly responsive to feedback inhibition from both dietary cholesterol and synthesized cholesterol. Feedback regulation is mediated by changes in the activity of 3-hydroxy-3-methylglutaryl-CoA reductase (HMG-CoA reductase), which reduces 3-hydroxy-3-methylglutaryl-CoA (HMG-CoA) to mevalonate. This reaction is the rate-limiting step of de novo cholesterol biosynthesis. HMG-CoA, when generated in the mitochondria through the action of 3-hydroxy-3-methylglutaryl-CoA synthase (choice B), serves as a source of ketone body production by serving as a substrate for 3-hydroxy-3-methylglutaryl-CoA lyase (choice C). Reactions involving squalene production (choice E) or of squalene (choice A) are not regulated.

305. (B) Fructose is a major carbohydrate of many fruits and vegetables and is used as a sweetener. In non-hepatic cells fructose can enter the glycolytic pathway by being phosphorylated to fructose-6-phosphate by hexokinase. However, hepatic glucokinase is specific for glucose and will not phosphorylate fructose. In the liver fructose is phosphorylated to fructose-1-phosphate by fructokinase. Fructose-1-phosphate is then hydrolyzed to dihydroxyacetone phosphate and glyceraldehyde by fructose-1-phosphate aldolase. Lack of fructose-1-phosphate aldolase leads to fructose intolerance. The disorder is characterized by an accumulation of fructose-1-phosphate and a depletion of ATP in the liver. The inability of hepatocytes to regenerate the ATP utilized to generate fructose-1-phosphate leads to a reduction in normal cellular processes and ultimately cellular damage. In particular the lowered activity of ATP-dependent cation pumps leads to osmotic lysis. A lack of fructokinase (choice A) leads to the disorder known as essential fructosuria. The remaining enzymes (choices C, D, and E) pertain to enzymes of glucose metabolism, and as such do not impact the utilization of fructose, which must first be converted to glucose to be utilized for energy.

306. (D) Glucagon is released from the pancreas in response to low blood glucose and stimulates hepatocytes to synthesize glucose for delivery to the blood. Therefore, it would be counterproductive for hepatocytes to divert any of the gluconeogenically derived glucose into glycogen. This is accomplished by inhibition of glycogen synthase. Glucagon exerts its effects on the liver through the glucagon receptor. When glucagon binds, the receptor activates adenylate cyclase leading to increased production of cAMP. In turn, cAMP activates cAMP-dependent protein kinase (PKA) which then phosphorylates a number of substrates. One of the substrates of PKA is glycogen synthase/phosphorylase kinase. Therefore, there would not be a decrease in the level of phosphorylated phosphorylase kinase (choice C). In turn, synthase/phosphorylase kinase phosphorylates glycogen phosphorylase and glycogen synthase.

Therefore, there is no increase in the level of dephosphorylated glycogen synthase (choice B). The effects of phosphorylation on glycogen synthase activity are inhibitory and on phosphorylase activating. In addition PKA itself can phosphorylate glycogen synthase. The net effect is an increase in the rate of glucose phosphorolysis from glycogen and a reduced incorporation of glucose into glycogen. An additional PKA substrate is phosphoprotein phosphatase inhibitor-1, and therefore there would not be a decrease in the level of the phosphorylated form of this enzyme (choice A). Glucagon has no effect on the level of phosphoprotein phosphatase (choice E).

307. (D) In the genetic disorder known as Tay–Sachs disease, ganglioside GM_2 is not catabolized. As a consequence, the ganglioside concentration is elevated many times higher than normal. The functionally absent lysosomal enzyme is β-N-acetylhexosaminidase. The elevated GM_2 results in irreversible brain damage to infants, who usually die before the age of 3 years. Under normal conditions, this enzyme cleaves N-acetylgalactosamine from the oligosaccharide chain of this complex sphingolipid, allowing further catabolism to occur. The cause of most lipidoses (lipid storage diseases) is similar. That is, a defect in catabolism of gangliosides causes abnormal accumulation. None of the other choices (A, B, C, and E) result in lipidotic disorders.

308. (B) In fasting or diabetes, lipolysis predominates in adipocytes because of the inability of these cells to obtain glucose, which is normally used as a source of glycerol 3-phosphate. Glycerol 3-phosphate is necessary for the esterification of fatty acids into triacylglycerides. Circulating fatty acids become the predominant fuel source, and β-oxidation in the liver becomes substantially elevated. This leads to an increased production of acetyl-CoA. Although gluconeogenesis is increased (choice C) in the liver as a result of the persistent elevation of glucagon levels, this pathway does not supply acetyl-CoA for the production of ketone bodies. The increased gluconeogenesis predisposes oxaloacetate and reduces (not increases, choice E) the flow of acetyl-CoA through the citric acid cycle. As a consequence, acetyl-CoA is diverted to the formation of ketone bodies. The persistently elevated levels of glucagon also increase the levels of cAMP in responsive tissues, such as adipocytes (choice D). This effect in adipocytes leads to persistently increased release of fatty acids to the circulation. Since skeletal muscle lacks receptors for glucagon, there is no diabetes-mediated increase in muscle metabolism, and thus no elevation in acetyl-CoA levels in skeletal muscle (choice A).

309. (A) Erythrocytes are the specialized oxygen-transporting cells of the body. As such they are continuously exposed to an oxidizing environment. These conditions can have profound effects on membrane lipids as a consequence of their attack by peroxides (particularly H_2O_2) prevalent in this environment. During the reduction of H_2O_2 catalyzed by glutathione peroxidase, glutathione acts as the donor of the necessary reducing equivalents generating oxidized glutathione. Glutathione (GSH) is a tripeptide of the structure, γ-glutamylcysteinylglycine, where the cysteine sulfhydryl side chains can form a disulfide bond between two molecules (designated as GSSG). To again perform the role of cofactor for glutathione peroxidase, the disulfide bond of GSSG must be reduced. This reaction is catalyzed by glutathione reductase which requires NADPH as a cofactor. Therefore, in order to maintain normal red cell membrane structure, erythrocytes utilize the pentose phosphate pathway for the generation of large amounts of NADPH. Erythrocytes are enucleate and therefore do not synthesize DNA and have no need for ribose-5-phosphate (choice B). Production of 2,3-bisphosphoglycerate (choice C) occurs through a side reaction of glycolysis, not the pentose phosphate pathway. The pentose phosphate pathway does not generate ATP (choice D) or result in the reduction of hydrogen peroxide (choice E).

310. **(E)** The principal substrates of gluconeogenesis are pyruvate, lactate, and amino acids, with some glucose being synthesized from the glycerol backbone of triacylglycerides. Lactate (choice A) is oxidized to pyruvate (choice D) and so feeds into gluconeogenesis in the same manner as that of pyruvate. Pyruvate cannot be freely converted into phosphoenolpyruvate (choice C) by pyruvate kinase, the glycolytic enzyme. Therefore, it undergoes a carboxylation step within the mitochondria, catalyzed by pyruvate carboxylase, to yield oxaloacetate (OAA). Oxaloacetate is then transported from the mitochondria to the cytoplasm in the form of malate (choice B) or aspartate, where it is reconverted to OAA. Cytoplasmic OAA is then converted into phosphoenolpyruvate (PEP) in a reaction catalyzed by PEP carboxykinase. The degradation products of most of the amino acids feed into pyruvate or TCA cycle intermediates, which ultimately lead to the generation of OAA. Therefore, OAA is considered the central molecule of gluconeogenesis.

311. **(D)** Ketogenesis occurs in the liver from acetyl-CoA during high rates of fatty acid oxidation and during early starvation. The principal ketone bodies are acetoacetate and β-hydroxybutyrate, which are reversibly synthesized in a reaction catalyzed by β-hydroxybutyrate dehydrogenase. The liver delivers β-hydroxybutyrate to the circulation where it is taken up by non-heptatic tissue for use as an oxidizable fuel. The brain will derive much of its energy from ketone body oxidation during fasting and starvation. Within extrahepatic tissues β-hydroxybutyrate is converted to acetoacetate by β-hydroxybutyrate dehydrogenase. Acetoacetate is reactivated to acetoacetyl-CoA in a reaction catalyzed by succinyl-CoA-acetoacetate-CoA-transferase (also called acetoacetate:succinyl-CoA CoA transferase), which uses succinyl-CoA as the source of CoA. This enzyme is not present in hepatocytes. The acetoacetyl-CoA is then converted to two moles of acetyl-CoA by the thiolase reaction of fatty acid oxidation. Each of the other enzyme choices (A, B, C, and E) are found within hepatocytes.

312. **(A)** Untreated diabetes leads to high blood glucose levels (hyperglycemia: choice D) and glucosuria (choice B), as glucose exceeds the kidney threshold and spills into the urine. At the same time that blood glucose levels are high, the lack of insulin leads to a favoring of lipolysis and consequent ketogenesis by the liver. The high level of ketogenesis by the liver produces ketonemia (high blood levels of ketone bodies: choice E) and ketonuria (ketone bodies in the urine: choice C). Insulin injections help to reduce these symptoms and allow diabetic persons to live relatively normal lives. However, insulin injections when blood glucose levels are low, as well as overdoses of insulin, can cause severe hypoglycemia. If blood glucose levels fall below 80 mg/100 ml, insulin shock occurs. When blood levels fall below 20 mg/100 ml, convulsions and coma occur because of the deprivation of glucose to the brain. IV glucose injections can reverse insulin shock.

313. **(C)** Phytanic acid is a methylated fatty acid byproduct of the catabolism of phytol, a constituent of chlorophyll. Phytanic acid is found in the milk and fats of ruminants. The normal pathway of phytanic acid oxidation in humans involves an α-hydroxylation followed by dehydrogenation and decarboxylation, and is termed α-oxidation, as opposed to the more common β-oxidation pathway of linear fats. The absence of the α-hydroxylating enzyme leads to the accumulation of large amounts of phytanic acid, leading to severe neurological complications associated with Refsum's disease. None of the other pathways (choices A, B, D, and E) are affected in Refsum's disease.

314. **(E)** Biotin serves as an intermediate carrier of CO_2 during carboxylations catalyzed by acetyl-CoA carboxylase, propionyl carboxylase, and pyruvate carboxylase. This vitamin is present in the prosthetic groups of these enzymes. Biotin is made from intestinal bacteria and is also obtained from a wide variety of foods. Avidin, a protein present in egg whites, tightly binds biotin in the gut, preventing its absorption. In individuals who consume large quantities of raw eggs, this leads to a toxic reaction due to biotin's role in carboxylation reactions. Biotin is not involved in the processes of decarboxylation (choice A), acetylcholine synthesis (choice B), coenzyme A synthesis (choice C), or transaminations (choice D). Therefore, an avidin-induced reduction in biotin absorption would not impact those processes.

315. (A) The α-amino group of many amino acids is transferred to α-ketoglutarate to form glutamate, which is then oxidatively deaminated to ammonium ion. A similar transamination reaction yields alanine from pyruvate during degradation of amino acids. The prosthetic group of all transaminases is pyridoxal phosphate, which is derived from pyridoxine. During transamination, the aldehyde group of pyridoxal phosphate forms a Schiff's-base linkage with the α-amino group of amino acids, ultimately transferring the amino group to either an α-ketoglutarate or pyruvate. Vitamin B_1 (choice B) is involved in oxidation-reduction reactions and the transketolase reaction. Vitamin B_{12} (choice C) is necessary for conversion of homocysteine to methionine and in the process of converting propionyl-CoA to succinyl-CoA. Vitamin B_2 (choice D) is involved in oxidation-reduction reactions. Biotin (choice E) is necessary for carboxylation reactions.

316. (E) Cyanide causes a rapid inhibition of the mitochondrial electron transport chain at the cytochrome oxidase step which constitutes complex IV of this process. Complex IV is composed of three atoms of copper and the hemes of cytochromes *a* and a_3. Cyanide binds to the Fe^{3+} in the heme of the cytochromes preventing oxygen from reacting with them. None of the other complexes or coenzymes (choices A, B, C, and D) are sites for cyanide interaction.

317. (B) LDLs are the primary carriers of blood cholesterol. Routine plasma lipid measurements are carried out after a 12-hr fast. In this way, the major endogenous plasma lipoproteins, VLDLs (choice E), and the major exogenous plasma lipoproteins (chylomicrons: choice A) have been cleared from the blood of normal individuals. LDLs, which are the end products of VLDL delipidation, and HDLs (choice C), which are protein rich, are the only lipoproteins circulating after a 12-hr fast. LDLs are rich in cholesterol, being composed of about 45% cholesterol or cholesterol esters. In both dietary and familial hypercholesterolemia, circulating LDL levels are increased. IDLs (choice D) represent an intermediate in the pathway of delipidation of VLDLs, and their concentration would be minimal following a 12-hr fast.

318. (A) Lovastatin is a fungal HMG CoA reductase inhibitor and is therefore useful for inhibiting *de novo* cholesterol biosynthesis. However, along the pathway to cholesterol biosynthesis, following the HMG CoA reductase–catalyzed step, important isoprenoid compounds are produced. These isoprenoid compounds are required not only for cholesterol biosynthesis, but also for the synthesis of dolichol (important for the synthesis of N-linked glycoproteins), coenzyme Q, the side chain of heme A, and in the prenylation (lipid modification) of certain membrane associated proteins. Therefore, chronic suppression of *de novo* cholesterol biosynthesis by use of the fungal-based inhibitors of HMG CoA reductase such as lovastatin can lead to toxicity. The amount of reduction in cholesterol afforded by lovastatin treatment (or use of other related statins), would not be sufficient to significantly impair membrane integrity and transport functions (choice E) or the production of bile acids (choice D). Lovastatin has no neurological impact (choice C) and does not build up in hepatocytes (choice B).

319. (C) Fatty acids destined for the oxidation pathway are activated by acetylation to coenzyme A. This activation is catalyzed by fatty acyl-CoA ligase (also called thiokinase or acyl-CoA synthetase) which utilizes the energy of ATP hydrolysis (to AMP and PP_i) to drive the reaction in the forward direction. The coupling of pyrophosphorylase-catalyzed hydrolysis of PP_i affords sufficient energy to ensure the reaction proceeds. The equivalent of two moles of ATP are thus required to regenerate ATP from the AMP generated in this reaction.

320. **(C)** Carbohydrates attached to asparagine residues have a common inner-core structure. Such a block of oligosaccharides is built up and carried to the asparagine of proteins on a lipid carrier. That carrier is dolichol phosphate, an aliphatic chain composed of isoprene units. *N*-acetylglucosamine is the sugar residue directly bonded to dolichol phosphate and then transferred to the asparagine side chain. Each of the remaining compounds represent either activated sugars (choices A and E) or modified sugars (choices B and D) that can be intermediates in the glycosylation process, but do not constitute a carrier (such as dolichol) of the activated core of the N-linked glycosylation process.

321. **(C)** As electrons flow through the various carrier proteins of the oxidative-phosphorylation chain, protons are pumped out of the inner mitochondrial space into the outer mitochondrial space (between the inner and outer mitochondrial membranes). This leads to a chemiosmotic (electrochemical) potential difference across the inner mitochondrial membrane. This electrochemical potential difference is what drives the activity of the membrane-associated ATP synthase to phosphorylate ADP yielding ATP. ATP export (choice A) from the mitochondria is not coupled to ATP synthesis and is the function of ATP/ADP translocate (also called adenine nucleotide transporter). Oligomycin (choice B) binds to ATP synthase and inhibits the passage of protons through ATP synthase, not the export of ATP. Transport of electrons through the complexes of oxidative-phosphorylation is coupled to the generation of a high concentration of H^+ outside the inner mitochondrial membrane, not a low concentration (choice D). ATP synthase is a complex of proteins embedded in the inner mitochondrial membrane, not as a soluble complex inside the matrix (choice E).

322. **(A)** During ethanol clearance in any individual, including alcoholic persons, ethanol is first converted to acetaldehyde by the action of alcohol dehydrogenase, and then to acetate by the action of acetaldehyde dehydrogenase. Both of these enzymes require the oxidized form of NAD^+ to function. During alcohol oxidation, the level of the reduced form of nicotinamide adenine dinucleotide (NADH) increases greatly in the liver, leading to an overload of the shuttle normally used to regenerate NAD^+. This causes the level of NAD^+ to be the bottleneck in the removal of alcohol from the body. The levels of alcohol dehydrogenase (choice D) may be somewhat higher than normal in chronically alcoholic persons. Nevertheless, NAD^+ is still the rate-limiting factor in the oxidation of ethanol. Although necessary for ethanol metabolism, acetaldehyde dehydrogenase (choice E), like alcohol dehydrogenase, would not function at any level if not for the presence of NAD^+. As indicated, the cofactor required by both enzymes of alcohol metabolism is NAD^+, therefore FAD (choice B) and $NADP^+$ (choice C) play no role in the process.

323. **(B)** Farber's lipogranulomatosis is characterized by painful and progressively deformed joints and progressive hoarseness due to involvement of the larynx. Subcutaneous nodules form near the joints and over pressure points. Granulomatous lesions form in these tissues and there is an accumulation of lipid-laden macrophages. Significant accumulation of ceramide and gangliosides is observed, particularly in the liver. If these compounds accumulate in nervous tissue there may be moderate nervous dysfunction. The illness often leads to death within the first few years of life, although milder forms of the disease have been identified. Metachromic leukodystrophy (choice A) is a disorder of myelin metabolism. It is characterized by the accumulation of galactosyl sulfatide (cerebroside sulfate). Symptoms may appear at any age and include mental regression, urinary incontinence, blindness, loss of speech, peripheral neuropathy, and seizures. Sandhoff–Jatzkewitz disease (choice C) is a disorder related to Tay–Sachs disease. It is characterized by a defect in the degradation of GM_2 gangliosides with symptoms of severe mental retardation, blindness, and early mortality. Fucosidosis (choice D) is characterized by the accumulation and excretion of glycoproteins, glycolipids, and oligosaccharides containing fucoside moieties. Symptoms of fucosidosis include psychomotor retardation, dystosis multiplex (a term referring to multiple skeletal abnormalities), growth retardation, and coarse facial features. Gaucher's disease (choice E) is characterized by an accumulation of glucosylceramide (glucocerebroside). Several forms of the disease have been identified and vary in severity. Typical symptoms include hepatosplenomegaly, bone lesions, and central nervous system involvement. Occasionally the lungs and other organs may be involved.

324. **(C)** Farber's lipogranulomatosis results from the defective function of acid ceramidase. Three biochemical pathways have been identified for the synthesis of ceramides: (1) a brain-specific ceramide synthetase; (2) microsomal synthesis from fatty acyl-CoA derivatives and sphingosine; and (3) the reversal of the reaction catalyzed by ceramidases (enzymes responsible for the degradation of ceramide). Acid ceramidase catalyzes the conversion of ceramides to sphingosine and a fatty acid. Tay–Sachs disease results from a deficiency in hexosaminidase A (choice A). Sphingomyelinase (choice B) deficiencies lead to Niemann–Pick disease. Deficiency in galactocerebrosidase (choice D) results in Krabbe's disease (also termed globoid leukodystrophy). Arylsulfatase A deficiency leads to metachromic leukodystrophy (choice E).

325. **(D)** Glycolysis is the only major source of ATP in erythrocytes, since they lack mitochondria. In order for glycolysis to continue uninterrupted, NADH must constantly be reoxidized to NAD^+ so that glyceraldehyde 3-phosphate may be oxidized. Conversion of pyruvate to lactate by lactate dehydrogenase accomplishes this. The excess lactate diffuses into the liver, where it is converted to glucose via gluconeogenesis. Besides the generation of ATP, erythrocytes must have a functioning mechanism for the generation of NADPH which is used by glutathione reductase to reduce oxidized glutathione (GSSG → GSH). This reaction is necessary so that erythrocytes can scavenge reactive oxygen species. The direction of the pertinent reaction, catalyzed by glucose-6-phosphate dehydrogenase, is $NADP^+ \rightarrow NADPH$, not the reverse as in choice A. Conversion of $FADH_2$ to FAD (choice B) would be coupled to a reduction reaction as in choice A. The reaction in choice C is principally carried out in the reverse direction to that shown, and is important for transporting cytoplasmic reducing equivalents into the mitochondria. Since erythrocytes lack mitochondria, this reaction is not carried out in these cells. The reaction in choice E is also written in the reverse direction relative to its major function, which is to metabolize ethanol. This latter reaction occurs primarily in the liver.

326. **(D)** Increases in either hydrogen ion concentration (choice C), CO_2 partial pressure, (choice E), or 2,3-BPG all lead to a decreased affinity of Hb for O_2. Conversely, decreases in these factors lead to an increased affinity of O_2 for Hb. A decrease in pH changes the charge on histidine residues in Hb, favoring the release of O_2. Binding of 2,3-BPG to deoxyhemoglobin causes the cross-linking of the β-chains (choice B), leading to a stabilization of the deoxygenated form of Hb and a lowered affinity for O_2. CO_2 can bind to the un-ionized α-amino groups on the terminal ends of Hb. This results in charged carbamino derivatives, which form salt bridges (choice A). The salt bridges further reduce the affinity of Hb for O_2.

327. **(B)** Numerous severe disorders are associated with the inability to properly degrade the complex carbohydrate moieties of glycosaminoglycans, proteoglycans, and glycoproteins. These disorders fall into a broad category of diseases termed the lysosomal storage diseases. Several of the lysosomal storage diseases result in hepatosplenomegaly, renal dysfunction, and skeletal defects, and therefore these symptoms are not diagnostic in themselves of a particular lysosomal storage disease, but only indicative of such disorders. However, disorders such as Niemann–Pick disease (choice C) and Tay–

Sachs disease (choice D) are of such severity that early childhood mortality occurs and thus would not present in a 42-year-old patient. It is necessary to evaluate enzyme function in skin fibroblasts or white cells of the blood. Gaucher's disease is caused by a defect in glucocerebrosidase activity and hence an assayable decrease in the activity of this enzyme would be diagnostic of this disease. Fabry's disease (choice A) results from a defect in α-galactosidase A. Niemann–Pick disease (choice C) results from a defect in sphingomyelinase. Tay–Sachs disease (choice D) results from a defect in hexosaminidase A. Krabbe's disease (choice E) results from a defect in galactocerebrosidase.

328. (D) The biochemical deficiency of the enzyme HGPRT results in mental retardation and compulsive self-destructive behavior seen in Lesch–Nyhan syndrome. This X-linked recessive disease also results in gout because of elevated levels of urate. However, unlike gout alone, allopurinol treatment of patients with Lesch–Nyhan syndrome does not increase the rate of synthesis of purines because it does not lower the level of PRPP. In genetically normal individuals, HGPRT allows the salvage synthesis of guanosine 5′-monophosphate (GMP) or inosine 5′-monophosphate (IMP) from guanine or hypoxanthine plus PRPP, thus there is less catabolism of these nucleotides to uric acid and gout symptoms do not occur. None of the other alterations in nucleotide metabolic pathways listed (choices B, C, and E) lead to disease states. Allopurinol (choice A) works principally to inhibit xanthine oxidase–mediated catabolism of xanthine to urate.

329. (A) Catabolism of the amino acids takes place to supply the body with needed energy, particularly in the absence of adequate carbohydrate and lipid intake. The carbon atoms of the amino acid are utilized as fuel either by being diverted into glucose production (glucogenic amino acids) or ketone body production (ketogenic amino acids). Several amino acids are both glucogenic and ketogenic. Leucine and lysine are the two amino acids that are strictly ketogenic, being catabolized to acetoacetate and acetyl-CoA (leucine) and acetoacetyl-CoA (lysine). Valine is catabolized to acetoacetate and acetyl-CoA and so is strictly ketogenic, but isoleucine (choice B) is catabolized to acetyl-CoA and propionyl-CoA. The latter can provide carbons for net glucose synthesis, hence isoleucine is both ketogenic and glucogenic. Choices C and D include amino acids of both choices A and B, thus do not reflect strictly ketogenic amino acids. Tyrosine (choice E) is both ketogenic, being catabolized to acetoacetate and acetyl-CoA, and glucogenic, since fumarate is another by-product of its catabolism. Catabolism of tryptophan (choice E) yields alanine residues, which make it glucogenic, and acetoacetyl-CoA, which is ketogenic.

330. (C) Marfan syndrome results in cardiovascular, musculoskeletal, and ophthalmic abnormalities as a result of a defect in the fibrillin gene. Fibrillin is a structural protein of the 10-nm microfibrils of cells. This class of microfibrils is primarily associated with amorphous elastin and is thought to serve at least 3 functions: linking elastin to other matrix structures, serving as scaffolds for elastin deposition, and performing structural functions in tissues lacking elastin. Osteogenesis imperfects (OI) (choice A) consists of a group of at least 4 types (mild, extensive, severe, and variable). Symptoms of OI arise due to defects in two α-collagen genes, the COL1A1 and COL1A2 genes. There have been over 100 mutations identified in these two genes. The mutations lead to decreased expression of collagen or abnormal proα1 proteins. The abnormal proteins associate with normal collagen subunits, which prevents the triple helical structure of normal collagen to form. The result is degradation of all the collagen proteins both normal and abnormal. Cutis laxa (choice B) is a disorder affecting connective tissue either through defective elastin metabolism or collagen metabolism. The latter mechanism is due to poor copper distribution as in occipital horn syndrome. However, cutis laxa is not X-linked as is occipital horn syndrome. Occipital horn syndrome (choice D), a disorder that manifests with symptoms similar to cutis laxa, results from defects in copper metabolism. The molecular basis for Ehlers–Danlos syndrome (choice E), which comprises at least 10 defined types of related symptoms, is heterogeneous. These related disorders are due to either defects in type III collagen metabolism, lysyl hydroxylation, or N-terminal procollagen protease.

331. (B) The synthesis of AMP from IMP and the salvage of IMP via AMP catabolism have the net effect of deaminating aspartate to fumarate. This process has been termed the purine nucleotide cycle. This cycle is very important in muscle cells. Increases in muscle activity create a demand for an increase in the TCA cycle, to generate more NADH for the production of ATP. However, muscle lacks most of the enzymes of the major anapleurotic reactions. Muscle replenishes TCA cycle intermediates in the form of fumarate generated by the purine nucleotide cycle. Choices A and C constitute pathways that do not involve nucleotides. There is no HGPRT or ADA cycle and hence, choices D and E do not represent real biological pathways.

332. (D) During the process of glycolysis two reactions are coupled to the phosphorylation of ADP to yield ATP, termed substrate-level phosphorylations. These two reactions are catalyzed by phosphoglycerate kinase and pyruvate kinase. The former enzyme phosphorylates ADP in the process of converting 1,3-bisphosphoglycerate to 3-phosphoglycerate, and the latter during the conversion of phosphoenolpyruvate (PEP) to pyruvate. Of the compounds listed, only the hydrolysis of PEP yields sufficient energy to be coupled to ADP phosphorylation. Hydrolysis of glucose-1-phosphate (choice A) does not occur. It is used as a substrate for glycogen metabolism, or is converted to glucose-6-phosphate by phosphoglucomutase and oxidized in the glycolytic pathway. 2,3-Bisphosphoglycerate (choice B) is formed from a side reaction of glycolysis within erythrocytes. Hydrolysis to 3-phosphoglycerate by 2,3-bisphosphoglycerate phosphatase does not yield ATP. Glycerol-3-phosphate (choice C) is not hydrolyzed, but is an intermediate in the synthesis of triacylglycerols or in the transfer of reducing equivalents from the cytosol to the mitochondria. Glucose-6-phosphate (choice E) serves as an entry point to glycolysis, and in this capacity is not hydrolyzed. When the liver is stimulated to deliver glucose to the blood, the phosphate is removed by glucose-6-phosphatase and no energy is generated.

333. (A) Phosphoglucose isomerase catalyzes the reversible conversion of fructose 6-phosphate to glucose-6-phosphate in both glycolysis and gluconeogenesis. In fact, most of the steps of glycolysis are simply reversed in gluconeogenesis. However, the three regulatory steps in the conversion of glucose to pyruvate are not reversible. These steps are: (1) glucose → glucose 6-phosphate (choice C), which is catalyzed by hexokinase, (2) fructose-6-phosphate → fructose-1,6-diphosphate (choice D), which is catalyzed by phosphofructokinase, and (3) phosphoenolpyruvate → pyruvate, which is catalyzed by pyruvate kinase. The reversal of these steps in gluconeogenesis requires the enzymes glucose 6-phosphatase and fructose-1,6-bisphosphatase for the formation of glucose and fructose-6-phosphate, respectively. The formation of phosphoenolpyruvate from pyruvate is more complicated in that these four steps are involved: (1) pyruvate carboxylase catalyzes the conversion of pyruvate to oxaloacetate, (choice B), (2) oxaloacetate is reduced to malate by mitochondrial malate dehydrogenase, (3) malate is reconverted to oxaloacetate by extramitochondrial malate dehydrogenase, and (4) oxaloacetate is transformed to phosphoenolpyruvate by GTP-dependent phosphoenolpyruvate carboxykinase (choice E).

334. (B) The formation of glycosylated hemoglobin occurs spontaneously (i.e., nonenzymatically through a reaction known as the Amadori rearrangement) in red blood cells. The amino terminal groups of the β-chains of hemoglobin complex with the aldehyde groups of glucose to form an amino ketone linkage. This form of hemoglobin is known as HbA_{1c}. Measurement of the circulating level of glycosylated hemoglobin is a diagnostic tool used to determine the relative length of hyperglycemia and can be used as a measure of treatment effectiveness. Glucose does not form covalent bonds with any of the other choices (A, C, D, and E).

335. (E) Patients with hereditary fructose intolerance have defective function in hepatic fructose-1-phosphate aldolase (also called aldolase B). This enzyme hydrolyzes fructose-1-phosphate to glyceraldehyde and dihydroxyacetone phosphate. The reaction is the second in the hepatic pathway of fructose metabolism, the initial one being the phosphorylation of fructose at the 1 position by fructokinase (choice B). When fructose is high in the diet (as in the consumption of large quantities of fruit) the capability to divert the fructose into the glycolytic pathway is severely impaired. Fructose becomes trapped in the liver as fructose-1-phosphate. Due to the lack of aldolase B, the capacity to phosphorylate fructose becomes limiting due to feedback inhibition of fructokinase, resulting in an elevation in serum fructose levels. Hepatic glucokinase (choice A) and aldolase A (choice D) are not involved in the metabolism of fructose. An allergic reaction (choice C) would not manifest with elevated serum fructose, hyperbilirubinemia, or hyperlacticacidemia.

336. (A) Fructose enters the liver and is phosphorylated to fructose-1-phosphate by fructokinase. This reaction requires ATP. The inability to further metabolize fructose in patients lacking aldolase B essentially traps hepatic energy in the form of fructose-1-phosphate. Gluconeogenesis requires a large input of energy and would be severely impaired by the trapping of phosphate energy in fructose. Since lactate is a major gluconeogenic substrate, the impaired ability to carry out gluconeogenesis would lead to hyperlacticacidemia. In the absence of aldolase B, fructose would not be metabolized by pyruvate, therefore, one would not have elevated levels of pyruvate (choice B). A vitamin insufficiency capable of leading to an inhibition of pyruvate dehydrogenase (choice C) would require a longer period of development than that seen in the patient. Additionally, symptoms would be more characteristic of beriberi, reflecting a niacin deficiency (choice E), than those of hyperbilirubinemia and hyperlacticacidemia. As indicated in the answer to 335, an allergic reaction (choice D) would not lead to the symptoms observed.

337. (C) In order for carbon atoms to be diverted into the gluconeogenic pathway, they must arrive in a form other than acetyl-CoA. Although acetyl-CoA enters the TCA cycle and intermediates from this cycle can be diverted into gluconeogenesis (oxaloacetate and malate), by the time the two carbons of acetyl-CoA have reached the point of these two TCA-cycle intermediates, there has been the release of two carbon atoms in the form of CO_2 (at the isocitrate dehydrogenase and α-ketoglutarate dehydrogenase catalyzed steps). The ketones acetoacetate (choice E) and β-hydroxybutyrate (choice B) are utilized by non-hepatic tissues as an energy source through a reversal of the process by which they were generated in the liver. The product of this reversal is acetyl-CoA, which then feeds into the TCA cycle for oxidation. The reduced electron carriers generated in the TCA cycle then provide the necessary energy to fuel the production of ATP in the oxidative–phosphorylation pathway. Cholesterol (choice D) is not degraded by the body, and as such has no means to supply carbon atoms to the gluconeogenic pathway. Fatty acids with an even number of carbon atoms, such as palmitate (choice A), are oxidized to acetyl-CoA, and therefore cannot provide carbons to gluconeogenesis. Fatty acids with odd numbers of carbon atoms have as an end product of oxidation propionyl-CoA. The propionyl-CoA is converted to succinyl-CoA, which enters the TCA cycle after the decarboxylation steps, and therefore can provide carbon atoms for net glucose synthesis. When stored triacylglycerides are hydrolyzed in response to hormonal signals, the glycerol backbone enters the blood and is transported to the liver, phosphorylated, and converted to dihydroxyacetone phosphate, which can then enter the gluconeogenic pathway.

338. **(E)** In infants, the supply of glycogen lasts less than 6 hours and gluconeogenesis is not sufficient to maintain adequate blood glucose levels. Normally, during periods of fasting (in particular during the night) the oxidation of fatty acids provides the necessary ATP to fuel hepatic gluconeogenesis as well as ketone bodies for non-hepatic tissue energy production. In patients with MCAD deficiency there is a drastically reduced capacity to oxidize fatty acids. This leads to an increase in glucose utilization with concomitant hypoglycemia. The deficit in the energy production from fatty acid oxidation, necessary for the liver to use other carbon sources, such as glycerol and amino acids, for gluconeogenesis further exacerbates the hypoglycemia. Normally, hypoglycemia is accompanied by an increase in ketone formation from the increased oxidation of fatty acids. In MCAD deficiency there is a reduced level of fatty acid oxidation, hence near normal levels of ketones are detected in the serum. None of the other choices (A, B, C, and D) reflect symptoms related in any way to MCAD deficiency and are not in themselves indicative of any specific disorder per se.

339. **(B)** One mechanism by which initiation of translation in eukaryotes is effected is by phosphorylation of a ser(S) residue in the α subunit of eIF-2. The factor eIF-2 requires activation by interaction with GTP. The energy of GTP hydrolysis is used during translational initiation, thereby allowing eIF-2 to have GDP bound instead of GTP. In order to reactivate eIF-2, the GDP must be exchanged for GTP. This requires an additional protein of the guanine–nucleotide exchange factor (GEF) family known as eIF-2B. The phosphorylated form of eIF-2, in the absence of the eIF-2B, is just as active an initiator of translation as the non-phosphorylated form. However, when eIF-2 is phosphorylated, the GDP-bound complex is stabilized and exchange for GTP is inhibited. When eIF-2 is phosphorylated it binds eIF-2B more tightly thus slowing the rate of exchange. It is this inhibited exchange that affects the rate of initiation. Within reticulocytes the phosphorylation of eIF-2 is the result of an activity called heme-controlled inhibitor (HCI). The presence of HCI was first seen in an in vitro translation system derived from lysates of reticulocytes. When heme is limiting it would be a waste of energy for reticulocytes to make globin protein, since active hemoglobin could not be generated. Therefore, when the level of heme falls, HCI becomes activated, leading to the phosphorylation of eIF-2 and reduced globin synthesis. Removal of phosphate is catalyzed by a specific eIF-2 phosphatase which is unaffected by heme. There is no effect of heme levels on RNA polymerase activity (choice A), or peptidyltransferase activity (choice C). No tRNA-specific degrading enzymes (choice D) are present in cells. There is no heme-controlled phosphatase activity (choice E) in any cell.

340. **(A)** Epinephrine binds to specific α- or β-type adrenergic receptors on hepatocytes or β-type receptors on skeletal muscle cells. Upon binding to either receptor type, intracellular changes take place to effect alterations in glycogen metabolism. Activation of β-adrenergic receptors leads to increased accumulation of cAMP, which in turn activates PKA leading to changes in the level of phosphorylation of numerous enzymes including those involved in glycogen metabolism. Glycogen breakdown is increased by the PKA-mediated phosphorylation and activation of synthase/phosphorylase kinase. Synthase/phosphorylase kinase then phosphorylates both phosphorylase and glycogen synthase. The phosphorylation of phosphorylase increases its activity such that an increase in glucose phosphorolysis from glycogen occurs. Conversely, phosphorylation of glycogen synthase reduces its activity, preventing glucose incorporation into glycogen. Glycogen synthase is also phosphorylated by PKA. Concomitant phosphorylation and activation of protein phosphatase inhibitor-1 leads to an inhibition of protein phosphatase-1, preventing removal of the newly incorporated phosphates thereby maintaining the altered activity of both enzymes. When α-adrenergic receptors are activated by epinephrine binding an increase in phospholipase C activity occurs. This enzyme hydrolyzes membrane phosphoinositides yielding diacylglycerol (DAG) and inositol trisphosphate (IP_3). IP_3 interacts with intracellular receptors leading to the release of intracellular stores of Ca^{2+}. The increased Ca^{2+} binds to the calmodulin subunit of phosphorylase kinase and activates it in the absence of phosphorylation. The net result is an increased rate of glycogen breakdown. Retinoic acid (choice B) binds to intracellular receptors which then interact with DNA to regulate gene expression. Insulin (choice C) binds to a transmembrane receptor, but stimulates glycogen accumulation, not breakdown. Parathyroid hormone (choice D) and thyrotropin (choice E) do not affect glycogen metabolism directly through activation of their cognate receptors.

341. (D) HDLs are synthesized de novo in the liver and small intestine, as primarily protein-rich disc-shaped particles. These newly formed HDLs are nearly devoid of any cholesterol and cholesteryl esters. HDLs are converted into spherical lipoprotein particles through the accumulation of cholesteryl esters. Any free cholesterol present in chylomicron remnants and VLDL remnants (IDLs) can be esterified through the action of the HDL-associated enzyme, lecithin–cholesterol acyltransferase (LCAT). LCAT is synthesized in the liver and so named because it transfers a fatty acid from the C-2 position of lecithin to the C-3-OH of cholesterol, generating a cholesteryl ester and lysolecithin. The activity of LCAT requires interaction with apo-A-I, which is found on the surface of HDLs. Cholesterol-rich HDLs return to the liver, where they are endocytosed, a process mediated through an HDL-specific apo-A-I receptor or through lipid–lipid interactions. Macrophages also take up HDLs through apo-A-I receptor interaction. HDLs can then acquire cholesterol and apo-E from the macrophages. Cholesterol-enriched HDLs are then secreted from the macrophages. HDLs also acquire cholesterol by extracting it from cell surface membranes. This process has the effect of lowering the level of intracellular cholesterol, since the cholesterol stored within cells as cholesteryl esters will be mobilized to replace the cholesterol removed from the plasma membrane. The cholesterol esters of HDLs can also be transferred to VLDLs and LDLs through the action of the HDL-associated enzyme, cholesterol ester transfer protein (CETP, also identified as apo-D). This has the added effect of allowing the excess cellular cholesterol to be returned to the liver through the LDL-receptor pathway as well as the HDL-receptor pathway. VLDLs (choice B) are synthesized in the liver for transport of fatty acids (in the form of triacylglycerols) to nonhepatic tissues. Cholesterol represents only 15 to 20% of the total lipid content of VLDLs when they leave hepatocytes. As VLDLs circulate in the plasma, the loss of fatty acids changes them to IDLs (choice C), and finally to LDLs (choice A), which return to the liver. As indicated above, HDLs transfer cholesterol to IDLs and LDLs in order for it to be transported to the liver. Chylomicrons (choice E) are lipoproteins that carry dietary lipid through the body. As pointed out, HDLs transfer cholesterol to chylomicron remnants which then transport the cholesterol to the liver.

342. (B) Two familial syndromes directly involve defects in LCAT. Familial LCAT deficiency is characterized by near complete absence of the enzyme activity from the plasma. Fish eye disease is characterized by an absence of LCAT activity toward high-density lipoproteins (HDLs) but presence of activity toward low-density lipoproteins (LDLs). Clinical features of familial LCAT deficiency include corneal opacities, anemia, and proteinuria. Due to the lack of LCAT activity, the plasma level of esterified cholesterol is lower than normal and phosphatidylcholine (the principal source of fatty acid for esterification to cholesterol) levels are higher than normal. The profile of all classes of plasma lipoproteins in patients with familial LCAT deficiency is abnormal. Familial hypercholesterolemia (choice A) is characterized by reduced LDL clearance which leads to severe hypercholesterolemia. Major clinical symptoms are arterial deposition of LDL-cholesterol which leads to atherosclerosis and coronary artery disease. Deposition of LDL-cholesterol is also seen in tendons and skin resulting in xanthomas. Wolman's disease (choice C) is cholesterol ester storage disease that leads to massive accumulation of cholesteryl esters and triglycerides in most tissues. This disease is almost always fatal within the first year of life and thus would not be present in a 28-year-old. Bassen–Kornzweig syndrome (choice D) also identified as abetalipoproteinemia, is due to a defect in apo-B expression. Clinical symptoms include retinitis pigmentosa, ataxic neuropathy and erythrocytes appear thorny (acanthocytosis). Familial hypertriacylglycerolemia (choice E), also identified as hyperlipoproteinemia type IV, is a form of lipoprotein lipase deficiency. The defect leads to increased levels of circulating VLDLs and is associated with glucose intolerance and hyperinsulinemia. This disorder is frequently associated with type 2 diabetes.

343. (B) Several proteins of the clotting cascade are posttranslationally modified by a vitamin K–dependent reaction that incorporates carboxy groups onto the R-groups of intrachain glutamates generating γ-carboxyglutamate residues (gla residues). Proteins of the cascade so modified include prothrombin, factors VII, IX, and X, as well as protein S. The incorporation of gla residues is absolutely required for biological activity of these factors. The gla residues allow the clotting factors to chelate calcium ions. Because the carboxylation reaction requires vitamin K, agents that competitively block vitamin K action, such as warfarin and dicumarol, act as anticoagulants. Hydroxyproline (choice A) and hydroxylysine (choice E) are found in the collagens. Many proteins are phosphorylated and this occurs primarily at serine residues (choice C). Acetylation of N-terminal residues of proteins is a common post-translational modification, and if this occurred when methionine remained as the N-terminal amino acid, N-acetylmethionine would be seen (choice D).

344. (E) Enzymes that are destined for the lysosomes (lysosomal enzymes) are directed there by a specific carbohydrate modification. During transit through the Golgi apparatus a residue of N-acetylglucosamine-1-phosphate is added to carbon 6 of one or more specific mannose residues that have been incorporated into these enzymes. The N-acetylglucosamine is activated by coupling to UDP, and is transferred by an N-acetylglucosamine phosphotransferase, yielding N-acetylglucosamine-1-phosphate-6-mannose-protein. A second reaction removes the N-acetylglucosamine, leaving mannose residues phosphorylated in the 6 position. A specific mannose-6-phosphate receptor is present in the membranes of the Golgi apparatus. Binding of mannose-6-phosphate to this receptor targets proteins to the lysosomes. Defects in the proper targeting of glycoproteins to the lysosomes can also lead to clinical complications. Deficiencies in N-acetylglucosamine phosphotransferase lead to the formation of dense inclusion bodies in fibroblasts. Two disorders related to deficiencies in the targeting of lysosomal enzymes are termed I-cell disease (mucolipidosis II) and pseudo-Hurler polydystrophy (mucolipidosis III). I-cell disease is characterized by severe psychomotor retardation, skeletal abnormalities, coarse facial features, painful restricted joint movement, and early mortality. Pseudo-Hurler polydystrophy is less severe; it progresses more slowly, and afflicted individuals live to adulthood. Each of the other choices (A, B, C, and D) represent other potential pathways that are not affected in the processing, delivery, or presentation of lysosomal enzymes or the receptors that recognize the properly processed enzymes.

345. (A) Although multiorgan involvement, liver and spleen enlargement and skeletal abnormalities are common to all the mucopolysaccharidotic (MPS) diseases, each encompasses features that allow for specific diagnosis. Hurler's syndrome is characterized by progressive multiorgan failure and premature death. Hallmark features include enlargement of the spleen and liver, severe skeletal deformity, and coarse facial features (which are associated with the constellation of defects referred to as dystosis multiplex). The disease results from a defect in α-L-iduronidase activity, which leads to intracellular accumulations of heparan sulfates and dermatan sulfates. The accumulation of these GAGs in Hurler's syndrome patients severely affects development of the skeletal system leading, primarily, to defective long bone growth plate disruption. Sanfilippo syndrome (choice B) comprises four recognized types characterized by severe central nervous system degeneration with only mild involvement of other organ systems. Symptoms do not appear until two to six years of age. Hunter's syndrome (choice C) has features similar to that of Hurler's with a lack of corneal clouding. Additionally, symptoms progress slower, with onset of symptoms occurring between two and four years of age. Morquio's syndrome (choice D) comprises two related disorders, both of which are characterized by short-trunk dwarfism, fine corneal deposits, and a skeletal dysplasia (spondyloepiphyseal) distinct from other MPS. Maroteaux–Lamy syndrome (choice E) encompasses symptoms similar to Hurler's but with normal mental development.

346. (A) In the reversible formation of glycine from serine, the side chain β-carbon of serine is transferred as a methylene group to tetrahydrofolate (H_4folate) to form N^5,N^{10}-methylene-H_4folate, which plays a central role in one-carbon metabolism. The reaction is catalyzed by serine transhydroxymethylase, which is a pyridoxal phosphate–requiring enzyme. N^5,N^{10}-methylene-H_4folate can be reduced to N^5-methyl-H_4folate which is necessary for methionine synthesis. Thus, serine is the major source of one-carbon units for tetrahydrofolate derivatives. None of the other amino acids (choices B, C, D, and E) directly participates in the one-carbon pool.

347. (D) β-Endorphin is the only protein derived from the POMC gene. The POMC gene encodes an mRNA that can be processed to yield at least eight separate proteins with distinct activities. Several act as hormones [adrenocorticotropic hormone (ACTH), β- and γ-lipotropins, α- and β-melanocyte–stimulating hormones (MSH), and corticotropin-like intermediary peptide (CLIP)] while others serve as neurotransmitters or neuromodulators (β-endorphin and met-enkephalin). The location of expression of the POMC gene dictates which of the biologically active proteins are made. Oxytocin (choice A) is derived from prepro-oxytocin, a protein that is processed into oxytocin and neurophysin I. Cholecystokinin (choice B) is an intestinal peptide hormone. Atrial natriuretic factor (choice C) is produced in the atria of the heart. Bradykinin (choice E) is derived from a plasma glycoprotein identified as high molecular weight (HMW) kininogen through the action of active plasma kallikrein.

348. (C) Deficiency in α-keto acid decarboxylase leads to maple syrup urine disease, named because the odor of urine from patients resembles that of maple syrup or burnt sugar. Plasma levels of leucine, isoleucine, valine, and their α-keto acids are elevated. The defect is evident within the first week following birth. Diagnosis prior to this time is only possible by enzymatic analysis. Extensive brain damage results and infants die within the first year. Phenylketonuria (PKU) (choice A) is characterized by excess production of alternative catabolites of phenylalanine (phenylpyruvate), phenylacetate, and phenyllactate). This disorder leads to mental retardation if left untreated. Routine neonatal screening for PKU is now compulsory. Alkaptonuria (choice B) is characterized by the darkening, upon exposure to air, of urine from afflicted individuals. As the name implies, isovaleric acidemia (choice D) is elevated serum levels of isovaleric acid, a by-product of leucine catabolism. Symptoms are evident following ingestion of protein-rich foods. Homocystinurias (choice E) are defects in methionine catabolism, evidenced by elevated levels of homocystine in the urine. Clinical symptoms include thromboses, osteoporosis, and frequently mental retardation.

349. (D) Heparin is a naturally occurring sulfated glycosaminoglycan (GAG) that plays an important role in the regulation of blood coagulation. It is found primarily in granules of mast cells and is released when these cells are stimulated. Heparan sulfates present on the surfaces of vascular endothelial cells also have limited antithrombic activity. Heparin binds to the major thrombin inhibitor, antithrombin III, resulting in an altered conformation of antithrombin III. The altered conformation has a higher affinity for thrombin (as well as for the activated forms of factors IX, X, XI, and XII) resulting in a reduced capacity of thrombin to convert fibrinogen to fibrin. Hyaluronate (choice A) predominates in synovial fluid and vitreous humor. Keratan sulfate (choice B) is found in cornea and bone and in aggregates with chondroitin sulfates in cartilage. Dermatan sulfates (choice C) are found in skin, heart valves, and vessels. In addition to cartilage, chondroitin sulfates (choice E) are found in bone and heart valves. None of these GAGs exhibit antithrombic activity.

350. (A) Gout is characterized by elevated levels of uric acid in the blood and urine. Uric acid is the end-product of purine catabolism and excess production results from a variety of metabolic abnormalities that lead to overproduction of purines via the de novo pathway. Uric acid is very insoluble and when generated in large amounts will precipitate as uric acid crystals in the joints of the extremities and in renal interstitial tissue. These deposits are gritty or sandy in nature and thus are termed tophaceous deposits. Lesch–Nyhan disease (choice B) is due to loss of hypoxanthine–guanine phosphoribosyltransferase activity. Characteristic symptoms include severe mental retardation and self-mutilation. A much less severe symptom associated with Lesch–Nyhan disease is hyperuricemia, which leads to gouty episodes. However, other symptoms are of such severity that patients die very early in life. Deficiency in glucose-6-phosphatase results in von Gierke's disease (choice C). Clinical symptoms of von Gierke's disease include fasting hypoglycemia, lactic acidemia, and mild gouty episodes. The hyperuricemia of von Gierke's disease is seldom severe enough to lead to the level of gouty deposits observed in this patient. Purine nucleotide phosphorylase (choice D) and adenosine deaminase (choice E) deficiencies result in various degrees of immune dysfunction and are not associated with gouty episodes.

351. (C) The first reaction of de novo pyrimidine biosynthesis is catalyzed by aspartate transcarbamoylase. This reaction is also the rate-limiting step in this pathway. PRPP synthetase (choice A) catalyzes the production of PRPP (used in the synthesis of purines and pyrimidines) from ribose-5-phosphate and ATP. PRPP amido transferase (choice B) is an enzyme of the de novo purine biosynthesis pathway. OMP decarboxylase (choice D) catalyzes the decarboxylation of OMP, yielding UMP. Ribonucleotide reductase (choice E) is required for the reduction of ribonucleotides to deoxyribonucleotides.

352. (D) Nitric oxide (NO) is generated from arginine in a reaction catalyzed by NO synthase (NOS). The other product of the reaction is citrulline. None of the other amino acids (choices A, B, C, and E) are substrates for NOS.

353. (E) Calcitriol [1,25-$(OH)_2$-D] is the hormonally active form of vitamin D and functions in concert with parathyroid hormone (PTH) and calcitonin to regulate serum calcium and phosphorous levels. The major function of calcitriol is the induction of synthesis of an intestinal calcium-binding protein, calbinden, which facilitates intestinal absorption of calcium. Oral administration of calcitriol will increase intestinal calcium uptake, but the hormone does not enter the peripheral circulation in significant amounts. Therefore, patients with renal osteodystrophy may need intravenous administration of calcitriol. Calcitonin (choice A) acts to block bone resorption when there are sufficient levels of calcium in the serum. PTH (choice B) acts to increase bone resorption, in concert with calcitriol, when serum calcium levels fall. Growth hormone (choice C) does not influence calcium homeostasis and would therefore not be useful in the treatment of renal osteodystrophy. Antidiuretic hormone (choice D) is responsible for renal water readsorption in response to increased extracellular Na^+ concentrations which lead to increased plasma osmolarity.

354. (B) Primary aldosteronism (Conn's syndrome) leads to elevated production of aldosterone and the symptoms presented by the patient. This disorder is due to small adenomas of the glomerulosa cells of the kidney. The associated hyperkalemia, hypertension, and hypernatremia lead to a reduction in renin release from the juxtaglomerulosa cells. Renin is required for the conversion of angiotensinogen (released from the liver) to angiotensin I (which is in turn converted to angiotensin II by converting enzyme), and so reduced levels of renin lead to reduced levels of angiotensin II. Androstenedione (choice A), is produced from pregnenolone via the 17α-hydroxylase pathway of androgen synthesis in the adrenal cortex or of estrogen synthesis in the ovary. Androstenedione is derived from DHEA (choice D) and is converted to estradiol (choice C) in the ovary or to testosterone (choice E) in the testis. Estrogens are responsible for maturation of the ovaries and testosterone maturation of sperm. None of these steroids regulate sodium or potassium and would therefore not lead to the symptoms presented if elevated or reduced.

355. (B) Tyrosine is the precursor for each of these neurotransmitters. Tyrosine hydroxylase converts tyrosine to dopa, which is in turn converted to dopamine, then to norepinephrine, and finally epinephrine. None of the other amino acids (choices A, C, D, and E) can serve as precursors for these neurotransmitters.

356. (C) Prolactin is necessary for initiation and maintenance of lactation. Physiological levels act only on breast tissue primed by female sex hormones. Endocrine dysfunction leading to excessive prolactin production is associated with breast enlargement and impotence in males. Excessive production of growth hormone (choice A) leads to gigantism if it occurs prior to epiphysial plate closure. If excessive release occurs following epiphysial plate closure acromegaly results, with characteristic facial changes (protruding jaw, enlarged nose) and enlarged feet, hands, and skull. Excessive production of gonadotropin-releasing hormone (choice B) would lead to increased production of luteinizing hormone (LH), follicle-stimulating hormone (FSH), and chorionic gonadotropin (hCG), with consequent effects on the female reproductive system. Excessive production of corticotropin-releasing hormone (choice D) would result in an increase in ACTH production which would lead to enhanced glucocorticoid and mineralocorticoid production. Excessive production of melanocyte-stimulating hormone (choice E) would lead to hyperpigmentation of the skin.

357. (A) Huntington's disease (HD) is an autosomal dominant disorder leading to progressive memory loss, personality changes, and peculiar motor problems such as involuntary movements of the arms and legs. The disease results from the expansion of a CAG triplet in the amino terminus of the HD protein, referred to as huntingtin. The repeats number from 10 to 30 in normal chromosomes and from 36 to 121 on the HD chromosomes. There is a general correlation between the length of the repeat and the age of onset of symptoms. Cystic fibrosis (CF) (choice B) is due primarily to a common mutation (in 70% of cases) that deletes three nucleotides in exon 10 of the CF gene which codes for the cystic fibrosis transmembrane conductance receptor (CFTR). Over 600 other mutations have been identified in the CF gene. Duchenne's muscular dystrophy (DMD) (choice C) results from deletions in one or more of the exons of the DMD gene which encodes the protein referred to as dystrophin. Menkes disease (choice D) is due to defects in copper absorption leading to defective function of numerous enzymes that need copper as a cofactor. Familial hypercholesterolemia (choice E) results from defects in the gene encoding the LDL receptor. These defects encompass insertions and deletions that can be found throughout the length of the LDL-receptor gene.

358. (C) The rate-limiting step in glycolysis occurs at the reaction catalyzed by phosphofructokinase-1 (PFK-1). This enzyme catalyzes the phosphorylation of fructose-6-phosphate to fructose-1,6-bisphosphate. PFK-1 is controlled by numerous allosteric effectors that act in either a positive or negative manner. The reaction depicted by choice A is catalyzed by glucokinase/hexokinase. This reaction is regulated by product inhibition, but does not constitute a rate-limiting step in glycolysis. The reactions catalyzed by phosphoglucose isomerase (choice B), fructose-1,6-bisphosphate aldolase or aldolase A (choice D), and triose phosphate isomerase (choice E) are freely reversible and are therefore not regulated reactions of glycolysis.

359. (E) Adenosine deaminase (ADA) catalyzes the deamination of adenosine to inosine during the catabolism of purines. Loss of ADA leads to significantly elevated levels of phosphorylated deoxyadenosine (in particular deoxyadenosine triphosphate, dATP). Levels of dATP in ADA deficiency can reach 50 times normal. High concentrations of dATP inhibit ribonucleotide reductase, which is required for the generation of deoxynucleotides from ribonucleotides. The inhibition of ribonucleotide reductase leads to severely impaired cellular DNA synthesis. Since lymphocytes must be able to proliferate dramatically in response to antigenic challenge, the loss of ADA activity results in a near complete lack of immune function. Purine nucleoside phosphorylase (PNP) (choice A) is also a purine catabolic enzyme which converts inosine to hypoxanthine and guanosine to guanine. Deficiency in PNP leads to a mild immunodeficiency. Orotic acid decarboxylase (choice B) catalyzes the decarboxylation of OMP to UMP. Deficiency in this enzyme results in orotic aciduria, type II. Aspartate transcarbamoylase (ATC) (choice C) is a component of a multifunctional enzyme which catalyzes the rate-limiting reaction of pyrimidine biosynthesis. No known deficiencies in this enzyme have been identified, likely due to the embryonic lethality predicted if the enzyme were defective. Hypoxanthine–guanine phosphoribosyl transferase (HGPRT) (choice D) catalyzes the salvage of hypoxanthine to IMP and guanine to GMP. Deficiency in HGPRT results in Lesch–Nyhan syndrome.

360. (D) DNA fingerprinting refers to the process of using polymorphic repeat sequences to establish a unique pattern of DNA fragments for any given individual. The polymorphic repeats that are identifiable by the fingerprinting technique are hypervariable repeats such as variable number tandem repeats (VNTRs). The bands are detected by Southern blotting enzyme-digested chromosomal DNA and probing the blot with various different VNTR probes. Hybridization (choice A) refers to the specific association of complimentary strands of DNA to one another. DNA footprinting (choice B) refers to the identification of sequences of DNA to which specific proteins bind, thereby rendering the DNA at that site resistant to digestion by DNA degrading nucleases. The PCR (choice C) uses synthetic oligonucleotides to direct the enzymatic amplification of specific sequences of DNA. The generation of a DNA library (choice E) refers to the establishment of a complete collection of cloned fragments of DNA, either from genomic sources or cDNA.

361. (D) The first reaction of heme biosynthesis takes place in the mitochondrion and involves the condensation of glycine and succinyl-CoA to yield δ-aminolevulinic acid (ALA). This reaction is catalyzed by ALA synthase and represents the rate-limiting step of heme biosynthesis. Once made, ALA is transported to the cytosol where ALA dehydratase (choice A) catalyzes the condensation of two moles of ALA to form porphobilinogen. Porphobilinogen (PBG) deaminase, also termed uroporphyrinogen I synthetase, (choice B) catalyzes the condensation of four moles of porphobilinogen yielding hydroxymethylbilane. Ferrochetalase (choice C) is a mitochondrial enzyme that catalyzes the final reaction of heme biosynthesis, which is the insertion of iron into the ring system of protoporphyrin IX. Uroporphyrinogen decarboxylase (choice E) catalyzes the decarboxylation of type III uroporphyrinogen yielding coproporphyrinogen III.

362. (B) The polyamines comprise spermine and spermidine. These compounds are derived from methionine and L-ornithine. None of the other amino acids (choices A, C, D, and E) can serve as precursors for polyamine biosynthesis.

363. (C) Zellweger syndrome is the most severe of a group of diseases that result from defective assembly of the peroxisomes, leading to the characteristic symptoms observed in the patient. This syndrome is apparent at birth and leads to death within the first year. The cause of Zellweger syndrome is a failure to import newly synthesized peroxisomal proteins into peroxisomes. Neonatal adrenoleukodystrophy (choice A), infantile Refsum's disease (choice B), and hyperpipecolic acidemia (choice D) are all much less severe disorders of the group that result from peroxisome dysfunction. Affected individuals with these latter disorders can survive into the third or fourth decade, albeit with deficits in vision, hearing, and cognitive function. It is suspected that the reduced severity of these three disorders, relative to Zellweger, relates to retention of partial gene function as opposed to complete loss. RCDP (choice E) is related to peroxisomal dysfunction at the level of their distribution and structure. The phenotype of RCDP differs from that of Zellweger syndrome in that patients have striking shortening of the proximal limbs, coronal clefts of vertebral bodies, and severely abnormal endochondrial bone formation.

364. (A) Apoprotein B-48 is found exclusively associated with chylomicrons and no other lipoprotein particle. Apo-B-48 is synthesized from an mRNA that is transcribed from the apo-B-100 gene. Following transcription the mRNA is edited within the intestinal epithelium yielding the B-48 transcript. Apo(a) (choice B) is an apoprotein found disulfide bonded to apo-B-100. This then forms a complex with LDL, generating a novel lipoprotein particle identified as lipoprotein(a), Lp(a). Lp(a) has a strong resemblance to plasminogen and its presence in the circulation is highly correlated with premature coronary artery disease. Apo-E (choice C) is found in chylomicrons, VLDLs, LDLs, IDLs, and HDLs. It is necessary for interaction of lipoprotein with the LDL-receptor (which is also referred to as the apo-B-100/apo-E receptor). Apo-C-II (choice D) is present in chylomicrons, VLDLs, LDLs, IDLs, and HDLs and is necessary for the activation of endothelial cell lipoprotein lipase. Apo-D (choice E) is found exclusively with HDLs and is also called cholesterol ester transfer protein (CETP).

365. (D) The non-oxidative portion of the pentose phosphate pathway performs carbohydrate remodeling reaction, interconverting 3, 4, 5, 6, and 7 carbon sugars. Transaldolase catalyzes the interconversion of erythrose-4-phosphate and fructose-6-phosphate into glyceraldehyde-3-phosphate and sedoheptulose-7-phosphate. Ribulose-5-phosphate 3-epimerase (choice A) interconverts ribulose-5-phosphate and xylulose-5-phosphate. Ribose-5-phosphate ketoisomerase (choice B) catalyzes the interconversion of ribulose-5-phosphate and ribose-5-phosphate. Transketolase (choices C and E) catalyzes the interconversion of xylulose-5-phosphate and ribose-5-phosphate into sedoheptulose-7-phosphate and glyceraldehyde-3-phosphate, as well as the interconversion of xylulose-5-phosphate and erythrose-4-phosphate into glyceraldehyde-3-phosphate and fructose-6-phosphate.

366. (C) Acromegaly results when there is an excess production of growth hormone after epiphysial closure and cessation of long bone growth. Excessive production of insulin-like growth factor II (choice A) could lead to abnormal neonatal development since it is expressed only during this period. Excessive production of gonadotropin-releasing hormone (choice B) would lead to increased production of luteinizing hormone (LH), follicle-stimulating hormone (FSH), and chorionic gonadotropin (hCG), with consequent effects on the female reproductive system. Excessive production of corticotropin-releasing hormone (choice D) would result in an increase in ACTH production, which would lead to enhanced glucocorticoid and mineralocorticoid production. Excessive production of thyroid-stimulating hormone (choice E) would lead to increased release of the thyroid hormones, leading to multisystemic involvement such as rapid heart rate, nervousness, inability to sleep, weight loss, excessive sweating, and sensitivity to heat.

367. (C) Transferrin is a glycoprotein synthesized in the liver having a central role in the body's metabolism of iron. Each mole of transferrin can transport two moles of Fe^{3+} in the circulation to sites where iron is required. Free iron is toxic, but when associated with transferrin this toxicity is greatly diminished. When bound to transferrin, iron can be directed to cells where it is needed. Many cells have transferrin receptors and upon binding, the transferrin–receptor complex is internalized. The acidic pH of the lysosome causes the iron to dissociate from transferrin. Iron-free transferrin is then recycled to the cell surface along with its receptor, where it then re-enters the circulation. Ceruloplasmin (choice A) is the major copper carrier of the body and is also synthesized in the liver. Metallothioneins (choice B) are found in many cells and can bind copper, zinc, cadmium, and mercury. Ferritin (choice D) is an intracellular iron-binding protein. It does not play a role in iron metabolism or transport, and its function is to prevent ionized iron (Fe^{2+}) from reaching toxic levels within cells. Haptoglobin (choice E) is a plasma glycoprotein that binds extracorpuscular (free) hemoglobin. This function of haptoglobin is to prevent free hemoglobin from being lost through the kidneys, since the haptoglobin-hemoglobin complex is too large to pass through the glomerulus.

368. (E) Synthesis of the prostaglandins (PGs), thromboxanes (TXs), and leukotrienes (LTs) occurs from arachidonic acid, which is liberated from membrane phospholipids following activation of various receptors (e.g., epinephrine, bradykinin, thrombin). PGs and TXs are synthesized by the cyclic pathway, LTs by the linear pathway. The initial step of PG and TX synthesis is catalyzed by the enzyme prostaglandin endoperoxide synthase. This enzyme possesses two activities, cyclooxygenase and peroxidase. It is the cyclooxygenase activity that is the target of the NSAIDs. Phospholipase A_2 (choice A) is the enzyme responsible for the release of arachidonic acid from membrane phospholipids. This enzyme is inhibited by the anti-inflammatory steroids. HMG CoA reductase (choice B) is the rate-limiting enzyme of cholesterol biosynthesis. Lipoxygenase (choice C) catalyzes the initial step in leukotriene synthesis from arachidonate. Once formed, prostaglandins are rapidly inactivated in order to limit their effects. 15-Hydroxyprostaglandin dehydrogenase (choice D) is the principal enzyme responsible for this rapid inactivation process.

369. (A) Menkes' disease is an X-linked recessive disorder that is manifest by a defect in copper absorption. This defect leads to dysfunction of numerous enzymes that need copper as a cofactor, leading to the typical symptoms observed in this patient. In fact, Menkes' is also referred to as steely hair disease, because of the characteristic brittleness of the hair, which is easily broken. Hemochromatosis (choice B) is the term applied when organ structure and function are impaired by the presence of excess amounts of iron. The liver, heart, pancreas, skin, joints, and endocrine organs are the principal tissues affected by iron accumulation. Symptoms include cirrhosis, cardiomyopathy, arthritis, abnormal skin pigmentation, and hypogonadism, as well as diabetes mellitus. Refsum's disease (choice C) results from a defect in the metabolism of phytanic acid, a plant lipid which must be oxidized by a separate pathway from that of animal fats. Cardinal symptoms include retinitis pigmentosa, peripheral neuropathy, and cerebellar ataxia. Gilbert syndrome (choice D) results from a defect in bilirubin metabolism. It is typically diagnosed in young adults and is characterized by mild, chronic, and unconjugated hyperbilirubinemia without associated hemolysis. Crigler–Najjar syndrome type I (choice E) is also due to defective bilirubin metabolism as a result of a loss of UDP-glucuronosyltransferase (UGT) activity. UGT is required to transfer two moles of glucuronic acid to bilirubin, generating bilirubin–diglucuronide, which makes bilirubin much more water soluble and therefore facilitates its excretion. Crigler–Najjar syndrome results in nonhemolytic icterus (jaundice) within the first few days of life and is generally fatal during neonatal life due to severe kernicterus.

370. (B) Porphobilinogen (PBG) deaminase (also referred to as uroporphyrinogen I synthase) catalyzes the conversion of four moles of porphobilinogen to hydroxymethylbilane. Porphobilinogen is the product of the δ-aminolevulinic acid (ALA) synthase. Therefore, a deficiency in PBG deaminase would lead to an elevation in the excretion of ALA and PBG. All products of the heme biosynthesis pathway from porphobilinogen on would be produced at extremely reduced levels due to a deficiency in PBG deaminase. This would include hydroxymethylbilane (choice C), type III uroporphyrinogen (choice D), which is produced from hydroxymethylbilane, coproporphyrinogen III (choice A), which is produced from type III uroporphyrinogen, and protoporphyrin IX (choice E), which is produced in several steps from coproporphyrinogen.

371. (E) Phosphorylase kinase (also referred to as phosphorylase/synthase kinase, because it can phosphorylate both glycogen phosphorylase and glycogen synthase) contains calmodulin as a subunit. The presence of calmodulin allows phosphorylase kinase to be activated in the absence of a cAMP-mediated phosphorylation cascade. This is important when muscle is stimulated by epinephrine binding to α-adrenergic receptors (this function is diagrammed in Figure 3–7) or by acetylcholine release at the neuromuscular junction. Each of these events leads to increases in intracellular Ca^{2+}. Each of the other proteins (choices A, B, C, and D) are independent activities not associated with phosphorylase kinase.

372. (A) Ornithine transcarbamoylase and carbamoyl phosphate synthetase I are the two enzymes of the urea cycle that are found in the mitochondria. Arginase (choice B), argininosuccinase (choice C) and argininosuccinate synthetase (choice D) are all found in the cytoplasm.

373. (B) The enzymes ferrochetalase and δ-aminolevulinic acid (ALA) synthetase are extremely sensitive to lead poisoning, which leads to severe anemia and excretion of high levels of coproporphyrinogen and ALA. None of the other enzymes (choices A, C, D, and E) of heme biosynthesis are affected by lead ingestion.

374. (B) Carbohydrate modification of proteins occurs by attachment of the carbohydrates to either hydroxyl groups (e.g., serine and threonine or hydroxylysines in collagen), termed O-linked glycoproteins, or amino groups (of asparagine), termed N-linked glycoproteins. The processing of both types of glycoproteins begins in the endoplasmic reticulum (choice D) either while the proteins are being synthesized (O-linked) or following completion of synthesis (N-linked). However, the terminal modifications to the carbohydrates occurs as the proteins progress through the Golgi apparatus to the cell surface. Carbohydrate modification only occurs in the endoplasmic reticulum and golgi, not in the mitochondria (choice A), at the plasma membrane (choice C), or in the lysosomes (choice E).

375. (E) Several enzymes of the blood clotting cascade (e.g., factors II, VII, IX, X, and protein C) bind calcium and are thus activated following cleavage of their zymogen forms. The ability of these proteins to bind calcium requires post-translationally modified glutamate residues. The modification is a γ-carboxylation yielding γ-carboxyglutamate (gla) residues. The carboxylation reaction has an absolute requirement for vitamin K as a cofactor. None of the other amino acid modifications (choices A, B, C, and D) requires vitamin K as a cofactor. Hydroxylation of proline (choice A) and lysine (choice D) is carried out by enzymes that require vitamin C as a cofactor.

376. (C) Steroid hormones are lipophilic and hence freely penetrate the plasma membrane of all cells. Within target cells, steroid hormones interact with specific receptors. These receptor proteins are composed of two domains; a hormone-binding domain and a DNA-binding domain. Following hormone–receptor interaction the complex is activated and enters the nucleus. The DNA-binding domain of the receptor interacts with specific nucleotide sequences termed hormone response elements (HREs). The binding of steroid–receptor complexes to HREs results in an altered rate of transcription of the associated gene(s). The effects of steroid–receptor complexes on specific target genes can be either stimulatory or inhibitory with respect to the rate of transcription. Complexes of steroid with receptor have no direct effect on DNA replication (choice A), post-transcriptional processing of RNA (choice B), translation (choice D), or post-translational events (choice E).

377. (A) When fatty acids are destined for oxidation they must first be activated by acetylation to coenzyme A to yield fatty acyl-CoAs. The biosynthesis of coenzyme A requires pantothenic acid (vitamin B_5) as a portion of the molecule. Therefore, fat oxidation requires vitamin B_5 as a cofactor. The synthesis of fatty acids begins with activated acetate (acetyl-CoA) and thus also requires vitamin B_5 as a cofactor. Additionally, fatty acid synthase (the multifunctional enzyme of fatty acid synthesis) contains an acyl carrier domain harboring a 4′-phosphopantetheine moiety derived from vitamin B_5. Thiamine (choice B), biotin (choice C), and cobalamin (choice D) are not involved in either biosynthesis or oxidation of fatty acids. Riboflavin (choice E) is necessary for fatty acid oxidation, but not for synthesis.

378. (B) Several amino acids required for human protein synthesis can be produced by normal metabolic pathways, provided sufficient precursors are made available in the diet. However, several amino acids are absolutely required in the diet because humans cannot synthesize them and are hence essential amino acids. Methionine is one of the essential amino acids, in particular large amounts are required to produce cysteine (a nonessential amino acid), if cysteine is not supplied in adequate amounts in the diet. All of the other amino acid choices (A, C, D, and E) are not essential.

379. (D) Glucose-6-phosphatase is required by the liver for it to supply the rest of the body with glucose that has been produced by hepatic gluconeogenesis or released from stored hepatic glycogen. A deficiency in glucose-6-phosphatase leads to the most common of the glycogen storage diseases, von Gierke's disease. This glycogen storage disease results from excess hepatic glucose-6-phosphate allosterically activating the β form of glycogen synthase, leading to increased conversion of glucose into glycogen. Glucagon (choice A) is released in response to reduced levels of blood glucose. Since a deficiency in glucose-6-phosphatase would hinder release of glucose from the liver, there would be an increase in the release of glucagon, not a decrease. Although a reduced level of circulating blood glucose could negatively affect skeletal muscle glucose utilization, the enzyme defect does not itself lead to decreased muscle glycogen production (choice B). The reduced delivery of glucose from the liver could lead to hypoglycemia, not hyperglycemia (choice C). Since the defect is not in the enzymes of glycogen synthesis, the character of glycogen (i.e., its level of branching) would not be affected (choice E).

380. (E) During starvation the ability of the liver to supply the brain with needed glucose diminishes. This leads to a shift in hepatic metabolism to that of increased fatty acid oxidation to produce large amounts of acetyl-CoA that can be diverted into ketone body production. The ketone bodies are then delivered to the blood and used by the brain (and other peripheral tissues) as an energy source. The brain cannot use fatty acids for energy production (choice A). Delivery of fatty acids from adipose tissue to the liver would accelerate during fasting and starvation as a source of acetyl-CoA for ketone body production. Fasting and starvation would lead to a depletion of hepatic glycogen stores (choice B), therefore this would not serve as a source for glucose delivery to the blood. Amino acids (choice C) are not themselves used directly as sources of energy, but are oxidized into compounds that can be. The brain does not store glucose in the form of glycogen (choice D).

381. (A) The major substrates of gluconeogenesis are pyruvate and lactate. During gluconeogenesis lactate is oxidized to pyruvate. For pyruvate to be converted back to glucose it must first be carboxylated to oxaloacetate, since a reversal of the pyruvate kinase reaction of glycolysis cannot occur to convert the pyruvate to phosphoenolpyruvate. The carboxylation of pyruvate is catalyzed by the mitochondrial enzyme pyruvate carboxylase. The activity of pyruvate carboxylase is absolutely dependent upon the presence of acetyl-CoA, which allosterically activates the enzyme. Of the enzymes listed, only pyruvate carboxylase and phosphoenolpyruvate carboxykinase (choice D) are involved in gluconeogenesis. Acetyl-CoA carboxylase (choice B) is involved in fatty acid synthesis and is not regulated by acetyl-CoA. Pyruvate kinase (choice C) is a glycolytic enzyme and is inhibited by acetyl-CoA, not activated by it. Pyruvate dehydrogenase (choice E) is the entry point for pyruvate into the TCA cycle. It is also inhibited by acetyl-CoA via the acetyl-CoA–mediated activation of pyruvate dehydrogenase kinase, an enzyme that phosphorylates and inactivates pyruvate dehydrogenase.

382. (B) Carbonic anhydrase catalyzes the following reaction:

$$CO_2 + H_2O \leftrightarrow H_2CO_3$$

This reaction is freely reversible and proceeds in one direction or the other dependent upon the relative partial pressures of CO_2 and O_2. In the lungs, where the partial pressure of O_2 is high, the O_2 leaves the alveoli and enters erythrocytes of the blood. There it is bound by hemoglobin for transport to the peripheral tissues. When O_2 is bound, hydrogen ions dissociate from hemoglobin and are titrated by bicarbonate ions to form carbonic acid: H_2CO_3. The increase in carbonic acid results in the carbonic anhydrase reaction proceeding to the right, relative to the equation above. The CO_2 thus formed flows out of the erythrocytes due to the relatively low partial pressure of CO_2 in the lungs. The CO_2 is then expelled from the lungs upon expiration. When erythrocytes enter the relatively high partial pressure of CO_2 in the tissues, the reverse process occurs, leading to release of the hemoglobin bound O_2. Ionization of carbonic acid (choice A), protonation of hemoglobin (choice C), carbamoylation of hemoglobin (choice D), and transport of chloride ion (choice E) all occur spontaneously, thus requiring no enzymes.

383. (E) Muscle cells lack glucose-6-phosphatase, and this prevents any glucose that is released from stored glycogen from leaving the muscle cell and entering the blood. During the normal process of glycogen breakdown a free molecule of glucose is released each time a limit dextrin is acted upon by the debranching enzyme. However, this free glucose is rapidly phosphorylated by the high activity of skeletal muscle hexokinase and trapped within the cell for oxidation. Muscle cells contain all of the other enzyme choices (A, B, C, and D) none of which would allow these cells to deliver free glucose to the blood.

384. (B) During strenuous physical exercise, the rate of production of pyruvate via glycolysis exceeds the capacity of the citric acid cycle to use it, and pyruvate accumulates. NADH also accumulates, and glycolysis cannot continue unless NAD^+ is regenerated. This is accomplished by the conversion of pyruvate to lactate by lactate dehydrogenase, which uses NADH as a cofactor and produces NAD^+. Pyruvate and lactate diffuse out of muscle into blood and are taken up by the liver, where lactate is converted to pyruvate, which is in turn converted to glucose. During strenuous (anaerobic) exercise), the $NAD^+/NADH$ ratio is kept relatively constant through the linked activities of glyceraldehyde-3-phosphate dehydrogenase and lactate dehydrogenase, therefore NAD^+ (choice A) would not increase. As indicated, some pyruvate exits muscle cells and enters the blood, thus increasing (not decreasing) its relative concentration in that compartment (choice C). Anaerobic exercise inhibits the TCA cycle, so citrate would not accumulate (choice D). Exercise depletes the level of ATP, it does not increase it (choice E).

385. (C) Dietary triacylglycerols are hydrolyzed in the intestines by pancreatic lipase and pancreatic phospholipase A_2. The resultant free fatty acids and monoacylglycerols enter intestinal epithelial cells, where the triacylglycerols are reformed. These triacylglycerols are packaged into chylomicrons and delivered to the circulation via the lymphatic system. Chylomicrons are therefore the molecules produced by the body to deliver dietary triacylglycerols to the circulation. VLDLs (choice A) are generated in the liver for transport of hepatic triacylglycerols to peripheral tissues. HDLs (choice B) are synthesized by the liver and intestine and are primarily involved in reverse cholesterol transport. LDLs (choice D) are by-products of intestinal VLDLs. Albumin (choice E) does not transport triacylglycerols, but individual fatty acids.

386. (E) Rifamycin (rifampicin) is an inhibitor of transcription. It specifically blocks initiation of transcription by interfering with formation of the first phosphodiester bond in the RNA chain. The other antibiotics listed are all inhibitors of protein synthesis. All of the other antibiotics listed (choices A, B, C, and D) inhibit the process of translation by different mechanisms.

387. (D) Fatty acids are activated to the coenzyme A derivatives at the outer mitochondrial membrane (catalyzed by enzyme 1 in Figure 3–8), but are oxidized inside the mitochondria. Long-chain fatty acyl-CoA molecules do not cross the mitochondrial membrane. A special transport system involving carnitine is used for movement of the activated fatty acids into the mitochondria. The fatty acyl moiety is transferred from the CoA to carnitine in a reaction catalyzed by carnitine acyltransferase I (enzyme 2 in Figure 3–8). Acyl carnitine thus formed is shuttled across the inner mitochondrial membrane (via enzyme 3 in Figure 3–8), where the fatty acyl group is transferred back to a coenzyme A molecule within the mitochondrial matrix. The latter reaction is catalyzed by carnitine acyltransferase II (enzyme 4 in Figure 3–8). Medium-chain fatty acyl-CoAs can cross the mitochondrial membrane and do not require the carnitine transport system for entry into the mitochondria. The compound(s) at point A are ATP and CoA, point B is carnitine, point C is acylcarnitine, point D is carnitine, and E is acylcarnitine. Therefore, the requirements for carnitine occur on either side of the inner mitochondrial membrane at points B and D, which occur during the translocation process. All other combinations (choices A, B, C, and E) have a compound or compounds other than or in addition to carnitine.

388. (B) Osteogenesis imperfecta consists of a group of at least four types (mild, extensive, severe, and variable). The disorder is characterized by brittle bones and abnormally thin sclerae, which appear blue owing to the lack of connective tissue. The symptoms arise due to defects in two α-collagen genes, the COL1A1 and COL1A2 genes. There have been over 100 mutations identified in these two genes. The mutations lead to decreased expression of collagen or abnormal proα1 proteins. The abnormal proteins associate with normal collagen subunits, which prevents the triple helical structure of normal collagen to form. The result is degradation of all the collagen proteins, both normal and abnormal. Marfan syndrome (choice A) results in cardiovascular, musculoskeletal, and ophthalmic abnormalities. Hallmark clinical manifestations are aortic dilation, mitral valve prolapse, dissecting aneurysms, arachnodactyly, and ectopia lentis. Ehlers–Danlos syndrome (choice C) comprises at least 10 defined types of a related disorder. Characteristic clinical features are easy bruising, markedly soft hyperextensible skin, extreme joint hypermobility, and the formation of thin, atrophic, "cigarette-paper" scarring following injury. Scurvy (choice D), which is caused by a deficiency in vitamin C, is characterized by decreased wound healing and hemorrhaging, anemia, osteoporosis, soft swollen gums, and easily bruised skin. Occipital horn syndrome (choice E), a disorder that manifests with symptoms similar to other collagen metabolism disorders, results from defects in copper metabolism. Clinical features include loose skin and joints, hernias, and abnormally shaped bones.

389. (A) Defective biosynthesis of α-collagen accounts for the clinical symptoms and signs observed with osteogenesis imperfecta. Marfan syndrome results from a defect in fibrillin (choice B) synthesis. Fibrillin is a component of the 10-nm microfibrils of the extracellular matrix. The biosynthesis of the intermediate filaments cytokeratin (choice C), vimentin (choice D), and desmin (choice E) are all unaffected with osteogenesis imperfecta.

390. (A) A Lineweaver–Burk plot (Figure 3–9) can be used to directly determine the K_m from the value of the X-axis (point A in Figure 3–9). This point represents the negative inverse of the K_m ($-1/K_m$). The value v_1/V_{max} (choice B) is only a portion of the derivation of the Michaelis–Menton equation. The equilibrium constant for a single order reaction is given by k_1/k_{-1} (choice C). The value for the slope of the line in Figure 3–9 (point C) is K_m/V_{max} (choice D). The inverse value of V_{max} (choice E) can be obtained from the Y-axis (point B in Figure 3–9).

391. (C) Any condition that results in elevated levels of purine nucleotides is likely to cause hyperuricemia. HGPRT is a salvage pathway enzyme that catalyzes the condensation of hypoxanthine or guanine with PRPP to yield IMP or GMP. In this way, purine bases, which become available in the diet or by virtue of nucleic acid degradation, can be recycled into the corresponding nucleotides and used for nucleic acid biosynthesis. If this salvage is blocked, the purine bases are degraded further to uric acid. Xanthine oxidase (choice A), adenosine deaminase (choice B), and purine nucleoside phosphorylase (choice D) are all purine degradative enzymes. The absence of any of these enzymes would prevent the formation of uric acid. PRPP aminotransferase (choice E) is the enzyme that catalyzes the committed step in purine biosynthesis. Its absence would result in lower levels of purines and would not result in elevated uric acid levels.

392. (D) Cockayne syndrome results in patients harboring a defect in the ability to repair UV damaged DNA. In particular, the defect is pronounced at the level of the repair of transcriptionally active genes, as opposed to overall excision repair in the total genomic DNA. Defects, if observed, in the other processes (choice A, B, C, and E) do not result in symptoms of Cockayne syndrome.

393. (A) Arsenate replaces the P_i that normally reacts with glyceraldehyde-3-phosphate (choice C) to form 1,3-bisphosphoglycerate. Instead, an unstable intermediate, 1-arseno-3-phosphoglycerate, is produced and immediately hydrolyzes to 3-phosphoglycerate (choice D). NADH is formed as usual (choice B). Thus glycolysis proceeds in the presence of arsenate, but the ATP usually produced in the conversion of 1,3-bisphosphoglycerate to 3-phosphoglycerate is lost. Since glycolysis proceeds, pyruvate is formed (choice E).

394. (B) The molar ratio of adenosine in any molecule of double-stranded DNA will be equivalent to that of thymidine, since these two nucleotides hydrogen bond to form base-pairs. Therefore, the total amount of the DNA accounted for in A-T base-pairs would be 40%. Since guanosine and cytidine hydrogen bond to form base-pairs, they too contribute an equivalent molar ratio in double-stranded DNA. In double-stranded DNA with 40% A-T composition, the molar ratio of cytidine would be half of the remaining 60% of the DNA, or 30%. No other molar ratio (choices A, C, D, and E) could account for the amount of cytidine in a double-stranded DNA with 20% adenosine.

395. **(D)** In cardiac and skeletal muscle, high-energy phosphate is stored through the transfer of a phosphate from ATP to creatine generating creatine phosphate. Creatinine is a non-enzymatic metabolite of creatine phosphate. When measured in the serum, levels of creatinine are remarkably constant from day to day and are proportional to muscle mass. In renal dysfunction the clearance of creatinine will be impaired and its levels will therefore rise in the serum. Although creatine is synthesized in the liver (choice A) from guanidoacetate, which is produced in the kidneys (choice B), it is not used by these two tissues, nor by the lung (choice C) or adipose tissue (choice E). Once synthesized, creatine is transported to cardiac and skeletal muscle where it is phosphorylated and stored for future energy needs.

396. **(D)** Li–Fraumeni syndrome (LFS) is a rare inherited form of cancer that involves breast and colon carcinomas, soft-tissue sarcomas, osteosarcomas, brain tumors, leukemia, and adrenocortical carcinomas. These tumors develop at an early age in LFS patients. The tumor suppressor gene found responsible for LFS is p53. Mutant forms of p53 are found in approximately 50% of all tumors. The normal p53 protein functions as a transcription factor that can induce either cell cycle arrest or apoptosis (programmed cell death) in response to DNA damage. Huntington's disease, HD (choice A) is an autosomal dominant disorder resulting from expansion of the triplet CAG within the huntingtin gene. The exact function of the huntingtin protein is still unclear. Symptoms of HD include personality changes, memory loss, and involuntary leg and arm movements (chorea). The average age of onset is 37 years. Crouzon syndrome (choice B) is characterized by craniosynostosis (mid-face hypoplasia and ocular proptosis) and is the result of a mutation in one of the receptors for fibroblast growth factor (FGFR2). Creutzfeld–Jakob disease (CJD) (choice C) encompasses three forms—infectious, sporadic, and inherited—with the vast majority of cases being sporadic. Clinical abnormalities of CJD are confined to the central nervous system and result from a pathogenic protein identified as prion protein (PrP). Prader–Willi syndrome (PWS) (choice E) is a relatively common cause of genetic obesity and mental retardation. Symptoms of severe hypotonia and poor suckling are evident at birth. PWS is caused by a deletion of a portion of the long arm of chromosome 15 [del(15q11-q13].

397. **(C)** Hereditary orotic aciduria results from a defect in the de novo synthesis of pyrimidines. The defect is in the bifunctional enzyme that catalyzes the last two steps in the de novo pathway, conversion of orotic acid to OMP and OMP to UMP. Administration of uridine allows afflicted individuals to produce sufficient levels of cytidine nucleotides via the salvage pathways. Treatment with uridine leads to a return of normal blood hemoglobin levels, and bone marrow will become normoblastic. Treatment with cytidine (choice B) has some limited ability to ameliorate symptoms of the disease, but not to the extent of uridine administration. None of the other nucleosides (choices A, D, and E) can be salvaged into cytidine or uridine nucleotides, and are therefore of no clinical value in the treatment of hereditary orotic aciduria.

398. **(B)** Transcription occurs in the 5′ to 3′ direction, and during this process RNA polymerase will move in the 3′ to 5′ direction relative to the template DNA strand. Therefore, the correct transcriptional product from the DNA template begins with its 5′ ribonucleotide corresponding to the complementary deoxyribonucleotide of the 3′ end of the template. None of the other RNA strands (choices A, C, D, and E) could be products generated from the template shown.

399. **(A)** Translation begins at AUG codons that usually reside near the 5′-end of the mRNA. Therefore, translation of the correct RNA product would begin two nucleotides from the 5′ end at the first AUG codon. This would result in the translation of a protein of four amino acids. None of the other choices (B, C, D, and E) translate into a four-unit amino acid chain.

400. **(E)** When epinephrine stimulates adipocytes, the immediate response is the activation of adenylate cyclase, which in turn leads to an increase in cAMP. Increased levels of cAMP lead to activation of PKA, which in adipocytes will phosphorylate and activate hormone-sensitive lipase. When hormone-sensitive lipase is active it removes fatty acids in a step-wise manner from stored triacylglycerides. The released fatty acids then enter the blood and are bound by albumin for transport to peripheral tissues including the liver. Lipoprotein lipase (choice A) is present on the surfaces of vascular endothelial cells and is activated by apolipoprotein C-II present in VLDLs and chylomicrons. Epinephrine is a stimulus that leads to energy consumption and therefore would not lead to an increase in triacylglyceride synthesis (choice B). When triacylglyceride breakdown is activated in adipocytes, the glycerol backbone is released as free glycerol, not glycerol-3-phosphate (choice C) to the blood and delivered to the liver for gluconeogenesis. Fatty acids released from adipose tissue are transported in the blood bound to albumin, not within any lipoprotein particle (choice D).

401. **(C)** Numerous cancers are caused by the loss of function of tumor suppressor genes. Li–Fraumeni syndrome (LFS) is a rare form of inherited cancer that involves breast and colon carcinomas, soft-tissue sarcomas, osteosarcomas, brain tumors, leukemia, and adrenocortical carcinomas. These tumors develop at an early age in LFS patients. The tumor suppressor gene found responsible for LFS is p53. Mutant forms of p53 are found in approximately 50% of all tumors. The normal p53 protein functions as a transcription factor that can induce either cell cycle arrest or apoptosis (programmed cell death) in response to DNA damage. Familial adenomatous polyposis (FAP) (choice A) is a rare inherited form of colon cancer. Germline mutations in the adenomatous polyposis coli (APC) gene are responsible for FAP. Wilms' tumor (choice B) is a form of childhood kidney cancer. The gene responsible for this disease has been identified and is called WT1 (Wilms' tumor 1). All cases of neurofibromatosis (choice D) arise by inheritance of a mutant allele. Roughly 50% of all affected individuals carry new mutations which appear to arise paternally, possibly reflecting genomic imprinting. The gene responsible for type 1 neurofibromatosis is termed NF1. Germline mutations at the NF1 locus result in multiple abnormal melanocytes (café-au-lait spots) and benign neurofibromas. Some patients also develop benign pheochromocytomas and CNS tumors. A small percentage of patients develop neurofibrosarcomas which are likely to be Schwann cell derived. Retinoblastoma (choice E) is a tumor of retinal cells which develops in children between birth and four years of age. The gene responsible is termed the retinoblastoma susceptibility gene (RB) and the protein product pRB.

402. **(E)** The extrinsic pathway is initiated at the site of injury in response to the release of tissue factor (factor III). Tissue factor is a cofactor in the factor VIIa–catalyzed (lower case "a" refers to the active form of the coagulation factors) activation of factor X. The formation of a complex between factor VIIa and tissue factor is believed to be a principal step in the overall clotting cascade. Evidence for this stems from the fact that persons with hereditary deficiencies in the components of the contact phase of the intrinsic pathway do not exhibit clotting problems. Factor VIIa, a γ-glutamate (gla residue) containing serine protease, cleaves factor X to factor Xa in a manner identical to that of factor IXa of the intrinsic pathway. The activation of factor VII occurs through the action of thrombin or factor Xa. The ability of factor Xa to activate factor VII creates a link between the intrinsic and extrinsic pathways. An additional link between the two pathways exists through the ability of tissue factor and factor VIIa to activate factor IX. Fibrinogen (choice A) is cleaved by thrombin (factor IIa), yielding fibrin monomers that polymerize to form a fibrin clot. The activation of factor VIII (choice

B) to factor VIIIa occurs in the presence of minute quantities of thrombin. Factor VIIIa is required for the activation of factor X, which represents the convergence of the intrinsic and extrinsic pathways. The activation of factor X to Xa requires assemblage of the tenase complex (Ca^{2+} and factors VIIIa, IXa, and X) on the surface of activated platelets. As the concentration of thrombin increases, factor VIIIa is ultimately cleaved by thrombin and inactivated. This dual action of thrombin upon factor VIII acts to limit the extent of tenase complex formation, and thus the extent of the coagulation cascade. Factor IX (choice D) functions only in the intrinsic cascade. When activated, factor IXa aids in the activation of factor X by functioning in the tenase complex as described above. Protein S (choice C) is a cofactor for protein C. Protein C is itself activated by thrombin and when active cleaves factors VIIIa and Va, thus limiting the extent of the coagulation cascade.

403. (A) The amino groups of amino acids are converted to urea for excretion via the urea cycle. The liver is the only organ capable of carrying this out. The human liver produces some 20 to 30 g of urea each day. Synthesis of gangliosides (choice B), which are components of all mammalian plasma membranes, can be carried out in all cells. Nucleotide biosynthesis (choice C) is also carried out by most cells, as is use of medium-chain fatty acids as an energy source (choice D). Glycogen can be degraded not only in the liver but also chiefly in muscle (choice E).

404. (D) Biotin is not required for these reactions. Formation of acetyl-CoA from pyruvate is catalyzed by the enzymes of the pyruvate dehydrogenase complex.

$$\text{pyruvate} + \text{CoA} + \text{NAD}^+ \rightarrow \text{acetyl-CoA} + \text{CO}_2 + \text{NADH}$$

As can be seen from the reaction, the stoichiometric cofactors are CoA and NAD^+ (choice A). In addition, pyruvate dehydrogenase requires thiamine pyrophosphate (choice C), dihydrolipoyltransacetylase requires lipoic acid (choice E), and dihydrolipoyl dehydrogenase requires FAD (choice B).

405. (E) Niacin (nicotinic acid) is required for the synthesis of NAD^+. Its deficiency results in pellagra, a disease characterized by psychic disturbances, diarrhea, and dermatitis. A diet rich in niacin will prevent the disease. A deficiency in vitamin D (choice A) leads to rickets in children and osteomalacia in adults. Riboflavin (choice B) deficiencies are rare, but can occur in chronic alcoholics due to their poor dietary habits. Vitamin A (choice C) deficiencies lead to night blindness. Thiamine (choice D) deficiency leads to beriberi and the related disorder Wernicke–Korsakoff syndrome, which occurs frequently in chronic alcoholism.

406. (B) The major mechanism for the inhibition of the extrinsic pathway occurs at the tissue factor—factor VIIa—Ca^{2+}–Xa complex. The protein, lipoprotein-associated coagulation inhibitor (LACI, formerly named anticonvertin), specifically binds to this complex. LACI is composed of 3 tandem protease inhibitor domains. Domain 1 binds to factor Xa and domain 2 binds to factor VIIa only in the presence of factor Xa. Antithrombin III (choice A) is the most important of four thrombin regulatory proteins. This is because antithrombin III can also inhibit the activities of factors IXa, Xa, XIa, and XIIa. The activity of antithrombin III is potentiated in the presence of heparin. Heparin binds to a specific site on antithrombin III, producing an altered conformation of the protein, and the new conformation has a higher affinity for thrombin as well as its other substrates. This effect of heparin is the basis for its clinical use as an anticoagulant. The naturally occurring heparin activator of antithrombin III is present as heparan and heparan sulfate on the surface of vessel endothelial cells. It is this feature that controls the activation of the intrinsic coagulation cascade. Protein C (choice C) is activated by thrombin when thrombin is bound to thrombomodulin. Active protein C functions with its cofactor, protein S, to degrade factors VIIIa and Xa. High molecular weight kininogen, HMWK (choice D) is important for initiation of the intrinsic pathway. When prekallikrein, HMWK, factor XI, and factor XII are exposed to a negatively charged surface, they become active. This is termed the contact phase. Exposure of collagen to a vessel surface is the primary stimulus for the contact phase. In addition to antithrombin III, thrombin activity is also inhibited by α_2-macroglobulin (choice E).

407. (C) When receptor–ligand interaction stimulates the activity of PLCγ, an increase in membrane associated phospholipid degradation occurs. The action of PLCγ is to hydrolyze polyphosphoinositides, in particular phosphatidylinositol-4,5-bisphosphate, PIP_2. The hydrolytic products of PLCγ action on PIP_2 is the release of inositol-1,4,5-trisphosphate (IP_3) and diacylglycerol (DAG). IP_3 interacts with intracellular membrane receptors resulting in the release of stored Ca^{2+}. DAG, in concert with Ca^{2+}, activates a specific kinase termed PKC (calcium, phospholipid-dependent kinase) that phosphorylates many substrates. As indicated, activation of PLCγ increases, not decreases (choice A), the release of membrane inositol lipids. PLCγ has no direct effect on the activity of adenylate cyclase (choice B) or on the activity of phosphodiesterase (choice D). The effect of PLCγ-mediated release of IP_3 is increased release of intracellular stores of calcium, not an increase in its uptake (choice E).

408. (B) When fatty acids are released from adipose tissue they are transported in the blood bound to albumin. VLDLs (choice A) are synthesized by the liver as a means to transport de novo synthesized fatty acids, in the form of triacylglycerides, to peripheral tissues. B_2-microglobulin (choice C) is involved in immune function. Chylomicrons (choice D) are synthesized in the intestine as a means to deliver dietary lipid to the body. α_2-Macroglobulin (choice E) is an antiprotease that functions to regulate the activities of a number of proteinases, such as thrombin, of the coagulation cascade.

409. (D) Approximately 5% of the entire genome encodes the messenger RNA (mRNA) genes, the remainder being composed of moderately to highly repetitive elements. These repetitive elements comprise the long interspersed elements (LINEs), short interspersed elements (SINEs), variable number tandem repeats (VNTRs), simple sequence repeats (SSRs), and the highly repetitive tandem repeats, such as those found near the centromeres.

REFERENCES

Devlin TM. *Textbook of Biochemistry: With Clinical Correlations,* 4th edition. New York: John Wiley & Sons, 1997

Murray RK, ed. *Harper's Biochemistry,* 24th edition. Stamford, CT: Appleton & Lange, 1996

Subspecialty List: Biochemistry

Question Number and Subspecialty

283. Blood
284. Kinetics
285. Integration of metabolism
286. Blood
287. Vitamins
288. Vitamins
289. Integration of metabolism
290. Vitamins
291. Muscle contraction
292. Lipid metabolism and disease
293. Carbohydrate metabolism
294. Carbohydrate metabolism
295. Molecular biology
296. Nucleotide metabolism
297. Integration of metabolism
298. Proteins
299. Carbohydrate metabolism
300. Carbohydrate metabolism
301. Molecular biology
302. Lipid metabolism
303. Diabetes
304. Lipid metabolism
305. Carbohydrate metabolism
306. Carbohydrate metabolism
307. Lipid metabolism and disease
308. Diabetes
309. Blood
310. Carbohydrate metabolism
311. Ketogenesis
312. Diabetes
313. Lipid metabolism and disease
314. Vitamins
315. Vitamins
316. Oxidative phosphorylation
317. Lipoproteins
318. Cholesterol metabolism
319. Lipid metabolism
320. Glycoproteins
321. Integration of metabolism
322. Alcohol metabolism
323. Lipid metabolism and disease
324. Lipid metabolism and disease
325. Blood
326. Blood
327. Lipid metabolism and disease
328. Genetic disorders
329. Ketogenesis
330. Genetic disorders
331. Nucleotide metabolism
332. Carbohydrate metabolism
333. Carbohydrate metabolism
334. Diabetes
335. Carbohydrate metabolism
336. Carbohydrate metabolism
337. Carbohydrate metabolism
338. Genetic disorders
339. Blood
340. Molecular biology
341. Lipid metabolism
342. Lipid metabolism and disease
343. Blood
344. Genetic disorders
345. Genetic disorders
346. Amino acids
347. Molecular biology
348. Genetic disorders
349. Blood
350. Genetic disorders
351. Nucleotide metabolism
352. Amino acids
353. Calcium–phosphate metabolism
354. Hormones
355. Hormones
356. Hormones

357. Genetic disorders
358. Carbohydrate metabolism
359. Immunodeficiency
360. Molecular biology
361. Blood
362. Amino acids
363. Genetic disorders
364. Lipid metabolism
365. Carbohydrate metabolism
366. Hormones
367. Iron metabolism
368. Inflammation
369. Genetic disorders
370. Genetic disorders
371. Molecular biology
372. Urea cycle
373. Lead intoxication
374. Molecular biology
375. Vitamins
376. Hormones
377. Vitamins
378. Amino acids
379. Carbohydrate metabolism
380. Integration of metabolism
381. Carbohydrate metabolism
382. Oxygen transport
383. Carbohydrate metabolism
384. Carbohydrate metabolism
385. Lipid metabolism
386. Molecular biology
387. Lipid metabolism
388. Genetic disorders
389. Genetic disorders
390. Kinetics
391. Genetic disorders
392. Genetic disorders
393. Carbohydrate metabolism
394. Molecular biology
395. Muscle metabolism
396. Genetic disorders
397. Genetic disorders
398. Molecular biology
399. Molecular biology
400. Lipid metabolism
401. Genetic disorders
402. Blood
403. Hepatic metabolism
404. Vitamins and cofactors
405. Vitamins
406. Blood
407. Lipid metabolism
408. Lipid metabolism
409. Molecular biology

CHAPTER 4

Microbiology

Questions

William W. Yotis, PhD

DIRECTIONS (Questions 410 through 546): Each of the numbered items or incomplete statements in this section is followed by answers or by completions of the statement. Select the ONE lettered answer or completion that is BEST in each case.

410. A medical student has been immunized with hepatitis B virus (HBV) recombinant vaccine. The curve in Figure 4–1 represents the production of protective antibodies to the viral component present in the recombinant vaccine. This viral component most likely is

(A) RNA genome of HBV
(B) nucleocapsid proteins of HBV
(C) viral core antigen (HBcAg)
(D) viral surface antigen (HBsAg)
(E) viral e antigen (HBeAg)

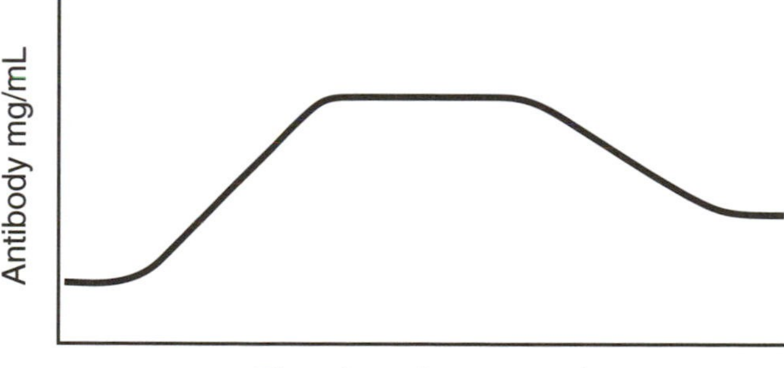

Figure 4–1

411. A banker has been told by his physician that the rash on his arm is due to delayed type hypersensitivity. If this is actually the case, which one of the following statements is accurate?

(A) This type of allergy usually occurs after inhalation of grass pollens.
(B) This allergy is due to IgE absorbed on mast cells.
(C) This allergy does not cause tissue damage.
(D) Delayed-type hypersensitivity is suppressed by antihistaminic drugs.
(E) Delayed-type hypersensitivity can be transferred passively to volunteers by sensitized lymphocytes.

412. Alpha interferon causes antiviral resistance by inducing formation of antiviral proteins in the cell that

(A) interfere with adsorption of virus to other cells
(B) block transcription of viral nucleic acid
(C) prevent penetration of virus
(D) inhibit viral uncoating
(E) block translation of viral mRNA

413. Ada had a catheter placed in her urethra. One week later she is experiencing suprapubic flank pain with urinary urgency and frequency. She has also chills and fever. After examining Ada and evaluating the sediment of her centrifuged urine, she is informed by her physician that she has acute ascending pyelonephritis. If the diagnosis is accurate and Ada's urine is cultured, what organism most likely will be isolated?

(A) *Escherichia coli* with pili
(B) *Clostridium difficile*
(C) *Staphylococcus aureus*
(D) *Pseudomonas aeruginosa*

414. Romeo, a 27-year-old electrician, has a sore throat with chills and fever. Within a week his throat has definitely improved, but he still has a fever and malaise. Suddenly he noticed that his urine is gray-brown, and he visits his physician. If the doctor thinks that Romeo has acute glomerulonephritis, which one of the following tests is most likely to verify this diagnosis?

(A) serum level of IgE
(B) serum level of anti-DNA antibodies
(C) evaluation of the number of T cells
(D) serum level of antistreptolysin O antibodies
(E) serum level of anti-H antibodies

415. A 22-year-old man complains to his family physician of fatigue, night sweats, and a dry unproductive cough. Until the past few months, he had apparently been in good health. A CBC and differential blood count reveal that he is lymphopenic. X-ray examination reveals an interstitial pneumonia. Skin test reactions to a battery of materials are normal. The next step in evaluating this patient's illness should be

(A) identification of the organism that is causing the pneumonia
(B) nitroblue tetrazolium reduction assay
(C) CH_{50} assay
(D) intracellular killing assay
(E) chemotaxis assay

416. Cultures of two streptomycin-sensitive strains of *Escherichia coli* are mixed together. Streptomycin is added, and the mixture is incubated. After two hours, the mixture is plated on a medium containing streptomycin. A few streptomycin-resistant colonies develop. This is probably an example of

(A) transduction by bacteriophage
(B) genetic transformation
(C) conjugation via sex pilus bridge
(D) spontaneous chromosomal mutation
(E) genetic complementation

417. A two-year-old girl with recurrent pulmonary infections has been brought to the hospital with meningitis by her mother. Gram stain of the spinal fluid reveals numerous polymorphonuclear neutrophils and gram-positive cocci in grape-like clusters. The drug of choice to be employed until the antibiotic sensitivity report is received from the laboratory is

(A) penicillin
(B) methicillin
(C) streptomycin
(D) ampicillin
(E) chloramphenicol

418. Which of the following statements concerning the Ouchterlony diagram in Figure 4–2 is true?

(A) line 1 will contain Ag ab and Ab b only
(B) line 2 will contain Ag ac and Ab b
(C) the spur will contain Ab a and Ag ab
(D) the spur will contain Ag ac and Ab a
(E) the spur will contain Ag ab and Ab b

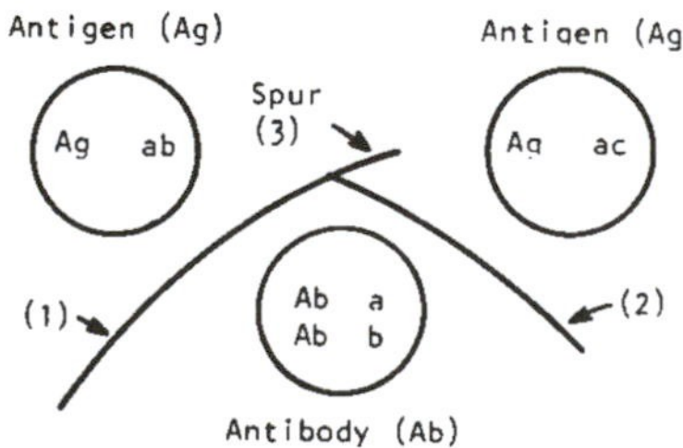

Figure 4–2

419. Figure 4–3 depicts an electrophoretic pattern of serum proteins. This electrophoretic design is likely to be obtained from a nine-month-old infant with

(A) Bruton's disease
(B) Graves' disease
(C) Goodpasture's syndrome
(D) Addison's disease
(E) myasthenia gravis

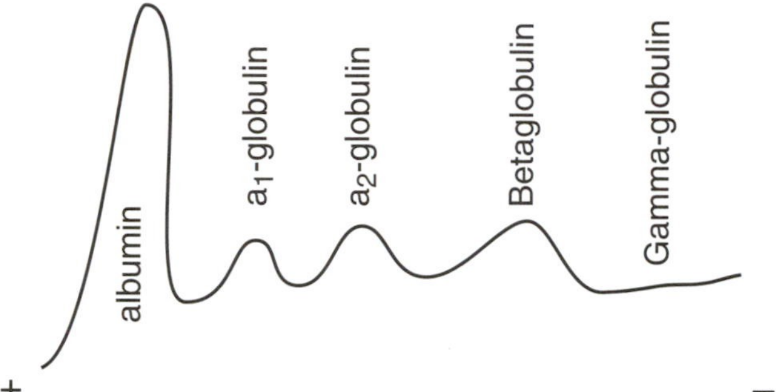

Figure 4–3

420. Mr. T., a 19-year-old college student, is experiencing intense burning during urination, and discharges a thick creamy urethral exudate. The exudate is composed of polymorphonuclear leukocytes with many intracellular, gram-negative, kidney-shaped diplococci. There are no lesions on the genital organ area. The most likely presumptive diagnosis is

(A) trichomoniasis
(B) syphilis
(C) gonorrhea
(D) lymphogranuloma venereum
(E) chancroid

421. Which one of the following approaches is likely to prevent future infection of Mr. T.?

(A) prophylactic use of 100 units oral penicillin
(B) vaccination with heat-killed germs
(C) frequent washing of the genital area
(D) use of condoms
(E) immunization with the appropriate toxoid

422. A boy is unprovokedly attacked and bitten on the shoulder by a fox and suffers a slight wound. In addition to flushing the wound, cleaning it surgically, and giving antitetanus prophylaxis and antibiotics as indicated, the physician should immediately

(A) order a search for the attacking fox for autopsy
(B) start rabies vaccine
(C) start rabies vaccine and give antirabies serum
(D) observe the boy very carefully
(E) report the incident to the state epidemiologist

423. Chlamydiae and rickettsiae are correctly described as

(A) being spread by the bite of an infected arthropod
(B) resistant to the usual broad-spectrum antibiotics
(C) containing either RNA or DNA, but not both
(D) obligate parasites of living cells
(E) dividing solely by binary fission

424. A laboratory worker has been diagnosed as having tuberculosis. He has been ill for 10 months with symptoms that include a productive cough, intermittent fever, night sweats, and a weight loss of 27.3 kg (60 lb). Numerous acid-fast bacilli are seen in a sputum examination, and more than fifty colonies of organisms grow out in culture. In a situation such as this, those contacts who have a positive skin test but no other signs of disease should

(A) receive prophylactic isoniazid (INH)
(B) receive a full course of INH and ethambutol
(C) be checked periodically by x-ray
(D) be immunized with bacillus Calmette–Guérin (BCG) vaccine
(E) be vaccinated with purified protein derivative (PPD)

425. A football player had gonococcal urethritis, and was treated with the appropriate doses of penicillin and probenecid. Three weeks later he had a relapse of gonococcal urethritis, and his physician administered another dose of penicillin. Within two minutes following the injection the football player experienced respiratory difficulties and collapsed. The most likely explanation for the difficulties in breathing and collapse is that

(A) the patient developed gonococcal pneumonia
(B) he might be reinfected
(C) the gonococcus that caused the initial infection became resistant to penicillin
(D) the patient developed hypersensitivity to penicillin
(E) he may have nongonococcal urethritis

426. Ultraviolet light is used as an antimicrobial physical agent because it

(A) disrupts the bacterial cell membrane
(B) removes free sulfhydryl groups
(C) is a common protein denaturant
(D) causes the formation of pyrimidine dimers
(E) acts as an alkylating agent

427. A five-year-old girl undergoing chemotherapy developed a disseminated varicella-zoster infection. The most likely reason for this viral infection is

(A) outgrowth of virus from varicella-zoster immunization
(B) hypogammaglobulinemia
(C) synergism between varicella-zoster and chemotherapy
(D) deficiency in the third component of complement
(E) T-cell deficiency

428. A zookeeper who had two seizures and is now semicomatose is brought to the hospital. His cerebrospinal fluid has normal glucose and protein levels, but 40 lymphocytes per cubic mm. A spherical, enveloped, double-stranded DNA virus has been isolated from clinical specimens and established as the etiological agent of the viral infection. The most likely virus involved is

(A) St. Louis encephalitis
(B) echovirus
(C) herpesvirus
(D) poliovirus
(E) rabies virus

429. Which of the following statements concerning Figure 4–4 (showing the frequency of serologic reactivity after exposure to *Coccidioides immitis*) is true?

(A) curve A represents the results of the precipitin assays
(B) curve B shows the results of the complement fixation assays
(C) curve C depicts the data of skin testing
(D) curve C shows the results of complement fixation assays
(E) curve A represents the results of agglutination assays

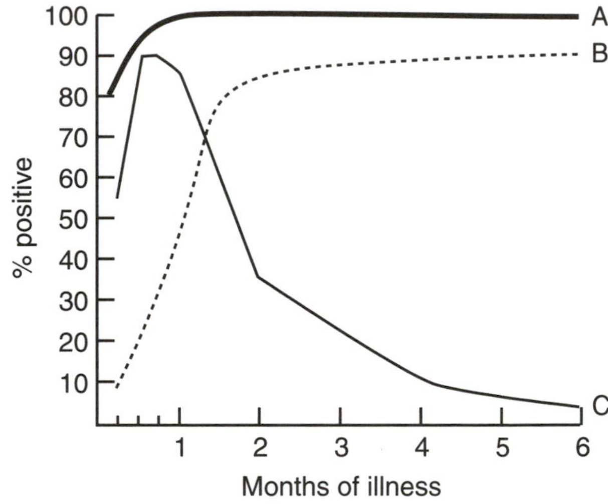

Figure 4–4

430. Tetracycline antibiotics specifically inhibit protein synthesis in prokaryotes because they

(A) bind to prokaryotic and not eukaryotic DNA-directed RNA polymerase
(B) are transported by prokaryotes but not eukaryotes

(C) bind to prokaryotic but not eukaryotic membranes
(D) inhibit initiation of protein synthesis, which specifically requires formyl-methionyl tRNA
(E) bind to prokaryotic but not eukaryotic ribosomes

431. Figure 4–5 shows a quantitative precipitin curve of an antigen-antibody reaction. According to the figure which one of the following statements is correct?

(A) point D represents the area of antigen destruction
(B) point B shows that there is no antibody formation
(C) point C indicates that there is little, if any, free antigen and antibody in the reaction tube

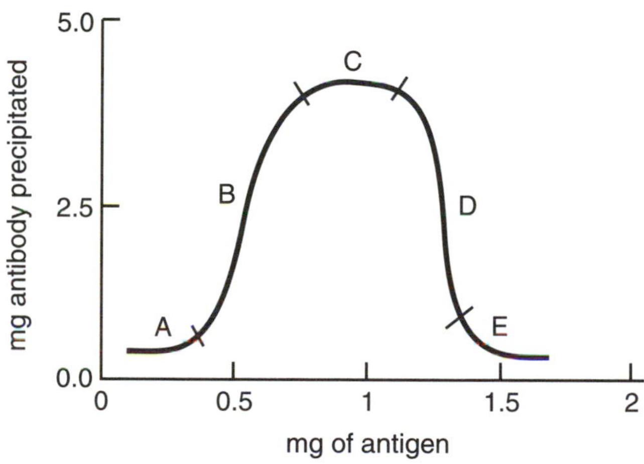

Figure 4–5

(D) point A shows antigen excess
(E) point E indicates antibody excess

432. A newborn boy appears to be lethargic and septic. A spinal tap was performed, and a Gram stain of the centrifuged spinal fluid revealed gram-positive bacilli resembling diphtheroids. Cultures of the spinal fluid on sheep blood agar plates, at a temperature of 22 to 25°C, yielded gram-positive, catalase-positive, hemolytic rods that had a tumbling motion. Proper treatment with penicillin cleared the infection. The most likely organism that caused this disease is

(A) *Bacillus cereus*
(B) *Bordetella pertussis*
(C) *Neisseria meningitidis*
(D) *Listeria monocytogenes*
(E) *Corynebacterium diphtheriae*

433. The antiphagocytosis property of group A streptococci is associated with

(A) M protein
(B) hyaluronidase
(C) streptolysin O
(D) streptolysin S
(E) DNAse

434. Secretory IgA consists of IgA dimer, secretory component (SC), plus

(A) paraprotein
(B) J chain
(C) SC epitope
(D) γ-chain
(E) ε-chain

435. Antigens can best be processed for presentation by

(A) macrophages
(B) Kupffer cells
(C) B cells
(D) young erythrocytes
(E) suppressor T cells

436. A medical student spending his summer in a dense forest as a tree cutter was bitten by infected ticks. In a week he developed a high fever, headache, muscular aches, nausea, and splenomegaly. Five days later his symptoms subsided. However, one week later all his previous symptoms returned. During the next nine days he went through a recovery and another relapse followed by a final recovery. The overall temperature curve of his illness is shown in Figure 4–6. The most likely etiological agent is

(A) *Treponema carateum*
(B) *Treponema pertenue*
(C) *Borrelia burgdorferi*
(D) *Borrelia recurrentis*
(E) *Leptospira interrogans*

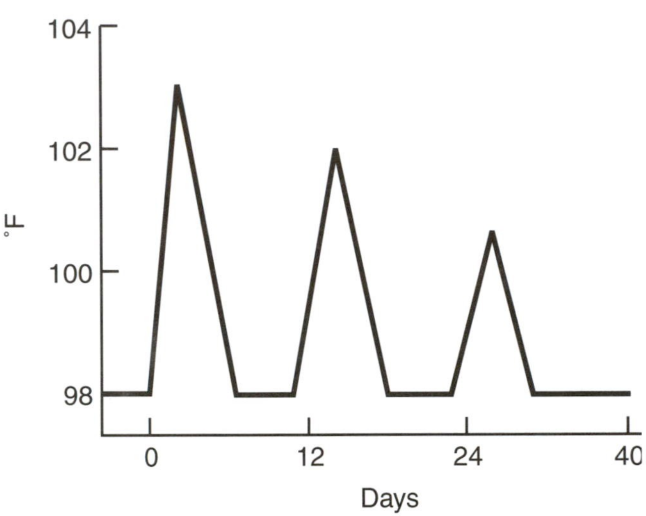

Figure 4–6

437. A seven-year-old boy has a thick gray pseudomembrane over his tonsils and throat, and a clinical diagnosis of diphtheria is made. Which of the following is the most immediate course of action?

(A) performance of a spinal tap
(B) culture of a throat specimen on blood agar
(C) acid-fast stain of a throat specimen
(D) oral administration of sulfonamides
(E) injection of diphtheria antitoxin

438. Which of the following modes of pathogenesis is most compatible with diphtheria?

(A) tumor necrosis factor production
(B) possession of capsule by the etiological agent
(C) lysis of natural killer T lymphocytes by bacterial envelope enzymes
(D) production of exotoxin by the causative agent
(E) immune complex formation

439. Patients with X-linked infantile agammaglobulinemia are known to

(A) exhibit profound deficiencies of cell-mediated immunity
(B) have very low quantities of immunoglobulin in their serum
(C) have normal numbers of B lymphocytes
(D) have a depletion of lymphocytes in the paracortical areas of lymph nodes
(E) be particularly susceptible to viral and fungal infections

440. During a routine pelvic examination, a woman is found to have vesicular lesions on the vagina. The patient states that she had similar lesions 12 months previously. The causative agent is most likely to be

(A) echovirus
(B) coxsackievirus
(C) rubella virus
(D) herpes simplex virus
(E) measles virus

441. Antibodies against acetylcholine neural receptors are thought to be involved in the pathogenesis of

(A) myasthenia gravis
(B) multiple sclerosis
(C) acute idiopathic polyneuritis
(D) Guillain–Barré syndrome
(E) postpericardiotomy syndrome

442. A seven-month-old child is hospitalized for a yeast infection that does not respond to therapy. The patient has a history of acute pyogenic infections. Physical examination reveals that the spleen and lymph nodes are not palpable. A differential WBC count shows 95% neutrophils, 1% lymphocytes, and 4% monocytes. A bone marrow specimen contains no plasma cells or lymphocytes. X-ray reveals absence of a thymic shadow. Tonsils are absent. These findings are most compatible with

(A) multiple myeloma
(B) severe combined immunodeficiency disease
(C) X-linked agammaglobulinemia
(D) Wiskott–Aldrich syndrome
(E) chronic granulomatous disease

443. Figure 4–7 represents the

(A) O antigen of *Salmonella typhimurium*
(B) peptidoglycan of *Staphylococcus aureus*
(C) C substance of *Streptococcus pneumoniae*
(D) peptidoglycan of *Mycoplasma pneumoniae*
(E) H antigen of *Salmonella typhimurium*

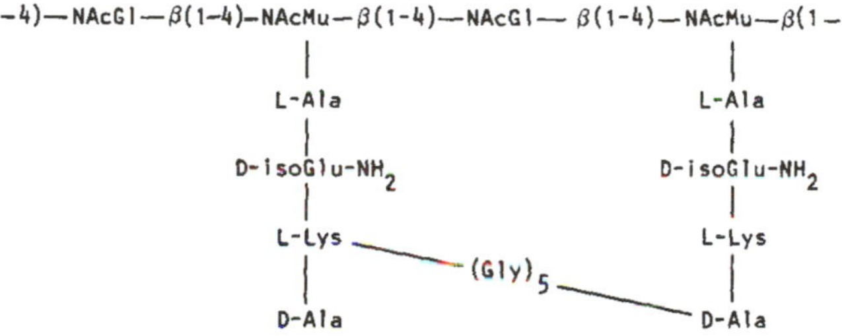

Figure 4–7

444. Immunity to whooping cough is

(A) usually acquired during the third month of infancy
(B) acquired by active immunization
(C) rarely acquired by natural infection with *Bordetella pertussis*
(D) conferred by antibody production to the Vi antigen of *Bordetella pertussis*
(E) of lifelong duration

445. A mother has been told that her three-year-old child has an inherited deficiency in the inhibitor of the first component of complement. This deficiency is likely to lead to which one of the following conditions?

(A) bacteremia
(B) an increased susceptibility to pyogenic infections
(C) angioedema
(D) enhancement of antibody production
(E) decreased production of anaphylatoxins

446. A rabbit is repeatedly injected with a hapten. Two weeks later, its serum is subjected to a gel diffusion assay with the hapten and a carrier protein. It would be expected that

(A) no precipitin line will be present
(B) a line of identity between the serum and carrier protein will be detected
(C) a line of identity between serum and both the carrier and the hapten will be present
(D) a line of partial identity between serum, carrier, and hapten will be detected
(E) a line of nonidentity between serum, carrier, and hapten will be detected

447. Structural integrity of the bacterial cell depends primarily upon the

(A) cell membrane
(B) capsular polysaccharides
(C) lipoproteins
(D) cell surface proteins
(E) peptidoglycan layer

448. Oncogenes

(A) are genes that may cause cancer
(B) have copies in viruses
(C) may code for products that are essential for normal cell function
(D) may code for cellular surface receptors
(E) all of the above

449. The infectiveness of *Chlamydia trachomatis* has been related to its

(A) elementary body (EB)
(B) capsule
(C) cell wall
(D) reticulate body (RB)
(E) phagosome

450. A 19-year-old man who had not been vaccinated for any viral infection had fever and anorexia for three days. Then he developed a tender swelling of the parotid glands, which became very painful. The pain was exacerbated with fluid intake. Hemagglutination inhibition assays indicated a fourfold rise in antibody production against the etiological agent. Which one of the following statements is correct about the etiological agent?

(A) this virus is susceptible to antiviral therapy
(B) the virus has been attenuated and used as a vaccine
(C) this virus does not cause any complications
(D) the genome of this virus is composed of DNA
(E) this virus is transmitted to humans by insects

451. Diphtheria toxin mediates

(A) dissociation of eukaryotic ribosomal subunits
(B) inhibition of peptide bond formation
(C) hydrolysis of messenger RNA
(D) adenosine diphosphate ribosylation of eukaryotic elongation factor 2
(E) destruction of the endoplasmic reticulum

452. A six-year-old girl has been having recurrent pyogenic bacterial infections. The latest one has been caused by *Neisseria meningitidis*. The results of her diagnostic tests are as follows:

TEST	RESULT
White cell count	Normal
T-cell count	Normal
Production of IgM to polysaccharides	Normal
Production of anti-DNA antibodies	Not detected
Levels of complement components C3 and C5 to 8	Low
Levels of thyroid-stimulating hormone	Normal
Levels of immunoglobulins	Normal
Intracellular killing of microbes by neutrophils	Normal

These results are consistent with a diagnosis of

(A) Graves' disease
(B) Wiskott–Aldrich syndrome
(C) deficiency in the opsonization of microbes by phagocytes
(D) systemic lupus erythematosus
(E) chronic granulomatous disease

453. High molecular weight substances that possess both immunogenicity and specificity are termed

(A) simple haptens
(B) determinant groups
(C) adjuvants
(D) antigens
(E) complex haptens

454. A laboratory test used to identify *Staphylococcus aureus* is based on the clotting of plasma. The microbial product that is responsible for this activity is

(A) coagulase reactive factor
(B) coagulase
(C) prothrombin
(D) thrombin
(E) plasmin

455. The Well–Felix reaction is correctly described as

(A) useful in the diagnosis of rickettsial diseases

(B) based on the agglutination of species of *Salmonella* by the patient's convalescent serum
(C) a test to detect antiviral antibodies
(D) based on scrotal swelling in a male guinea pig infected with the organism
(E) positive for Q fever when *Proteus* OXK is agglutinated

456. Which one of the following is the best neutrophil and macrophage attractant?

(A) C5a
(B) variable region of the heavy chain of IgG
(C) J chain
(D) HLA-A
(E) HLA-B

457. The most common medium used for the cultivation of fungi is

(A) tellurite medium
(B) SS agar
(C) Lowenstein–Jensen medium
(D) selenite F medium
(E) Sabouraud's glucose agar

458. Congenital rubella syndrome is most prominent in an infant when a pregnant woman becomes infected

(A) during the first trimester of pregnancy
(B) one week before a full-term delivery
(C) one month before a full-term delivery
(D) hours before childbirth
(E) during the third trimester of pregnancy

459. The tolerance of facultative anaerobic bacteria to superoxide and hydrogen peroxide is due to

(A) cytochrome oxidase
(B) presence of superoxide dismutase and catalase
(C) absence of catalase
(D) presence of peroxidase
(E) inability to form oxygen

460. A burn patient developed a wound infection, and a bacteriologic culture of the site indicates a gram-negative rod that is oxidase positive and produces a bluish-green pigment. The organism was relatively resistant to antibiotics, but susceptible to ticarcillin, gentamicin, and tobramycin. The organism is likely to be identified as

(A) *Escherichia coli*
(B) *Klebsiella pneumoniae*
(C) *Proteus mirabilis*
(D) *Serratia marcescens*
(E) *Pseudomonas aeruginosa*

461. Acute glomerulonephritis is a sequela of a previous infection by

(A) any M type of group A streptococci
(B) a few M types of group A streptococci
(C) only lysogenic group A streptococci
(D) all of the Lancefield groups of streptococci
(E) only encapsulated strains of *Streptococcus pneumoniae*

462. *Cryptococcus neoformans* differs from other pathogenic fungi in that it

(A) has a capsule
(B) is an intracellular parasite
(C) has septate hyphae
(D) reproduces by binary fission
(E) is dematiaceous

463. *Diphyllobothrium latum* causes anemia by

(A) its blood-sucking activities
(B) the production of a toxin that affects hematopoiesis
(C) competition with the host for vitamin B_{12}
(D) occlusion of the common bile duct
(E) inhibition of the absorption of iron

464. Which of the following zoonotic diseases is usually transmitted to humans by the bite of an arthropod vector?

(A) anthrax
(B) brucellosis
(C) salmonellosis
(D) plague
(E) leptospirosis

465. Ms. Y. is sneezing and has a runny nose and watery eyes every summer. Her physician is convinced that Ms. Y. is suffering from an allergy and performs some skin tests. The results of these tests are shown below:

ALLERGEN USED FOR TESTING	RESPONSE TO ALLERGEN (WHEAL DIAMETER IN MM)
cat dander	1
house dust	4
Kentucky blue grass	13
pollen	7
fungal spores	6
solvent-only control	5

Which one of the test allergens is most likely to be inducing the symptoms of Ms. Y.?

(A) mold
(B) cat dander
(C) house dust
(D) Kentucky blue grass
(E) pollen

466. Which one of the following substances is most likely to prevent the attachment of the mold allergen to the sensitized mast cells of Ms. Y.?

(A) corticosteroids
(B) complement
(C) IgG anti-mold
(D) epinephrine
(E) cromolyn sodium

467. A 64-year-old alcoholic man has fever, chills, cough, and pleuritic pain. His sputum is a dark brown color, and upon cultivation on blood agar produces alpha hemolytic colonies. These colonies are composed of gram-positive, optochin positive cocci. The microbes most likely are

(A) *Staphylococcus aureus*
(B) *Streptococcus pneumoniae*
(C) *Neisseria meningitidis*
(D) *Streptococcus pyogenes*
(E) *Enterococcus faecalis*

468. According to Figure 4–8 the rate of growth of the bacterial culture for which it was obtained reaches its maximum rate of growth between

(A) noon and 1:00 p.m.
(B) 2:00 p.m. and 3:00 p.m.
(C) 3:00 p.m. and 4:00 p.m.
(D) 4:00 p.m. and 5:00 p.m.
(E) 3:00 p.m. and 5:00 p.m.

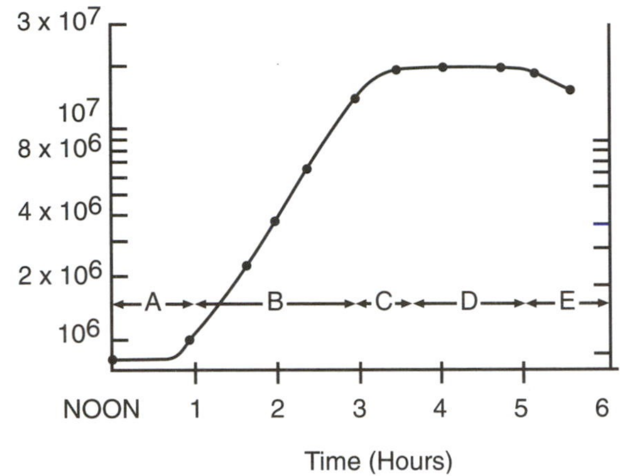

Figure 4–8

469. A 33-year-old woman may be suffering from a B-cell deficiency. What is the best method for assessing the total number of B lymphocytes of this patient?

(A) quantitative immunoglobulin levels
(B) Fc receptor assay
(C) E rosette assay
(D) surface immunoglobulin (sIg) assay
(E) phytohemagglutinin A (PHA) mitogenicity

470. Functional assessment of T lymphocytes includes

(A) E rosette assay
(B) sIg evaluation
(C) transformation of lymphocytes by PHA
(D) serum immunoglobulin determination
(E) enumeration of y-bearing cells

471. A 21-year-old man has Lyme disease. Which one of the following statements concerning Lyme disease is correct?

(A) It is transmitted by mites.
(B) It is caused by *Leptospira interrogans.*
(C) It is a disease in which the serum levels of IgM correlate with disease activity.
(D) It has not been associated with arthritis.
(E) It does not respond to tetracycline treatment early in the acute illness.

472. A gram-negative bacterium is isolated from a patient's cerebrospinal fluid (CSF). It grows on enriched chocolate agar, but does not grow on blood agar, except adjacent to a streak of staphylococci. The organism most probably is

(A) *Neisseria meningitidis*
(B) *N. gonorrhoeae*
(C) *H. influenzae*
(D) *S. pneumoniae*
(E) *Listeria monocytogenes*

473. A laboratory worker died within a day following an accidental ingestion of a very small amount of a bacterial toxin. This toxin had the lowest 50% lethal dose (LD50), and was most likely produced by

(A) *Salmonella typhi*
(B) *Yersinia pestis*
(C) *Clostridium tetani*
(D) *Clostridium botulinum*
(E) *Corynebacterium diphtheriae*

474. The most common cause of bacterial meningitis in newborns is

(A) *S. aureus*
(B) *E. coli*
(C) *S. pyogenes*
(D) *N. meningitidis*
(E) *S. pneumoniae*

475. *Helicobacter pylori*

(A) is usually found in the oral cavity
(B) produces an abundant amount of coagulase
(C) appears to be important in the pathogenesis of peptic ulcer
(D) is an obligate intracellular parasite
(E) does not induce specific antibodies in gastritis patients

476. The immunoglobulin which passes the placental barrier in humans is

(A) IgM
(B) IgD
(C) IgE
(D) IgA
(E) IgG

477. A 27-year-old man was treated with penicillin for gonorrhea. Thirty-five days later he was reinfected with the same germ, and his physician administered an intramuscular dose of penicillin. Two minutes following the injection of penicillin the patient had respiratory difficulties and became unconscious. This reaction was most likely mediated by

(A) activation of the classical complement pathway
(B) activation of the alternate complement pathway
(C) IgG
(D) IgD
(E) IgE

478. A urine sample containing viable *E. coli* is inoculated into an appropriate medium to 500 cells per mL. Assuming the generation time of *E. coli* cells in this medium is 20 minutes, the number of viable cells per mL after three hours of incubation will be

(A) 8000
(B) 32,000
(C) 16,000
(D) 64,000
(E) 256,000

479. Viruses are attractive vectors for gene therapy because

(A) they infect cells with much lower efficiency compared to chemical or physical means of gene transfer
(B) the genes inserted into viruses may be expressed in a regulated way
(C) adenovirus vectors cannot be used to target gene transfer into cells of the respiratory tract
(D) retrovirus vectors can be produced in extremely small quantities from producer cell lines
(E) they work only in non-human diseases with multiple affected genes

480. An experiment is performed in which lawn bacteria is plated onto a nutrient plate and "replica plated" to four media, each containing an antibiotic. Results are shown in Figure 4–9.

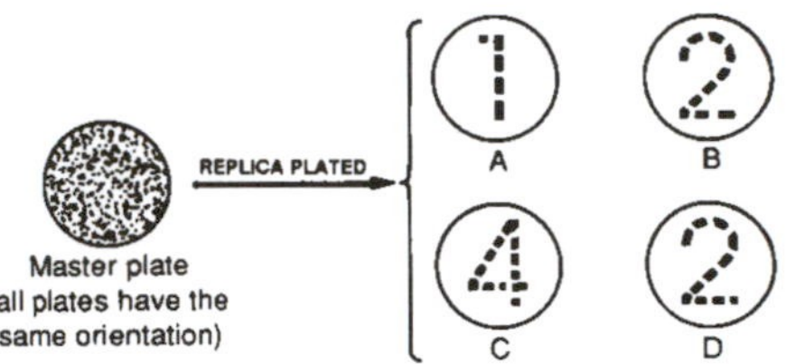

Figure 4–9

Which of the following statements is true concerning the interpretation of this experiment?

(A) Plates B and D likely contain the same antibiotics.
(B) Lamarckian theory is not supported.
(C) Plates B, C, and D all contain different antibiotics.
(D) The replica plate technique is an inappropriate method to answer questions about spontaneous mutation.
(E) Mutation is not likely to occur in bacteria.

481. Four hours after eating fried rice, a man develops diarrhea, vomiting, and nausea. Which of the following microorganisms is MOST likely involved?

(A) *Clostridium tetani*
(B) *Bacillus cereus*
(C) *Salmonella enteritidis*
(D) *Clostridium botulinum*
(E) *Proteus mirabilis*

482. X-linked agammaglobulinemic patients are most likely to present with repeated infections involving

(A) viruses
(B) fungi
(C) intracellular bacteria
(D) extracellular bacteria
(E) *Pneumocystis carinii*

483. Recent experiments in gene therapy have taken the approach of expressing TNF (tumor necrosis factor) in TIL (tumor-infiltrating lymphocytes). It is hoped that this approach will

(A) generate high serum levels of endotoxin
(B) allow the TIL to return to the tumor and produce locally high levels of TNF
(C) stimulate T-cell proliferation
(D) lyse tumor cells due to retrovirus infection
(E) stimulate natural killer (NK) cell activity

484. A two-year-old boy who has not been vaccinated against any germ is experiencing severe spasms in the muscles of the jaw and face. These spasms do not allow the child to open his mouth. Laboratory tests established that a bacterial toxin was responsible for this boy's symptoms. The toxin involved was most likely produced by

(A) cholera toxin
(B) clostridial alpha toxin
(C) diphtherial toxin
(D) botulinum toxin
(E) tetanus toxin

485. A college freshman has the typical symptoms of infectious mononucleosis. The most sensitive means of confirming this infection is

(A) antibody to hemagglutinin
(B) antibody to neuraminidase
(C) heterophile antibody that reacts with antigens on sheep erythrocytes
(D) antibody that reacts with Epstein–Barr virus–associated nuclear antigen
(E) nucleic acid hybridization assays for the presence of Epstein–Barr viral nucleic acid

486. Prokaryotes differ from eukaryotes in that prokaryotes have

(A) peptidoglycan
(B) sterols in their membrane
(C) 2 to 4 chromosomes
(D) endoplasmic reticulum
(E) larger (80s) ribosomes than eukaryotes

487. A hemagglutination assay was performed with a sample of influenza virus. A fixed number of chicken red blood cells were mixed with increasing dilutions of the influenza virus. The results of the assay are shown in Figure 4–10. The hemagglutination titer of the virus was

(A) 20
(B) 40
(C) 80
(D) 160
(E) 320

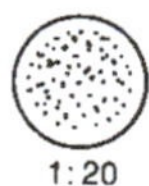
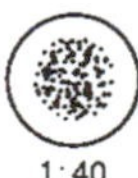
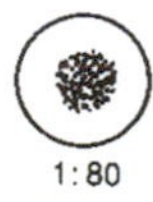
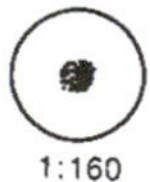
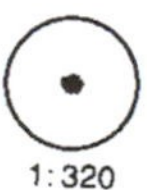

Figure 4–10

488. The AIDS virus (HIV) differs from the RNA tumor viruses in that it

(A) does not require T_4 receptor protein for adsorption to host cells
(B) contains two copies of single-stranded RNA in its virion
(C) contains the *gag* gene
(D) contains the *pol* gene
(E) lyses the host cells

489. The spread of herpesvirus type 1 occurs primarily by

(A) breast milk
(B) blood
(C) frozen plasma
(D) direct personal contact
(E) contaminated syringes

490. A 24-year-old construction worker who had four injections of the DPT (diphtheria, pertussis, and tetanus) vaccine in his first year of life and boosters at ages five and 19 received a deep laceration while excavating a building's foundation. The preferred treatment would be

(A) streptomycin
(B) human tetanus immune globulin, because it will stimulate his anamnestic response
(C) equine tetanus immune globulin, because it will passively immunize him
(D) tetanus toxoid, because it will stimulate his anamnestic response
(E) penicillin

491. A 19-year-old student who spent a month removing bushes along the North Atlantic coast found a tick attached to his leg, and he crushed the tick with his fingers. A few days later he developed fever, chills, fatigue, and headache. In the area where he was bitten by the tick he noticed a spreading, circular rash with a clear center. The most likely diagnosis is

(A) trench fever
(B) Q fever
(C) rickettsial pox
(D) epidemic typhus
(E) Lyme disease

492. The structure in Figure 4–11 represents

(A) azidothymidine (AZT), which inhibits the AIDS virus reverse transcriptase
(B) dideoxyinosine, which inhibits poliovirus replication
(C) idoxuridine, which inhibits herpesvirus thymidine kinase
(D) acyclovir, which inhibits the herpesvirus-encoded DNA polymerase
(E) enviroxine, which inhibits rhinoviruses

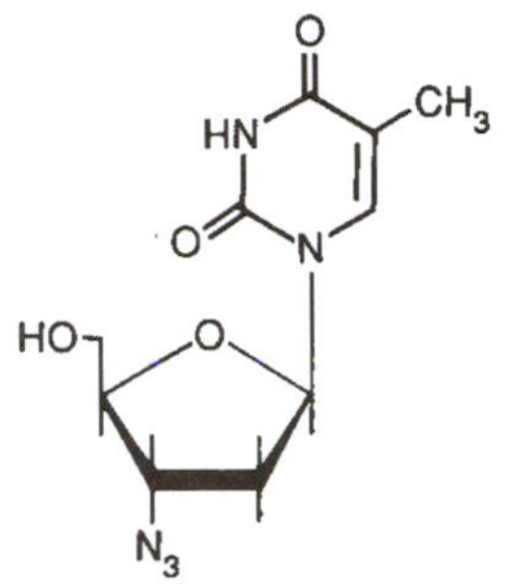

Figure 4–11

493. A middle-aged nurse was providing voluntary medical services in a very poor area, where she was bitten by an infected arthropod vector and developed epidemic typhus. Which one of the following vectors transmitted the disease?

(A) louse
(B) mite
(C) mosquito
(D) flea
(E) tick

494. The pneumococcal antigen that reacts with a nonantibody serum globulin present in inflammatory states is

(A) capsular polysaccharide
(B) penicillin-binding protein 2
(C) C substance (phosphocholine-containing teichoic acid)
(D) pneumolysin
(E) purpura-producing principle

495. A correct characteristic of the members of the genus *Neisseria* is that they are

(A) diplococci
(B) gram-positive cocci
(C) oxidase-negative cocci
(D) acid-fast rods
(E) optochin-sensitive, gram-negative diplococci

496. A young child developed staphylococcal scalded syndrome. Which one of the following toxins is most likely responsible for this syndrome?

(A) toxic shock syndrome toxin
(B) erythrogenic toxin
(C) exfoliatin
(D) alpha toxin
(E) staphylococcal toxins A through D

497. You are faced with the problem of controlling a virus infection in a community and are told that it has been determined it is a togavirus (arborvirus). You know then that your problem most likely is one of

(A) stopping the spread by respiratory droplets and dust of a virus that enters by the respiratory tract
(B) preventing the use of arbovirus carriers as food handlers
(C) improving the treatment of sewage
(D) stopping spread by reducing the close contact of children in schools
(E) identifying and controlling an insect vector and identifying and controlling an animal reservoir

498. Diagnosis of syphilis can be made using the treponemal and nontreponemal serological tests. Which one of the following statements concerning the Venereal Diseases Regional Laboratory (VDRL) test is correct?

(A) It is a widely used nontreponemal test.
(B) It is not useful for screening large numbers of people for syphilis.
(C) It does not require diphosphatidyl glycerol (cardiolipin) as an antigen.
(D) It is basically a complement fixation test.
(E) It cannot be used to follow the efficiency of penicillin treatment.

499. Jacklyn, a fashion model, had several teeth extracted because she had periodontal abscesses. Three months later, she developed a fever of 39.8°C and lower abdominal pain. Anaerobic cultures of the biopsy material showed small spidery colonies in two to three days. The colonies contained Gram-positive, non–acid-fast rods, and branching filaments, while pus from a liver abscess contained yellow granules. Administration of six million units of penicillin daily for two months brought complete remission of Jacklyn's illness. The most likely causative agent of her disease is

(A) *Histoplasma capsulatum*
(B) *Mycobacterium kansasii*
(C) *Actinomyces israelii*
(D) *Mycobacterium tuberculosis*
(E) *Nocardia asteroides*

500. *M. pneumoniae* (Eaton agent) is an infectious agent that

(A) lacks steroids in its cytoplasmic membrane
(B) contains muramic acid in its cell wall
(C) contains only DNA
(D) causes primary atypical pneumonia
(E) is susceptible to penicillin

501. A gardener pricked his toe while cutting rose bushes. Four days later, a pustule that changed to an ulcer developed on his toe. Then three nodules formed along the local lymphatic drainage. The most likely agent is

(A) *Trichophyton rubrum*
(B) *Aspergillus fumigatus*
(C) *Candida albicans*
(D) *Sporothrix schenckii*
(E) *Cryptococcus neoformans*

502. The genome of which virus is a circular molecule of DNA having the structure diagrammed in Figure 4–12

(A) papillomavirus
(B) hepatitis A virus
(C) Epstein–Barr virus
(D) J.C. virus
(E) hepatitis B virus

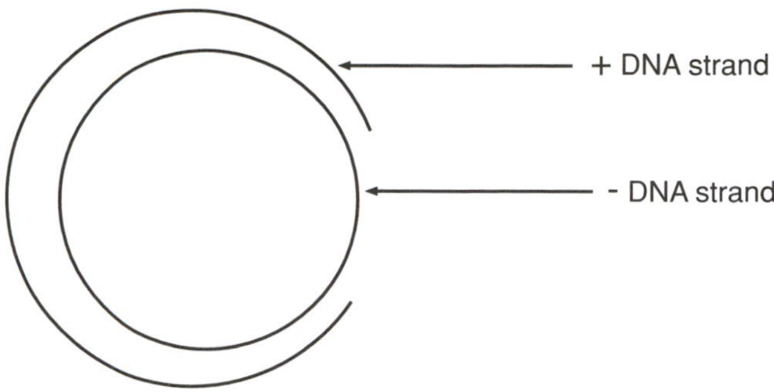

Figure 4–12

503. A 19-year-old girl has smooth, annular, scaly, erythematous, vesicular lesions on her leg. Assuming that you suspect tinea corporis, what would be the most suitable laboratory diagnostic approach?

(A) silver staining of tissue scraping
(B) acid-fast staining on the vesicular fluid
(C) culture of the vesicular fluid on agar
(D) digestion of tissue biopsies with 10 to 25% KOH
(E) serology for *Blastomyces dermatitidis*

504. The cause of antigenic drift of influenza viruses is

(A) mixing of the double-stranded DNA genome
(B) reassortment of genome segments during mixed infections
(C) phenotypic mixing
(D) accumulated point mutations in the hemagglutinin gene
(E) phenotypic masking

505. A 46-year-old cattle rancher develops a low-grade fever 5 days after his 20th high school reunion, which included a rabbit hunt. Standard febrile agglutinin titrations reveal low levels of antibodies to the following organisms: *Francisella tularensis, Brucella suis, Brucella abortus, Salmonella typhi,* and *Proteus* OX-19. The differential diagnosis should include

(A) tularemia
(B) brucellosis
(C) typhoid fever
(D) Rocky Mountain spotted fever
(E) tularemia, brucellosis, typhoid fever, and Rocky Mountain spotted fever

506. The "virus" responsible may be just infectious protein with no nucleic acid for

(A) subacute sclerosing panencephalitis
(B) distemper
(C) herpes encephalitis
(D) progressive multifocal leukoencephalopathy
(E) Creutzfeldt–Jacob disease

507. Plasmid-encoded genes

(A) specify multiple drug resistance
(B) cannot encode enterotoxins of *E. coli*
(C) have not been associated with bacteriocin production
(D) cannot specify exotoxin production
(E) cannot encode for resistance to bacteriophage

508. The cellular oncogene involved in the chromosomal translocation that is characteristic of many Burkitt's lymphomas is

(A) V-abl
(B) V-ras
(C) C-myc
(D) V-fms
(E) V-src

509. A child has fever, conjunctivitis, coryza, and sore throat. The clinical laboratory has isolated a non-enveloped, icosahedral DNA virus shown in Figure 4–13. This microorganism most likely is

(A) poxvirus
(B) parvovirus
(C) adenovirus
(D) herpesvirus
(E) hepadnavirus

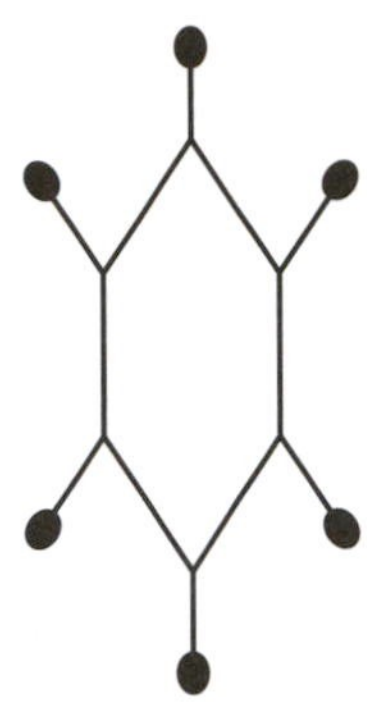

Figure 4–13

510. An infant has congenital syphilis, which can best be detected by

(A) x-rays
(B) use of Wassermann complement fixation test
(C) dark-field examination
(D) FTA-ABA IgM test
(E) silver nitrate staining of spirochetes

511. A 21-year-old man has been skin tested and had a positive test to purified protein derivative (PPD). This indicates that he has

(A) active tuberculosis
(B) been exposed to *Mycobacterium tuberculosis*
(C) received BCG vaccine
(D) provided sound information on his health status
(E) proper B-cell function

512. Amantadine is often useful in the treatment of infections by

(A) herpes simplex virus
(B) rabies virus
(C) Epstein–Barr virus

(D) influenza virus
(E) rhinovirus

513. Immunologic suppression for transplantation

(A) cannot occur by lymphoid irradiation
(B) can occur by antilymphocyte globulin
(C) cannot be achieved by cyclosporine administration
(D) is not likely to respond to steroid administration
(E) is facilitated by gamma-interferon administration

514. The genome of this virus is a linear double-stranded DNA, which contains a virus encoded protein that is covalently cross-linked to each 5′ end of the linear genome. It is

(A) herpes simplex virus
(B) varicella-zoster virus
(C) adenovirus
(D) SV40
(E) vaccinia virus

515. Immune complexes

(A) do not contain complement
(B) are the key players in delayed hypersensitivity
(C) are not involved in serum sickness
(D) have not been implicated in lupus erythematosus
(E) play a role in acute poststreptococcal glomerulonephritis

516. Desirable properties of a vector plasmid for use in molecular cloning include

(A) low copy number
(B) selectable phenotype
(C) non-autonomous replication
(D) multiple sites for restriction enzymes
(E) incorporation into host cell chromosome

517. *Legionella pneumophila*

(A) cannot survive for months in tap water at 25°C
(B) is not the major cause of legionellosis in humans
(C) is easily demonstrable in Gram stains of clinical specimens
(D) has been found in air-conditioning systems
(E) is the cause of trench fever

518. A patient is complaining of a sore throat. Physical examination of the throat indicates severe redness and an exudate; lymphadenopathy is also evident. This triggers consideration of

(A) throat culture
(B) bacitracin discs
(C) blood agar
(D) penicillin
(E) all of the above

519. Which one of the following is the most likely penicillin-binding bacterial component?

(A) porin
(B) transpeptidase
(C) alanine racemase
(D) mucopeptide
(E) glycine pentapeptide

520. Which of the following is a T-cell–dependent antigen?

(A) polymerized flagellin
(B) poly-D amino acids
(C) pneumococcal polysaccharides
(D) albumin
(E) endotoxin

521. Which one of the following viruses lacks RNA-dependent RNA polymerase as a structural component of the virion?

(A) respiratory syncytial virus
(B) rabies virus
(C) influenza virus A
(D) retrovirus
(E) influenza virus B

522. A 19-year-old man has tuberculosis. Numerous acid-fast bacilli are seen in his sputum, and more than 70 colonies of *Mycobacterium tuberculosis* developed on the Lowenstein–Jensen medium. The individuals who have come into contact with this patient should

(A) not be checked periodically by sputum culture
(B) not be checked periodically by x-ray
(C) be immunized by BCG vaccine
(D) receive a full course of ethambutol and INH
(E) receive prophylactic isoniazid (INH)

523. Judging from the graph in Figure 4–14, which microorganism is likely to be the causative agent of food poisoning characterized by diarrhea, abdominal cramps, and severe vomiting?

(A) *Salmonella typhimurium*
(B) *Vibrio parahaemolyticus*
(C) *Yersinia enterocolitica*
(D) *Campylobacter jejuni*
(E) *Staphylococcus aureus*

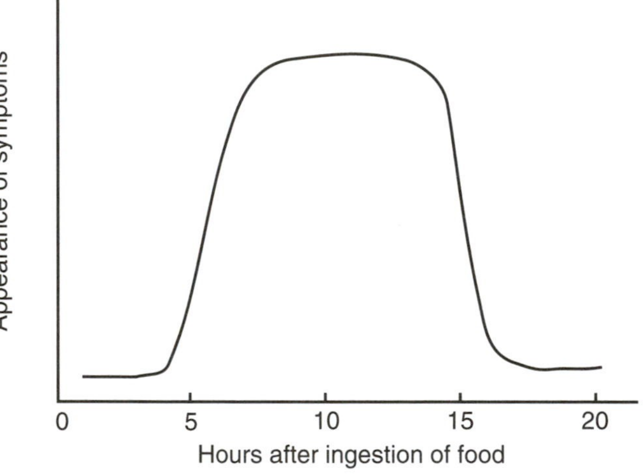

Figure 4–14

524. The hypervariable regions of immunoglobulin IgG are located

(A) on the Fab piece of IgG
(B) at the carboxyl-terminal end of IgG
(C) at the J region of IgG
(D) within the Fc region of IgG
(E) on the constant region of IgG

525. A boy with diphtheria, who has not been immunized against this disease, is given diphtheria antitoxin. Administration of the antitoxin may lead to

(A) elevation in the concentration of serum complement
(B) production of antibodies against diphtheria
(C) development of serum sickness in 4 to 10 days
(D) elimination of the need for immunization with the diphtheria toxoid
(E) lifelong immunity against diphtheria

526. A virus that is not inactivated by mild detergents that solubilize phospholipid membranes is

(A) poliovirus
(B) eastern equine encephalitis virus
(C) variola virus
(D) mumps virus
(E) cytomegalovirus

527. A viral genome which does not replicate in the cytoplasm of the infected cell is found in

(A) poliovirus
(B) rabies virus
(C) mumps virus
(D) cytomegalovirus
(E) rubella virus

528. Poliovirus type 2 has been isolated from the stool of a 55-year-old patient who has been clinically diagnosed as having poliomyelitis. There have been no previous cases of polio reported. However, an infant grandchild was vaccinated about three weeks prior to onset of the disease. How can the laboratory determine whether the isolated virus is related to the vaccine strain or a wild-type virus?

(A) Inoculate the virus into mice to determine whether it kills them.
(B) Determine the cytopathic effects of the virus.

(C) Do neutralization studies using the infant's serum.
(D) Stain the virus with fluorescent antibody.
(E) Do oligonucleotide mapping of the unknown virus and compare with maps of wild-type and vaccine strains.

529. Radioimmunoassay is used to

(A) establish the heterogeneity of an antigen
(B) demonstrate cross-reactions between antigens
(C) demonstrate the homogeneity (purity) of an antigen
(D) quantitate an antigen
(E) identify the isotype of an antibody

530. Two days following surgery to repair a defective valve, a patient developed an acute infection caused by a penicillin-resistant strain of *Staphylococcus aureus.* Figure 4–15 shows the penicillin molecule. Select the most likely numbered site of penicillinase action.

(A) 1
(B) 2
(C) 3
(D) 4
(E) 5

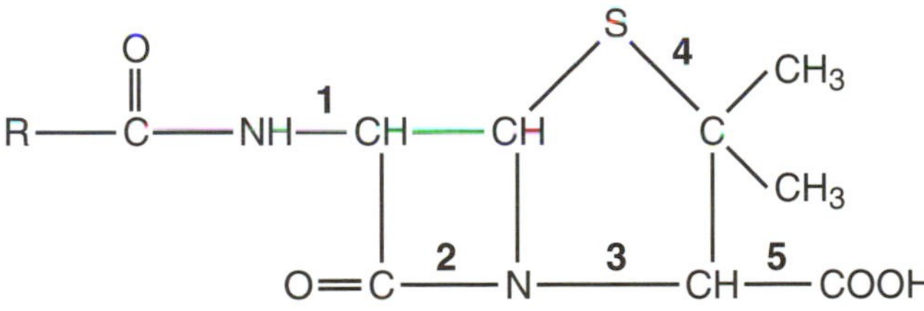

Figure 4–15

531. The laboratory diagnosis of tinea pedis (athlete's foot), caused by *Trichophyton rubrum,* may be made by finding characteristic conidia in cultures of skin scrapings. Which one of the drawings in Figure 4–16 shows the characteristic conidia of *Trichophyton rubrum?*

(A) 1
(B) 2
(C) 3
(D) 4
(E) 5

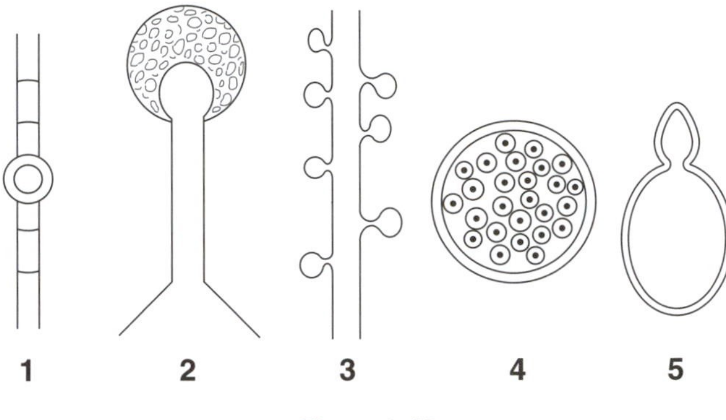

Figure 4–16

532. A 25-year-old male patient comes to your office experiencing inability to swallow and speech difficulty. The patient was in perfect health prior to the consumption of home-canned green beans. He also stated that the can was swollen at the ends prior to its being opened. Which of the following is the most likely method of treatment?

(A) administration of staphylococcal enterotoxin antiserum
(B) penicillin administration
(C) immunization with *S. aureus* enterotoxin toxoid
(D) administration of trivalent botulinum antitoxin
(E) placement of the patient in a hyperbaric oxygen chamber

533. A patient has been given an antifungal agent to inhibit the biosynthesis of fungal ergosterol. The agent given most likely is

(A) amphotericin B
(B) griseofulvin
(C) flucytosine
(D) nystatin
(E) ketoconazole

534. A 5-year-old child with a history of recurrent pulmonary infections has been brought to the emergency room in respiratory distress. A Gram stain reveals numerous polymorphonuclear neutrophils and gram-positive cocci in grape-like clusters in his sputum. The antibiotic to be employed until antibiotic sensitivity tests are reported is

(A) penicillin
(B) methicillin
(C) streptomycin
(D) ampicillin
(E) kanamycin

535. Scott, a 10-year-old boy, was camping on the East Coast during the summer when he was bitten by ticks. Seven days later he developed myalgia, a temperature of 102°C, macules, and petechiae. The rashes appeared first on his arms and legs, then spread over his body, and Scott became delirious. Scott's pediatrician conducted the appropriate laboratory tests and became convinced that Scott had

(A) Q fever
(B) Rocky Mountain spotted fever
(C) epidemic typhus
(D) rickettsial pox
(E) scrub typhus

536. Which one of the following tests provided the most reliable information to establish the diagnosis of Scott's illness?

(A) complement fixation
(B) Weil–Felix reaction
(C) culture on Saboraud's agar
(D) Gram stain
(E) culture on blood agar

537. It can be safely stated that the etiological agent of Scott's disease

(A) cannot be seen with a light microscope
(B) has a cell wall resembling the cell wall of gram-negative bacteria
(C) replicates with a distinct intracellular cycle
(D) lacks a cell wall
(E) is resistant to tetracycline

538. Miss T., upon her return from vacation in a tropical area with poor sanitary conditions, became ill. She experienced lower abdominal pain, colitis, tenesmus, flatulence, and bloody diarrhea caused by a protozoa. The most likely diagnosis is

(A) acute amoebic dysentery
(B) malaria
(C) trypanosomiasis
(D) trichomoniasis
(E) toxoplasmosis

539. The etiological agent of Miss T.'s disease is usually transmitted by the ingestion of

(A) larvae
(B) ova
(C) sporozoites
(D) gametocytes
(E) cysts

540. The drug(s) of choice for the treatment of Miss T.'s illness is(are)

(A) metronidazole and iodoquinol
(B) chloroquine
(C) stibogluconate
(D) sulfonamide and pyrimethamine
(E) trimethoprim and sulfamethoxazole

541. Mr. X. has been feasting on raw oysters for the past nine months. This 26-year-old man has been healthy all of his life. Suddenly he developed fatigue, loss of appetite, nausea, vomiting, abdominal pain, and fever. Following a careful evaluation, his doctor informed him that he is suffering from a viral infection. This infection was caused by a small (20 to 30 nm), non-enveloped, single-stranded RNA virus. This virus most likely is

(A) adenovirus
(B) hepatitis B virus
(C) rhinovirus
(D) rotavirus
(E) hepatitis A virus

542. Diagnosis of the causative agent of Mr. X.'s illness can best be made by

(A) detection of IgM antibodies against the specific virus
(B) detection of IgA antibodies against the specific virus
(C) assays for specific viral cytopathic effects
(D) detection of Negri bodies in Mr. X.'s tissues
(E) a positive Tzanck smear

543. Mr. X.'s viral infection can best be prevented by

(A) interferon
(B) immunization with the specific subunit vaccine
(C) immunization with HBcAg
(D) immunization with the specific inactivated virus
(E) administration of human gamma globulin

544. Neutrophils from a 3-year-old child who has been suffering from repeated staphylococcal infections, show normal phagocytosis. However, intracellular killing of staphylococci by the neutrophils is severely impaired. Myeloperoxidase activity of neutrophils is normal. The child has no history of streptococcal infection. The most likely disease affecting this patient is

(A) severe combined immunodeficiency disease (SCID)
(B) systemic lupus erythematosus (SLE)
(C) rheumatoid arthritis
(D) Graves' disease
(E) chronic granulomatous disease

545. The reason why the child described in the previous question has no history of streptococcal infection is

(A) he has been injected with pooled human gamma globulin
(B) he has been administered antistreptolysin O
(C) he has been immunized with CRP
(D) streptococci are catalase negative
(E) phagocytosis plays a minor role in the killing of streptococci

546. The diagnosis of the disease affecting the 3-year-old boy described in question 544 is made by the

(A) mixed lymphocyte reaction
(B) nitroblue tetrazolium test
(C) Coombs' test
(D) methyl red test
(E) India ink test

Answers and Explanations

410. (D) The envelope of hepatitis B virus (HBV) contains an antigen known as HBsAg (hepatitis B surface antigen). This antigen is of importance because production of antibodies to HBsAg indicates immunity against hepatitis B virus, which resulted either from infection or vaccination with HBsAg. Treatment of HBV with a nonionic detergent removes the envelope and produces the viral core, which contains the hepatitis B core antigen (HBcAg). Antibodies to HBcAg are not protective (choice C). Treatment of the viral core with strong detergents results in the release of a soluble core antigen called hepatitis virus antigen e (HBeAg). Production of antibody to HBeAg signals active disease during which the patient is infectious (choice E). The RNA genome (choice A), or the nucleocapsid proteins of HBV (choice B) are not protective.

411. (E) Delayed-type hypersensitivity is mediated by helper CD4 lymphocytes, not antibody (choice B). Thus it can only be transferred by sensitized CD4 helper lymphocytes. Sensitization occurs via such substances as poison ivy, poison oak, some cosmetics, topically applied sulfonamides, or other drugs and simple chemicals, such as nickel, formaldehyde, and others, but not inhalation of grass pollens (choice A). Part of the tissue destruction seen in tuberculosis is due to delayed type hypersensitivity, so this type of hypersensitivity reaction may lead to tissue damage (choice C). Administration of antihistaminic drugs, epinephrine, or cromolyn sodium is used for the treatment of anaphylactic reactions resulting from type I hypersensitivity, but not delayed-type hypersensitivity (choice D).

412. (E) Alpha interferons inhibit the translation of viral mRNA. Interferon activates cellular genes that code for antiviral proteins. The main target is the translational step in viral replication, which is blocked by two mechanisms—a protein kinase that is activated by dsRNA and inactivates initiation factor EF-2 by phosphorylation, and a nuclease, also activated by dsRNA, which destroys mRNA. Alpha interferon does not interfere with adsorption of virus to the host cells (choice A), the penetration of virus into host cells (choice C), viral uncoating (choice D), or block transcription of viral nucleic acid (choice B).

413. (A) Piliated strains of *Escherichia coli* move up the urethra to infect the bladder and kidney. Infections of the kidney cause pyelonephritis. The vast majority of cases of bacterial pyelonephritis, cystitis, and other urinary tract infections are caused by *E. coli.* Introduction of catheters into the urethra has been associated with the occurrence of urinary tract infections. *Clostridium difficile* is the cause of pseudomembranous colitis (choice B). *Staphylococcus aureus* is usually the cause of boils, skin sepsis, postoperative wound infections, scalded skin syndrome, food-borne infection, septicemia, endocarditis, toxic shock syndrome, osteomyelitis, and pneumonia (choice C). *Pseudomonas aeruginosa* is usually the cause of infections of skin and burns. It is also the major pathogen in cystic fibrosis, and can cause urinary infections, but not as commonly as *E. coli* (choice D).

414. (D) Acute glomerulonephritis appears as a complication only after pharyngeal infection with Group A *Streptococcus pyogenes.* Patients with poststreptococcal acute glomerulonephritis develop high levels of antibodies against streptolysin O of *S. pyogenes.* Thus, the titer of antibodies to streptolysin O can be important in the diagnosis of poststreptococcal acute glomerulonephritis. Determination of serum levels of IgE can be important in the diagnosis of immediate-type hypersensitivity, or in certain parasitic infections (choice A). Serum levels of antibodies against DNA may be of value in the diagnosis of lupus erythematosus (choice B). Estimation of the number of T cells is useful for the diagnosis of T-cell immunodeficiencies (choice C). *Streptococcus pyogenes* do not possess flagella, thus it lacks flagellar antigen H, which would be required for the production of anti-H antibodies (choice E).

415. (A) The patient described in the question probably has AIDS. Such individuals will be lymphopenic and have greatly reduced immunity. AIDS victims commonly develop *Pneumocystis carinii* pneumonia. The most important evaluative procedure for the patient described is determining the cause of the pneumonia so the problem can be corrected. Identifying the infecting organism may assist in the overall diagnosis. Choices B through E involve innate immunity, either complement activity or phagocytic cell functions, and would not be of much diagnostic assistance.

416. (D) The key feature in the problem described is that *two* streptomycin sensitive *E. coli* were mixed together and a *few* streptomycin-resistant colonies developed after exposure to streptomycin. This result indicates that no genetic exchange involving streptomycin resistance occurred between the two *E. coli* strains, and that we are dealing with spontaneous chromosomal mutation. Transduction by bacteriophage involves the transfer of genetic material from one bacterial cell to another by bacteriophage (choice A). In transformation, naked or soluble DNA from a streptomycin-resistant culture is used to transform a streptomycin-sensitive culture to streptomycin resistance (choice B). In conjugation, a piece of chromosome is mobilized by an F factor and antibiotic resistance is transferred from a streptomycin-resistant donor to a streptomycin-sensitive recipient. The net result is recombination and development of streptomycin-resistant colonies (choice C). Complementation is a genetic test of gene function and gene products which involves introducing two mutations to see if the wild-type phenotype is produced. Complementation does not involve recombination, but depends on the interaction of the products of genes (choice E).

417. (B) The child appears to be suffering from meningitis due to *S. aureus,* which should always be assumed to be a β-lactamase–producing organism until the laboratory reports its antibiotic sensitivity. Methicillin is a β-lactamase–resistant penicillin that would be the drug of choice among those listed (choices A, C, D, and E). It is also bactericidal and is not associated with toxicity, which is a feature of streptomycin and chloramphenicol. Other antibiotics that might be used include the cephalosporins, gentamicin, or vancomycin, which may be injected intrathecally.

418. (E) In the Ouchterlony diagram, each antibody will react with its homologous determinant group on the antigen molecule. Thus antibodies a and b will react with antigen ab, but only antibody a will react with antigen ac. Antibody b will diffuse through the line of precipitate formed by antibody a and antigen ac to bind to epitope band and precipitate with antigen ab, forming the spur at position 3. Line 1 will contain both antibodies. The spur (3) will contain antibody b, not antibody a. Line 2 will contain antigen ac and antibody a only.

419. (A) Bruton's disease is an X-linked congenital agammaglobulinemia. Thus, electrophoresis of the serum of infants, after the passively transferred maternal antibodies have been eliminated, reveals the absence or very low levels of gamma globulin. In contrast to Bruton's disease all the other diseases listed will reveal a gamma globulin peak. Goodpasture's syndrome and Addison's disease are caused by autoantibody production to basement membrane of kidney and adrenal cortex, respectively (choices C and D). Myasthenia gravis involves autoantibody production to acetylcholine receptor of the neuromuscular junctions (choice E). Graves' disease is caused by autoantibody production to thyroid-stimulating hormone receptors (choice B).

420. (C) The most important presumptive diagnostic test for gonorrhea is the demonstration of gram-negative, kidney-shaped diplococci inside polymorphonuclear leukocytes, obtained from a thick creamy urethral exudate. Patients with gonorrhea experience an intense burning sensation during urination. Individuals with trichomoniasis discharge a watery foul-smelling urethral exudate, and staining of this discharge reveals pear-shaped trophozoites that have a jerky motion (choice A). Primary syphilis produces painless ulcers on the genital organs, anal area, or mouth. These ulcers have well-defined raised borders, and a clean, hard base (hard chancre). The primary lesions usually contain spirochetes which cannot be demonstrated by conventional stains. However the spirochetes can be visualized by silver stain, with immunofluorescence, or with a dark-field microscope (choice B). Lymphogranuloma venereum, caused by *Chlamydia trachomatis* immunotypes L1 to L3, produces abscesses in the lymph nodes. Diagnosis depends on the demonstration of cytoplasmic inclusions, which are visualized with Giemsa stain, or immunofluorescence (choice D). Chancroid, caused by *Hemophilus ducrei,* produces sharply circumscribed, nonindurated, painful ulcers. These ulcers are usually found in the genitalia and perianal regions. The ulcers have a soft base and thus are called soft chancres. Bacteria in chancres can be visualized by Gram stains, which reveal gram-negative rods (choice E).

421. (D) Prevention of gonorrhea rests on the use of safe, properly worn condoms, and immediate treatment of symptomatic patients as well as their sexual partners. Ceftriaxone is the best treatment for uncomplicated cases of gonococcal infections. Since 1976, penicillinase-producing strains of *Neisseria gonorrhoeae* have been isolated that show a high level of resistance to penicillin. Thus, use of 100 units penicillin will be of little if any value for the prevention of gonorrhea (choice A). There are no vaccines composed of either killed germs or toxoids available for the prevention of gonorrhea (choices B, E). Frequent washing of the genital areas is not likely to prevent gonorrhea (choice C).

422. (C) If exposure to rabies virus appears definite, as in this case, treatment with human diploid cell live-derived vaccine and hyperimmune antirabies gamma globulin should be started immediately. Serum antibodies provide an immediate barrier to the growth of virus; meanwhile, antibodies are elicited by the vaccine. If the level of exposure is minimal (e.g., no skin puncture) and the animal probably is not rabid, vaccine is not recommended. Ordering a search for the attacking fox for autopsy to determine if it has rabies is like searching for a needle in a haystack, and thus not the best approach to address a possible rabies infection, which requires immediate actions (choice A). Initiation of rabies vaccine will lead to production of antibodies against the rabies virus, but it will require approximately two weeks to develop protective antibodies. By that time, severe damage may have already occurred (choice B). Postexposure immunization and human rabies immunoglobulin is the best approach. Observation of the patient (choice D) or reporting of the incident to the state epidemiologist (choice E) do not address the real needs of an individual running the risk of rabies.

423. (D) Chlamydiae and rickettsiae are the largest of the obligate intracellular parasites. They are bacterialike in that they have a cell wall, contain both DNA and RNA (choice C), and are susceptible to certain antibiotics (e.g., tetracyclines and chloramphenicol) (choice

B). Most rickettsiae are spread by arthropod vectors; chlamydiae are spread by direct contact or by the respiratory route (choice A). In addition, chlamydiae divide by binary fission and by an unequal divisional process involving elementary and reticulate body formation (choice E).

424. (A) Exposure to the TB bacillus does not assure disease, but a positive skin test makes the diagnosis more likely. Chemoprophylaxis with isoniazid (INH) would be the treatment of choice for contacts of actively infected persons. Ethambutol is very effective against most mycobacteria, but would be used in the therapy of TB, not in prophylaxis (choice B). The skin test is the most sensitive index of infection, and for individuals who have already shown a positive response, x-ray would not add much information. Sequential x-rays months apart might indicate if the lesion were increasing in size, but that is certainly not a high-priority procedure for the persons described in the question (choice C). Immunization with the live attenuated TB strain bacillus Calmette–Guérin (BCG) would be pointless, as the contacts have already experienced an infection with *M. tuberculosis* (choice D). Immunization with purified protein derivative does not induce protection against tuberculosis. It is used to determine exposure to *Mycobacterium tuberculosis* (choice E).

425. (D) The most acute form of hypersensitivity is systemic anaphylaxis during which there is constriction of the bronchioles and hypotension. Anaphylaxis is mediated by such pharmacologically active substances as histamine, the slow-reacting substance, eosinophil chemotactic factor of anaphylaxis, serotonin, prostaglandins, and thromboxanes. Penicillin is known to be a sensitizing allergen. The patient was sensitized when he was given his first injection of penicillin to treat his urethritis. During the next three weeks IgE formed and attached to receptors on the surface of mast cells. When the physician reinjected penicillin, it combined with the IgE, and the mast cells released pharmacologically active substances, inducing constriction of bronchioles and collapse. Gonococcal pneumonia is an extremely rare infection caused by *N. gonorrhoeae* (choice A). Nongonococcal urethritis and reinfection of the urethra with penicillin-sensitive or -resistant strains of *N. gonorrheae* do not cause bronchoconstriction or collapse (choices B, C, and E).

426. (D) The mode of action of ultraviolet light on microorganisms is related to its absorption by the DNA. This absorption leads to the formation of covalent bonds between adjacent pyrimidine bases. These pyrimidine dimers alter the form of the DNA and thus interfere with normal base pairing during the synthesis of DNA. Disruption of the bacterial cell membrane, removal of free sulfhydryl groups, protein denaturation, and addition of alkyl groups to cellular components are induced by detergents, heavy metals, heat or alcoholic compounds, and ethylene oxide or formaldehyde, respectively (choices A, B, C, and E).

427. (E) An undesirable side effect of chemotherapy used to treat malignancies is the destruction of T cells, which play a key role in the development of immunity against viral infections. This is especially true for viral diseases in which the etiological agent remains dormant in the body. Varicella-zoster is an excellent example of such a virus. Thus, flare-ups of varicella-zoster infections are well known occurrences in cancer patients who receive chemotherapy. The varicella-zoster virus is a single entity. It is a medium-sized (100 to 200 nm) double-stranded DNA virus of the herpesvirus group, with only one serological type. Primary infection with the varicella-zoster virus causes chicken pox. Immunity develops, but the virus remains in the body. Immunosuppression by chemotherapy reactivates the varicella-zoster virus and causes shingles (choices A and C). Deficiency in the third component of complement is associated with enhanced susceptibility to pyogenic extracellular bacterial, but not viruses (choice D). Hypogammaglobulinemia has not been shown to cause disseminated varicella-zoster infection (choice B).

428. (C) Herpes B virus is a spherical, enveloped, double-stranded DNA virus that causes a rare and often fatal encephalitis. Persons in close contact with monkeys (such as zookeepers) or tissue culture workers are at high risk for herpes B virus infection. St. Louis encephalitis virus is a small (40 nm) spherical, enveloped, RNA flavivirus. Severe headache, vomiting, and nuchal rigidity are common symptoms, with tremors, convulsions, and coma developing in severe cases (choice A). The poliovirus and the echovirus are small (20 to 30 nm), non-enveloped, single-stranded viruses. Poliovirus causes flaccid paralysis, while echovirus usually induces a flu-like infection (choices D and B). Rabies virus is a single-stranded RNA, bullet-shaped, enveloped virus. The pathognomonic symptoms of rabies are salivation, hydrophobia, and coma (choice E).

429. (B) Curve B depicts the frequency of serologic reactivity following exposure to *Coccidioides immitis* determined by the complement fixation test. Curve A shows the frequency in serologic reactivity following exposure to *C. immitis* determined by the skin test. The skin test becomes positive approximately two weeks after the onset of coccidioidomycosis, precedes the appearance of precipitating complement-fixing antibodies, and tends to remain positive indefinitely (choices A and E). Curve C depicts the frequency of serologic reactivity following exposure to *C. immitis* determined by precipitin test. Precipitin antibodies can be detected in 90% of patients about two weeks after the appearance of the symptoms and disappear in approximately four to five months. Thus, a positive precipitin test suggests active primary or reactivated coccidioidomycosis (choices C and D).

430. (B) The specificity of the tetracycline antibiotics is attributable to an energy-dependent transport system present in prokaryotes, but not in eukaryotic cells. This transport system results in accumulation of the drug inside the bacterial cell, where it binds to the ribosome and interferes with binding of aminoacyl-tRNA to the acceptor site. Tetracyclines bind to the bacterial ribosome, but not to DNA-directed RNA polymerase, or prokaryotic membranes (choices A and C). Tetracyclines do not inhibit initiation of protein synthesis, which specifically requires formylmethionyl tRNA (choice D). Both prokaryotic and eukaryotic cells bind tetracyclines. However, the prokaryotic cells have much more effective tetracycline transport systems than eukaryotic cells. Thus, prokaryotic cells accumulate higher intracellular concentrations of tetracyclines than eukaryotic cells, which induces a significant inhibition of protein synthesis only in prokaryote cells (choice E).

431. (C) Point C represents the zone of equivalence, that is, that point of the antigen-antibody reaction when optimal concentrations of antigen and antibody combine. Thus, there is little, if any, free antigen and antibody, and as a consequence maximal amounts of antigen and antibody will be found in the precipitate resulting from the antigen–antibody reaction. Points A and B represent areas in the antigen–antibody precipitin curve where there is an excess of antibody (choices B and D). Points D and E show areas in the precipitin curve where there is an antigen excess in the antigen–antibody reaction mixture (choices A and E).

432. (D) *Listeria monocytogenes* causes meningitis and sepsis in newborns and patients whose immune systems have been compromised by irradiation or chemotherapy. When this microbe is growing at a temperature of 22 to 25°C on blood agar it yields gram-positive rods, which move with a characteristic tumbling motion. A slight zone of hemolysis surrounds the colonies of *Listeria monocytogenes.* These characteristics are not applicable to *Bacillus cereus, Bordetella pertussis, Neisseria meningitidis,* or *Corynebacterium diphtheriae* (choices A, B, C, and E).

433. (A) Group A streptococci produce two antiphagocytic surface components—hyaluronic acid and M protein—which interfere with ingestion. The streptolysins O and S are able to kill phagocytic cells by membrane disruption (choices C and D). Other streptococcal extracellular products that may have a deleterious effect on leukocytes after phagocytosis include DNAse, proteinase, and RNAse (choice E). Hyaluronidase and streptokinase are virulence factors that may play a role in the organism's spread through the body (choice B).

434. (B) Immunoglobulin IgA is found in genital, intestinal, and respiratory secretions, and in saliva, tears, and colostrum. It inhibits contact of germs to mucous membranes. Secretory IgA consists of two heavy chains, two light chains, and a secretory component (sc), which allows IgA to pass to a mucosal surface, and suppresses degradation of IgA in the intestinal tract. Secretory IgA also contains a J (joining) chain. IgA contains a secretory component (sc) but not an sc epitope. An epitope is defined as the antigenic determinant of a molecule (choice C). The heavy chains for IgG are designated γ, for IgA are designated α, and for IgE are designated ε (choices C and D). IgA does not contain paraprotein (choice A).

435. (A) There is evidence that antigens must be metabolically processed by macrophages before they can be recognized by the T-helper cells. For example, T-helper cells from F_1 hybrids between two inbred strains ($P_1 \times P_2$) that have been sensitized on antigen-pulsed macrophages from one parent (P_1) will proliferate in response to a second challenge of the antigen only if F_1 macrophages or macrophages from P_1 are present. Kupffer cells, young erythrocytes, or suppressor T cells are not considered inducers of T-helper cell proliferation (choices B, D, and E). B cells may be involved in antigen processing, but are not the best antigen processors (choice C).

436. (D) The endemic form of relapsing fever is transmitted by ticks infected by *Borrelia recurrentis*. Relapsing fever begins with headache, high fever, muscle aches, and splenomegaly. It has a unique fever curve due to the emergence of various antigenic types of *B. recurrentis*. *Treponema carateum* is the cause of pinta, which is characterized by hyperpigmentation of the skin (choice A). *Treponema pertenue* is transmitted by contact with infected persons and is characterized by the development of cauliflower-like skin lesions (choice B). *Borrelia burgdorferi* causes a distinct spreading circular rash with a clear center, which is called erythema chronicum migrans (choice C). *Leptospira interrogans* is transmitted by rat urine and causes leptospirosis. This disease is associated with jaundice, uremia, and aseptic meningitis (choice E).

437. (E) A physician is justified in giving antitoxin on clinical evidence, or suspicion of diphtheria, without waiting for laboratory confirmation. The antitoxin dosage should be adjusted according to the weight of the patient and the severity of the infection. The antitoxin is given to neutralize free diphtheria exotoxin in the body fluids and timeliness is of extreme importance. Once the exotoxin has been bound by the body cells and exerted its influence, diphtheria antitoxin is of little value. *Corynebacterium diphtheriae* localizes in the throat, and thus spinal taps are useless (choice A). Tellurite agar, not blood agar, is used for the isolation of *C. diphtheriae* from throat swabs, because it is a selective medium for this germ, inhibiting the growth of other bacteria present in throat swabs (choice B). *C. diphtheriae* is not an acid-fast microbe. Methylene blue is used to stain smears for the bacteriological diagnosis of diphtheria (choice C). This initial treatment of choice for diphtheria is antitoxin. Treatment with penicillin G or erythromycin, but not sulfonamides, may be used. Penicillin G or erythromycin are not substitutes for diphtheria antitoxin (choice D).

438. (D) Diphtheria is typically a toxemic disease. The causative agent *C. diphtheriae* remains localized in the nose and throat where it produces diphtheria exotoxin, which has a selective action on certain organs, such as the heart, kidneys, adrenals, and diaphragm. The exotoxin inhibits protein synthesis by ADP ribosylation of elongation factor 2. Tumor necrosis factor is an inflammatory substance produced by macrophages, and as such may contribute in the pathogenesis of diphtheria, but does not explain the toxigenicity of *C.*

diphtheriae (choice A). *C. diphtheriae* has not been shown to possess a capsule that plays a major role in the pathogenesis of diphtheria (choice B). *C. diphtheriae* has not been shown to have any envelope enzymes that kill natural killer T lymphocytes (choice C). Immune complex formation has been shown to be involved in the pathogenicity of acute glomerulonephritis, type III hypersensitivity, and various autoimmune diseases, but not diphtheria (choice E).

439. (B) Bruton's hypogammaglobulinemia is a B-cell immunodeficiency disorder. Affected patients are deficient in B cells in the peripheral blood and in B-dependent areas of lymph nodes and spleen. Most of the serum immunoglobulins are absent, and the IgG level is < 200 mg/L. Recurrent pyogenic infections usually begin to occur at five to six months of age, when maternal IgG has been depleted. Individuals with Bruton's syndrome have normal T-cell–mediated immune responses (choice A). Patients suffering from X-linked hypogammaglobulinemia do not have normal numbers of B lymphocytes, because the pre–B cells from which B cells are produced fail to differentiate into B cells. This is due to a gene mutation in pre–B cells which does not allow pre–B cells to form tyrosine kinase (choice C). The number of lymphocytes in the paracortical areas of lymph nodes of patients with Bruton's syndrome is normal (choice D). Individuals with X-linked hypogammaglobulinemia have normally functioning T cells, and thus are not particularly susceptible to viral or fungal infections, which are dependent on proper T-cell–mediated immune responses (choice E).

440. (D) Recurrent vesiculating lesions in the genital region suggest human herpesvirus type II, although type I is seen in some cases. Rubella and measles are not closely associated with vesiculating genital lesions (choices C and E). Coxsackievirus and echovirus produce a wide variety of diseases, including meningitis, encephalitis, upper respiratory tract infections, and enteritis. A macular rash may accompany some of these conditions, but its presence has no particular diagnostic significance. Furthermore, they do not produce genital vesicular lesions (choices A and B).

441. (A) Anti-acetylcholine receptor antibodies are found in more than 90% of myasthenia gravis patients. If the clinical symptoms are suggestive of myasthenia gravis, this finding alone is often considered diagnostic. Multiple sclerosis patients tend to have high levels of measles virus antibodies in their spinal fluid. However, the role of this agent in the disease is undetermined (choice B). Guillain–Barré syndrome (also called acute idiopathic polyneuritis) is a demyelinating disease of peripheral nerves. It commonly occurs after a viral infection or an injection, such as influenza immunization. The disease seems to be caused by a T-cell response to nervous tissue (choices C and D). Postpericardiotomy syndrome is a term used to describe a disorder following surgery of the pericardium to remove cysts or tumors or to correct a malformation (choice E).

442. (B) The patient described has a profound deficiency of both the B-cell and T-cell components of the immune response (i.e., severe combined immunodeficiency disease). The dramatic absence of lymphocytes and lymphoid tissue would not be found in any of the other conditions listed. Multiple myeloma is a neoplasm of plasma cells characterized by excessive synthesis of myeloma proteins. Two-thirds of all myeloma proteins are IgG (choice A). X-linked agammaglobulinemia is a B-cell immunodeficiency disorder. Most serum immunoglobulins are absent, and the IgG level is < 200 mg/L. T cells are normal (choice C). Persons with Wiskott–Aldrich syndrome are not able to synthesize IgM against bacterial capsular polysaccharides and thus suffer from recurrent pyogenic infections. The IgG and IgA levels are normal. However, the T-cell immune responses are variable (choice D). Chronic granulomatous disease is the inability of the neutrophils to manifest intracellular microbicidal activity because they lack NADPH oxidase (choice E).

443. (B) Figure 4–7 represents the peptidoglycan of *S. aureus.* The O antigen of *Salmonella typhimurium* is the outer moiety of the endotoxin (lipopolysaccharide) of *S. typhimurium.* It does not have the N-acetyl glucosamine-N-acetyl muramic acid units, side peptides, or cross bridges of the bacterial peptidoglycan (choice A). The C substance of *Streptococcus pneumoniae* is part of the teichoic acid of *S. pneumoniae.* Pneumococci can be agglutinated with antisera against C substance, which is a polysaccharide (choice C). *Mycoplasma pneumoniae* does not have a cell wall and is therefore devoid of peptidoglycan (choice D). The H antigen of *S. typhimurium* is a flagellar protein, and not a part of the cell wall (choice E).

444. (B) Whooping cough can be prevented by vaccination with DPT (diphtheria, tetanus, pertussis) or DTaP (the acellular form of the pertussis vaccine). Immunization has drastically reduced the number of cases of whooping cough. The main immunogens used in the vaccines are either heat-killed cells (in DPT), or the toxoid of *Bordetella pertussis* (in DTaP). Immunity is not acquired by the third month of infancy, but it can be induced by infection. Protection against whooping cough, whether achieved by infection or immunization, is not of lifelong duration, because infections have occurred in persons who either have been previously infected or vaccinated (choices A, C, and E). *B. pertussis* does not possess Vi antigen, therefore immunity to whooping cough cannot be conferred by antibody production to V antigen (choice D).

445. (C) Deficiency in the inhibitor of the first component of complement (C1) is associated with angioedema, because this condition leads to the production of anaphylatoxins C3a, C4a, and C5a. These anaphylatoxins act on mast cells, which release large amounts of histamine. Production of histamine increases capillary permeability resulting in edema. Enhanced susceptibility to pyogenic infections has been attributed to C3 and C5 to C8 components of complement. Bacteremia is a term used to indicate the presence of bacteria in the blood. Thus it has nothing to do with the first component of complement (choice A). Inherited deficiencies of C3 and C5 to C8 have been associated with increased susceptibility to pyogenic infections, but not the first component of complement (choice B). Complement can act synergistically with antibody to modify its action, but not its production (choice D). The conversions of the third (C3) and fifth (C5) components of complement by the C3 and C5 convertases to C3a and C5a anaphylatoxins lead to the increased production of anaphylatoxins (choice E) seen with C1 inhibitor deficiency.

446. (A) By definition a hapten is a substance of low molecular weight that by itself does not elicit the formation of antibodies. However, when attached to a carrier protein, antibody production becomes possible. The hapten-carrier approach has been employed to produce antibodies against penicillin, steroids, nucleotides, lipids, and even 2,4-dinitrophenol. Since the rabbit has been repeatedly injected with the hapten only, the serum cannot be expected to have antibodies against the hapten. It is clear that when the serum is subjected to a gel diffusion assay with the hapten and a carrier protein not used to complex the hapten during immunization, no antigen-antibody precipitin lines of either identity, partial identity, or nonidentity can be expected to form (choices B, C, D, and E).

447. (E) Structural integrity of the bacterial cell is provided by the peptidoglycan layer, which constitutes an integral part of the bacterial cell wall. The main function of the cytoplasmic membrane is to control movement of nutrients into and out of the bacterial cell (choice A). Capsular polysaccharides, lipoproteins, or surface proteins are components of the bacterial cell, but their key functions are not protection of cellular integrity (choices B, C, and D).

448. (E) Although we know that oncogenes are normal cellular genes, their discovery came from studies involving a virus that caused tumors in chickens. This virus is a retrovirus, or RNA tumor virus. The oncogenes have copies in viruses (V-onc), and cells (C-onc, or proto-oncogenes). These oncogenes are involved with the production of molecules essential to normal cell development and function. For example, they may code for proteins which can be tyrosine kinases, such as the src gene of the Rous sarcoma virus, or the abl gene of the Abelson murine leukemia virus. They may code for guanine nucleotide binding proteins (the H-ras gene of the Harvey sarcoma virus). They may code for chromatin-binding proteins, such as the myc gene of the MC29 myelocytomatosis virus, or the fos gene of FBJ osteosarcoma virus. Finally, the oncogenes may code for cellular surface receptors (the epidermal growth factor receptor). The oncogenes are switched off or downregulated, in normal cells.

449. (A) *Chlamydia trachomatis* forms a small (0.2 to 0.4 μm) spherical elementary body (EB). The EB is the infective form of *C. trachomatis* and is responsible for binding and entrance of the organism into host cells. *C. trachomatis* cells lack capsules and cell walls (choices B and C). The reticulate body (RB) of *C. trachomatis* is a larger (0.6 to 1 μm) circular–oval structure. It is the reproductive form of *C. trachomatis* (choice D). The phagosome is a vesicle in the phagocytic cells where digestion of microbes occurs (choice E).

450. (B) This patient has mumps, which can be prevented by immunization with a live attenuated vaccine. Immunization usually produces lifelong protection against mumps. The key diagnostic feature of mumps is tender swelling of the parotid glands, either bilateral or unilateral. Usually fever and anorexia precede the disease. The swelling of the parotid glands is accompanied by pain that is intensified by drinking citrus juices. There are no known antiviral agents to treat mumps (choice A). Two important complications of mumps are orchitis, which can lead to sterility, and meningitis (choice C). Mumps is an enveloped, non-segmented, single-stranded RNA virus of negative polarity. The envelope of the virus has spikes which contain hemagglutinin and neuraminidase on each spike. The diagnosis of mumps is made clinically, however confirmation rests on demonstration of a fourfold rise in antibody using hemagglutinin inhibition tests (choice D). The mumps virus is transmitted by respiratory droplets (choice E).

451. (D) Diphtheria toxin is an exotoxin produced by toxigenic strains of *Corynebacterium diphtheriae.* The toxin consists of two subunits, A and B. Subunit A is a toxigenic moiety that enzymatically ribosylates the elongation factor 2 (EF-2) of the eukaryotic cell. The modification of EF-2 results in the inhibition of protein synthesis and eventual death of the host cell. Subunit B is a receptor-binding component of the toxin. Magnesium deficiency causes dissociation of ribosomal subunits (choice A). Certain antibiotics such as chloramphenicol and puromycin inhibit peptide bond formation (choice B). Hydrolysis of mRNA occurs via various mRNA enzymes (choice C). Diphtheria exotoxin has not been shown to be involved in the destruction of endoplasmic reticulum (choice E).

452. (C) The diagnostic tests ordered by the physician are consistent with a deficiency in the C3, C5 to C8 components of complement. Individuals with these deficiencies have recurrent pyogenic infections, and show enhanced susceptibility to meningococcal infections. All other choices are not consistent with the laboratory findings. Graves' disease involves autoantibody production to thyroid-stimulating hormone receptors (choice A). Wiskott–Aldrich syndrome is associated with recurrent pyogenic infections, but is due to an inability of plasma cells to produce IgM against bacterial polysaccharides, and it occurs only in male infants (choice B). Lupus erythematosus involves production of anti-DNA antibodies (choice D). Chronic granulomatous disease entails a defect in the intracellular killing of microbes by neutrophils (choice E).

453. (D) Antigens have the ability to induce an immune response (immunogenicity) and also react specifically with the products of that response, either humoral antibodies or specifically sensitized lymphocytes. Haptens, whether simple or complex, are partial or incomplete antigens. They have specific reactivity but are not immunogenic by themselves (choices A and E). Determinant groups are the portions of the antigen molecule that determine its specificity (choice B). Adjuvants are substances that have the ability to enhance the immune response to antigens without necessarily being antigenic themselves. For example, *Bordetella pertussis* will cause the host to produce large amounts of IgE antibodies to antigens that normally would not induce the production of this antibody at all. Similarly, presence of mycobacterial cells in a vaccine will encourage the development of cell-mediated immunity to other antigens in the vaccine (choice C).

454. (B) In a laboratory test used to identify *S. aureus,* coagulase reacts with a prothrombin-like compound in plasma to produce an active enzyme (a complex of thrombin and coagulase) that converts fibrinogen to fibrin. This activity of *S. aureus* has a very high correlation with the organism's virulence, although coagulase-negative organisms may cause less severe disease. Coagulase reactive factor is a plasma protein with which coagulase reacts. This protein is presumably a modified derivative of prothrombin (choice A). Prothrombin is the substrate from which coagulase splits a number of amino acids to convert it to thrombin (choice C). Thrombin is the proteolytic enzyme that converts fibrinogen to fibrin, forming the plasma clot (choice D). Plasmin is a plasma protein associated with the destruction of a plasma clot (choice E).

455. (A) The Weil–Felix reaction, which is based on the agglutination of different strains of *Proteus vulgaris* by serum from patients with rickettsial diseases, is a useful diagnostic test. The Weil–Felix reaction uses *P. vulgaris* cells as antigens, not *Salmonella* cells, because *P. vulgaris* has common antigens with rickettsia, while *Salmonella* does not (choice B). The Weil–Felix reaction does not detect viral antibodies. It is used to detect antibodies against *Rickettsia* (choice C). Another test, rarely used in diagnosis of rickettsial diseases today, is the Neill–Mooser reaction, in which viable murine typhus organisms are injected into laboratory animals. Scrotal swelling is the end point of this test (choice D). Q fever does not induce the production of *Proteus* agglutinins. OXK agglutination suggests a diagnosis of scrub typhus (choice E).

456. (A) C5a is a component of complement. Activation of complement by endotoxin, or antigen–antibody complexes produces C5a, which is a neutrophil and macrophage attractant. The variable region of the heavy chain of IgG is not known as the best neutrophil or macrophage attractant (choice B). The J moiety of IgM and IgA does not possess chemotactic properties for neutrophils and macrophages (choice C). HLA-A and HLA-B are genes for the human leukocyte antigens (HLA), and they control the synthesis of class I antigens (choices D and E).

457. (E) Cultivation of fungi requires a medium that is adjusted to the optimal pH of growth for fungi, a pH of 4.0 to 5.0. Such a medium is the one developed by Sabouraud. Tellurite medium is used for the selective isolation of *Corynebacterium diphtheriae,* which is not as sensitive to the concentration of tellurite incorporated into the medium as other bacteria that may be encountered in specimens submitted for the microbiologic diagnosis of diphtheria (choice A). The SS medium is used to isolate bacterial species belonging to the genera *Salmonella* and *Shigella* (choice B). Lowenstein–Jensen medium is used for the cultivation of *Mycobacterium tuberculosis* and other mycobacteria (choice C). Selenite medium is employed to increase the number of *Salmonella* species that may be present in small numbers in fecal or other clinical specimens (choice D).

458. (A) The route of infection of rubella virus is the respiratory tract, with spread to lymphatic tissue and then to the blood (viremia). Maternal viremia is followed by infection of the placenta, which leads to congenital rubella. Many organs of the fetus support the multiplication of the virus, which does not seem to destroy the cells, but reduces the rate of growth of the infected cells. This leads to fewer than normal numbers of cells in the organs at birth. Therefore, the earlier in pregnancy infection occurs, the greater chance for the development of abnormalities in the infected fetus. Many maternal infections that occur during the first trimester of pregnancy result in such fetal defects as pulmonary stenosis, ventricular septal defect, cataracts, glaucoma, deafness, mental retardation, and other maladies.

459. (B) Superoxide, which is bactericidal, is generated during electron transport and in the autoxidation of hydroquinones, leukoflavins, ferredoxins, and flavoproteins. Superoxide dismutase, however, forms oxygen and hydrogen peroxide from superoxide radicals. When catalase is present, it destroys the bactericidal hydrogen peroxide, because catalase hydrolyzes hydrogen peroxide to water and oxygen. Thus, the presence of both enzymes allows aerobes, facultative anaerobes, and aerotolerant microbes to survive when they grow in the presence of oxygen. Obligate anaerobic bacteria generally lack superoxide dismutase or catalase or both and thus cannot grow in the presence of oxygen. Oxidase is an enzyme that oxidizes a substrate by the addition of oxygen or the removal of hydrogen. It cannot oxidize the bactericidal radical superoxide (choice A). Catalase is an enzyme that converts the bactericidal substance hydrogen peroxide to water and oxygen. It has no effect on the microbicidal action of superoxide. Bacteria that lack catalase are likely to be suppressed by hydrogen peroxide (choice C). Peroxidase is an enzyme which catalyzes the dehydrogenation of a substrate in the presence of hydrogen peroxide, which acts as hydrogen acceptor and becomes converted into two molecules of water. Thus, possession of peroxidase in a given microbe will allow it to grow in the presence of hydrogen peroxide, but not in the presence of superoxide (choice D). There are no known pathogenic bacteria that cannot form oxygen (choice E).

460. (E) *P. aeruginosa* is a gram-negative, oxidase-positive, aerobic rod that produces a green-blue pigment called pyocyanin. This microorganism has been associated frequently with wound infections in burn patients, and it is the second leading cause of burn infections after *S. aureus. P. aeruginosa* tends to develop resistance to various antibiotics. However, it may respond to ticarcillin, gentamycin, tobramycin, piperacillin, or azlocillin. *E. coli, K. pneumoniae, P. mirabilis,* and *S. marcescens* may cause urinary or pulmonary tract infections, but are not considered leading causes of burn infections. Furthermore, these bacteria are oxidase negative and do not produce blue-green pigments (choices A, B, C, and D).

461. (B) There are two nonsuppurative sequelae of group A streptococcal disease; rheumatic fever and acute glomerulonephritis. Although rheumatic fever can follow pharyngeal infection with practically any group A streptococcal organism, the majority of nephritogenic strains belong to only six or seven M types. Types 1, 4, 12, 25, and 49 are the most commonly associated with acute glomerulonephritis. The preceding streptococcal infection need not be restricted to the upper respiratory tract to trigger this condition, and streptococcal erysipelas is a frequent cause.

462. (A) *C. neoformans* is the only encapsulated yeast that is pathogenic for humans. Visualization of a capsule around yeast cells in an India ink preparation of spinal fluid is diagnostic for cryptococcal disease, although soluble capsular antigen could also be detected by countercurrent immunoelectrophoresis or latex agglutination. This organism is considered to be an opportunistic pathogen, as over 80% of the individuals who become clinically ill are immunosuppressed in some way or have compromised respiratory functions. The organism is abundant in pigeon excreta-contaminated soil, which is most probably the source of human infections. *Histoplasma capsulatum* may occur as an oval budding yeast inside macrophages (choice B), and may exist in the soil as a mold that has septate hyphae (choice C). In general, fungi reproduce sexually by mating and forming sexual spores, or by forming asexual spores called conidia. The majority of medically important fungi reproduce by asexual spores (choice D). Fungi that contain brown-black pigments in their cell walls are called dematiaceous fungi. *C. neoformans* does not possess these pigments (choice E).

463. (C) *D. latum,* also known as the fish or broad tapeworm, is the biggest worm and can reach 10 m in size. Humans acquire the infection by eating raw fish containing the larvae of the tapeworm. The worm attaches to the small intestine and causes abdominal discomfort. Nausea, diarrhea, weight loss, and pernicious anemia can result. The anemia is induced by the tapeworm's tendency to compete with humans for vitamin B_{12}, which it easily accumulates from the intestinal contents. *D. latum* does not possess blood-sucking organs (choice A). No one has demonstrated that *D. latum* toxin affects hematopoiesis (choice B) or the absorption of iron (choice E). *Schistosoma mansoni* tends to block the common bile duct (choice D).

464. (D) Plague, a zoonotic disease caused by the bacillus *Yersinia pestis,* is transmitted to humans from its animal reservoir (rats in urban plague, squirrels and other wild animals in sylvatic plague), by fleas (e.g., *Xenopsylla cheopis,* the rat flea). Anthrax is an industrial disease, usually acquired by wool and leather workers. The spores contaminate the hides and raw wool and are inhaled by the workers during processing (choice A). Brucellosis and salmonellosis are acquired by ingestion of contaminated foods (choices B and C). Humans may develop leptospirosis if they come in contact with groundwater that has been contaminated with urine from rodents who are harboring the agent in their normal flora, or through a subclinical infection. This disease occurs usually in campers and hunters. Veterinarians are particularly prone to develop zoonotic infections because of their constant contact with infected animals (choice E).

465. (D) Mrs. Y. is suffering from allergic rhinitis. The diagnosis of this allergy is made on the basis of clinical symptoms and the performance of a skin test, as well as a radioallergosorbent test (RAST). In a skin test, a battery of potential allergens are injected separately subcutaneously, and the area of the wheal and flare reaction is measured. The allergen which induces the greatest wheal and flare reaction when compared to solvent is usually the one which causes the allergy. In this case injection of Kentucky blue grass yielded the biggest wheal and flare reaction, and thus this is the allergen which caused rhinitis in Ms. Y. Allergens such as mold, cat dander, house dust, and pollen gave wheal and flare reactions which were either below or slightly above the skin test values of the allergen solvent. Therefore they are not likely to be causing allergy in Ms. Y. (choices A, B, C, and E).

466. (C) The IgG anti-mold–blocking antibody will combine with the mold allergen and will not permit the mold allergen to reach the IgE anti-mold on the surface of the mast cells, thus inhibiting the allergic reaction. Corticosteroids suppress inflammation, but will not prevent the attachment of the mold allergen to the sensitized mast cells by Ms. Y. (choice A). Complement is not fixed by IgE allergen complexes and plays no role in the attachment of mold allergen to sensitized mast cells (choice B). Epinephrine reverses constriction of bronchioles and bronchi, and also has no effect on the attachment of mold allergen to sensitized mast cells (choice D). Cromolyn sodium stabilizes the membrane of mast cells and thus prevents release of histamine from mast cells (choice E).

467. (B) The main symptoms of pneumonia caused by *Streptococcus pneumoniae* are fever, chills, and cough that produces a dark brown sputum. Alcoholism predisposes an individual to pneumonia because it reduces phagocytic activity, and promotes aspiration of microbes. In addition to *S. pneumoniae, S. pyogenes, Staphylococcus aureus,* and *Neisseria meningitidis* can cause pneumonia. However, the other microbes do not produce alpha hemolysis and are not sensitive to optochin.

468. (B) By definition, the rate of growth of bacteria represents the change in the bacterial cell numbers over the change in time. From the choices given, the maximum rate of growth occurs between 2 p.m. and 3 p.m., where within one hour the number of bacteria has increased approximately threefold. Between noon and 1 p.m., 3 to 4 p.m., and 3 to 5 p.m., there is no increase in the number of cells and the rate of growth is zero.

$$\frac{2\times10^7-2\times10^7}{5-4}=0$$

469. (D) The best method for assessing the total number of B lymphocytes is performance of a surface immunoglobulin assay, because B lymphocytes have immunoglobulin on their surface. Quantitative immunoglobulin levels reflect the secretory activity of B lymphocytes, and could be misleading as to the actual number of such cells; for example, in multiple myeloma or other B-cell malignancies, one would expect to find a marked hypergammaglobulinemia (choice A). B cells are not the only cells that have receptors for the Fc fragment of immunoglobulin. Phagocytic cells also have such receptors and thus could be included in an Fc receptor assay (choice B). E rosetting is a property of T lymphocytes, as is PHA mitogenic response; hence neither of these assays would be appropriate for the enumeration of B lymphocytes (choices C and E).

470. (C) PHA induces mitosis in thymus-derived lymphocytes (T cells). Mitosis is detected in the assay by measuring the amount of radioactive thymidine that is incorporated into the T cells during a 24-hour period of incubation with this nucleotide. The E rosette assay measures the number of T lymphocytes but does not indicate their functional status (choice A). Both sIg and serum immunoglobulin determinations would measure B-cell functions (choices B and D). Enumeration of y-bearing cells also would not give any information on their functional status (choice E).

471. (C) Lyme disease is a recently discovered illness caused by *Borrelia burgdorferi*. The disease produces a unique annular skin lesion called erythema chronicum migrans (ECM). Diagnosis of the disease may be assisted by correlating the serum levels of IgM with Lyme disease activity, because these patients develop IgM antibodies to *B. burgdorferi* three to six weeks after infection. Lyme disease is transmitted by tick, not mite bites (choice A). Lyme disease is caused by *B. burgdorferi*, not *Leptospira interrogans*, the organism that causes leptospirosis (choice B). Certain patients develop neurologic and cardiovascular symptoms and arthritis (choice D). Tetracyclines are the drugs of choice for the treatment of Lyme disease during its acute phase (choice E).

472. (C) The organisms of the genus *Haemophilus* are small, gram-negative, non-motile, non–spore-forming bacilli with complex growth requirements. *H. influenzae* requires a heat-stable factor found in blood (X factor), which can be replaced by hematin, and nicotinamide adenine dinucleotide (V factor), which can be added to the medium as a supplement, or can be supplied by other microorganisms, such as staphylococci (satellite phenomenon). *N. meningitidis, N. gonorrhoeae, S. pneumoniae,* and *Listeria monocytogenes* are able to synthesize hematin and nicotinamide adenine dinucleotide, and thus they will grow in culture media which do not contain these nutrients. They also do not need to rely on the production of hematin and nicotinamide adenine dinucleotide by *S. aureus* to grow (choices A, B, D, and E). In contrast to *H. influenzae, Streptococcus pneumoniae* is a gram-positive, lancet-shaped diplococcus, not a gram-negative bacterium (choice D). *Listeria monocytogenes* is a gram-positive rod (choice E).

473. (D) By definition, LD50 is the dose of a microbe or its products that will kill 50% of the species into which it is injected. *Clostridium botulinum* produces one of the most powerful known bacterial toxins. It has been stated that the LD50 of *C. botulinum* exotoxin for humans is approximately 1 μg. *Salmonella typhi* and *Yersinia pestis* are gram-negative bacteria, and as such produce endotoxins which have very high LD50s (choices A and B). *Clostridium tetani* and *Corynebacterium diphtheriae* produce exotoxins which have an LD50 6 to 10 times higher than *Clostridium botulinum* (choices C and E).

474. (B) *Escherichia coli* as well as group B streptococci are the primary etiological agents of neonatal meningitis, because these germs constitute approximately 30% of the vaginal flora of pregnant women. Babies are infected during passage through the birth canal. *S. aureus, S. pyogenes, N. meningitidis* and *S. pneumoniae* are not normal flora of the vagina, and thus are not likely to infect a baby during delivery (choices A, C, D, and E).

475. (C) Evidence now shows that *H. pylori* is associated with the pathogenesis of peptic ulcer. It is found in almost all patients with duodenal ulcers and more than 80% with stomach ulcers. *H. pylori* is a newly discovered curved and spiral-shaped gram-negative bacterium found in the human gastric mucosal layer, but not in the oral cavity (choice A). *H. pylori* produces an abundant amount of urease. It does not produce coagulase, which is elaborated by *S. aureus* (choice B). *H. pylori* is not an obligate intracellular parasite because it can be cultured on a number of artificial media in two to seven days (choice D). Patients infected with *H. pylori* develop IgM, IgG, and IgA, which can be used in its diagnosis (choice E).

476. (E) There are five known classes of immunoglobulins: IgG, IgA, IgM, IgD, and IgE. IgG is the major immunoglobulin that is found in human serum and the only one that has been shown to pass the placental barrier in humans. IgM possesses higher agglutinating and complement-fixing capacity than IgG. IgM has a molecular weight of 900,000. Carbohydrates constitute 7 to 11% of the total weight of IgM (choice A). IgD constitutes a minor portion of serum immunoglobulins (1%). It contains higher amounts of carbohydrate (13%) than the other immunoglobulins, but it is an important B-cell receptor. No other biological functions have been described for IgD (choice B). IgE is the immunoglobulin that has been associated with anaphylactic hypersensitivity. IgE has a molecular weight of 190,000 to 200,000, contains 11 to 12% carbohydrate, and constitutes 0.002% of the total serum immunoglobulin (choice C). IgA is the major immunoglobulin of extracellular secretions. It has a molecular weight of 160,000 to 440,000, has modest agglutinating capacity, and its carbohydrate content is two to three times higher (7.5%) than that of IgG (choice D).

477. (E) Anaphylaxis triggered by penicillin is an immediate hypersensitivity reaction, which is typically mediated by IgE antibodies. IgE antibodies bind to specific Fc receptors on the surface of mast cells and basophils. Upon cross-linking of the IgE antibodies with their specific antigen (penicillin in this case), mast cells and basophils release histamine within minutes along with other pharmacologically active shock mediators which produce the characteristic symptoms of anaphylaxis. Activation of either the classical or the alternate complement pathway do not play any meaningful role in anaphylaxis (choices A and B). IgG and IgD are not involved in anaphylactic reactions (choices C and D).

478. (E) Bacteria divide by splitting into two equal parts (binary fission). The time required for bacteria to undergo binary fission is called the generation time. The given generation time of *E. coli* is 20 minutes. Thus, within three hours (180 minutes), *E. coli* will have undergone nine divisions. Therefore, the number of *E. coli* per mL if we start with 500 bacteria will be as follows: 1000 in 20 minutes, 2000 in 40 minutes, 4000 in 60 minutes, 8000 in 80 minutes, 16,000 in 100 minutes, 32,000 in 120 minutes, 64,000 in 140 minutes, 128,000 in 160 minutes, and 256,000 in 180 minutes.

479. (B) Gene therapy may be useful for acquired diseases such as cancer or infectious diseases. One of the problems encountered in gene therapy is the need of introducing the desired gene into the host cells. Viruses with weak pathogenic potential, capable of entering into host cells have been found to be useful gene carriers. One of the reasons viruses are attractive vectors in gene therapy is that the genes inserted into viruses can be expressed in a regulated way. Viruses infect cells with a much higher efficiency compared to chemical or physical means of gene transfer (choice A). Adenovirus vectors may be used to target gene transfer into cells of the respiratory tract (choice C). Retrovirus vectors can be produced in large quantities from producer cell lines (choice D). The concept of gene therapy is based on the assumption that definitive treatment for any genetic disease should be possible by directing treatment to the site of the defect itself, the mutant gene, and not to the secondary effects of that mutant gene. Since there are many hereditary diseases that are caused by defects in a single gene, there are many potential applications of this type of therapy to the treatment of human diseases (choice E).

480. (A) Mutation occurs in bacteria as in all other cells (choice E). After the initial observation that bacterial populations contain mutants (such as a mutant that is resistant to an antibiotic), the question is whether the mutation is *directed* (induced by the antibiotic) or *random* (spontaneous). This question is most easily answered by the use of the *replica plate technique* (choice D). A velveteen pad is used to press on the colonies of the master plate and then pressed to plates A, B, C, and D. When the bacteria are replica plated to plates A, B, C, and D, each containing a given antibiotic, the resistant colonies always appear in the same places. This is indeed the case in plates B and D, which contain the same antibiotic. This implies that resistant colonies existed before exposure to antibiotic. Hence, mutation is spontaneous. The Lamarckian theory states that acquired characteristics may be transmitted to descendants (choice B).

481. (B) The clinical features of food poisoning due to *B. cereus* include an incubation period of two to eight hours during which nausea, vomiting, and diarrhea develop. Usually eating food containing preformed enterotoxin of *B. cereus* is the source of food poisoning. *B. cereus* grows in the gastrointestinal tract, leading to the production of enterotoxin that causes diarrhea and vomiting. *Clostridium tetani* causes a disease that is characterized by convulsive toxin contractions of voluntary muscles, leading to lockjaw, and opisthotonos (the spine and extremities are so bent that the body rests on the head and the heels) (choice A). The incubation period of tetanus is five days to several weeks. Gastroenteritis caused by *S. enteritis* has an incubation period of 10 to 48 hours; vomiting is rare, but there is diarrhea and low-grade fever. The organisms grow in the gut, leading to superficial infection with little invasion and no enterotoxin production (choice C). Diplopia, dysphagia, dysphonia, and respiratory distress are the clinical features of food poisoning caused by *C. botulinum* (choice D). *P. mirabilis* is a normal inhabitant of the gut, and it may cause occasional urinary tract infections when the bacteria leave the intestinal tract. Diarrhea, vomiting, or nausea are not pathognomonic features of urinary tract infections (choice E).

482. (D) Individuals who have been diagnosed as X-linked agammaglobulinemic lack B lymphocytes and are not able to produce immunoglobulins. The lack of immunoglobulins in X-linked agammaglobulinemia renders individuals susceptible to a succession of infectious diseases caused by extracellular bacteria. These infections may be partially controlled by the injection of specific gamma globulin as a supportive therapy. X-linked agammaglobulinemic patients have T cells that are the key players in cell-mediated immunity associated with graft rejection, intracellular parasites, viruses, and fungi. *P. carinii* is now considered a fungus, causing infections in immunocompromised patients, such as those with AIDS (choices A, B, C, and E).

483. (B) Tumor necrosis factor (TNF) is cytotoxic to certain tumor cells. Recent experiments in gene therapy have taken the approach of expressing TNF in tumor-infiltrating lymphocytes (TIL), with the hope of allowing the TIL to return to the tumor and produce a high concentration of TNF and kill the tumor cells. Tumor necrosis factor (TNF) is a mediator of endotoxin-induced shock and is involved in inflammation, but does not generate high levels of endotoxin (choice A). There is no evidence to support that TNF stimulates T cell proliferation (choice C). TNF is cytotoxic to certain tumor cells, but it does not lyse tumor cells by retroviral participation (choice D). NK cells can destroy tumor cells, however, they cannot be stimulated by TNF (choice E).

484. (E) Tetanus toxin produced by *Clostridium tetani* is a protease that often first affects the masseter muscles. Patients so affected cannot open their mouths and have what is called trismus. Trismus provides an explanation for the term *lockjaw* used to describe tetanus. Cholera toxin causes fluid and electrolyte loss that leads to severe diarrhea (choice A). The clostridial alpha toxin kills cells and produces necrosis (choice B). Diphtheria toxin is an inhibitor of protein synthesis affecting heart, kidney, and other cells. Protein synthesis is inhibited because diphtheria exotoxin ribosylates elongation factor 2 (EF-2) (choice C). Botulinum toxin cleaves the proteins involved in the release of acetylcholine. This leads to paralysis of ocular, pharyngeal, and respiratory muscles (choice D).

485. (E) Infectious mononucleosis is caused by Epstein–Barr virus (EBV), which is a member of the herpesviruses. Nucleic acid hybridization assays for EBV DNA are the most sensitive means of diagnosing infectious mononucleosis. Hemagglutinins and neuraminidases are associated with orthomyxoviruses and paramyxoviruses (choices A and B). The majority of infectious mononucleosis patients develop what is known as heterophile antibody, antibodies that cross-react with unrelated antigens, such as those found on sheep and horse erythrocytes. The heterophile antibody test is used for the diagnosis of infectious mononucleosis, but since it is not a very specific test, it is not as good as the nucleic acid hybridization assays for the presence of Epstein–Barr viral nucleic acid (choice C). Important antigens that also may be used, but which are less sensitive for diagnostic purposes, include the viral capsid protein (VCA), the early proteins (EA), and the Epstein–Barr virus–associated nuclear antigen (EBNA). Infectious mononucleosis patients develop antibody titers exceeding 1:320 and 1:20 against VCA and EA, respectively, during the acute phase of infectious mononucleosis. Antibodies to EBNA develop 1 to 2 months after acute infection (choice D).

486. (A) Prokaryotes are distinguished from eukaryotes in that the prokaryotes have peptidoglycan in their cell walls. Sterols and endoplasmic reticulum are features of eukaryotic cells (choices B and D). Bacteria generally contain a single circular chromosome (choice C). The prokaryotic ribosome has a sedimentation constant of 70 Svedberg units, not 80 (choice E).

487. (C) The ability of certain viruses, such as influenza, mumps, and parainfluenza viruses, to agglutinate red blood cells is used to diagnose these viruses. In general, chicken or human type O red blood cells are employed for the identification of influenza and other viruses. Red blood cells have receptors for the surface component of the influenza virus called hemagglutinin. This hemagglutinin is a glycoprotein. In a hemagglutination assay, a fixed number of red blood cells is mixed with increasing dilutions of the influenza virus. Following incubation at 4°C for two hours, the tubes containing the red blood cells and the virus are examined for hemagglutination. Cells agglutinated by the virus form a lattice that covers the entire bottom of the test tube (virus dilutions 1:20; 1:40; 1:80). The hemagglutination titer of the virus is the highest dilution of virus that forms a lattice. In this case, the hemagglutination titer is 1:80. Unagglutinated cells form a dark bottom (virus dilutions 1:160; 1:320) (choices D and E).

488. (E) An important difference between the AIDS (HIV) virus and the RNA tumor viruses is that HIV lyses the host cells, while RNA tumor viruses transform the cells they invade, but they lack cytolytic activity. The tropism of the HIV virus for T_4 lymphocytes depends on the presence of the T_4 protein on the surface of the lymphocytes. This protein serves as the receptor for the adsorption of the HIV virus to T_4 lymphocytes. The HIV virus is a member of the retroviruses (choice A). The genomic RNA molecule of HIV contains the *gag, pol,* and *env* genes. Thus, the HIV virus does not differ from RNA tumor retroviruses (choices C and D). HIV contains one copy, not two, of single-stranded RNA in its virion (choice B).

489. (D) Transmission of herpes simplex virus type 1 occurs primarily by direct contact. Breast milk, blood, frozen plasma, or contaminated syringes have been implicated in the transmission of AIDS virus (HIV), but are not considered the primary vehicles of herpes simplex virus type 1 transmission (choices A, B, C, and E).

490. (D) Since there are memory lymphocytes primed by a previous tetanus toxoid injection, booster immunization with tetanus toxoid will lead to rapid production of adequate levels of protective antibody. This is the routine procedure followed by physicians for trauma patients who have been vaccinated against tetanus and received booster immunization within the last 5 to 7 years. The antibody titer to tetanus toxoid remains at protective levels for 5 to 10 years. Aminoglycosides such as streptomycin or penicillin will not be effective against the spores or vegetative cells of *Clostridium tetani* (choices A and E). Human tetanus immune globulin will only provide antibodies to tetanus exotoxin for a short time and cannot induce an anamnestic response because an injection of tetanus exotoxin or toxoid is required (choice B). Individuals who have been vaccinated against tetanus require injections of the tetanus toxoid to induce rapid production of adequate levels of protective antibody. Treatment with equine tetanus immunoglobulin, which will only provide antitetanus antibody for a short time, is not the preferred method of treatment for this patient (choice C).

491. (E) This patient's symptoms point to a diagnosis of Lyme disease, caused by *Borrelia burgdorferi,* and transmitted to humans by ticks that harbor this organism. The initial symptoms of Lyme disease are fever, chills, fatigue, and headache, but the pathognomonic feature is a spreading, circular rash with a clear center. The rash begins three to 18 days after the tick bite and is called erythema chronicum migrans. Q fever, epidemic typhus, rickettsial pox, and trench fever do not produce erythema chronicum migrans (choices A, B, C, and D).

492. (A) The antiviral drug currently used against the immunodeficiency virus is AZT, or 3-azido-3-deoxythymidine (azidothymidine). Its structure is shown in Figure 4–11. The structures of related compounds idoxuridine (choice C) and dideoxyinosine (choice B) are shown below in Figure 4–17. Acyclovir (choice D) and enviroxine (choice E) differ chemically from the structure depicted in Figure 4–11.

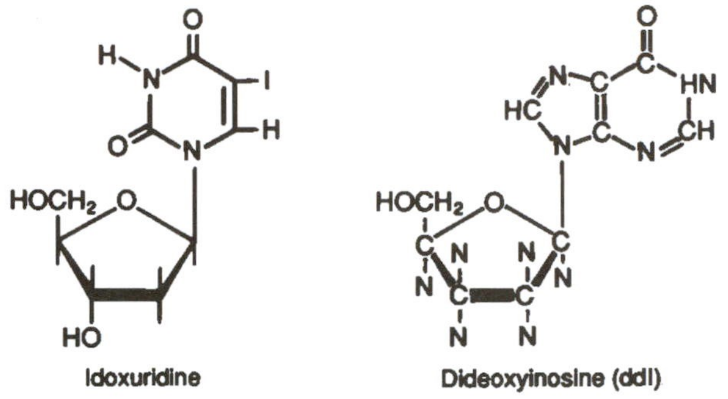

Figure 4–17

493. (A) Epidemic typhus is caused by *Rickettsia prowazeki.* It is transmitted from one individual to another by bites of the human body louse. The louse becomes infected when it takes a meal from an individual that harbors *R. prowazeki.* The mite is the biological vector of rickettsial pox and another rickettsial disease called scrub typhus (choice B). Mosquitoes transmit such diseases as malaria, yellow fever, St. Louis encephalitis, eastern equine encephalitis, western equine encephalitis, California encephalitis, and other diseases (choice C). Fleas transmit endemic typhus and plague (choice D). Ticks are the biological vectors of many diseases, such as Lyme disease, Rocky Mountain spotted fever, and tularemia (choice E).

494. (C) C substance, or C polysaccharide, which is a species-specific teichoic acid polymer containing phosphocholine as a major determinant, precipitates with a nonspecific serum beta globulin called C-reactive protein (CRP). Levels of CRP, which is not an antibody, are elevated in individuals with a wide variety of acute inflammatory diseases. The high CRP levels may be used as an indication of an individual with an inflammatory disease. The C substance–CRP precipitate activates complement via the classic pathway, and it may function as an opsonin to facilitate the phagocytosis early in pneumococcal infections. Capsular polysaccharides are the subunits which constitute the bacterial capsule. They are usually carbohydrates composed of pentoses or hexoses (choice A). Penicillin-binding proteins are cell membrane proteins which interact with penicillin. Alteration in the structure of these proteins may lead to resistance to penicillins and related antibiotics (choice B). Pneumolysin is an enzyme found in *Streptococcus pneumoniae* which under proper conditions may lyse pneumococci (choice D). Purpura-producing principle is a substance produced by *Haemophilus aegyptius* which causes purpuric fever, a disease of children that can produce purpura and shock (choice E).

495. (A) *Neisseria* species are gram-negative cocci usually seen in pairs (diplococci with adjacent flattened sides). All species of *Neisseria* are oxidase-positive diplococci (choice C). *S. pneumoniae* is a gram-positive lancet-shaped diplococcus which is optochin sensitive (choice A). *S. aureus, S. pneumoniae* and *S. pyogenes* are examples of gram-positive cells (choice B). Mycobacteria are acid-fast bacilli (choice D). There are no known pathogenic optochin-sensitive gram-negative diplococci (choice E).

496. (C) Exfoliatin toxin is produced by certain strains of *Staphylococcus aureus* belonging to phage group II. This exotoxin divides the epidermis between the stratum granulosum and the stratum spinosum. The end-result of exfoliatin action is the exfoliation of the skin, known as the staphylococcal scalded skin syndrome. The toxic shock syndrome toxin (TSST) causes multisystem involvement with shock which can be lethal. TSST is a super antigen that releases large concentrations of IL-1, IL-2, and tumor necrosis factor (TNF) (choice A). Erythrogenic toxin is produced by *Streptococcus pyogenes* and is associated with scarlet fever (choice B). Alpha toxin is produced by *S. aureus* and causes necrosis and hemolysis of blood cells (choice D). Staphylococcal enterotoxins A through F are responsible for food poisoning (choice E).

497. (E) Togaviruses contain viral species that cause encephalitis. They are transmitted via mosquito vectors with birds serving as reservoirs of infection. Western and eastern encephalitis viruses cause infections that have high mortality in children and in aged individuals. These viruses enter the bloodstream from insect inoculation. The virus is removed by the reticuloendothelial cells and multiplies in the spleen and lymph nodes. From these tissues, a secondary viremia is established, spreading the virus to the central nervous system by passage through the blood–brain junction (virus grows through the vascular endothelium or in some way is passively transported across the blood–brain barrier). The brain and spinal cord become edematous and show vascular congestion and small hemorrhages. There are no human vaccines, and control is limited to controlling the insect vectors (choices A, B, C, and D).

498. (A) The most widely used nontreponemal test for syphilis is the glass slide flocculation Venereal Disease Research Laboratory (VDRL), or the card rapid plasma reagin (RPR) test. In the VDRL test, the antigen employed is an alcoholic extract of beef heart containing cardiolipin (diphosphatidyl glycerol), which also appears to be a component of the cytoplasmic membrane of *Treponema pallidum* that causes syphilis (choice C). The VDRL is a rapid serological test which is very useful for screening large numbers of people for syphilis (choice B). The VDRL is a slide flocculation, and not a complement fixation test (choice D). The VDRL titer reflects the activity of the disease. Such titers reach a level of 1:32 or higher in secondary syphilis. A persistent fall in titer following penicillin or other antibiotic treatment indicates an adequate response to therapy (choice E).

499. **(C)** The detection of yellow sulfur granules in pus obtained from the liver abscess suggests hepatic actinomycosis, because the sulfur granules represent colonies of *Actinomyces israelii* or other oral *Actinomyces* species. The *Actinomyces* associated with hepatic actinomycosis, which may follow teeth extractions, especially in patients with paradental abscesses, are usually *A. israelii, A. bovis,* or *A. odontolyticus.* All these fail to grow aerobically, but can be cultured anaerobically on brain heart infusion agar where in two to three days at 37°C, *A. israelii* produces small, white, spidery colonies containing gram-positive rods and filaments. In pus, *A. israelii* is found as sulfur granules representing colonies of the microorganism. When the sulfur granules are washed, crushed between two glass slides, and Gram stained, under the microscope they show a twisted aggregation of filaments which break up into bacilli, cocci, or small gram-positive, non-acid-fast filaments. *Mycobacterium tuberculosis, M. kansasii,* and *Nocardia asteroides* are aerobic, acid-fast microorganisms. *A. israelii* and *N. asteroides* are sensitive to penicillin, while *M. tuberculosis, M. kansasii,* and the fungus *Histoplasma capsulatum* are resistant to it (choices A, B, D, and E).

500. **(D)** *M. pneumoniae* is the causative agent of primary atypical pneumonia, which was initially described by Eaton, giving rise to the eponym *Eaton agent. M. pneumoniae* requires sterols for growth, usually in the form of cholesterol that is incorporated into the cell membrane (choice A). *M. pneumoniae* lacks muramic acid in its cell wall as do all microorganisms belonging to genus *Mycoplasma* (choice B). Similarly, and in harmony with other species of the genus, *Mycoplasma pneumoniae* contains both DNA and RNA (choice C). *M. pneumoniae* is completely resistant to penicillin, which inhibits cell wall synthesis, because *M. pneumoniae* does not have a cell wall (choice E).

501. **(D)** *S. schenckii* is found on thorns, and it is introduced into the skin of extremities through trauma. A regional lesion begins as a pustule, abscess, or ulcer, and then nodules and abscesses are formed along the lymphatics. The history and the symptoms described in this patient are consonant with a diagnosis of sporotrichosis. *T. rubrum* is the cause of dermatophytosis ringworm of skin, scalp, and especially nails. The nails thicken and are discolored (choice A). *A. fumigatus* and *C. albicans* are associated with deep opportunistic infections in immunocompromised patients such as AIDS patients. Aspergillosis is basically a pulmonary infection. Candidiasis can be associated with pathological conditions of the mucous membranes of the respiratory, genital, and gastrointestinal tract, where it is found as a normal inhabitant (choices B and C). *C. neoformans* is the cause of meningitis (choice E).

502. **(E)** The genome of hepatitis B virus is composed of a circular, double-stranded DNA. It has a negative strand of 3200 nucleotides and another positive, incomplete strand of 1700 to 2600 nucleotides. Papilloma and polyomaviruses belong to the family of *Papoviridae,* which lacks envelopes and have a double-stranded, circular DNA genome. Both strands are complete and thus differ from the genome of hepatitis B virus that has one incomplete positive strand (choice A). Hepatitis A virus, the cause of infectious hepatitis, has a linear single-stranded RNA genome, and as such it is a member of the enteroviruses (choice B). Epstein–Barr virus (EBV) is a member of the herpesviruses and as such has a double-stranded, linear DNA genome. EBV has been associated with infectious mononucleosis, Burkitt's lymphoma, and nasopharyngeal carcinoma (choice C). J.C. virus is a member of the polyomaviruses (choice D).

503. **(D)** The most appropriate laboratory diagnostic procedure for cases of suspected tinea corporis is digestion of tissue biopsies with 10 to 20% KOH and a search for hyaline, branched septate hyphae on squamous epithelial cells. A 10 to 20% potassium hydroxide solution dissolves the tissue without destroying the fungal cytology, thus allowing easy visualization of the fungal cells. Silver staining is used for the detection of spirochetes (choice A). Acid-fast stain is employed for the identification of mycobacteria (choice B). Culture of the vesicular fluid on nutrient agar does not permit growth of the fungal cells. Fungi are grown on Sabouraud's nutrient agar, which contains peptones, carbohydrates, vitamins, minerals, and water, and it has a pH of 5.3, which is optimal for fungal growth (choice C). Serology for *B. dermatitidis* is inappropriate, because *T. rubrum* is the causative agent of tinea corporis. Furthermore, serology is of marginal value for the diagnosis of tinea corporis (choice E).

504. (D) The cause of antigenic drift of influenza viruses is accumulated point mutations in the hemagglutinin gene. The genome of the influenza virus is composed of segmented, single-stranded RNA. Influenza virus has a lipid envelope where its important antigens are localized. The virus-encoded surface glycoproteins hemagglutinin and neuraminidase undergo frequent variation independent of each other. Minor antigenic alterations are called *antigenic drift,* while major antigenic variations are termed *antigenic shift.* Antigenic drifts can be diagnosed by amino acid changes in the hemagglutinin glycoprotein molecule and are the results of the accumulations of point mutations in the hemagglutinin gene. Antigenic shifts are due to reassortment of the eight RNA segments of the viral genome. This occurs when persons are infected with two influenza viruses, i.e., a human influenza virus to which the person has partial immunity and an animal influenza virus possessing different hemagglutinins and neuraminidases (choice B). Mixing of the double-stranded DNA genome has nothing to do with the antigenic drift of influenza virus, that has an RNA genome (choice A). Phenotypic mixing involves changes in the appearance of neurominidase and hemagglutinin spikes resulting from mixing of spikes. There is no alteration in the genetic makeup or sequence of the amino acids in the spikes (choice C). The proteins surrounding the RNA influenza virus genome (capsids) may be encoded by the genomes of the human and animal viruses (phenotypic masking). This situation can be detected by antigenic analysis (choice E).

505. (E) The history of the patient described in the question would require careful consideration of all of the diseases listed, and the serology would not serve to rule out any. In the acute phase of the illness, an elevation of antibodies specific for the causative agent might not occur. Usually the rise in antibody levels does not occur until the second or third week of the infection, thus the significance of paired (acute and convalescent) serum samples, which allow the observation of an increase in the antibody specific for the causative agent of the infection. Identifying the cause of most bacterial infections is ideally accomplished by culture of the organism. Serology is used to confirm these identifications and is also used when the agent is slow growing or very expensive to culture, or when the agent cannot be grown at all.

506. (E) Creutzfeldt–Jakob disease is a degenerative central nervous system disease. The etiological agent does not seem to be a conventional virus, but infectivity is related to a proteinaceous macromolecule that appears to be devoid of any nucleic acid. This macromolecule is resistant to formaldehyde. It is inactivated by autoclaving, iodine disinfectants, ether, acetone, 6 M urea, 10% sodium dodecyl sulfate, or 0.5% sodium hypochloride. Subacute sclerotizing panencephalitis is currently believed to be caused by measles virus, or a defective variant of the measles virus (rubeola virus) (choice A). Distemper is a canine viral infection. It is caused by an RNA virus that is a member of the paramyxoviridal family (choice B). Herpes encephalitis is a DNA virus that is well characterized (choice C). Progressive multifocal leukoencephalopathy has been associated with the J.C. virus, which is a member of the polyomaviruses (choice D).

507. (A) Plasmid-encoded genes specifies a variety of functions that include multiple drug resistance. The heat-labile and heat-stable enterotoxins of *E. coli* are plasmid encoded (choice B). Bacteriocinogens are a group of plasmids that specify the production of the bactericidal proteins known as bacteriocins (choice C). The gene for exfoliative toxin, an exotoxin responsible for the staphylococcal scalded skin syndrome, is also located on a plasmid (choice D). Plasmids contain genes which encode for the resistance to bacteriophages (choice E).

508. **(C)** Burkitt's lymphoma is associated with Epstein–Barr virus (EBV), which is a member of the herpesviruses. In this herpetic virus lymphoma, under the influence of EBV, an oncogene called *c-myc,* which is usually located on the eighth chromosome of B lymphocytes, is translocated to chromosome 14 of B lymphocytes at the region of immunoglobulin heavy chain genes. This translocation places the *c-myc* gene side by side to an active promoter, and high levels of *c-myc* RNA are formed. The oncogenes, or transforming genes *v-abl* and *v-fms,* have been associated with the Abelson murine leukemia virus. They appear to be involved in the synthesis of proteins p160 and gp180 (choices A and D). The *v-ras* oncogene has been linked to Harvey murine sarcoma virus that causes sarcoma and leukemia in rats. The *v-ras* oncogene is involved in the production of a protein known as p21 (choice B). The *v-src* oncogene has been connected with the Rous sarcoma virus, which is the etiological agent of chicken sarcoma. The product of the *v-src* oncogene appears to be a protein known as pp60 (choice E).

509. **(C)** Adenoviruses are the only ones that produce spikes extending from each one of the vertices of the capsid. These microbes are DNA, non-enveloped, icosahedral viruses. Adenoviruses cause upper respiratory infections associated with coryza, sore throat, fever, and conjunctivitis.

510. **(D)** The best way to detect congenital syphilis is by the use of fluorescent treponema antibody-absorption-IgM (FTA-ABA-IgM). All newborn infants of mothers with reactive VDRL, or reactive FTA-ABA tests, will themselves have reactive tests, whether or not they have actually acquired syphilis, because of the passive placental transfer of maternal immunoglobulins. However, if IgM antisyphilitic antibody is present in the infant's serum, it will reflect fetal antibody production in response to intrauterine infection (congenital syphilis) because *maternal* IgM antibody does not penetrate a healthy placenta. X-rays will not reveal congenital syphilis in an infant (choice A). Use of the Wassermann complement fixation test is not as specific as the FTA-ABA-IgM test for the detection of congenital syphilis (choice B). It is difficult to detect *T. pallidum* in infants by dark-field examinations or by silver staining. Furthermore, sampling of an infant's blood or other body fluids entails risk for the infant (choices C and E).

511. **(B)** A positive PPD skin test indicates that the individual has experienced mycobacterial infection at some time. A positive PPD skin test is usually obtained in individuals who have been vaccinated with the attenuated strain of *Mycobacterium bovis* produced by Calmette–Guérin, who named the vaccine bacillus–Calmette–Guérin (BCG). However, as has been indicated above, any individual who had contact with *M. tuberculosis* usually gives a positive PPD test (choice C). The PPD skin test does not necessarily indicate current disease or give any information on the health status of the individual (choices A and D). The PPD skin test may be used to assess proper T-cell function, but not B-cell function (choice E).

512. **(D)** Amantadine (generic name) or Symmetrel (trade name) inhibits an early event in the multiplication cycle of influenza virus, as well as arenaviruses. It blocks the uncoating process. Mutations in the M protein genes result in the development of drug-resistant mutants. The drug is not used extensively in the United States because it seems impractical to control this type of infectious disease that is not ordinarily fatal. To protect individuals at high risk, and in those in whom the infection is potentially dangerous, the choice is between this drug and the influenza vaccine. In most cases, the vaccine is usually preferred. Acyclovir is used to shorten the duration of herpes simplex virus episodes and also to limit the duration of viral shedding (choice A). There are no antiviral drugs for rabies (choice B). Acyclovir has slight antiviral action for Epstein–Barr virus (choice C). There is no antiviral agent against rhinovirus (choice E).

513. (B) There are various ways by which immunologic suppression for transplanted tissue can occur. One of these ways is administration of antilymphocyte globulin. Other means used to obtain immunologic suppression for transplantation include destruction of B and T lymphocytes by irradiation (choice A). Cyclosporin is also used to achieve immunologic suppression for transplantation. It is thought to inhibit interleukin-2 which drives antigen activated cells to proliferate (choice C). Steroid administration is an effective means to suppress the immune system (choice D). Suppression of transplanted tissue cannot be obtained by interferon administration, because interferon inhibits translation of viral mRNA (choice E).

514. (C) Adenoviruses do not have an envelope. Their linear, double-stranded DNA is enclosed within a capsid with icosahedral symmetry. Spikes project from each of the 12 vertices. The viral DNA contains a virus-encoded protein that is covalently cross-linked to each 5′ end of the linear adenovirus genome. Herpesviruses and varicella-zoster virus belong to the same family of herpes viridae and have a linear, double-stranded DNA genome, in which the complementary strands are not covalently cross-linked at the termini of the genome (choices A and B). SV40 virus is a member of the polyoma group of viruses, and possesses a circular, double-stranded DNA genome (choice D). Finally, the genome of the vaccinia virus has linear, double-stranded DNA with inverted terminal repeats (choice E).

515. (E) Acute poststreptococcal glomerulonephritis is related to deposition of antigen–antibody complexes on the glomerular basement membrane. The complexes are composed of antigen, antibody, and complement. Acute poststreptococcal glomerulonephritis occasionally follows infection with group A streptococci that possess type 49, 12, 4, or 2 M protein. Immune complexes are composed of antigen–antibody-complement complexes. Thus, immune complexes contain complement (choice A). Immune complexes are not the key players in delayed hypersensitivity. Delayed-type hypersensitivity is induced by CD4 T lymphocytes which have been exposed to an antigen, and release lymphokines upon second exposure to the same antigen (choice B). Any foreign substance against which the host can produce antibody can cause this disease, although horse serum historically has been the culprit. The immune complexes in serum sickness may localize in the vascular bed, producing vasculitis, or may cause arthritis (choice C). Immune complexes have also been associated with lupus erythematosus. Lupus erythematosus is one of the most significant complications of autoimmune disease, and occurs as a result of DNA/anti-DNA antibody complexes (choice D).

516. (B) To be useful as a cloning vector, a plasmid should possess several properties. It should code for one or more selectable markers (such as antibiotic resistance) to allow identification of transformants and to allow maintenance of the plasmid in a bacterial population. A vector plasmid should have a high, not a low, copy number. With high copy numbers, large amounts of a specific segment of foreign DNA can be obtained readily in pure form (choice A). A plasmid vector should have autonomous, not non-autonomous replication. Autonomous replication is necessary and allows a high copy number of plasmids to be obtained (choice C). Also, a vector plasmid should contain single sites for restriction enzymes in regions of the plasmid that are not essential for replication. Single sites for restriction enzymes allow for insertion of foreign DNA molecules that have been cleaved with the restriction enzymes (choice D). Plasmids by definition are pieces of DNA which replicate autonomously in the host cell cytoplasm, without incorporation into host cell chromosome (choice E).

517. **(D)** *Legionella pneumophila* is spread from water reservoirs, contaminated air-conditioning units, nebulizers filled with water, or evaporative condensers. The organism can survive for over a year in tap water at room temperature (23 to 25°C) (choice A). Legionellosis, or legionnaire's disease, was first detected in 1976 when an outbreak of deadly pneumonia occurred in over 200 persons attending an American Legion convention. Epidemiologic investigations showed that the disease was caused by a gram-negative rod that was named *L. pneumophila* (choice B). *L. pneumophila* is difficult to stain with Gram stain or other common bacterial stains. It will stain faintly gram-negative when safranin is left on for an extended period. The organism can be demonstrated by the direct fluorescent antibody procedure or by the silver impregnation method (choice C). The cause of trench fever is *Bartonella quintana* (previously known as *Rochalimaea quintana*), not *L. pneumophila* (choice E).

518. **(E)** The physical examination supports a provisional diagnosis of streptococcal pharyngitis. This is a common infection caused by group A, β-hemolytic streptococci, which are usually susceptible to penicillin and bacitracin. Laboratory diagnosis of group A streptococcal pharyngitis is based on blood agar cultures, bacitracin sensitivity tests, and various serologic assays.

519. **(B)** Penicillins and cephalosporins inhibit bacterial growth by binding to transpeptidase. This binding leads to interference with bacterial cell wall synthesis and subsequent lysis of the bacterial cell. Porins are cell membrane proteins which form channels in cell membranes, and thus play a role in the regulation of the entrance of small, hydrophilic molecules into the bacterial cell (choice A). Alanine racemase converts L-alanine to D-alanine and amino acid, which is a constituent of the bacterial cell wall (choice C). Mucopeptide constitutes the major component of the bacterial cell wall and is composed of N-acetylglucosamine-N-acetylmuramic acid (choice D). Glycine pentapeptide serves as the bridging moiety that cross-links the side chains of amino acids attached to muramic acid of the mucopeptide of *Staphylococcus aureus* (choice E).

520. **(D)** Antigens, such as albumin, which do not have repeating antigenic determinants, belong to a group of antigens which require the participation of T cells to generate antibodies to them. Polymerized flagellin, long chains of D-amino acids, pneumococcal polysaccharides, endotoxins and other large polymers having repeating antigenic determinants are T-independent antigens (choices A, B, C, and E).

521. **(D)** The retroviruses carry a reverse transcriptase, an RNA-directed DNA polymerase. The negative-stranded, single-stranded RNA viruses (the first three responses listed) must all carry RNA-dependent RNA polymerase as a structural component because their negative-stranded RNA cannot serve directly as messenger RNA (choices A, B, C, and E).

522. **(E)** Exposure to *M. tuberculosis* does not assure contraction of it. Thus, chemoprophylaxis with isoniazid (INH) should be the treatment of choice for contacts of actively infected persons. Individuals receiving INH should be checked periodically by sputum cultures and by x-rays (choices A and B). Immunization with the live attenuated tuberculosis strain bacillus Calmette–Guérin (BCG) would be pointless because the contacts have already experienced infection with *M. tuberculosis* (choice C). Ethambutol is very effective against most mycobacteria, but it is used in the therapy of tuberculosis, not in prophylaxis (choice D).

523. **(E)** The short incubation of four hours indicates staphylococcal food poisoning. This is a situation arising from the ingestion of preformed staphylococcal enterotoxin which induces symptoms within one to six hours following consumption of contaminated food, including diarrhea, abdominal cramps, and severe vomiting. These symptoms last for six to 12 hours, and complete recovery usually occurs in less than one day. The incubation periods for *Salmonella typhimurium, Vibrio parahaemolyticus, Yersinia enterocolitica,* and *Campylobacter jejuni* are 8 to 12, 24 to 96, 24 to 48, and 72 to 168 hours, respectively. These longer incubation periods in comparison to the incubation period of staphylococcal food intoxication are due to the need for these bacteria to invade the human intestinal tract, and then multiply and form the toxins responsible for the infective form of food poisoning (choices A, B, C, and D).

524. (A) If an IgG molecule is treated with papin, two identical Fab fragments are produced. The two Fab fragments constitute the hypervariable regions of the antibody molecule that carry the antigen binding sites. The hypervariable regions of IgG are located at the amino-terminal end of the molecule, not the carboxy terminal end of IgG, not within the Fc region of IgG, or the constant region of IgG (choices B, D, and E). Only IgA and IgM have J chains (choice C).

525. (C) Administration of diphtheria antitoxin quickly provides large amounts of preformed antibodies. These antibodies will neutralize unbound diphtheria exotoxin in body fluids, and thus reduce tissue damage. Diphtheria antitoxin is produced in horses, sheep, or goats. Persons sensitive to horse, sheep, or goat proteins may develop type III hypersensitivity reactions, a good example of which is serum sickness. Administration of diphtheria antitoxin most likely will combine with diphtheria exotoxin and complement, and thus will decrease, not increase, the concentration of serum complement (choice A). Injection of diphtheria antitoxin can lead to production of antibody against serum proteins of the animal used to produce diphtheria antitoxin, but not antibodies against diphtheria (choice B). Administration of diphtheria antitoxin does not eliminate the need for immunization with diphtheria toxoid. Because the protection afforded by antitoxin is of short duration, and prolonged protection against diphtheria is achieved by vaccination with diphtheria toxoid, diphtheria antitoxin alone will not confer lifelong immunity (choices D and E).

526. (A) Poliovirus is not enveloped and therefore is not inactivated by mild detergents that solubilize the phospholipid viral membranes. Eastern equine encephalitis virus, variola virus, mumps virus, cytomegalovirus, and rubella virus are all enveloped viruses, and thus are inactivated by mild detergents, which solubilize the phospholipid-containing viral envelope (choices B, C, D, and E).

527. (D) Cytomegalovirus has a viral genome which does not replicate in the cytoplasm of the infected cell. Poliovirus, rabies virus, mumps virus, and rubella virus each has a genome which replicates in the cytoplasm of the infected cell (choices A, B, C, and E).

528. (E) To determine whether the poliovirus is a wild-type virus or if it is related to that used for vaccination, it will be necessary to prepare oligonucleotide maps of the isolated virus and compare them to those of the wild-type and vaccine strains. Many viruses may kill mice; thus, one cannot determine whether poliovirus strains are related or unrelated by mouse lethality studies (choice A). Cytopathology cannot be used for definitive diagnosis of poliovirus strains or other types of viruses (choice B). Viral neutralization assays using the grandchild's serum will only indicate whether the grandchild has been exposed to and vaccinated for the polioviruses in question, but will not establish whether the poliovirus isolated from the stool of the grandfather is related to the poliovirus used to vaccinate his grandchild (choice C). Staining of the virus with fluorescent antibody may detect the presence of poliovirus, but will not establish whether the poliovirus is a wild-type virus or if it is related to that used for vaccination (choice D).

529. (D) Radioimmunoassays are the most sensitive and versatile tests for the quantitation of antigens or haptens. Radioimmunoassay is particularly useful in the measurement of serum levels of many hormones, drugs, and other biologic materials. The method is based on competition for specific antibody between the labeled (known) and unlabeled (unknown) concentration of the antigen or haptens. Radioimmunoassays are not normally used to establish the heterogeneity of an antigen, to demonstrate cross-reactions between antigens, to demonstrate purity of antigens, or to identify the isotypes of an antibody (choices A, B, C, and E).

530. (B) An important part of the penicillin molecule is the beta lactam group. This group is composed of two carbon and two hydrogen atoms at the top of the group. The bottom part of the group contains one carbon which is linked to one nitrogen atom and one oxygen atom. Penicillinase breaks the bond between the bottom carbon and nitrogen atom, and destroys the antibacterial activity of penicillin, along with that of cephalosporin, which also possesses a β-lactam group.

531. (C) The laboratory diagnosis of tinea pedis (athlete's foot) caused by *Trichophyton rubrum* depends on the demonstration of typical pear-shaped microconidia, which develop on white-red colonies of *T. rubrum.* Number 1 shows a chamydospore (choice A), number 2 a sporangiospore of *Rhizopus* (choice B), number 4 a spherule filled with endospores of *Coccidioides immitis* (choice D), and number 5 a budding yeast cell of *Blastomyces dermatiditis* (choice E).

532. (D) The patient described in this question is showing the typical symptoms of botulism, which is commonly caused by types A, B, or E *Clostridium botulinum* toxin. Therefore, early administration of potent botulinum antitoxin containing antibodies to toxins A, B, and E constitutes the most appropriate type of treatment. Administration of staphylococcal enterotoxin antiserum could have been helpful if the patient were suffering from staphylococcal food poisoning, but he is not (choice A). Immunization with staphylococcal enterotoxin toxoid, administration of penicillin, or placing this patient in a hyperbaric chamber are all useless (choices B, C, and E).

533. (E) Ketoconazole inhibits the biosynthesis of ergosterol by blocking demethylation at the C14 site of the ergosterol precursor, lanosterol. This results in the accumulation of lanosterol-like sterols in the cell, which alters the properties of the cell membrane, and permits the leakage of potassium ions. Amphotericin B and nystatin impair the permeability of the cell membrane by directly complexing with the membrane sterol (choices A and D). The target of griseofulvin is microtubules (choice B). Flucytosine (5′-fluorocytosine) is incorporated into RNA after being deaminated and then phosphorylated. It also interferes with DNA synthesis because it is a non-competitive inhibitor of thymidylate synthetase (choice C).

534. (B) The child described appears to be suffering from meningitis due to *S. aureus,* which should always be considered a beta lactamase producing germ until the laboratory reports its antibiotic sensitivity. Methicillin is a β-lactamase–resistant penicillin, and it would be the antibiotic of choice among those listed. Other antibiotics that might be used are cephalosporins or vancomycin, but not penicillin, streptomycin, ampicillin, or kanamycin (choices A, C, D, and E).

535. (B) The patient had contracted Rocky Mountain spotted fever, because it is transmitted by tick bites, and is characterized by high fever, myalgia, macules, and petechiae. The rash appears first on the arms and feet, and then spreads to the trunk. Q fever is an influenza-like illness which progresses to a pneumonitis. It is not associated with rash, and it is transmitted by respiratory droplets, not arthropod vector bites (choice A). Epidemic typhus is transmitted by lice, not ticks, and is characterized by a maculopapular rash that begins in the trunk, not the arms and legs. It is associated with severe meningoencephalitis and delirium (choice C). Rickettsial pox is transmitted by mite bite, and is a mild illness characterized by moderate fever, headache, and a vesicular rash which forms an eschar (choice D). Scrub typhus is also transmitted by mite bite, and is characterized by mild fever, a rash, which may have an eschar, and lymphadenopathy (choice E).

536. (A) The most reliable test for the diagnosis of Rocky Mountain spotted fever is the complement fixation test employing specific antigens of the etiological agent *Rickettsia rickettsii.* The Weil–Felix reaction employs *Proteus vulgaris,* OX-2, OX-19, and OX-K to test for antibody production to rickettsia. The reason why *P. vulgaris* can be used instead of rickettsia in the Weil–Felix agglutination reaction is because rickettsia and *P. vulgaris* have common antigens. Since the cultivation and handling of rickettsia is difficult and dangerous, *P. vulgaris* provides convenient, safe antigens for the presumptive diagnosis of rickettsial diseases. However, patients infected with *P. vulgaris* will also give positive results (choice B). The Gram stain will only reveal the presence of small gram-negative rods, and thus cannot be very useful for the diagnosis of Rocky Mountain spotted fever (choice D). The etiological agent *Rickettsia rickettsii* cannot be cultured on Sabouraud's or blood agar plates (choices C and E).

537. (B) Rickettsia are gram-negative short rods, and as such have a cell wall that resembles that of gram-negative bacteria. The cell size of rickettsia is 0.6×0.3 microns. The limit of resolution of the light microscope is 0.2 microns, thus rickettsia can be seen with a light microscope (choice A). Rickettsia replicate by binary fission. *Chlamydia* replicate with a distinct intracellular cycle (choice C). Rickettsia have cell walls that resemble the cell wall of gram-negative bacteria (choice D). Tetracyclines and chloramphenicol are the drugs of choice for the treatment of Rocky Mountain spotted fever (choice E).

538. (A) The most likely diagnosis of the patient's illness is acute amoebic dysentery, because the classical symptomatology of acute amoebic dysentery is lower abdominal pain, cramping, colitis, tenesmus, flatulence, and bloody diarrhea. Malaria is characterized by periodic fever, fatal cerebral episodes, lysis of red blood cells, and nephritis due to immune complex formation, and is transmitted by mosquito bites (choice B). Trypanosomiasis is transmitted by bites of the tsetse fly and the trypanosomes initially cause chancres at the site of the bite. Then the trypanosomes reach the central nervous system, and the patient has lassitude, develops sleeping episodes, and tissue wasting or even death can occur (choice C). Trichomoniasis is limited to the vagina and is associated with a watery, foul smelling, abundant greenish-gray discharge (choice D). Toxoplasmosis is a mild influenza-like disease with possible lymph node enlargement, and may be severe in immunocompromised patients. Congenital infections can damage the eyes or brain and may be fatal (choice E).

539. (E) Cysts are the infective form of *Entamoeba histolytica* and are transmitted by ingestion of infected food or drink. Ingestion of ova is the mode of transmission of such organisms as *Enterobius vermicularis, Ascaris lumbricoides, Trichuris trichiura* and others, but not *Entamoeba histolytica* (choice B). Larval penetration of the skin is the mode of transmission for hookworms, *Strongyloides* and *Schistosoma* (choice A). Sporozoites are the infective stage of malaria parasites spread to humans by mosquito bites (choice C). The gametocyte is the infective stage of malaria parasites for mosquitoes (choice D).

540. (A) The drugs of choice for acute amoebic dysentery are metronidazole and iodoquinol. Chloroquine is normally used for the treatment of malaria (choice B). Stibogluconate is recommended for the treatment of leishmaniasis (choice C). Sulfonamide and pyrimethamine is used for the treatment of toxoplasmosis (choice D). Trimethoprim and sulfamethoxazole are the drugs of choice for the treatment of pneumonia caused by *Pneumocystis carinii* (choice E).

541. (E) Hepatitis virus A is a small (20 to 30 nm), non-enveloped, single-stranded RNA virus. The virus is transmitted via the fecal–oral route, usually by eating contaminated foods, such as oysters grown in polluted waters. The symptoms of hepatitis A infection include fatigue, loss of appetite, nausea, vomiting, abdominal pain, fever, and jaundice. The urine excreted from patients with jaundice may be dark and the feces pale. Adenovirus is a non-enveloped, double-stranded, linear DNA virus. It is transmitted by respiratory secretions, and it causes pharyngitis, conjunctivitis, keratoconjunctivitis, pneumonia, and gastroenteritis (choice A). Hepatitis B is an enveloped, partially double-stranded DNA virus with a circular genome. It is transmitted by infected blood or blood products, sexually, or congenitally (choice B). Rhinoviruses are members of the picornaviruses. Rhinoviruses cause the common cold, and are isolated from people with mild upper respiratory tract infections (choice C). Rotavirus is a member of the reoviruses. Its genome is quite unusual in that it is composed of double-stranded RNA consisting of 10 segments. Rotavirus causes diarrhea in children mostly under the age of six (choice D).

542. (A) Diagnosis of Mr. X.'s infectious hepatitis can best be made by the demonstration of a fourfold rise of IgM against hepatitis A virus. Patients with hepatitis virus A do not show any meaningful rise of IgA (choice B). Hepatitis virus does not induce any pathognomonic cytopathic effects (choice C). The detection of Negri bodies is useful in the diagnosis of rabies, not hepatitis virus A (choice D). A positive Tzanck test is useful for the diagnosis of herpes virus, not hepatitis virus A (choice E).

543. (D) Hepatitis virus A infection can best be prevented by immunization with the intact inactivated virus. Interferons act only in the early phase of a viral infection limiting the spread of virus, and are not recommended for long-term protection against viral diseases (choice A). Immunization with a subunit vaccine is used to prevent hepatitis virus B infection, not hepatitis virus A infection (choice B). Hepatitis B core antigen (HBcAg) is not effective for vaccination, even against the hepatitis B virus from which it is derived (choice C). Administration of human gamma globulin may provide only passive immunity, which will be of short duration, and thus it is not the best way to prevent hepatitis A viral infection (choice E).

544. (E) This patient has chronic granulomatous disease. Children with this disease suffer chronic suppurative infections caused most frequently by *Staphylococcus aureus.* The cause of chronic granulomatous disease is a genetic defect in NADPH-oxidase. Neutrophils contain myeloperoxidase, which utilizes hydrogen peroxide and halide ions to produce hypochlorite, which is highly microbicidal. Because of the defective NADPH-oxidase, the patient's phagocytes cannot generate sufficient hydrogen peroxide, thus the myeloperoxidase–hydrogen peroxide and halide system cannot function normally. Neutrophils from these patients can phagocytize bacteria and fungi normally, but they cannot kill them because of the defective myeloperoxidase–hydrogen peroxide–halide system. Severe combined immunodeficiency disease (SCID) is characterized by the absence of T and B cells, absence of thymus, and a lack of lymphocyte proliferative response to mitogens, antigens, and allogeneic cells in vitro (choice A). Systemic lupus erythematosus is an autoimmune disease (type III hypersensitivity or immune-complex disease). Patients with lupus erythematosus produce anti-DNA antibodies (choice B). Rheumatoid arthritis is another autoimmune disease. Patients with this disease produce IgM autoantibodies to the Fc moiety of IgG (choice C). Patients with Graves' disease produce autoantibodies to thyroid stimulating hormone receptors (choice D).

545. (D) Streptococcal infections in chronic granulomatous disease are rare, because the defective myeloperoxidase–hydrogen peroxide–halide system can use hydrogen peroxide accumulated by phagocytosed streptococci, which are catalase negative and cannot convert hydrogen peroxide to water and oxygen. Administration of pooled gamma globulin or antistreptolysin is likely to provide only brief, but not chronic, protection against streptococci (choices A and B). C-reactive protein (CRP) is a beta serum globulin which reacts with the C carbohydrate of the cell wall of *Streptococcus pneumoniae.* It is not an antibody and thus will not provide even brief protection against streptococci (choice C). Phagocytosis plays a major, not a minor, role in the killing of streptococci (choice E).

546. (B) The diagnosis of chronic granulomatous disease is made by the inability of phagocytes to reduce the dye nitroblue tetrazolium (NBT). During phagocytosis in normal phagocytes, when reactive oxygen intermediates are produced, the yellow dye is converted to purple-blue formazan. In patients with chronic granulomatous disease during phagocytosis, reactive oxygen intermediates are not produced and NBT remains yellow. The mixed lymphocyte reaction is used to test the responsiveness of recipient lymphocytes to antigens present on donor cells (choice A). The Coombs' test is used to detect antibody on a patient's erythrocytes. If antibodies are attached, the erythrocytes will be agglutinated by antihuman immunoglobulin (choice C). The methyl red test is designed to detect use of a carbohydrate by bacteria (choice D). The India ink test is used to demonstrate the capsule of *Cryptococcus neoformans* (choice E).

REFERENCES

Brooks GF, Butel JS, Morse SA. *Jawetz, Melnick, and Adelberg's Medical Microbiology,* 21st edition. Stamford, CT: Appleton & Lange, 1998

Joklik WK, Willett HP, Amos BD, Wilfert CM. *Zinser Microbiology,* 20th edition. Norwalk, CT: Appleton & Lange, 1992

Levinson WE, Jawetz E. *Medical Microbiology & Immunology,* 5th edition. Stamford, CT: Appleton & Lange, 1998

Murray PR, Rosenthal KS, Kobayashi GS, Pfaller MA. *Medical Microbiology,* 3rd edition. St. Louis: Mosby-Year Book, 1998

Roitt I, Brostoff J, Male D. *Immunology,* 5th edition. London, UK: Mosby-Year Book, 1998

Subspecialty List: Microbiology

Question Number and Subspecialty

410. Virology
411. Immunology
412. Virology
413. Pathogenic bacteriology
414. Pathogenic bacteriology
415. Virology
416. Microbial genetics
417. Pathogenic bacteriology
418. Antigen–antibody reactions
419. Immunology
420. Pathogenic bacteriology
421. Pathogenic bacteriology
422. Virology
423. Pathogenic bacteriology
424. Tuberculosis
425. Immunology
426. Microbial physiology
427. Immunology
428. Virology
429. Mycology
430. Microbial physiology
431. Antigen–antibody reactions
432. Pathogenic bacteriology
433. Microbial physiology
434. Immunology
435. Immunology
436. Pathogenic bacteriology
437. Pathogenic bacteriology
438. Pathogenic bacteriology
439. Immune disorders
440. Virology
441. Immune disorders
442. Immune disorders
443. Microbial physiology
444. Immunology
445. Complement system
446. Antigen–antibody reactions
447. Microbial physiology
448. Oncogenes
449. Pathogenic bacteriology
450. Virology
451. Pathogenic bacteriology
452. Complement system
453. Antigenicity
454. Pathogenic bacteriology
455. Serology
456. Complement system
457. Mycology
458. Virology
459. Microbial physiology
460. Pathogenic bacteriology
461. Pathogenic bacteriology
462. Mycology
463. Parasitology
464. Pathogenic bacteriology
465. Immunology
466. Immunology
467. Pathogenic bacteriology
468. Microbial physiology
469. Immunology
470. Immunology
471. Pathogenic bacteriology
472. Pathogenic bacteriology
473. Toxins
474. Pathogenic bacteriology
475. Pathogenic bacteriology
476. Immunology
477. Immunology
478. Microbial physiology
479. Virology
480. Microbial physiology
481. Pathogenic bacteriology
482. Immunology
483. Immunology

484. Pathogenic bacteriology
485. Virology
486. Microbial physiology
487. Immunology
488. Virology
489. Virology
490. Pathogenic bacteriology
491. Pathogenic bacteriology
492. Virology
493. Vectors
494. C-reactive protein
495. Pathogenic bacteriology
496. Toxins
497. Virology
498. Serology
499. Mycology
500. Pathogenic bacteriology
501. Mycology
502. Virology
503. Mycology
504. Virology
505. Pathogenic bacteriology
506. Prions
507. Plasmids
508. Oncogenes
509. Virology
510. Virology
511. Tuberculosis
512. Syphilis
513. Immunology
514. Virology
515. Immunology
516. Plasmids
517. Pathogenic bacteriology
518. Pathogenic bacteriology
519. Antibodies
520. Immunology
521. Virology
522. Tuberculosis
523. Pathogenic bacteriology
524. Immunoglobulins
525. Pathogenic bacteriology
526. Virology
527. Virology
528. Virology
529. Miscellaneous
530. Antibiotics
531. Mycology
532. Pathogenic bacteriology
533. Mycology
534. Pathogenic bacteriology
535. Pathogenic bacteriology
536. Pathogenic bacteriology
537. Pathogenic bacteriology
538. Parasitology
539. Parasitology
540. Parasitology
541. Virology
542. Virology
543. Virology
544. Defective host defense
545. Defective host defense
546. Defective host defense

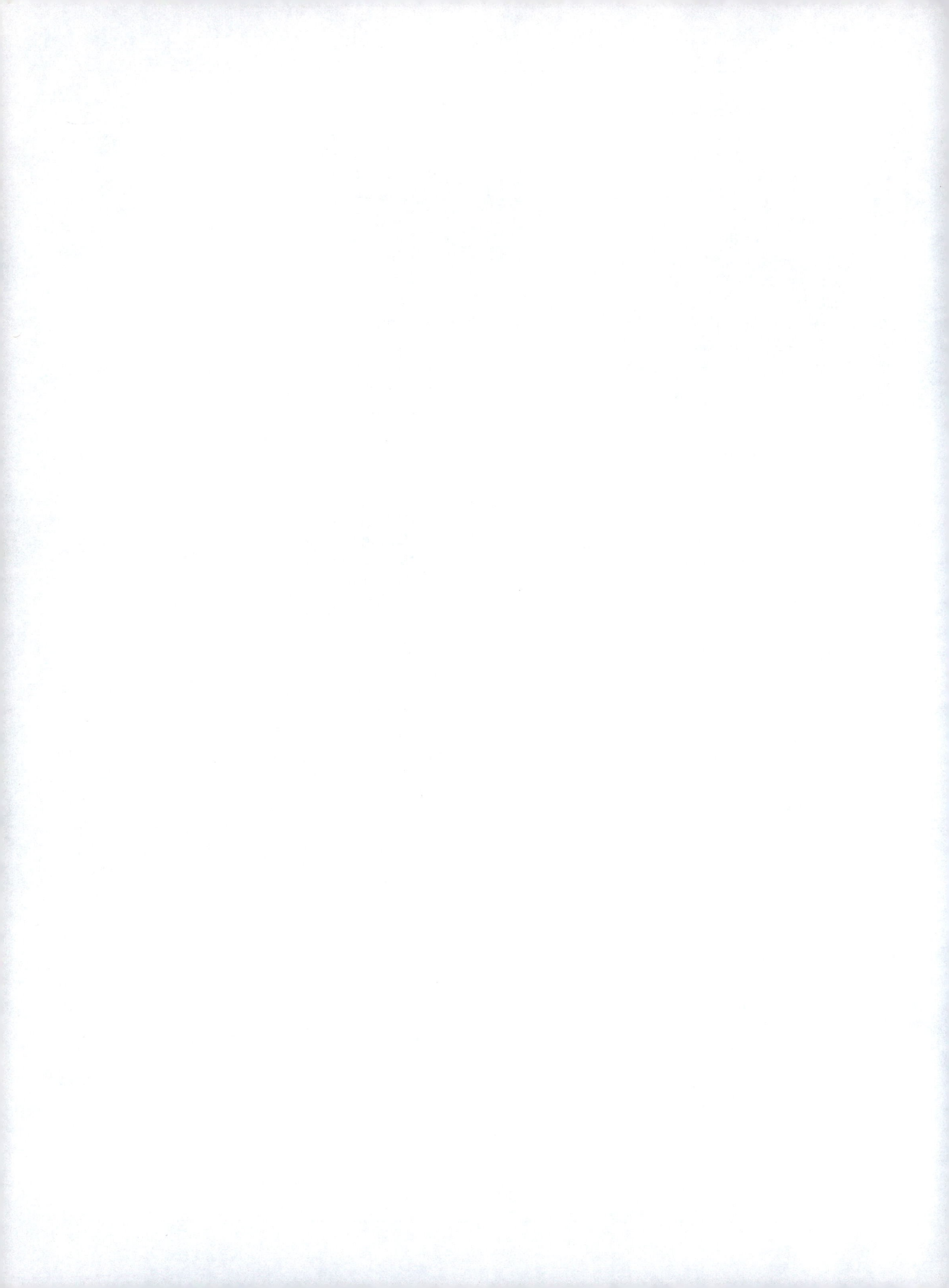

CHAPTER 5

Pathology
Questions

Thomas K. Barton, MD and Martin G. Lewis, MD, MBBS, FRC (Path)

DIRECTIONS: (Questions 547 through 673): Each of the numbered items or incomplete statements in this section is followed by answers or by completions of the statement. Select the ONE lettered answer or completion that is BEST in each case.

547. A 50-year-old white female complains of a lump in her thyroid gland. A fine needle aspiration of this lump is reported as medullary carcinoma. Which tumor-associated marker is most likely to be elevated in her serum?

(A) CA 125
(B) calcitonin
(C) CA 15-3
(D) alpha-fetoprotein
(E) human chorionic gonadotropin

548. A middle-aged woman suffers from weakness of her ocular and facial muscles, which worsens with repeated use. She has antibodies to acetylcholine receptors in her serum. The likely diagnosis is

(A) orbital inflammatory pseudotumor
(B) Parkinson's disease
(C) conjunctivitis
(D) myasthenia gravis
(E) polymyositis

549. A chronic demyelinating neurologic disorder of young adults that is characterized by plaques within the central nervous system and cerebrospinal fluid oligoclonal immunoglobulins is

(A) multiple sclerosis
(B) Huntington's disease
(C) pemphigus vulgaris
(D) amyotrophic lateral sclerosis
(E) spinocerebellar degeneration

550. The photomicrograph in Figure 5–1 depicts a diseased fallopian tube. What is the most likely diagnosis?

(A) chronic salpingitis
(B) endometriosis
(C) endosalpingiosis
(D) ectopic tubal pregnancy
(E) serous papillary carcinoma

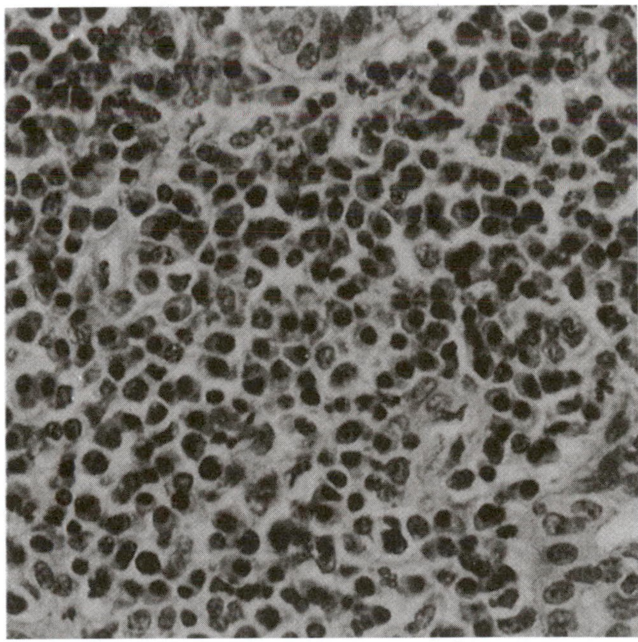

Figure 5–1

551. Extreme generalized edema with marked expansion of the extracellular fluid space within the subcutaneous tissues, visceral organs, and body cavities is called

(A) anasarca
(B) apoptosis
(C) angioedema
(D) hemochromatosis
(E) hyperthecosis

552. A patient who is allergic to penicillin is inadvertently given an injection of penicillin and immediately develops anaphylactic shock. This is an example of

(A) type I hypersensitivity
(B) type II hypersensitivity
(C) type III hypersensitivity
(D) type IV hypersensitivity
(E) type V hypersensitivity

553. An aspirate of joint fluid from a painful and inflamed metatarsophalangeal joint of the great toe reveals abundant needle-shaped, negatively birefringent crystals within neutrophils. The most likely diagnosis is

(A) acute bacterial pyarthrosis
(B) ochronosis
(C) gout
(D) calcium pyrophosphate deposition disease
(E) ganglion cyst

554. Metaplasia is defined as

(A) an increase in the size of cells
(B) an increase in the number of cells
(C) irregular, atypical proliferative changes in epithelial or mesenchymal cells
(D) replacement of one type of adult cell by another type of adult cell
(E) loss of cell substance, producing shrinkage of cell size

555. Niacin deficiency is associated with

(A) night blindness
(B) a bleeding diathesis
(C) altered formation of connective tissues
(D) neuromuscular and cardiac problems and edema
(E) dermatitis, diarrhea, and dementia

556. An adult with an untreated growth hormone-secreting microadenoma of the pituitary gland is likely to develop

(A) dwarfism
(B) Addison's disease
(C) hyperparathyroidism
(D) Cushing's disease
(E) acromegaly

557. A deficiency state caused by a lack of dietary vitamin C is termed

(A) beriberi
(B) scurvy
(C) pernicious anemia
(D) rickets
(E) marasmus

558. An individual with chronic hepatitis C viral infection has a chemistry profile performed. Which serum analyte is most likely to be decreased?

(A) gamma globulin
(B) alanine aminotransferase
(C) albumin
(D) lactate dehydrogenase
(E) aspartate aminotransferase

559. A young adult has been complaining of intermittent diarrhea, fever, and abdominal pain for several months. A radiograph of the small bowel reveals several separate areas of luminal narrowing. A photomicrograph of this patient's ileal biopsy is displayed in Figure 5–2. What is the diagnosis?

(A) abetalipoproteinemia
(B) Crohn's disease
(C) ulcerative enterocolitis
(D) carcinoid tumor
(E) adenocarcinoma

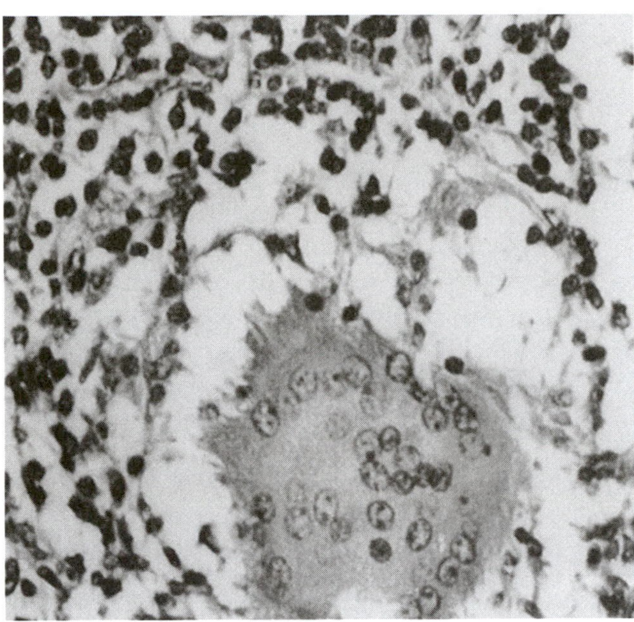

Figure 5–2

560. Patients with Sjögren's syndrome show an increased risk for the development of

(A) pleomorphic adenoma
(B) melanoma
(C) lymphoma
(D) esophageal carcinoma
(E) leukemia

561. The human embryo or fetus is most susceptible to malformation caused by environmental factors during

(A) days 1 to 15
(B) days 15 to 60
(C) the second trimester
(D) the third trimester
(E) delivery

562. The Philadelphia chromosome is most often associated with which disease?

(A) follicular lymphoma
(B) Burkitt's lymphoma
(C) Down syndrome
(D) acute lymphoblastic leukemia
(E) chronic myelogenous leukemia

563. DiGeorge's syndrome may be defined as

(A) a deficiency of T lymphocytes due to thymic hypoplasia
(B) a deficiency of B lymphocytes due to toxins
(C) an abnormal proliferation of atypical monocytes
(D) a deficiency of dietary fatty acids
(E) multiple mucosal neurofibromatous tumors

564. Diverticulosis occurs most frequently in the

(A) cecum
(B) ascending colon
(C) transverse colon
(D) descending colon
(E) sigmoid colon

565. Which of the following disease states characteristically produces the nephrotic syndrome?

(A) interstitial nephritis
(B) membranous glomerulonephritis
(C) unilateral hydronephrosis
(D) acute crescentic glomerulonephritis
(E) polycystic disease of the kidneys

566. A 56-year-old man dies in an ambulance while on the way to the hospital. His premortem chemistry studies are remarkable for an elevation of the MB isoenzyme of creatine phosphokinase. This laboratory finding would suggest acute damage to which organ?

(A) liver
(B) lung
(C) brain
(D) heart
(E) kidney

567. The most common cause of a pulmonary abscess is

(A) irritant gases
(B) alveolar proteinosis
(C) aspiration
(D) vasculitis
(E) cigarette smoking

568. What is the most likely diagnosis for the lesion pictured in the photograph in Figure 5–3?

(A) peptic ulceration
(B) adenocarcinoma
(C) adenomatous polyp
(D) Brunner gland adenoma
(E) leiomyoma

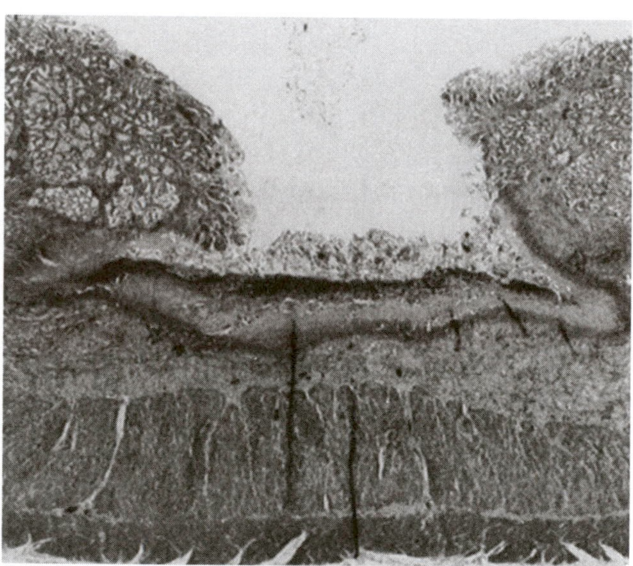

Figure 5–3

569. Auer rods are usually evident in the cytoplasm of

(A) silicotic pneumocytes
(B) neurons infected with rabies virus
(C) diabetic islet cells
(D) transformed urothelial cells
(E) myeloblasts

570. Which of the following tumors occurs mainly during adulthood?

(A) neuroblastoma
(B) retinoblastoma
(C) medulloblastoma
(D) nephroblastoma
(E) meningioma

571. A young black female has noticed a slowly growing firm nodule near the site of a recent earpiercing. Excision and microscopic examination of the nodule reveals it to be composed of densely collagenized fibrous tissue. The most probable diagnosis is

(A) teratoma
(B) hamartoma
(C) keloid
(D) dermoid cyst
(E) Brenner tumor

572. Which of the following neoplasms is benign?

(A) adenocarcinoma
(B) cystadenoma
(C) fibrosarcoma
(D) lymphocytic leukemia
(E) melanoma

573. The development of which of the following tumors is associated with the ingestion of aflatoxin?

(A) hepatocellular carcinoma
(B) pulmonary sarcomas
(C) chordomas of the lower spine
(D) uterine leiomyomas
(E) sebaceous carcinoma of the eyelid

574. An elderly male with congestive heart failure undergoes a thoracentesis, which yields about 200 mL of straw-colored watery fluid. A laboratory study of the fluid reveals:

Specific gravity	1.010
Total protein	0.4 g/dL
Cell count	Very rare mesothelial cell present
Fat stain	Negative

These pleural fluid findings are indicative of a(n)

(A) exudate
(B) empyema

(C) hemothorax
(D) transudate
(E) chylothorax

575. The characteristic inflammatory cell seen in the tissues in response to infection by *Salmonella typhi* is the

(A) polymorphonuclear leukocyte
(B) eosinophil leukocyte
(C) monocyte
(D) multinucleate giant cell
(E) plasma cell

576. What is the term used to describe an abnormal toxic yellow pigmentation found in the brains of neonates exposed to excessive unconjugated hyperbilirubinemia?

(A) kernicterus
(B) mucoviscidosis
(C) zellballen
(D) cholestasis
(E) sequestrum

577. A microscopic examination of a 20-hour–old myocardial infarct would be expected to demonstrate

(A) fibrosis and collagen deposition
(B) coagulative necrosis without many neutrophils
(C) abundant neutrophils and monocytes
(D) monocytes and neovascularization
(E) plasma cells and caseous necrosis

578. Which of the following statements is true regarding breast cancer?

(A) incidence is higher in Japan than in the United States
(B) there is a decreased incidence with early menarche or late menopause
(C) there is a decreased incidence with a high-fat diet
(D) there is a decreased incidence with atypical ductal or lobular hyperplasia
(E) there is an increased incidence with a family history of breast cancer

579. A rectal biopsy is the usual approach to the morphologic documentation of Hirschsprung's disease. Which of the following findings is considered diagnostic of Hirschsprung's disease on histologic examination of the rectal biopsy specimen?

(A) hypertrophy of the muscle coat of the wall of the rectum
(B) atrophy of the mucosal lining of the wall of the rectum
(C) absence of the nerve fibers that innervate the wall of the rectum
(D) absence of parasympathetic ganglion cells in the submucosal and myenteric plexus
(E) presence of multiple small polyps along the mucosal surface of the rectal wall

580. The most common cause of neonatal cholestasis is

(A) intrahepatic biliary atresia
(B) extrahepatic biliary atresia
(C) choledochal cyst
(D) primary biliary cirrhosis
(E) Budd–Chiari syndrome

581. With the TNM cancer staging system, the T component is defined as

(A) the time between diagnosis and definitive treatment
(B) the size or extent of the primary tumor
(C) the type of cells identified
(D) the treatment plan
(E) the presence of nodal metastases

582. An elderly alcoholic is found dead at home during the winter. The medical examiner feels that the likely cause of death is lobar pneumonia. At autopsy this diagnosis is confirmed and is said to be at the "red hepatization" stage. What pathologic process within the lung is responsible for the gross abnormality termed "red hepatization"?

(A) fibroblastic proliferation within the septal walls
(B) leukocytes, erythrocytes, and fibrin filling the alveolar spaces
(C) pleural deposits of fibrin and low molecular weight proteins
(D) desquamation of tracheal and bronchial epithelial cells
(E) alcoholic toxic necrosis of the pulmonary tissue

583. An x-ray of the pancreas displays numerous scattered abnormal small areas of calcification. The most likely histologic finding would be

(A) fat necrosis
(B) viral inclusion bodies
(C) lipofuscin pigmentation
(D) liquefaction necrosis
(E) melanin pigmentation

584. A genetic autosomal recessive disorder of copper metabolism characterized by hepatolenticular degeneration is

(A) Wilson's disease
(B) Reye's syndrome
(C) primary sclerosing cholangitis
(D) congenital hepatic fibrosis
(E) peliosis hepatis

585. The vegetation characteristically seen in acute rheumatic carditis most commonly occurs in

(A) the aortic sinuses of Valsalva
(B) the line of closure (free margins) of mitral valve
(C) the insertion of the chordae tendinae
(D) the mitral valve annulus
(E) just lateral to the coronary artery ostia

586. An autopsy heart specimen from a 58-year-old black male weighs 420 grams. There are no anomalous connections between the ventricles or between the atria. The cardiac chambers are not dilated and all the valves appear unremarkable. The atrial walls and the right ventricle wall are of normal thickness. The left ventricle wall is hypertrophied to a thickness of 1.7 cm. What is the most likely cause of these cardiac findings?

(A) chronic essential hypertension
(B) atrial septal defect
(C) congestive heart failure
(D) Chagas' disease
(E) tricuspid stenosis

587. A 36-year-old female has a known history of alpha-1-antitrypsin deficiency with a PiZZ genotype and micronodular cirrhosis. Her pulmonary reserve has been gradually decreasing over the past few years. What pathologic process is likely to be found on biopsy of her lung?

(A) pulmonary hamartomas
(B) chronic viral pneumonia
(C) intralobar sequestration
(D) alveolar proteinosis
(E) panacinar emphysema

588. Numerous previously healthy children in a day care center suddenly develop diarrhea. A culture of their stools is likely to grow which virus?

(A) variola
(B) parvovirus B19
(C) herpes simplex virus
(D) rotavirus
(E) cytomegalovirus

589. Opsonization of pathogenic bacteria may be mediated through which complement component?

(A) C8
(B) C1

(C) Factor B
(D) C4a
(E) C3b

590. The decedent had a short clinical history of prolonged vomiting and retching complicated by hematemesis. A significant postmortem finding is observed in the lower esophagus as a blood-coated longitudinal mucosal tear. What syndrome is likely to be cited on the autopsy report?

(A) Letterer–Siwe syndrome
(B) blind loop syndrome
(C) Mallory–Weiss syndrome
(D) Dubin–Johnson syndrome
(E) Conn syndrome

591. Saccular aneurysms of the thoracic aorta may be seen in tertiary syphilis. The usual pathogenic mechanism is

(A) medial cystic necrosis
(B) endarteritis obliterans of the vasa vasorum with subsequent mural ischemia
(C) intimal fibroplasia and lipid deposition
(D) immune complex formation and complement activation
(E) hypersensitivity reaction with multinucleate giant cells and fibrinoid mural necrosis

592. The bone marrow biopsy depicted in Figure 5–4 was obtained from an infant with hepatosplenomegaly and mental retardation. What is the pathologic basis of this disorder?

(A) exposure to excessive radiation during embryogenesis
(B) traumatic injury during delivery
(C) oncogenic viral integration into host's DNA initiates unregulated cellular proliferation
(D) deficient cellular immunity permits continued intracellular bacterial proliferation
(E) hereditary deficiency of catabolic enzyme leads to abnormal intracellular accumulation of lipids

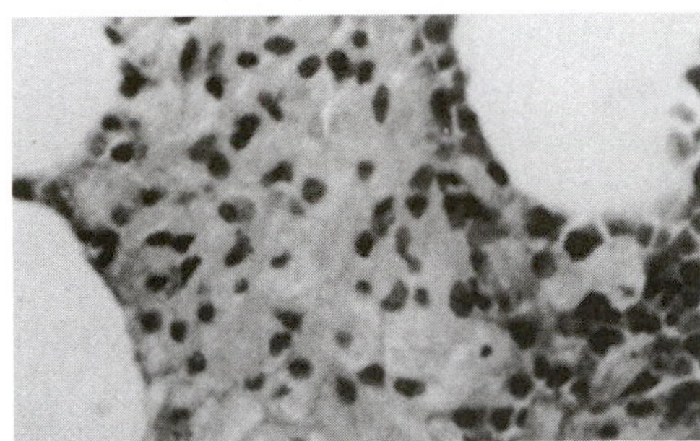

Figure 5–4

593. A 54-year-old male smoker has noticed a slowly enlarging mass over the past two years within his right parotid gland. At the time of surgical excision the mass measured 2.8 cm in diameter and was focally cystic. Microscopic examination revealed a tumor composed of benign papillary oncocytic epithelial fronds supported by benign lymphoid stroma. The most likely diagnosis is

(A) Warthin's tumor
(B) pleomorphic adenoma
(C) acute suppurative sialoadenitis
(D) mucoepidermoid carcinoma
(E) adenoid cystic carcinoma

594. A Pap smear reports low-grade squamous intraepithelial lesion with prominent koilocytosis. What is the most likely etiology?

(A) hereditary disorder of squamous epithelium
(B) normal intermenstrual reaction
(C) human papillomavirus
(D) protozoan infection or infestation
(E) hormonal imbalance

595. A 13-year-old boy has noticed slowly progressive enlargement of his left breast. Surgical removal of the button-shaped subareolar mass confirms the clinical suspicion of gynecomastia. What is the usual pathogenesis of these changes?

(A) dietary deficiency
(B) clonal neoplastic proliferation
(C) hyperestrinism
(D) ionizing radiation
(E) subacute inflammation

596. A 36-year-old male is now in his third year of steroid therapy since he was diagnosed with a systemic vasculitity. Prior to initiating treatment in the acute phase of the disorder he underwent a biopsy of a medium-sized artery. This biopsy specimen displayed fibrinoid necrosis of the media accompanied by a transmural acute inflammatory infiltrate. Significant negative clinical findings included a normal aortic arch, absence of giant cells in the artery biopsy, normal upper airway examination, and no history of tobacco use. What disorder best fits these findings?

(A) polyarteritis nodosa
(B) Takayasu's disease
(C) Kawasaki's disease
(D) giant cell arteritis
(E) thromboangiitis obliterans

597. The most frequent acute cause of death in fires is

(A) thermal burns
(B) hypovolemia
(C) vascular thrombosis
(D) smoke inhalation
(E) stroke

598. A 6.4 cm tumor is removed from the retroperitoneum. The frozen section report states that the tumor is malignant and appears to be derived solely from nonepithelial mesenchyme. Which entity would be compatible with this interpretation?

(A) serous cystadenoma
(B) hepatoma
(C) hemangioma
(D) liposarcoma
(E) chondroma

599. The critical pathologic finding that defines the Budd–Chiari syndrome is

(A) malignant transformation of the biliary epithelium
(B) agenesis of a hepatic lobe
(C) congenital inability to fully metabolize bilirubin
(D) dietary deficiency of an essential nutrient
(E) occlusion of the hepatic venous drainage

600. An elderly male expires after a four-day hospital course with a clinical diagnosis of adult respiratory distress syndrome. At autopsy a pathologic diagnosis of diffuse alveolar damage is rendered. What are the expected microscopic findings on examination of the autopsy lung tissue?

(A) alveolar hyaline membrane formation
(B) eosinophilic inflammatory infiltrates
(C) pulmonary vasculature occluded by microthrombi
(D) pleural effusion and fibrous pleuritis
(E) hemorrhagic infarction

601. Mutations in the retinoblastoma gene which result in growth of a retinoblastoma is an example of tumorigenesis through

(A) viral integration into the host DNA
(B) trisomy of chromosomes
(C) inactivation of a tumor suppressor gene
(D) activation of an oncogene or proto-oncogene
(E) chemical alteration of host DNA

602. A young adult has self-limited episodes of cutaneous vesicle formation around the lips. A diagnostic Tzanck smear of vesicle fluid is displayed in Figure 5–5. What is the etiology of these lesions?

(A) dietary deficiency
(B) reactivation of viral infection
(C) neoplastic process
(D) autoimmune disorder
(E) hereditary disorder

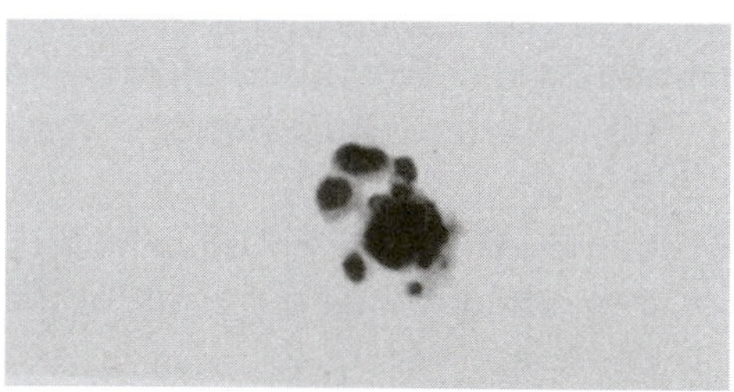

Figure 5–5

603. Epidermal growth factor accelerates the healing of certain wounds. After binding to a transmembrane receptor this polypeptide exerts its action through activation of a cytoplasmic

(A) adenylate cyclase
(B) tyrosine kinase
(C) guanylate cyclase
(D) kallikrein
(E) lysosomes

604. Liquefaction necrosis is most likely to follow an infarct in which organ?

(A) lung
(B) small bowel
(C) kidney
(D) brain
(E) spleen

605. A 42-year-old male seeks medical attention for a skin disorder characterized by the recent appearance of numerous large fluid-filled cutaneous blisters. A diagnosis of pemphigus vulgaris is made. What pathologic process produces these fluid-filled lesions?

(A) local ischemia
(B) dietary deficiency
(C) induced by chemical toxin
(D) psychiatric condition
(E) autoimmune disorder

606. Which morphologic observation is a reversible nonlethal cellular abnormality?

(A) karyorrhexis
(B) hydropic swelling
(C) pyknosis
(D) apoptosis
(E) rupture of the nuclear membrane

607. A 56-year-old male is noted to have episodic hypertension, a mass in his adrenal gland, and elevated catecholamines. The most likely diagnosis is

(A) pheochromocytoma
(B) ganglioneuroma
(C) adrenal cortical hyperplasia
(D) adrenal cortical carcinoma
(E) neuroblastoma

608. A 67-year-old female has lymphocytosis. The white blood count is elevated at 43,000 per μL with 92% of the cells appearing as small to medium-sized, mature, morphologically normal lymphocytes. Flow cytometry studies characterize almost all of the lymphocytes as CD5 positive, CD20 positive, κ light chain positive, and λ light chain negative. What is the most likely reason for her lymphocytosis?

(A) plasma cell leukemia
(B) reactive lymphocytosis
(C) adult T-cell leukemia
(D) Castleman's disease
(E) chronic lymphocytic leukemia

609. A tissue sample examined microscopically demonstrates an increase in size of individual cells but no increase in the number of cells. This is best described as

(A) hyperplasia
(B) hypoplasia
(C) hypertrophy
(D) metaplasia
(E) dysplasia

610. An autopsy heart from a four-year-old male with a premortem history of cyanotic congenital heart disease displays right ventricular hyperplasia, pulmonary stenosis, ventricular septal defect, and dextroposition of the aorta. What term best defines this disorder?

(A) tetralogy of Fallot
(B) transposition of the great arteries
(C) anomalous pulmonary venous drainage
(D) Ebstein malformation
(E) dextrocardia

611. The clinical presentation of osteogenesis imperfecta, type I, may include numerous childhood fractures, blue sclera, hearing abnormalities, and misshapen teeth. What pathologic alteration is responsible for these clinical findings?

(A) synthesis of abnormal type I collagen
(B) inability to metabolize vitamin D
(C) inadequate mineralization of bone matrix
(D) renal inability to conserve phosphorous
(E) abnormal intestinal receptors for calcium

612. The formation of a vascular thrombus is most likely in which clinical setting?

	PLATELET COUNT	COUMADIN THERAPY	LUMINAL BLOOD FLOW	ENDOTHELIAL DAMAGE
(A)	normal	yes	normal	none
(B)	low	yes	stasis	none
(C)	low	none	normal	none
(D)	normal	none	stasis	yes
(E)	low	yes	normal	yes

613. During an acute inflammatory reaction, endothelial membrane glycoproteins called cell adhesion molecules proliferate and may serve as attachment sites for the recruitment of phagocytic cells. Which substance is most likely to function as a cell adhesion molecule.

(A) histamine
(B) interleukin 1
(C) plasmin
(D) myeloperoxidase
(E) ELAM-1

614. Which site is the leading cause of female cancer deaths in the United States?

(A) breast
(B) lung
(C) colon
(D) uterus
(E) ovary

615. On physical examination a 17-year-old male is noted to have only minimal secondary sexual development, gynecomastia, and an eunuchoid tall habitus. His chromosome analysis is reported as 47,XXY. Which syndrome best defines these findings?

(A) Down syndrome
(B) Edwards' syndrome
(C) Klinefelter's syndrome
(D) Turner's syndrome
(E) multi-X syndrome

616. A 61-year-old man develops fulminant diarrhea following extensive antibiotic therapy for osteomyelitis. Endoscopic biopsies of his large bowel demonstrates pseudomembranous colitis. What organism is most likely to be isolated from his colon?

(A) *Helicobacter pylori*
(B) *Yersinia* species
(C) *Clostridium difficile*
(D) *Salmonella* species
(E) *Shigella* species

617. A 10-year-old female develops sudden onset of hematuria and hypertension. Two weeks previously she had a severe sore throat from which was cultured *Streptococcus pyogenes.* Her laboratory studies now demonstrate an elevated antistreptolysin, elevated antihyaluronidase, and elevated serum creatinine. The pathologic renal changes will be found at the

(A) distal convoluted tubule
(B) glomerulus
(C) afferent arteriole
(D) proximal convoluted tubule
(E) calyx

618. Multiple endocrine neoplasia, type IIA, is also termed Sipple syndrome. What abnormalities frequently constitute this hereditary disorder?

(A) medullary thyroid carcinoma, adrenal medullary hyperplasia or neoplasia, and parathyroid hyperplasia or neoplasia
(B) adrenal cortical hyperplasia or neoplasia, islet cell tumors, and neurofibromas
(C) adenomatous thyroid goiter, chondromas, and adrenal cortical adenomas or hyperplasia

(D) splenic adenomas, thrombocytopenia, and leukopenia
(E) adrenal cortical adenomas or hyperplasia, thyroid follicular adenomas, parathyroid adenomas

619. The most frequent cause of death in the five- to nine-year-old age range within the United States is

(A) malignant neoplasms
(B) congenital abnormalities
(C) heart disease
(D) infectious agents
(E) accidents and trauma

620. Fatal overdoses of acetaminophen are associated with

(A) pulmonary necrosis
(B) infarction of the spleen
(C) meningeal inflammation
(D) hepatic necrosis
(E) acute renal tubular necrosis

621. Which critical element defines the difference between type I and type II diabetes mellitus?

(A) age of patient
(B) degree of kidney dysfunction
(C) need for parenteral insulin
(D) presence of cerebral vascular hemorrhage
(E) ketoacidosis

622. The decedent has a five-year history of progressively worsening heart failure. An autopsy limited to the heart reveals extensive replacement of the myocardium by an acellular eosinophilic material. After congo red staining this substance displays apple green dichromism when examined under polarized light microscopy. What is this material?

(A) post infarctive cicatrix
(B) calcium salt deposition
(C) amyloid
(D) myocyte fibrinoid necrosis
(E) cholesterol

623. A 56-year-old male employed in a cottonmill has an asthmalike pulmonary disorder due to prolonged inhalation of cotton fibers. What term is used to describe this pneumoconiosis?

(A) silicosis
(B) stannosis
(C) byssinosis
(D) anthracosis
(E) berylliosis

624. Environmental exposure to vinyl chloride or thorium dioxide is associated with the later development of which tumor?

(A) liver cell carcinomas
(B) hepatic adenomas
(C) focal nodular hyperplasia
(D) hepatic fibromas
(E) hepatic angiosarcomas

625. A 21-year-old female presents with a six-hour history of left-sided lower abdominal pain and is hypotensive. A hemorrhagic mass is discovered in her left fallopian tube during laparoscopy. The tube is surgically excised. A photomicrograph of the tubal contents is displayed in Figure 5–6. What is the diagnosis?

(A) leiomyoma
(B) choriocarcinoma
(C) ectopic tubal pregnancy
(D) granular cell tumor
(E) chorioadenoma destruens

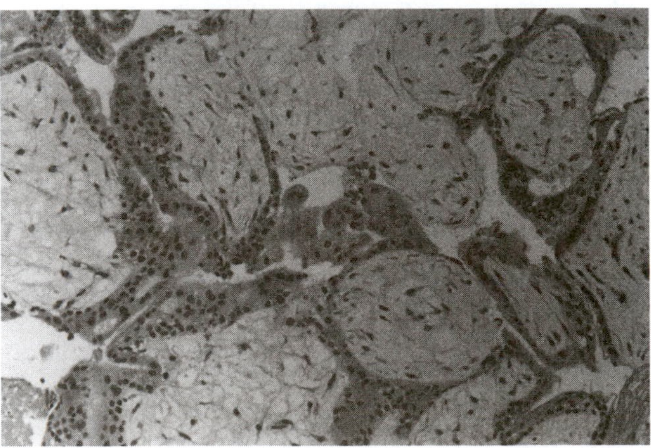

Figure 5–6

626. A one-year-old child has unilateral cryptorchidism. The pediatrician strongly recommends performing an orchiopexy. What long-term pathologic consequence of cryptorchidism would support recommending this surgical therapy?

(A) increased risk of testicular feminization syndrome
(B) increased risk of testicular infarction
(C) increased risk of testicular hemorrhage
(D) increased risk of testicular neoplasia
(E) increased risk of testicular infection

627. The distinguishing feature separating eclampsia from pre-eclampsia is

(A) convulsions
(B) hypertension
(C) edema
(D) proteinuria
(E) occurrence late in pregnancy

628. Hyperacute rejection of a renal transplant is frequently avoided by

(A) providing an ABO blood group compatible kidney
(B) long-term postoperative corticosteroid therapy
(C) providing a kidney compatible for HLA-A, HLA-B, and HLA-DR
(D) a preoperative dose of an immune suppressive drug
(E) intraoperative lymphocyte apheresis

629. A 13-year-old female presents with clinical symptoms suggestive of acute appendicitis. At surgery the appendix appears uninflamed and an alternative diagnosis of acute mesenteric adenitis with enterocolitis is made. What is the likely etiology of this entity?

(A) local vascular compromise
(B) bacterial infection
(C) viral infection
(D) fungal infection
(E) parasitic infection

630. A 34-year-old woman has a history of menorrhagia. Within the wall of her uterus are several solid whitish nodules. The histologic appearance of one of the nodules is depicted in Figure 5–7. What are these nodules?

(A) Krukenberg tumors
(B) leiomyomas
(C) adenomyosis
(D) ovarian ectopias
(E) metastatic malignancy

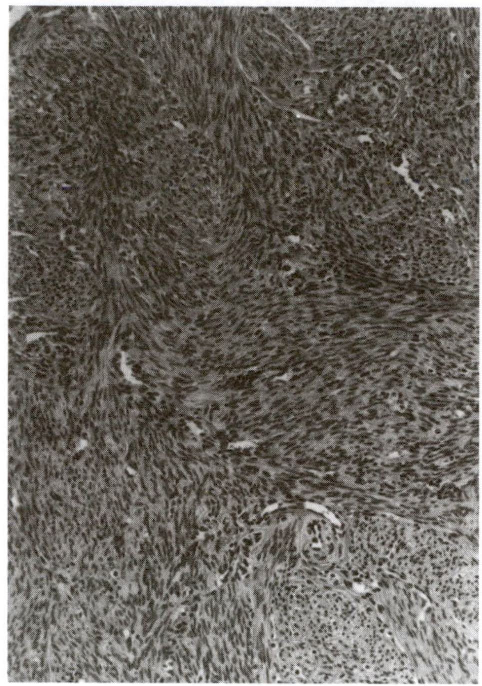

Figure 5–7

631. A newborn infant is diagnosed with Wiskott–Aldrich syndrome. What are the expected findings?

(A) hereditary immunodeficiency disorder with recurrent infections, thrombocytopenia, and eczema
(B) congenital viral infection with subsequent mental retardation and microcephaly
(C) constellation of unilateral renal agenesis, spina bifida, and pulmonary hypoplasia
(D) neonatal parasitic infection leading to diarrhea and dehydration
(E) left to right shunted congenital heart disease

632. A 55-year-old male has recently been discovered to be affected with Sezary syndrome. What is this disorder?

(A) gastric B-cell lymphoma
(B) large B-cell lymphoma arising from chronic lymphocytic leukemia
(C) leukemic variant of mycosis fungoides
(D) adult T-cell leukemia due to infection with HTLV-1
(E) lymphoma arising secondary to HIV-1 infection

633. A 69-year-old female complains of a recent erosive eczematous change on her left nipple. A biopsy demonstrates intraepidermal adenocarcinoma. This histologic finding would support a diagnosis of

(A) epidermolysis bullosa
(B) Paget's disease of the nipple
(C) dermatitis herpetiformis
(D) desmoid tumor
(E) Bowen's disease

634. Small cell undifferentiated pulmonary carcinoma is felt to arise from malignant transformation of which cell?

(A) Clara cell
(B) neuroendocrine cell
(C) metaplastic bronchial epithelial cell
(D) type I alveolar pneumocyte
(E) type II alveolar pneumocyte

635. Irreversibly postmitotic cells are permanent cells incapable of further mitotic division. A fatal injury to these cells lasts the lifetime of an individual. Which disorder is an example of fatal damage to irreversibly postmitotic type cells.

(A) bullet wound through the liver
(B) stroke
(C) esophageal erosion
(D) first degree thermal burn to skin
(E) solitary rectal ulcer syndrome

636. A 62-year-old female has a history of repeated urinary tract infections. Her physician requests a cystoscopy which reveals scattered soft yellow plaques in the bladder mucosa. A biopsy of a plaque contains a mixed chronic inflammatory infiltrate and numerous microcalcospherites. What disorder does this woman have?

(A) endometriosis
(B) exstrophy
(C) polypoid cystitis
(D) malakoplakia
(E) chronic interstitial cystitis

637. Gastric mucosal infection by which bacterial organism is associated with ulcer formation?

(A) *Helicobacter pylori*
(B) *Salmonella typhi*
(C) *Bartonella bacilliformis*
(D) *Brucellosis melitensis*
(E) *Pseudomonas aeruginosa*

638. In the United States, the major factor leading to the development of chronic pancreatitis is

(A) gallstones
(B) neoplasms at the ampulla of Vater
(C) chronic ethanol abuse
(D) diabetes mellitus
(E) viral infections

639. Which item best describes the pathogenesis of muscle spasms and seizures with *Clostridium tetani* infections.

(A) local wound infection erodes into subarachnoid space
(B) local wound infection produces systemic neurotoxin
(C) local wound infection is complicated by septicemia
(D) type III hypersensitivity reaction to tetanus toxoid
(E) superinfection by secondary organism

640. Your patient in the genetic disorders clinic has a confirmed diagnosis of alcaptonuria. He wants to know why his urine darkens rapidly if left standing open in the air.

(A) bacterial metabolism of excess tryosine
(B) oxidation of excess phenylalanine
(C) reduction of excess cystine
(D) precipitation of excess glycine
(E) oxidation of excess homogentisic acid

641. A nine-year-old girl living in rural South Carolina is noted by her physician to be anemic. An examination of her stool reveals hookworm eggs. Which nematode is she infected with?

(A) *Dracunculis medinensis*
(B) *Enterobius vermicularis*
(C) *Ascaris lumbricoides*
(D) *Entamoeba coli*
(E) *Necator americanus*

642. A 64-year-old male presents to his family physician with hematuria and flank pain. A radiology study identifies a renal mass. A photograph of this renal lesion's histology is displayed in Figure 5–8. What is the kidney mass?

(A) renal cell carcinoma
(B) angiomyolipoma
(C) transitional cell carcinoma
(D) oncocytoma
(E) xanthogranulomatous pyelonephritis

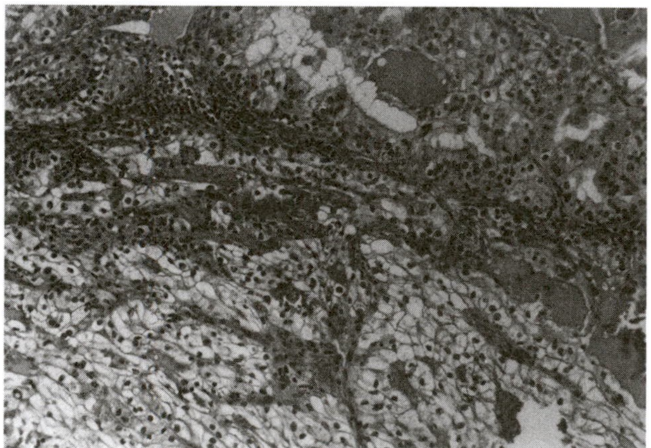

Figure 5–8

643. A 43-year-old female is found to have numerous bone marrow emboli within the pulmonary vasculature at autopsy. What is the likely premortem clinical history?

(A) acute leukemia
(B) idiopathic thrombocytopenia
(C) trauma
(D) pulmonary fibrosis
(E) anomalous venous drainage

644. A 21-year-old overweight female suffers from amenorrhea and hirsutism. On laparoscopic biopsy her ovary is enlarged due to the presence of a thickened cortex containing numerous benign small follicular cysts. These findings would be compatible with a diagnosis of

(A) hereditary multiple endocrine neoplasia, type 2B
(B) Stein–Leventhal syndrome
(C) pseudomyxoma peritonei
(D) hereditary multiple endocrine neoplasia, type 2A
(E) true hermaphrodite

645. The etiologic agent of lymphogranuloma venereum is

(A) *Chlamydia psittaci*
(B) *Rickettsia prowazekii*
(C) *Coxiella burnetii*
(D) *Borrelia burgdorferi*
(E) *Chlamydia trachomatis*

646. A 62-year-old man has Zollinger–Ellison syndrome. What is the etiology of his peptic ulceration?

(A) gastric mucosal atrophy
(B) antibodies to intrinsic factor
(C) vascular abnormality
(D) ectopic hypersecretion of gastrin
(E) pressure ulceration from bezoar

Questions 647 through 649

A 26-year-old female complains of the acute onset of anuria, purpura, and mental confusion. Her peripheral blood film displays marked thrombocytopenia and abundant schistocytes. Laboratory studies reveal elevations of bilirubin, creatinine, and lactose dehydrogenase. A skin biopsy shows numerous intravascular thrombi within the dermal microvasculature.

647. What is the likely diagnosis?

(A) May-Hegglin anomaly
(B) acute idiopathic thrombocytopenia purpura
(C) thrombotic thrombocytopenic purpura
(D) Glanzmann thrombasthenia
(E) Bernard–Soulier syndrome

648. The recommended treatment for this disorder is

(A) antibiotics
(B) immunosuppressive agents
(C) renal transplant
(D) plasmapheresis
(E) antiviral therapy

649. If appropriate and rapid treatment is instituted what is the expected one-year survival rate with this disorder?

(A) about 10%
(B) about 25%
(C) about 40%
(D) about 60%
(E) about 90%

Questions 650 and 651

A 14-year-old male of normal stature and intelligence has recently been told that he has icthyosis.

650. What histologic features evident on a skin biopsy would support this diagnosis?

(A) hyperpigmentation of the epidermal basal layer
(B) dermal fibrosis
(C) perivascular chronic inflammation
(D) increased thickness of stratum corneum
(E) subepidermal blister formation

651. This disorder is usually due to

(A) a hereditary condition
(B) a type IV hypersensitivity
(C) a bacterial infection
(D) a viral infection
(E) a hormonal imbalance

Questions 652 and 653

For the past six months a 67-year-old white female has been aware of a small flesh-colored papule on her lower eyelid. A photograph of this papule's microscopic anatomy is shown in Figure 5–9.

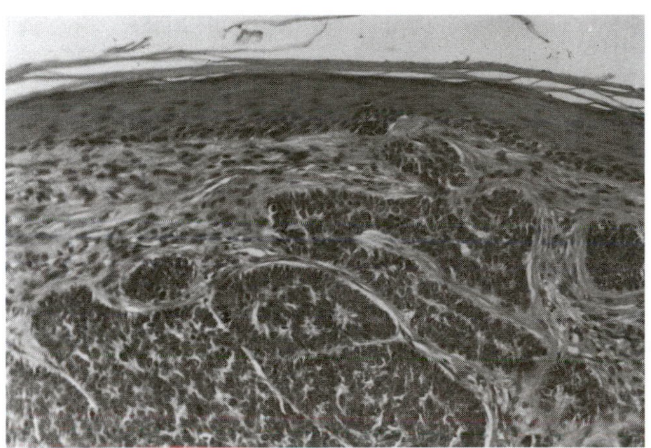

Figure 5–9

652. What is the appropriate diagnosis?

(A) verruca vulgaris
(B) molluscum contagiosum
(C) Bowen's disease
(D) epidermal cyst
(E) basal cell carcinoma

653. What is the primary pathologic process that leads to the development of this lesion?

(A) papillomavirus infection
(B) focal luminal occlusion with subsequent cyst formation
(C) actinic damage
(D) fungal infection
(E) poxvirus infection

Questions 654 and 655

A middle-aged female has a three-month history of fatigue and pruritis. A percutaneous liver biopsy reveals changes that are compatible with a diagnosis of primary biliary cirrhosis.

654. What is the most common etiology of this disorder?

(A) autoimmune disease
(B) follows viral infection
(C) alcohol abuse
(D) parasitic infection
(E) acquired vascular abnormality

655. Which serum chemistry panel typifies the later stages of this disorder?

	ALKALINE PHOSPHATASE	BILIRUBIN	CHOLESTEROL
(A)	decreased	decreased	decreased
(B)	decreased	elevated	decreased
(C)	decreased	decreased	elevated
(D)	decreased	elevated	elevated
(E)	elevated	elevated	elevated

Questions 656 and 657

A 53-year-old female has recently noticed a 2-cm firm nodule in her right breast during monthly self-examination. The histology of her breast biopsy tissue is displayed in Figure 5–10.

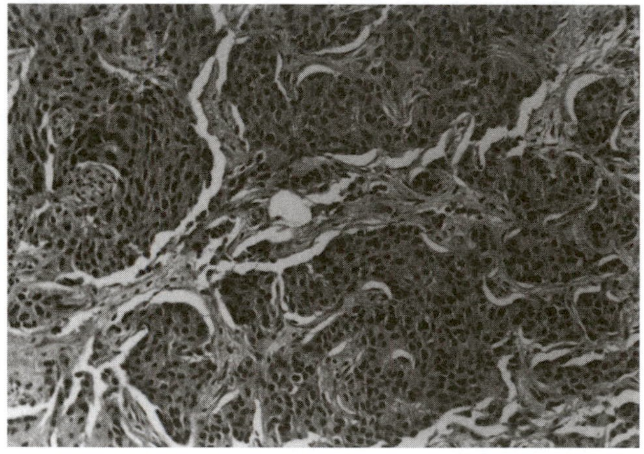

Figure 5–10

656. Identify a known risk factor that favors the development of this change

(A) early menopause
(B) Asian ethnicity
(C) late menarche
(D) family history of this disorder
(E) early age of first pregnancy and multiparity

657. Identify an adverse prognostic indicator that may be seen with this disorder.

(A) estrogen receptor positive
(B) well differentiated, grade I of III, histology
(C) low S phase
(D) progesterone receptor positive
(E) overexpression of NEU oncogene

Questions 658 and 659

An overweight 46-year-old male has complained of heartburn for the past two years. A biopsy of his lower esophagus is displayed in Figure 5–11.

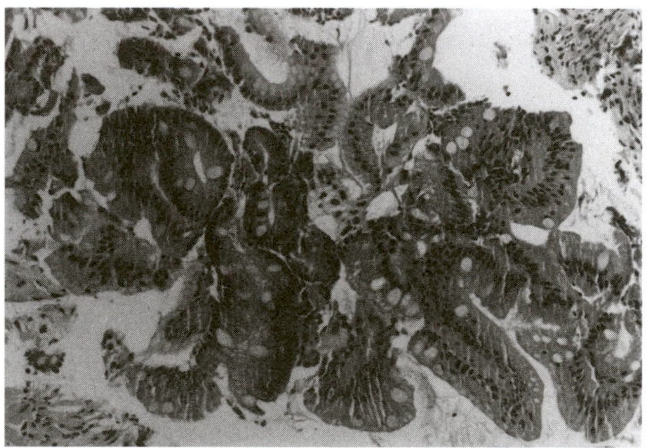

Figure 5–11

658. What is the diagnosis?

(A) Plummer–Vinson syndrome
(B) *Candida* esophagitis
(C) granulomatous esophagitis
(D) Barrett's esophagitis
(E) viral esophagitis

659. If left untreated this lesion may predispose to the development of

(A) squamous carcinoma
(B) fungal septicemia
(C) viral encephalitis
(D) adenocarcinoma
(E) esophageal varices

Questions 660 through 662

A two-year-old child has an abdominal mass discovered during a routine physical examination. The pediatrician suspects that the mass is a Wilms' tumor and refers the child to a regional medical center for further therapy.

660. During the course of this child's therapy the abdominal mass is excised and pathologic examination confirms the diagnosis of Wilms' tumor. What is the expected microscopic morphology of this neoplasm?

(A) malignant gland-forming epithelium with glycogen-containing clear cytoplasm and abundant vascularity
(B) malignant endothelial cells forming abortive vascular structures
(C) malignant osteoid or cartilage
(D) malignant adrenal neural crest cells
(E) malignant primitive renal tissue

661. If chromosomal analysis were performed on the surgical tissue the most likely abnormality would be

(A) trisomy
(B) translocation
(C) ring formation
(D) inversion
(E) deletion

662. The five-year survival rate of children with this tumor if given appropriate combined surgical, radiation, and antineoplastic therapies is about

(A) 90%
(B) 60%
(C) 40%
(D) 20%
(E) 5%

Questions 663 and 664

A six-year-old child has a long history of a hereditary bleeding disorder characterized by spontaneous nontraumatic hemorrhages into joint spaces, skeletal muscle, and mucous membranes. Laboratory studies reveal a normal prothrombin time, elevated partial thromboplastin time, very low factor VIII, normal factor X, normal factor XI, and normal platelet aggregation studies with ristocetin.

663. The likely diagnosis is

(A) hemophilia A
(B) hemophilia B
(C) von Willebrand's disease
(D) Christmas disease
(E) Rosenthal's syndrome

664. The usual mode of inheritance of this disorder is

(A) X-linked recessive
(B) X-linked dominant
(C) autosomal recessive
(D) autosomal dominant
(E) autosomal codominant

Questions 665 and 666

A 72-year-old man has radiographic evidence of multiple bony lytic areas. A fine-needle aspiration of one of these areas demonstrates clumps of atypical plasma cells. His lymph nodes are not enlarged. His total protein is elevated to 10.6 g/dL and his serum albumin is low.

665. What disease is most likely?

(A) metastatic melanoma
(B) mononucleosis
(C) metastatic adenocarcinoma
(D) multiple myeloma
(E) malignant lymphoma

666. A serum or urine electrophoresis will probably demonstrate

(A) bisalbuminemia
(B) hypogammaglobulinemia
(C) polyclonal hypergammaglobulinemia
(D) monoclonal paraprotein
(E) reduced alpha fractions

Questions 667 and 668

A 49-year-old female had a total hysterectomy five years ago for uterine prolapse. Her current vaginal Pap smear demonstrates clusters of benign glandular cells suggestive of vaginal adenosis.

667. Researching this patient's past history would likely reveal an in utero exposure to which agent?

(A) rubella virus
(B) radiation
(C) diethylstilbestrol
(D) aspirin
(E) methotrexate

668. The most serious long-term complication of vaginal adenosis is the potential to develop

(A) endometrial adenocarcinoma
(B) clear cell adenocarcinoma
(C) vaginal sarcomas
(D) uterine leiomyomas
(E) serous papillary carcinoma

Questions 669 through 671

A 14-year-old severely physically disabled individual is now on a respirator. His first four years of life were medically uneventful. During the last 10 years he has suffered from increasing symmetric muscle weakness which first affected the pelvic girdle and now involves almost all muscle groups. The calf portion of his legs several years ago appeared enlarged and on biopsy demonstrated fatty pseudohypertrophy with random alternating muscle fiber atrophy and hypertrophy.

669. The most likely diagnosis is

(A) poliomyelitis
(B) trichinosis
(C) cerebral palsy
(D) myositis ossificans
(E) muscular dystrophy

670. The disorder is

(A) a hereditary condition
(B) viral induced
(C) due to *Trichinella spiralis* infestation
(D) a neoplastic process
(E) secondary to neonatal trauma

671. Which serum chemistry panel typifies this disorder?

	CREATINE KINASE	ALDOLASE	LACTATE DEHYDROGENASE
(A)	elevated	elevated	elevated
(B)	normal	normal	normal
(C)	decreased	decreased	decreased
(D)	elevated	normal	low
(E)	low	normal	elevated

Questions 672 and 673

A 66-year-old male undergoes an elective right colectomy for stage III adenocarcinoma of the cecum.

672. What is the most likely set of preoperative laboratory findings?

	SERUM CEA	STOOL OCCULT BLOOD	HEMO-GLOBIN
(A)	normal	negative for blood	normal
(B)	normal	positive for blood	normal
(C)	normal	negative for blood	elevated
(D)	elevated	negative for blood	normal
(E)	elevated	positive for blood	low

673. Several months postoperatively if distant non-nodal metastases are discovered, which organ is likely to first be affected?

(A) brain
(B) lung
(C) adrenal
(D) appendix
(E) liver

Answers and Explanations

547. (B) Calcitonin is a hormone secreted by the parafollicular C cells of the thyroid gland. Medullary carcinoma arises from malignant transformation of these cells. CA 125 (choice A) is a tumor-associated glycoprotein which is frequently expressed by ovarian carcinomas. CA 15-3 (choice C) is a tumor-associated glycoprotein which is frequently expressed by breast carcinomas. Alpha-fetoprotein (choice D) may be elevated in the serum in association with hepatomas and gonadal tumors. Elevations of human chorionic gonadotropin (choice E) in the serum may be seen in normal pregnancies, gonadal tumors, and with choriocarcinomas.

548. (D) Myasthenia gravis is an autoimmune disease characterized by autoantibodies to acetylcholine receptors, and weakness of both facial and ocular muscles. Orbital inflammatory pseudotumor (choice A) is a benign mass lesion of the eye region not associated with muscle weakness and autoantibodies. Parkinson's disease (choice B) is a neurologic movement disorder which does not demonstrate either weakness or acetylcholine autoantibodies. Conjunctivitis (choice C) defines an inflammatory or infectious condition of the conjunctiva. Polymyositis (choice E) is a rheumatic disease of skeletal muscle.

549. (A) Multiple sclerosis is a chronic demyelinating neurologic disorder of young adults. Pathologic abnormalities associated with the disease include the formation of fibrous plaques within the central nervous system and the presence of cerebrospinal fluid oligoclonal immunoglobulins. Huntington's disease (choice B) is an autosomal dominant neuropathy. Early dementia and generalized involuntary movements characterize the disease. Pemphigus vulgaris (choice C) is an autoimmune blister-forming dermatologic condition with normal neurologic status. Amyotrophic lateral sclerosis (choice D) is a neurologic disease of unknown etiology which is characterized by degeneration of motor neurons and muscle wasting. Spinocerebellar degeneration (choice E) is a rare degenerative neurologic condition that affects the cerebellum and spinal cord.

550. (A) The photograph displays a benign reactive plasmacytic and lymphocytic chronic inflammatory infiltrate. This inflammatory pattern would be consistent with nonspecific chronic inflammation at various body sites. Chronic salpingitis is the only option listed which represents a chronic inflammatory disorder. The histology of endometriosis (choice B) features benign endometrial glands, benign endometrial stroma, and usually accompanying hemorrhage. Endosalpingiosis (choice C) is not a chronic inflammatory condition. Benign cervical glandular epithelium would be a necessary histologic attribute. Ectopic tubal pregnancy (choice D) would display chorionic villi and hemorrhage. The microanatomy of serous papillary carcinoma (choice E) is characterized by malignant glandular epithelium with a micropapillary architecture. Chronic inflammation, if present, is a minor secondary phenomenon.

551. (A) Anasarca is a term used to describe an extensive systemic transudative expansion of the extracellular fluid space within subcutaneous tissues, visceral organs, and body cavities. Reduced serum oncotic pressure is the usual etiology. Clinically, anasarca may be seen with nephrotic syndrome or cirrhosis. Apoptosis (choice B) defines a certain type of cell death which morphologically displays cytoplasmic eosinophilic fibrillary transformation. Angioedema (choice C) refers to the abnormal accumulation of extracellular fluid in the deeper dermis and subcutaneous fat. Body cavity spaces and visceral organs are not affected. Hemochromatosis (choice D) is a nonedematous disorder characterized by abnormal iron accumulation in skin and visceral organs. The term hyperthecosis (choice E) refers to an increase in ovarian stromal thecal cells.

552. (A) Type I hypersensitivity, or anaphylaxis, is an IgE-mediated reaction to a previously sensitizing antigen. Mast cells and basophils orchestrate this process through the release of preformed substances such as histamine, heparin, and chemotactic factors. Type II hypersensitivity (choice B) occurs as an antigen-antibody reaction on the surface of the host cell. A hemolytic transfusion reaction is an example of this type of immune injury. Type III hypersensitivity (choice C) uses circulating antigen–antibody complexes such as an Arthus reaction or serum sickness to produce immune injury. Type IV hypersensitivity (choice D) is a cell-mediated delayed reaction that usually involves a granulomatous inflammatory response. There is no hypersensitivity reaction yet defined as type V (choice E).

553. (C) Gout is a disease caused by elevated uric acid levels. Symptoms may include joint pain, joint effusions, renal calculi, and subcutaneous collections of uric acid crystals. Examination of fluid aspirated from an inflamed joint may reveal diagnostic needle-shaped urate crystals which are negatively birefringent when observed under polarized light microscopy. Acute bacterial pyarthrosis (choice A) should display neutrophils, necrotic debris, and perhaps, bacteria. Crystals would not be seen. Ochronosis (choice B) is a hereditary condition due to an inability to metabolize homogentisic acid. Clinically, there is pigmented arthritis, but joint crystals are not evident. Calcium pyrophosphate deposition disease (choice D) is a nonspecific crystalline deposit found in joints damaged by various etiologies. Pyrophospate crystals differ from urate crystals by their rhomboid shape and positive birefringence. A ganglion cyst (choice E) would reveal abundant mucoid debris and scant benign fibrous elements on aspiration. No crystals would be seen.

554. (D) Metaplasia is the replacement of one type of adult cell by another type of adult cell. Bronchial squamous metaplasia in response to cigarette smoke is a common example of this adaptive alteration. An increase in the size of cells (choice A) is termed hypertrophy. Hyperplasia is defined as an increase in the number of cells (choice B). Irregular, atypical proliferative changes in epithelial or mesenchymal cells (choice C) is a definition of dysplasia or neoplasia. Atrophy may be defined as a loss of cell substance producing shrinkage of cell size (choice E).

555. (E) Niacin deficiency, also known as pellagra, is associated with dermatitis, diarrhea, and dementia. Night blindness (choice A), with or without keratomalacia and papular dermatitis, suggests vitamin A deficiency. A bleeding diathesis (choice B) is likely to be due to a lack of vitamin K. This deficiency inhibits the formation of clotting factors II, VII, IX, and X. A deficiency of vitamin C, also termed scurvy, is associated with an altered formation of connective tissue (choice C). Polyneuropathy, cardiac problems, and edema (choice D) are seen with beriberi, a deficiency of thiamine.

556. (E) An untreated growth hormone-secreting microadenoma of the pituitary gland would be likely to produce acromegaly. The clinical features of acromegaly include osteoarthritis, diabetes, organomegaly, and atherosclerosis. Dwarfism (choice A) is a genetic disorder, usually of autosomal dominant inheritance. Addison's disease (choice B) is another term for adrenocortical insufficiency. Hyperparathyroidism (choice C) refers to an increased secretion of parathyroid hormone, not growth hormone. Cushing's disease (choice D) is defined as excess cortisol secretion.

557. (B) A lack of dietary vitamin C is termed scurvy. The disorder is characterized by formation of collagen that lacks tensile strength. Clinically, this alteration can be observed as tooth loss, joint hemorrhages, anemia, and poor wound healing. Beriberi (choice A) refers to a dietary lack of thiamine. Pernicious anemia (choice C) is usually caused by an autoimmune induced gastric atrophy with consequent inability to absorb dietary vitamin B_{12}. Rickets (choice D) is a deficiency of vitamin D occurring in children. Marasmus (choice E) refers to a lack of both essential elements and adequate calories.

558. (C) Hepatitis C viral infections commonly cause necrosis of hepatocytes. One of the major products synthesized by hepatocytes is albumin. As liver cells are damaged there is a concomitant reduction in the synthesis of albumin. Therefore, serum albumin levels are likely to decline during chronic hepatocellular injury. Gamma globulin (choice A) is increased in most chronic inflammatory states, especially with chronic hepatitis. Alanine aminotransferase (choice B), lactate dehydrogenase (choice D), and aspartate aminotransferase (choice E) are all enzymes normally found in liver cells. As liver cells die these enzymes leak from the necrotic cells into the bloodstream. An increased serum content of these enzymes is a useful laboratory method to detect hepatocellular injury.

559. (B) The photograph displays granulomatous inflammation characterized by multinucleate giant cell formation, lymphocytes, plasma cells, and monocytes. Of the listed choices, only Crohn's disease characteristically invokes a granulomatous inflammatory response. Abetalipoproteinemia (choice A) is a genetic disorder. Malabsorption without granulomatous inflammation is the typical clinical picture. Ulcerative enterocolitis (choice C) is a type of idiopathic inflammatory bowel disease. Granulomatous inflammation is not present. Carcinoid tumor (choice D) should display islands or ribbons of cohesive neoplastic epithelial cells. Granulomatous inflammation is not evident. A biopsy of ileal adenocarcinoma (choice E) would demonstrate malignant gland-forming epithelium without granulomatous inflammation.

560. (C) Sjögren's syndrome is an autoimmune disease in which there is immune-mediated destruction of lacrimal and salivary gland epithelium. One of the long-term risks of Sjögren's syndrome is an increased risk for developing malignant lymphoma. Pleomorphic adenoma (choice A) is a benign salivary gland tumor composed of both neoplastic epithelium and stroma. Its occurence is not associated with Sjögren's syndrome. Melanoma (choice B) is a malignancy of melanocytes unrelated to Sjögren's syndrome. The development of esophageal carcinoma (choice D) is associated with alcohol use, smoking, Barrett's metaplasia, and Epstein–Barr virus infections. Chronic Sjögren's syndrome is not known to cause an increased incidence of leukemia (choice E).

561. (B) The human embryo is most susceptible to malformations caused by environmental factors during days 15 to 60 of gestation. This period is referred to as the "organogenetic period" during which most of the major organ systems are organized and begin to grow. Environmental factors acting during the first two weeks after fertilization (choice A) usually lead to abnormalities of embryo implantation that result in complete fetal wastage rather than malformations. During the second trimester (choice C), third trimester (choice D), and at delivery (choice E) all of the major organ systems have already formed their requisite component structures and are unlikely to suffer subsequent malformation by environmental agents introduced at these times.

562. (E) Ninety percent of individuals with chronic myelogenous leukemia have an acquired Philadelphia chromosome abnormality consisting of a translocation between chromosomes 22 and 9. The translocation places the proto-oncogene *c-abl* from chromosome 9 next to the breakpoint cluster region *(bcr)* on chromosome 22. The unique gene sequence *bcr-abl* confers a growth advantage with subsequent clonal expansion. Follicular lymphoma (choice A) is associated with a translocation between chromosomes 14 and 18. Burkitt's lymphoma (choice B) is associated with a translocation of the *c-myc* oncogene from chromosome 8 to chromosome 14. Down syndrome (choice C) is due to a trisomy of chromosome 21. Acute lymphoblastic leukemia (choice D) does not have a known reproducible gross chromosomal derangement.

563. (A) DiGeorge's syndrome is a congenital deficiency of T lymphocytes due to thymic hypoplasia. Developmental failure of the third and fourth pharyngeal pouches is responsible for total or partial atresia of the thymus, parathroid, and thyroid. These gross structural abnormalities usually produce a clinical picture of poor T-cell–mediated immunity, tetany, and mental retardation. B lymphocytes are normal in number and function (choice B) with DiGeorge's syndrome. Atypical monocytic proliferation (choice C) is not a feature of DiGeorge's syndrome. The dietary fatty acids (choice D) are normal in DiGeorge's syndrome. Multiple mucosal neurofibromas (choice E) are seen with von Recklinghausen's disease, not DiGeorge's syndrome.

564. (E) The presence of multiple outpouchings of colonic mucosa through the muscularis propria into the adventitial subserosal fat is termed diverticulosis. It is common in developed countries with diets deficient in fiber. Diverticulosis occurs most frequently in the sigmoid. The most serious complication associated with chronic diverticulosis is inflammatory perforation leading to acute peritonitis. Colonic diverticulosis is rarely seen isolated to the cecum (choice A), ascending colon (choice B), transverse colon (choice C), or descending colon (choice D) unless there is pancolitic diverticulosis. If pancolitic diverticulosis is evident, the sigmoid would invariably be involved and be the site of most severe disease.

565. (B) The nephrotic syndrome includes proteinuria, edema, lipiduria, and hyperlipidemia. The key abnormality is pathologic leakage of protein through altered glomerular basement membranes. Membranous glomerulonephritis is a glomerular-focused renal disease which disrupts the microarchitecture of the glomerular basement membrane and evokes clinical expression of the nephrotic syndrome. Interstitial nephritis (choice A) affects the renal stroma and tubules. The lack of primary lesions in the glomeruli makes nephrotic syndrome an unlikely clinical correlate. Unilateral hydronephrosis (choice C) is usually seen with postrenal obstruction such as neoplasm or a stone. Since the other kidney is unaffected, nephrotic syndrome is not evident. Acute crescentic glomerulonephritis (choice D) usually produces a nephritic syndrome with hematuria and hypertension, rather than the nephrotic syndrome. Polycystic kidney disease (choice E) is tubulointerstitial nephropathy unassociated with the nephrotic syndrome.

566. (D) The decedent probably died from an acute myocardial infarct. An acute myocardial infarct results in cardiac myocyte necrosis. As these myocytes die, certain substances unique to cardiac muscle cells leak out into the bloodstream. The sudden appearance of these substances in the blood can serve as a useful laboratory marker for acute cardiac damage. The myocyte-derived substances most frequently tested for are the MB isoenzyme of the enzyme creatine phosphokinase and troponin. Liver (choice A) and lung (choice B) both lack significant creatine phosphokinase MB activity. Injury to the liver would produce elevations of certain transaminase enzymes and the fifth isoenzyme fraction of lactate dehydrogenase. Pulmonary injury would release the second isoenzyme fraction of lactate dehydrogenase. The brain (choice C) contains the BB, not the MB isoenzyme fraction, of creatine phosphokinase. The kidney (choice E) does not contain measurable quantities of the MB isoenzyme of creatine phosphokinase.

567. **(C)** Aspiration is the most common cause of pulmonary abscess formation. Alcoholics, epileptics, drug addicts, and neurologically compromised individuals are likely to aspirate. Cough, chest pain, fever, and the production of a large quantity of fetid sputum are the expected clinical signs of a pulmonary abscess. Irritant gases (choice A) are likely to produce acute diffuse pneumonitis, not a localized abscess. Alveolar proteinosis (choice B) is a diffuse pulmonary process in which there is abnormal accumulation of protein-rich fluid throughout the alveolar spaces. Vasculitis (choice D) may produce localized pulmonary lesions. They usually remain sterile, however, unless secondarily infected by an event such as aspiration or sepsis. Cigarette smoking (choice E) is likely to damage the lung through bronchial squamous metaplasia and emphysema. Abscess formation is not associated with chronic tobacco use.

568. **(A)** The photograph depicts a chronic peptic ulcer. There is loss of mucosal continuity, an ulcer bed with necrotic tissue, and fibrosis of the submucosa. Peptic ulcers are associated with increased gastic acid secretion and *Helicobacter pylori* mucosal infestation. Hemorrhage, perforation, and penetration may complicate an ulcer. Adenocarcinoma (choice B) may form an ulcer. Within the ulcer, however, there would be diagnostic malignant glandular epithelium. Adenomatous polyps (choice C) are not associated with gross ulcer formation. Histologically, there is an increased number of benign glandular elements. Brunner gland adenoma (choice D) frequently presents as a duodenal mass. The microanatomy reveals hyperplasia of submucosal Brunner glands. A leiomyoma (choice E) is a benign smooth muscle tumor. The photograph does not display a neoplasm.

569. **(E)** Auer rods are intensely azurophilic cytoplasmic inclusions frequently seen in leukemic myeloblasts. Most are rod-shaped and represent an aberrant form of myeloid primary granules. Their presence serves as a useful aid for the morphologic diagnosis of acute myeloblastic leukemia. Silicotic pneumocytes (choice A) are not myeloid derived and do not contain Auer rods. Neurons infected with rabies virus (choice B) may contain eosinophilic round cytoplasmic inclusions called Negri bodies that morphologically resemble red blood cells. Diabetic islet cells (choice C) and transformed urothelial cells (choice D) are not myeloid derived cells and do not contain Auer rods.

570. **(E)** Meningioma is a neoplasm that arises from the dura or its invaginations. Typically, it is a tumor that occurs in older adults. Neuroblastoma (choice A) is a malignant neoplasm formed by immature neuroepithelium. It is usually seen in infants and young children. Retinoblastoma (choice B) is a malignant neoplasm that arises from retinal neuroepithelium. It occurs in early childhood. Medulloblastoma (choice C) is a malignant neoplasm that is usually found in the cerebellum of children and adolescents. Nephroblastoma (choice D) is a malignant neoplasm of early childhood that arises from immature renal tissue.

571. **(C)** The described lesion is a keloid. Keloids are an example of excessive scar formation due to a relative abundance of collagen matrix ground substance which is laid down in a disorganized manner. Keloids most frequently occur in blacks and may recur after excision. A teratoma (choice A) is a neoplasm derived from germ cells and usually displays several types of partially mature tissue. They usually occur in the ovary, testicles, or mediastinum. A hamartoma (choice B) is a collection of several different types of adult tissue in an abnormal location. The lung is the most frequent site. A dermoid cyst (choice D) is a mature teratoma of the ovary. Excessive collagenization is not evident with this tumor. Brenner tumor (choice E) is a benign neoplasm of the ovary.

572. **(B)** Cystadenoma is a benign neoplasm with a gross cystic architecture. The microanatomy reveals adenomatous epithelium. Cystadenomas occur in several organs. Adenocarcinoma (choice A) is a malignant tumor composed of glandular epithelium. Fibrosarcoma (choice C) is a malignant neoplasm that is derived from fibrous mesenchyme. Lymphocytic leukemia (choice D) is a low-grade malignancy of mature lymphocytes. Melanoma (choice E) is a malignant neoplasm arising from melanocytes. The skin is the most frequent location.

573. **(A)** Aflatoxin is a known potent chemical carcinogen that can produce liver cell carcinoma in humans. It is a fungal derived contaminant of improperly stored foods. Pulmonary sarcomas (choice B) are rare tumors. Most occur sporadically. Radiation exposure is a known risk factor. Chordomas of the lower spine (choice C) are also rare. Their occurrence is not associated with aflatoxin exposure. Uterine leiomyomas (choice D) are benign tumors of smooth muscle origin. They occur more frequently in blacks and have no relation to aflatoxin. Sebaceous carcinoma of the eyelid (choice E) is a highly malignant rare tumor whose occurrence is unrelated to aflatoxin.

574. **(D)** Transudates are an ultrafiltrate of plasma that enter the extracellular space by either increased hydrostatic pressure or decreased colloid oncotic pressure. Transudates typically have a specific gravity below 1.010, less than 3 gm/dL of protein, minimal fibrin, and minimal cells. Clinically, transudates are seen with right heart failure, cirrhosis, kwashiorkor, and nephrotic syndrome. An exudate (choice A) is an extracellular fluid accumulation that has a specific gravity above 1.010, more than 3 gm/dL protein, a high content of fibrin, and many cells. Most exudates are inflammatory in nature. An empyema (choice B) is a collection of pus within the thoracic cavity with many neutrophils. Hemothorax (choice C) is a collection of blood within the thoracic spaces. An analysis would reveal many erythrocytes and a total protein of more than 3 gm/dL. A collection of fat-rich fluid within the thoracic cavity is called a chylothorax (choice E). The fat stain would be positive. Trauma, tuberculosis, and lymphoid malignancies are associated with chylothorax formation.

575. **(C)** Although most bacterial infections invoke a neutrophilic inflammatory response, *Salmonella* organisms are an exception in that the response typically is monocytic. This hematologic picture may be due to chemotactic factors produced by bacteria. The polymorphonuclear leukocyte (choice A) is the cell involved in most acute bacterial inflammatory reactions. *Salmonella* infections, however, are an exception to this rule. Eosinophils (choice B) are not seen in great numbers with *Salmonella* infections. Instead, parasitic and allergic reactions tend to recruit eosinophils. Multinucleate giant cells (choice D) are seen with cell-mediated immunity, some viral infections, and foreign body reactions. Plasma cells (choice E) are immunoglobulin-producing cells that are derived from stimulated lymphocytes and are outnumbered by monocytes in a typical *Salmonella* infection.

576. **(A)** Kernicterus is the morphologic term that describes toxic yellow discoloration seen in the brains of severely jaundiced neonates. The pigment is especially prominent in the basal ganglia, pontine nuclei, and cerebellar dentate nuclei. Mucoviscidosis (choice B) is another term for the genetic disorder cystic fibrosis. Zellballen (choice C) describes the nested microarchitecture of certain tumors of neuroendocrine derivation such as paragangliomas. Cholestasis (choice D) is seen as a brownish pigment that accumulates in liver cells when there is an impediment to the normal flow of bile. Sequestrum (choice E) is the fragment of necrotic bone that may be present within pus associated with acute hematogenous osteomyelitis.

577. **(B)** A 20-hour-old ischemic infarct of the myocardium should demonstrate coagulative necrosis without much of an inflammatory response. Fibrosis and collagen deposition (choice A) are late healing phenomena that do not begin until at least one week after the

infarct has occurred. Abundant neutrophils and monocytes (choice C) typically are seen about two to four days after an infarction. Monocytic infiltration and neovascularization (choice D) usually occur about three to six days after an infarction. Plasma cells and caseous necrosis (choice E) are not seen with ischemic myocardial damage. This pattern occurs with granulomatous inflammation.

578. **(E)** About one in 11 women in the United States will have breast cancer in her lifetime. A family history of breast cancer is a known risk factor for other female members of the family to develop breast cancer. The incidence of breast cancer is higher in the United States than in Japan (choice A). There is an increased incidence of breast cancer with early menarche or late menopause (choice B). A diet high in fat (choice C) is associated with a higher risk of developing breast cancer. Atypical hyperplasias (choice D) are strongly linked to an increased incidence of breast cancer.

579. **(D)** Hirschsprung's disease is caused by the congenital absence of parasympathetic ganglion cells in the submucosal and myenteric plexus. This presents clinically soon after birth as an inability to pass stool and abdominal distention. The diagnosis is usually confirmed by a full thickness colon biopsy showing disorganized nonmyelinated nerve fibers replacing the missing ganglion cells. Muscular hypertrophy (choice A) or atrophy (choice B) are not specific diagnostic findings with Hirschsprung's disease. In Hirschsprung's disease it is the ganglion cells, not the nerve fibers (choice C), which are missing. Mucosal polyp development (choice E) is not associated with Hirschsprung's disease.

580. **(B)** The most common cause of neonatal cholestasis is extrahepatic biliary atresia. This anatomic aberration may be due to intrauterine infections or inflammatory processes that retard the normal growth of bile ductules and ducts out from neonatal hepatocytes. Intrahepatic biliary atresia (choice A) is not as common as the extrahepatic variant in neonates. Choledochal cysts (choice C) are a rare cause of neonatal cholestasis. Primary biliary cirrhosis (choice D) is an autoimmune disease which occurs in adults. Budd–Chiari syndrome (choice E) is due to hepatic venous obstruction, rather than biliary obstruction.

581. **(B)** With the TNM international staging system for cancer, the letter T refers to the size or extent of the primary tumor, the letter N to the number and distribution of lymph node metastases, and the letter M to the presence of distant metastases. Values for these letters may be assigned by either pathologic or clinical examination. For each organ site, various combinations of T, N, and M values define stages I through IV. The time between diagnosis and definitive treatment (choice A), type of cells identified (choice C), or treatment plan (choice D) do not define the use of the letter T in the TNM staging system. The presence of nodal metastases (choice E) would define N1 or N2 in the TNM system, not the T value.

582. **(B)** Lobar pneumonia may progress through four stages: congestion, red hepatization, gray hepatization, and resolution. The second stage, red hepatization, is characterized grossly by a liver-like firm consistency to the lung due to filling of the alveolar spaces by erythrocytes, fibrin, and leukocytes. Fibroblastic proliferation (choice A), pleural deposits (choice C), tracheobronchial epithelial desquamation (choice D), and alcoholic toxic necrosis (choice E) are not pathologic processes that usually cause red hepatization.

583. **(A)** Fat necrosis is commonly associated with dystrophic calcific deposits. Acute pancreatitis allows digestive enzymes to leak out of damaged acinar cells. Liberated lipases act on the adjacent fat to precipitate calcific deposits which may be visualized by radiographic means. Viral infections (choice B) are rare in the pancreas. None are associated with calcium deposition. Lipofuscin (choice C) is a noncalcific degradation pigment that is not radiopaque. Liquefaction necrosis (choice D) is a peculiar form of cell death which is usually seen only in the brain and with abscesses. Calcification is not part of the process. Melanin (choice E) is a black pigment made by melanocytes that cannot be visualized radiographically.

584. (A) Wilson's disease is an autosomal recessive disorder of copper metabolism, probably due to defective biliary excretion of the metal. Cells of the liver and brain are particularly vulnerable to the toxic effects of excessive copper accumulation. Treatment with copper chelating agents, such as penicillamine or triethylene tetramine, have a dramatic beneficial effect. Reye's syndrome (choice B) is acute hepatic failure in infants following ingestion of aspirin. Primary sclerosing cholangitis (choice C) is due to chronic fibrosis of bile ductules. The etiology is obscure. Most of those affected also have ulcerative colitis. Congenital hepatic fibrosis (choice D) is a rare disorder of unknown etiology. It is most prevalent in India. Peliosis hepatis (choice E) demonstrates small blood-filled spaces within the liver. Steroid hormone usage is associated with its development in some instances.

585. (B) The vegetative lesions seen in rheumatic carditis most commonly occur along the line of closure of the mitral valve. Other features of rheumatic carditis may include fibrinous pericarditis and Aschoff nodules within the myocardium. Late sequelae may include valvular stenosis, valvular insufficiency, conduction defects, and adhesive pericarditis. The aortic sinuses of Valsalva (choice A), the insertion of the chordae tendinae (choice C), mitral valve annulus (choice D), and coronary artery ostia (choice E) are unlikely sites for the formation of rheumatic vegetative lesions.

586. (A) The heart demonstrates left ventricular hypertrophy. Chronic essential hypertension is the commonest etiology in the United States. Atrial septal defect (choice B) is an anomalous mural defect between the two atria. Congestive heart failure (choice C) is characterized by dilation of the cardiac chambers. Chagas' disease (choice D) is a protozoan infection of the heart that does not produce left ventricular hypertrophy. Tricuspid valvular stenosis (choice E) is usually caused by rheumatic carditis and is not associated with left ventricular hypertrophy.

587. (E) The genetic lack of antiprotease activity predisposes an individual to the early development of panacinar emphysema. Pulmonary hamartomas (choice A), chronic viral pneumonia (choice B), intralobular sequestration (choice C), and alveolar proteinosis (choice D), are all pulmonary disorders that are not related to hereditary antitrypsin deficiency.

588. (D) Epidemic rotavirus diarrhea is the correct choice. Other less likely etiologic agents that might fit this scenario would include Norwalk virus, adenovirus, calicivirus, and astrovirus infections. Variola (choice A) virus causes smallpox. Skin lesions, not diarrhea, typify this disease. Parvovirus B19 (choice B) infection may result in erythema infectiosum (fifth disease), transient aplastic crisis, and fetal hydrops. Herpes simplex virus (choice C) is a DNA virus seen with oral or genital cutaneous vesicle formation. Cytomegalovirus (choice E) infection is usually subclinical except in immunocompromised individuals.

589. (E) Opsonization is the binding of IgG or C3b to pathogenic bacteria. The opsonized bacteria are more readily phagocytized by neutrophils and macrophages which possess receptors for Fc and C3b. C8 (choice A) is part of the complement membrane attack complex and does not participate in opsonization. C1 (choice B) is an initial participant in the classical pathway. The C1 components do not opsonize bacteria. Factor B (choice C) is active through the alternative complement pathway. C4a (choice D) has anaphylactic properties rather than opsonizing abilities.

590. (C) The Mallory–Weiss syndrome consists of a clinical history of prolonged vomiting or retching, hematemesis, and longitudinal mucosal tears in the lower esophagus. Letterer–Siwe syndrome (choice A) is a malignant systemic disorder of Langerhans cells that usually affects infants and young children. Blind loop syndrome (choice B) is associated with nonhemorrhagic malabsorption with bacterial overgrowth. Dubin–Johnson syndrome (choice D) describes a genetic disorder of intermittent jaundice and black hepatocytic pigmentation. Conn syndrome (choice E) is another term for primary hyperaldosteronism. Adrenal cortical hyperplasia or adenoma are the usual anatomic findings.

591. (B) Syphilitic saccular aneurysms of the thoracic aorta result from endarteritis obliterans of the vasa vasorum with subsequent mural ischemic necrosis. Cystic medial necrosis (choice A) is a non-infectious disorder characterized by abnormally weak connective tissue in the aortic media and deposits of myxoid substances. Intimal fibroplasia and lipid deposition (choice C) are the early lesions of atherosclerosis. Immune complex formation and complement activation (choice D) may be seen with tertiary syphilis, but involve only the small vessels, without aneurysm formation. Hypersensitivity reactions, multinucleate giant cells, and fibrinoid necrosis (choice E) play no significant role in the development of syphilitic aortic aneurysms.

592. (E) The photomicrograph depicts macrophages filled with lipids from an infant with Gaucher's disease. The disease is due to a genetic lack of the catabolic enzyme glucocerebrosidase which fosters the abnormal accumulation of glucocerebroside within the reticuloendothelial cells and neurons. Gaucher's disease is not caused by radiation (choice A), trauma (choice B), viral infection (choice C), or deficient cellular immunity (choice D).

593. (A) The clinical history, surgical findings, and described microscopic pattern all support the diagnosis of Warthin's tumor, a benign neoplasm of the major salivary glands. Pleomorphic adenoma (choice B) is also a common benign neoplasm of the salivary glands. However, it differs from Warthin's tumor in several aspects. Pleomorphic adenoma is rarely cystic, usually lacks significant oncocytic epithelial elements, and the stroma is myxoid rather than lymphoid. Acute suppurative sialoadenitis (choice C) would have a more acute clinical history, pus may be observed at the time of surgery, and the histology would confirm an acute inflammatory process rather than neoplasm. Mucoepidermoid carcinoma (choice D) and adenoid cystic carcinoma (choice E) are both malignant neoplasms of the salivary gland. Neither displays the benign histology described for Warthin's tumor.

594. (C) A significant proportion of low-grade squamous intraepithelial lesions are the result of human papillomavirus infection. Viral subtypes 16 and 18 are more likely to progress to high-grade dysplasias. Koilocytosis is the usual morphologic marker of viral infection. It is unlikely that these changes would result from a hereditary disorder (choice A), normal intermenstrual reactions (choice B), a protozoan infection (choice D), or hormonal imbalances (choice E).

595. (C) Gynecomastia usually occurs in the setting of hyperestrinism. Puberty, cirrhosis, old age, certain pharmaceutical agents, and estrogen-secreting tumors may all induce gynecomastia. Dietary deficiency states (choice A) are not known at present to be agents of gynecomastia. The hyperplasia of ducts and periductular stroma seen with gynecomastia are not clonal (choice B). Ionizing radiation (choice D) and subacute inflammation (choice E) are not etiologic concerns in the formation of gynecomastia.

596. (A) Polyarteritis nodosa is a systemic vasculitis primarily seen in young adult males. Fibrinoid necrosis and acute inflammation are seen microscopically in the acute phase. Takayasu's disease (choice B) is characterized by fibrosis of the upper aorta. The classic patient is a Japanese female with HLA-DR4. Mucocutaneous lymph node syndrome (Kawasaki's disease) (choice C) is a childhood disorder with coronary vasculitis, cervical lymphadenopathy, and acute onset. Giant cell arteritis (choice D) is a granulomatous arterial inflammation seen in the elderly. The superficial temporal and intercranial arteries are preferentially involved. Thromboangiitis obliterans (choice E) is an occlusive disease of small arteries strongly related to cigarette smoking.

597. (D) The majority of people who die in fires succumb to smoke inhalation with subsequent anoxia. Thermal burns (choice A) are the second most common cause of acute fire deaths. Hypovolemia (choice B) may be fatal in a minority of fire deaths as thermally damaged skin weeps protein-rich fluid, but death occurs in a subacute or chronic time frame rather than acutely. Vascular thrombosis (choice C) and stroke (choice E) are rarely seen as cause of death in fires unless there is concomitant severe thermal damage.

598. (D) Liposarcoma is a malignant tumor derived from nonepithelial lipomatous mesenchyme. Serous cystadenoma (choice A) is a benign epithelial tumor. Hepatoma (choice B) is a malignant epithelial neoplasm of hepatocytic origin. Hemangioma (choice C) is a benign tumor composed of blood vessels. A chondroma (choice E) is a benign neoplasm derived from chrondrocytes.

599. (E) The Budd–Chiari syndrome is due to extensive occlusive fibrosis of the hepatic venous drainage. The clinical findings usually include ascites, hepatomegaly, and portal hypertension. The Budd–Chiari syndrome is unlikely to be caused by malignant biliary transformation (choice A), agenesis of a hepatic lobe (choice B), congenital disorders of bilirubin metabolism (choice C), or a dietary deficiency (choice D).

600. (A) Hyaline membranes are usually seen microscopically in lungs showing diffuse alveolar damage. Grossly, the lungs are heavy, wet, and meaty. The clinical course is termed adult respiratory distress syndrome and is characterized by relative unresponsiveness to oxygen therapy. Eosinophilic inflammatory infiltrates (choice B), vascular microthrombi (choice C), pleural effusions (choice D), and hemorrhagic infarction (choice E) are not typically seen with diffuse alveolar damage.

601. (C) The retinoblastoma gene is a tumor suppressor gene. If both copies of this gene are abnormal, there is a two-hundred–fold increase in the risk of retinoblastoma. Although tumorigenesis may occur through viral integration into host DNA (choice A), trisomy of chromosomes (choice B), activation of oncogenes (choice D), and chemical alterations of host DNA (choice E), these processes are not thought to be significant with retinoblastoma.

602. (B) The Tzanck smear demonstrates a multinucleate giant cell with the characteristic nuclear inclusions of herpes virus infection. After initial infection of epidermal and neural cells there is latency of virus within the neuronal cells. Recurrent crops of vesicles are due to viral reactivation by the neuronally infected cells. Dietary deficiencies (choice A), neoplasia (choice C), autoimmune diseases (choice D), and hereditary disorders (choice E) are not active contributors to formation of herpetic vesicles.

603. (B) Many growth factors, including epidermal growth factor, exert their influence through activation of cytoplasmic tyrosine kinase. Adenylate cyclase (choice A), guanylate cyclase (choice C), and kallikrein (choice D) are components of the acute inflammatory response. Lysosomes (choice E) are intracytoplasmic bodies with degrading enzymatic activity.

604. (D) Liquefaction necrosis is a peculiar pattern of postinfarctive stromal breakdown seen in the brain. Infarcts of the lung (choice A) and small bowel (choice B) usually produce hemorrhagic coagulative necrosis. Infarcts of the kidney (choice C) and spleen (choice E) usually produce non-hemorrhagic pale areas of coagulative necrosis.

605. (E) Pemphigus vulgaris is an autoimmune disorder. The autoantibodies are directed against keratinocyte antigens with subsequent dyshesion and fluid-filled blister formation. Local ischemia (choice A), dietary deficiencies (choice B), chemical toxins (choice C), and psychiatric conditions (choice D) are not thought to be the causative agent of pemphigus vulgaris.

606. **(B)** Hydropic swelling is a reversible non-lethal morphologic alteration which usually corresponds ultrastructurally to accumulation of excess fluids within the endoplasmic reticulum. Karyorrhexis (choice A), pyknosis (choice C), apoptosis (choice D), and rupture of the nuclear membrane (choice E) are all irreversible lethal morphologic abnormalities.

607. **(A)** Pheochromocytoma is a neoplasm of the adrenal medulla. Episodic hypertension and elevated catecholamines usually accompany the clinical finding of an adrenal mass. Ganglioneuroma (choice B) is a rare neoplasm of young children that is composed of both differentiated and immature neural elements. Adrenal cortical hyperplasia (choice C) and adrenal cortical carcinoma (choice D) are not usually associated with elevations of catecholamines. Neuroblastoma (choice E) is a childhood neoplasm composed of immature neural tissue.

608. **(E)** Chronic lymphocytic leukemia is a disease of the elderly with mature lymphocytosis, B-cell markers, light chain restriction, and expression of CD5. Plasma cell leukemia (choice A) would have different CD markers and appear morphologically as plasma cells rather than mature lymphocytes. It is a very rare entity. Reactive lymphocytosis (choice B) would demonstrate a mixed κ and λ pattern and different CD markers. Adult T-cell leukemia (choice C) would not demonstrate B-cell lymphocyte markers such as CD20. Castleman's disease (choice D) usually is defined by a histologically unique pattern of lymphadenopathy without a peripheral lymphocytosis.

609. **(C)** Hypertrophy is an increase in individual cell size without an increase in the number of cells. Left ventricular cardiac hypertrophy secondary to essential hypertension is a clinical example of this phenomenon. Hyperplasia (choice A) is an increase in the number of cells present with or without an increase in the size of individual cells. Hypoplasia (choice B) is a decrease in the number of cells evident. Metaplasia (choice D) is change of one adult cell type for another, such as respiratory squamous metaplasia occurring after chronic cigarette smoking. Dysplasia (choice E) is an abnormal maturation of cells which may be premalignant.

610. **(A)** Tetralogy of Fallot includes right ventricular hyperplasia, pulmonary stenosis, ventricular septal defect, and dextroposition of the aorta. It is a cyanotic congenital heart disorder with a dismal prognosis unless surgically corrected. Transposition of the great arteries (choice B) is a congenital heart disease defined as the aorta arising from the right ventricle and the pulmonary artery originating from the left ventricle. Anomalous pulmonary venous drainage (choice C) occurs when there is aberrant drainage of the pulmonary veins into the left atrium. The Ebstein malformation (choice D) is a congenital abnormality of the tricuspid valve and right ventricle. Dextrocardia (choice E) is a mirror image inversion of the heart.

611. **(A)** Osteogenesis imperfecta, type I, is a genetic disorder characterized by synthesis of an abnormal type I collagen. Frequent childhood fractures, blue sclera, poor hearing, and misshapen teeth may all occur clinically because of the abnormal collagen synthesis. Inability to metabolize vitamin D (choice B), inadequate mineralization of bone matrix (choice C), renal inability to conserve phosphorous (choice D), and abnormal intestinal receptors for calcium (choice E) are not the primary pathologic alteration responsible for this disorder.

612. **(D)** The formation of a vascular thrombus is most likely to occur clinically when there is stasis of the luminal blood flow, the presence of a hypercoagulable state, adequate or increased quantity of functioning platelets, and endothelial damage. Individuals who are likely to form thrombi, such as endocardial mural thrombi with atrial fibrillation, are usually treated with an anticoagulant such as coumadin to inhibit thrombogenesis. The choices indicating coumadin therapy (choices A, B, and E) are inprobable clinical settings for thrombus formation. Individuals with low platelet counts, normal luminal blood flow, and no endothelial damage (choice C) are unlikely to form thrombi.

613. (E) ELAM-1 is recognized as an endothelial cellular adhesion molecule. Its expression on the membrane assists in the recruitment of neutrophils during an acute inflammatory response. Other cellular adhesion molecules may include ELAM-2 and GMP-140. Histamine (choice A), interleukin 1 (choice B), plasmin (choice C), and myeloperoxidase (choice D) are not examples of cellular adhesion molecules.

614. (B) Lung carcinoma is the leading cause of cancer deaths among females in the United States. Carcinoma of the breast (choice A) and carcinoma of the colon (choice C) are the second and third most frequent fatal sites for females in the United States, respectively. Neither carcinoma of the uterus (choice D) nor carcinoma of the ovary (choice E) is the leading cause of female cancer deaths in the United States.

615. (C) Klinefelter's syndrome has a 47,XXY karyotype, testicular atrophy, eunuchoid tall habitus, gynecomastia, and a female distribution of hair. Down syndrome (choice A) is characterized by trisomy 21, congenital cardiac defects, epicanthic folds, mental retardation, dysplastic ears, and an increased risk of developing leukemia. Edwards' syndrome (choice B) is a trisomy of chromosome 18. Individuals with Edwards' syndrome may display mental retardation, micrognathia, rocker bottom feet, and prominent occiput. Turner's syndrome (choice D) has a 45,X karyotype, webbing of the neck, amenorrhea, streak gonads, short stature, and cardiac defects. Multi-X syndrome (choice E) is usually a phenotypically normal female.

616. (C) Antibiotic induced overgrowth of *Clostridium difficile* is frequently associated with the occurrence of pseudomembranous colitis. The bacterial organism mediates these pathologic changes via a potent toxin. Rapid laboratory tests are available to detect the toxin in feces. *Helicobacter pylori* (choice A) is associated with gastric ulcers. *Yersinia* species (choice B) are usually associated with ileal infections and mesenteric lymphadenitis. *Salmonella* species (choice D) and *Shigella* species (choice E) may both produce severe diarrhea. Neither, however, is commonly associated with pseudomembranous colitis.

617. (B) In postinfectious acute glomerulonephritis the major renal alterations are evident within the glomerulus. Hypercellularity and ultrastructural changes are morphologic correlates to the clinical observations of hematuria and hypertension. The other sites in the kidney such as the distal convoluted tubule (choice A), afferent arteriole (choice C), proximal convoluted tubule (choice D), and calyx (choice E) are not usually directly altered with acute postinfectious glomerulonephritis.

618. (A) Sipple syndrome (MEN IIA) may demonstrate medullary thyroid carcinoma, adrenal medullary hyperplasia or neoplasia, and parathyroid hyperplasia or neoplasia. The other options (choices B, C, D, and E) all offer collections of items that do not as a whole define the syndrome.

619. (E) Accidents and trauma comprise the most frequent cause of death within the United States in the age range of five to nine years old. Malignant neoplasms (choice A) is the second most frequent cause of death in this age range. Congenital anomalies (choice B) is the third most frequent cause of death in this age range. Neither heart disease (choice C) nor infectious agents (choice D) is the leading cause of deaths within this age group in the United States.

620. (D) Overdoses of acetaminophen overwhelm the liver's glutathione reductase capacity. The toxic metabolites that accumulate predictably produce hepatic necrosis. Pulmonary necrosis (choice A), infarction of the spleen (choice B), meningeal inflammation (choice C), and acute renal tubular necrosis (choice E) are not associated with acetaminophen overdoses.

621. (C) Type I diabetes mellitus is also called insulin-dependent diabetes mellitus. The need for parenteral insulin separates this entity from type II diabetes (non–insulin-dependent diabetes mellitus). Generally, type I diabetes is the more severe condition with an earlier age range (choice A) and more frequent complications (choices B, D, and E). Type I diabetes may be the result of viral or immune destruction of the pancreatic islet cells. Type II diabetes demonstrates a strong polygenic hereditary tendency.

622. (C) Amyloid is an acellular material that is eosinophilic. After congo-red staining there is apple-green dichromism when examined under polarized light microscopy. A post infarctive cicatrix (choice A) would also display a relatively acellular eosinophilic morphology. Congo-red staining would not be dichromic, however. Calcium salts (choice B) tend to be deeply basophilic, not eosinophilic, with routine stains. Myocyte fibrinoid necrosis (choice D) would be moderately cellular and eosinophilic. Congo-red dichromism is not evident. Cholesterol deposits (choice E) tend to dissolve out of tissues with routine processing agents and only empty outlines of where the crystals once were are present.

623. (C) The asthmalike pulmonary disorder that develops after long-term inhalation of cotton fibers is termed byssinosis. Silicosis (choice A) is a pneumoconiosis resulting from the inhalation of silica. Occupational exposure can be seen with mining, sandblasting, stone masonry, pottery manufacture, and glass making. Inhalation of tin fumes or debris may result in pulmonary stannosis (choice B). Anthracosis (choice D) is commonly seen in human lungs. Coal miners have a particularly severe form of the disorder. City dwellers and smokers tend to have more moderate disease. Berylliosis (choice E) is a pneumoconiosis seen with beryllium inhalation. Occupational exposure is usually through the production of fluorescent lighting.

624. (E) Environmental exposure to either vinyl chloride or thorium dioxide is associated with the later development of hepatic angiosarcoma. Liver cell carcinoma (choice A) is associated with cirrhosis, chronic viral hepatitis, and aflatoxin exposure. Hepatic adenomas (choice B) occur sporadically in the setting of exogenous steroid hormone usage. Focal nodular hyperplasia (choice C) and hepatic fibromas (choice D) do not at present have well defined antecedent environmental exposure histories.

625. (C) The photograph displays viable benign chorionic villi which are diagnostic of an ectopic tubal pregnancy. The clinical history of acute lower abdominal pain and hypotension are expected findings with an ectopic pregnancy. Leiomyomas (choice A) rarely occur in the fallopian tube. They are most commonly seen in the wall of the uterus. Bundles of benign smooth muscle cells would be seen microscopically. Choriocarcinoma (choice B) is a malignant neoplasm composed of gestational trophoblastic tissue. The photomicrograph displays benign chorionic elements. Granular cell tumor (choice D) is a neoplasm of neural type tissue. The photomicrograph is incompatible with this diagnostic consideration. Chorioadenoma destruens (choice E) is also referred to as invasive mole, and would display invasion of chorionic elements into the uterine, not tubal, muscular layers.

626. (D) Cryptorchidism is associated with increased risk for infertility and the development of testicular neoplasms. Testicular germ cell neoplasms are most likely to develop in undescended testes. Cryptorchidism is not usually associated with an increased risk for testicular feminization syndrome (choice A), infarction (choice B), hemorrhage (choice C), or infection (choice E).

627. (A) Convulsions are seen only with eclampsia and serve as a defining feature to separate eclampsia from pre-eclampsia. Hypertension (choice B), edema (choice C), and proteinuria (choice D) are seen in both eclamptic and preeclamptic individuals. Eclampsia and preeclampsia are both seen most commonly late in pregnancy (choice E).

628. (A) Hyperacute renal transplant rejection is due to incompatibilities of the ABO blood groups. In an incompatible transplant there is hyperacute rejection due to binding of naturally occurring circulating anti-A or anti-B to renal endothelium. Long-term postoperative corticosteroid therapy (choice B) may help prevent chronic rejection. A kidney that is compatible for HLA-A, HLA-B, and HLA-C (choice C) is less likely to experience acute or chronic rejection. A preoperative dose of an immune suppressive drug (choice D) and intraoperative lymphocyte apheresis (choice E) are both unlikely to alter the development of hyperacute, acute, or chronic transplant rejection.

629. (B) Mesenteric adenitis with enterocolitis is associated with *Yersinia* species infections. Clinically, the disorder closely mimics acute appendicitis, presenting as acute right lower quadrant abdominal pain, fever, and leukocytosis. If the patient comes to surgery, the appendix usually appears fairly normal, and instead there is striking enlargement of the mesenteric lymph nodes. The nodes display an acute necrotizing granulomatous pattern if examined histologically. Mesenteric adenitis is unlikely to be caused by local vascular insufficiency (choice A), viral infection (choice C), fungal infection (choice D), or parasitic infection (choice E).

630. (B) The photograph displays interweaving bundles of smooth muscle cells, which as a discrete myometrial nodule would define a leiomyoma. These are common tumors which may be asymptomatic or produce menorrhagia. The gross appearance is that of a solid white nodule. A Krukenberg tumor (choice A) is replacement of the ovary by metastatic gastrointestinal adenocarcinoma. Adenomyosis (choice C) may clinically and grossly mimic leiomyomas. Adenomyosis, however, has a triphasic microscopic appearance consisting of benign endometrial glands, benign endometrial stroma, and smooth muscle hypertrophy. Ovarian ectopia (choice D) is exceedingly rare and would not be compatible with the histology of the photomicrograph. The diagnosis of metastatic malignancy (choice E) is not supported by the photomicrograph of a benign process.

631. (A) Wiskott–Aldrich syndrome is a rare X-linked hereditary immunodeficiency disorder characterized by recurrent infections by pyogenic bacteria and opportunistic organisms, thrombocytopenia, and eczema. Bone marrow transplantation may be curative. The syndrome is not characterized by a congenital viral infection (choice B), renal agenesis and pulmonary hypoplasia (choice C), neonatal parasitic infection (choice D), or congenital heart disease (choice E).

632. (C) Sezary syndrome is the leukemic variant or phase of mycosis fungoides. Mycosis fungoides is a peripheral epidermotrophic T-cell lymphoma which afflicts middle-aged and elderly individuals. Most Sezary cells have a highly convoluted, cerebriform nucleus. Extranodal gastric B-cell lymphoma (choice A) does not define the Sezary syndrome. Large B-cell lymphoma arising in the setting of chronic lymphocytic lymphoma (choice B) is termed Richter syndrome. Adult T-cell leukemia due to HTLV-1 infection (choice D) and lymphoma that arises in HIV positive patients (choice E) do not define the Sezary syndrome.

633. (B) Paget's disease of the nipple usually presents as an ulcerated crusted lesion of one nipple. A biopsy specimen will reveal intraepithelial adenocarcinoma. On further examination the underlying breast tissue may show an intraductal or infiltrating ductal adenocarcinoma. Epidermolysis bullosa (choice A) is a benign dermatologic condition characterized by cutaneous blister formation with minor trauma. Dermatitis herpetiformis (choice C) is a gluten sensitivity related cutaneous disorder characterized by pruritic plaque formation. Desmoid tumor (choice D) is a form of fibromatosis usually occurring in the ventral abdominal subcutis. Bowen's disease (choice E) is another term for cutaneous squamous cell carcinoma in situ. It frequently occurs on sun-exposed aged skin.

634. (B) Small cell undifferentiated pulmonary carcinoma is closely linked to cigarette smoking. This highly lethal malignancy is thought to arise from neuroendocrine cells of the bronchial mucosa. Clara cells (choice A) may give rise to certain pulmonary adenocarcinomas. Metaplastic bronchial epithelium (choice C) is the likely source of squamous cell carcinoma. The alveolar pneumocytes (choices D and E) rarely sustain malignant transformation.

635. (B) A stroke produces variable lethal injury to neuronal irreversibly postmitotic cells. Adjacent neurons are incapable of mitotic activity to replace the neighboring dead neurons. Liver cells (choice A) are not irreversibly postmitotic cells and are fully capable of mitotic replacement of adjacent necrotic hepatocytes. The esophageal epithelium (choice C) is mitotically active and able to regenerate to heal erosive lesions. First-degree thermal burns (choice D) can be healed by ingrowth of nearby squamous epithelial cells. The colonic epithelium (choice E) is fully capable of mitotic activity.

636. (D) Malakoplakia is most frequent in middle-aged females with a clinical history of repeated bladder infections. The gross appearance is characterized by scattered soft yellow plaques in the bladder mucosa. Chronic inflammation with numerous microcalcospherites (Michaelis–Gutmann bodies) is present microscopically. Endometriosis (choice A) is not associated with bladder infections, appears red on gross exam, and microscopically would display a mixture of benign endometrial glands and stroma. Exstrophy (choice B) of the bladder refers to a birth defect in which the bladder mucosa is everted through an abdominal wall defect. Polypoid cystitis (choice C) is associated with indwelling urinary catheters. The bladder lesion is usually single, polypoid, and red. Chronic interstitial cystitis (choice E) is also called Hunner ulcer. The bladder mucosa is red, fibrotic, and may be ulcerated. Microcalcospherites are not part of the usual histology.

637. (A) Gastric mucosal infections with *Helicobacter pylori* are strongly linked to the development of ulceration. Antibiotic treatment which eliminates the bacteria is the usual treatment for gastric ulcers induced by *H. pylori. Salmonella typhi* (choice B), *Bartonella bacilliformis* (choice C), *Brucellosis melitensis* (choice D), and *Pseudomonas aeruginosa* (choice E) may all inflict variable pathogenic damage to the gastrointestinal tract. These organisms are not frequently associated, however, with gastric ulceration.

638. (C) Individuals with chronic pancreatitis may complain of abdominal pain and demonstrate pancreatic exocrine or endocrine dysfunction. Histologically, there is extensive fibrous and inflammatory atrophy of the pancreatic parenchyma. The leading cause of chronic pancreatitis in the United States is chronic ethanol abuse. Gallstones (choice A), neoplasms at the ampulla of Vater (choice B), diabetes mellitus (choice D), and viral infections (choice E) are all infrequent causes of pancreatitis in the United States.

639. (B) The muscle spasms and seizures that may result from *Clostridium tetani* infection are due to a systemic neurotoxin which is produced by the organism at a local wound site. The neurotoxin is believed to block the release of the inhibitory neurotransmitter glycine leading to muscular hyperactivity. The muscle spasms and seizures do not result from erosion of the organism into the subarachnoid space (choice A), complicating septicemia (choice C), a type III hypersensitivity reaction to tetanus toxoid (choice D), or a superinfection by a secondary organism (choice E).

640. (E) Alcaptonuria is an autosomal recessive genetic disorder caused by the absence of the degradative enzyme homogentisic acid oxidase. This deficiency results in the accumulation of homogentisic acid in cartilage, soft tissues, and urine. Oxidation by air of urinary homogentisic acid is evidenced by the formation of a dark pigment. The urinary pigment does not result from bacterial metabolism (choice A), excess phenylalanine (choice B), excess cystine (choice C), or excess glycine (choice D).

641. **(E)** Hookworms infect the human small bowel producing mucosal lacerations, blood loss, and subsequent anemia. In the United States the most common etiologic agent is *Necator americanus. Dracunculis medinensis* (choice A) is a tissue nematode found in the Middle East which causes subcutaneous ulcers and allergic reactions along the lower extremities. *Enterobius vermicularis* (choice B) is the intestinal nematode responsible for pinworm infection. *Ascaris lumbricoides* (choice C) is an intestinal nematode. Most infections with this roundworm are asymptomatic. *Entamoeba coli* (choice D) is nonpathogenic intestinal amoeba.

642. **(A)** The photograph shows a clear cell adenocarcinoma which is the most common histologic appearance for renal cell carcinoma. The patient's age, gender, and clinical presentation are typical for this malignant neoplasm. Angiomyolipoma (choice B) is a benign renal tumor which displays a mixture of blood vessels, smooth muscle, and mature fat on microscopic examination. Transitional cell carcinoma (choice C) usually arises in the renal pelvis and histologically is composed of anaplastic transitional cells without a clear cell adenocarcinoma component. Oncocytoma (choice D) is a benign renal neoplasm constructed by monomorphic cells with granular eosinophilic cytoplasm. Xanthogranulomatous pyelonephritis (choice E) is a benign inflammatory condition of the kidney which may produce a mass effect. The gross appearance, but not the microscopic appearance, may be confused with renal cell carcinoma.

643. **(C)** The most common cause of pulmonary bone marrow emboli is trauma. Long bone fractures and resuscitative efforts that fracture the ribs are likely premortem events. Dislodged marrow elements gain access to the venous circulation during trauma and the circulating marrow is then subsequently trapped in the narrowing pulmonary vasculature. Acute leukemia (choice A), idiopathic thrombocytopenia (choice B), pulmonary fibrosis (choice D), and anomalous venous drainage (choice E) are not usually associated with pulmonary bone marrow emboli.

644. **(B)** The Stein–Leventhal syndrome is seen as a constellation of polycystic ovaries, hirsutism, obesity, and amenorrhea. The pathogenesis probably relates to luteinizing hormone-dependent ovarian overproduction of androgens. It is a sporadic cause of female infertility in the United States. Multiple endocrine neoplasia, type 2B (choice A), consists of a possible combination of pheochromocytoma, medullary thyroid carcinoma, and mucosal neuromas. Pseudomyxoma peritonei (choice C) is a peritoneal collection of mucinous debris due to rupture of appendiceal or ovarian mucinous tumors. Multiple endocrine neoplasia, type 2A, (choice D) may display pheochromocytoma, thyroid medullary carcinoma, gliomas, and parathyroid hyperplasia. A true hermaphrodite (choice E) has both testicular and ovarian gonads.

645. **(E)** Lymphogranuloma venereum is a sexually transmitted disease caused by *Chlamydia trachomatis.* Inguinal lymphadenopathy due to a necrotizing granulomatous reaction evoked by the organism characterizes the acute phase of the disease. Ulcers and strictures may occur in the chronic phase. Antibiotics in the acute phase of the disease are curative. Infections with *Chlamydia psittaci* (choice A) may cause a pneumonic disorder in humans called psittacosis. *Rickettsia prowazekii* (choice B) is the etiologic agent of epidemic typhus. Q fever is caused by the rickettsial-like organism *Coxiella burnetii* (choice C). *Borrelia burgdorferi* (choice D) is the etiologic agent of Lyme disease.

646. **(D)** The peptic ulcerations that are seen in the Zollinger–Ellison syndrome are due to ectopic hypersecretion of gastrin. An islet cell tumor of the pancreas is the most frequent ectopic site. Gastric mucosal hypertrophy, not atrophy (choice A), is the expected result with an increased secretion of gastrin as is seen with Zollinger–Ellison syndrome. Antibodies to intrinsic factor (choice B) are seen with pernicious anemia and usually cause gastric mucosal atrophy and metaplasia. Vascular abnormalities (choice C) and pressure ulceration from bezoars (choice E) are not the etiology of the peptic ulcerations seen with the Zollinger–Ellison syndrome.

647. **(C)** Thrombotic thrombocytopenic purpura is an acute microangiopathic hemolytic anemia. The clinical picture usually includes mental alterations, anuria, mucosal bleeding, and purpura. An abnormal platelet aggregating substance is the likely initiating event. May Hegglin anomaly (choice A) is an inherited condition with thrombocytopenia and morphologically abnormal white blood cells. Hemolysis, acute onset, and mental aberrations do not typify this disorder. Acute idiopathic thrombocytopenia (choice B) does not have a hemolytic component, lacks renal failure, and would not display thrombi in the skin biopsy. Glanzmann thrombasthenia (choice D) and Bernard–Soulier syndrome (choice E) are hereditary disorders of platelet aggregation. Clinical symptoms of a coagulopathy usually occur in infancy.

648. **(D)** Therapeutic apheresis is the currently recommended treatment for thrombotic thrombocytopenic purpura. Plasmapheresis is performed daily for about a week in most instances. The cure rate with this therapy approaches 90%. Antibiotics (choice A), immunosuppressive agents (choice B), renal transplant (choice C), and antiviral therapy (choice E) are not the primary modalities used to treat thrombotic thrombocytopenic purpura.

649. **(E)** The recent use of therapeutic apheresis in the treatment of thrombotic thrombocytopenic purpura (TTP) is an encouraging development in medicine. Prior to the use of plasmapheresis about 90% of patients with TTP died acutely. The statistics are now reversed with about 90% of TTP patients surviving if given rapid and appropriate therapeutic apheresis. The other options of 10% (choice A), 25% (choice B), 40% (choice C), and 60% (choice D) are incorrect.

650. **(D)** Icthyosis is a hereditary condition characterized clinically by coarse fish-like scaly skin. The microanatomy demonstrates marked thickening of the stratum corneum. Basal hyperpigmentation (choice A), dermal fibrosis (choice B), perivascular chronic inflammation (choice C), and subepidermal blister formation (choice E) are not the histologic hallmarks of icthyosis.

651. **(A)** Icthyosis is a hereditary condition. The most common form of the disorder in the United States is inherited in an X-linked fashion. The disease is not caused by a hypersensitivity reaction (choice B), bacterial infection (choice C), viral infection (choice D), or a hormonal imbalance (choice E).

652. **(E)** The photograph displays the histology of a basal cell carcinoma. These tumors are slowly growing, appear as flesh- to pearl-colored cutaneous nodules, and arise principally on sun-exposed areas. The histologic pattern is one of infiltrating small dermal clusters of basophilic cells with peripheral basal orientation. Verruca vulgaris (choice A) is a cutaneous viral disorder with prominent papillomatosis. Molluscum contagiosum (choice B) is also a viral disorder. Molluscum bodies are the critical histologic finding. Bowen's disease (choice C) is another term used for cutaneous intraepidermal squamous cell carcinoma. An epidermal cyst (choice D) is a benign dermal collection of central keratotic debris with a peripheral cyst wall formed by benign, mature, stratified squamous epithelium.

653. **(C)** Basal cell carcinomas arise from actinically damaged skin. Areas of the body that are rarely exposed to ultraviolet light are unlikely to develop these tumors. Papillomavirus infection (choice A), luminal occlusion (choice B), fungal infection (choice D), and poxvirus infection (choice E) are not significant etiologic factors in the development of basal cell carcinoma.

654. (A) Primary biliary cirrhosis is an autoimmune disorder which occurs most frequently in middle-aged females. Autoantibodies against mitochondria are usually present. The clinical picture is nonspecific early in the disorder. Hyperbilirubinemia, steatorrhea, portal hypertension, and osteomalacia may be seen in the later stages of the disease. Viral infections (choice B), alcohol abuse (choice C), parasitic infections (choice D), and vascular abnormalities (choice E) all may mimic the clinical picture of primary biliary cirrhosis. They are not, however, the usual etiologic agent.

655. (E) In the later stages of primary biliary cirrhosis the serum chemistry studies will usually display a striking elevation of alkaline phosphatase, bilirubin, and cholesterol. This pattern of chemical abnormality suggests that there is intrahepatic obstruction of the biliary tract. It would be very unlikely that these three chemical studies would all be decreased (choice A) in the later stages of primary biliary cirrhosis. Usually these three tests are all elevated strikingly and in tandem with this disorder. An elevation of only one test (choices B and C), or of only two tests (choice D) would be very uncommon.

656. (D) The photograph reveals a poorly differentiated infiltrating ductal mammary adenocarcinoma. A family history of breast carcinoma puts other female relatives at increased statistical risk to develop breast cancer themselves. Early menopause (choice A) decreases the relative risk to develop breast cancer. Asians (choice B) are less likely to develop breast cancer than are Caucasians or blacks. Late menarche (choice C) decreases the relative risk to develop breast cancer. Both early age of first pregnancy and multiparity (choice E) decrease the risk of developing mammary carcinoma.

657. (E) Overexpression of NEU oncogene in invasive breast carcinoma is an adverse prognostic indicator. Breast cancers that are estrogen receptor positive (choice A), well differentiated (choice B), have a low S phase (choice C), and are progesterone receptor positive (choice D) are considered to have more favorable prognostic implications. Size of the primary breast carcinoma and the status of the axillary lymph nodes are also major factors that influence the prognosis of invasive ductal breast adenocarcinoma.

658. (D) Barrett's esophagitis is a metaplastic alteration of the lower esophagus in response to chronic acid reflux. The photograph displays the specialized type of Barrett's esophagitis, complete with numerous goblet mucous cells. Plummer–Vinson syndrome (choice A) describes the formation of a luminal web in the upper third of the esophagus. The microanatomy would display squamous epithelium, not metaplastic glandular epithelium. A photograph of *Candida* esophagitis (choice B) would not contain glandular epithelium. Squamous epithelium, yeast, and pseudohyphae would be expected instead. Granulomatous esophagitis (choice C) and viral esophagitis (choice E) would not be characterized by metaplastic glandular epithelium. Giant cells or inclusion bodies may be seen depending on the etiology.

659. (D) Long-standing Barrett's metaplasia substantially increases the risk of developing adenocarcinoma in the lower esophagus. Most lesions pass through a dysplasia stage from which the carcinoma later arises. Frequent endoscopic monitoring of a Barrett's esophagus may identify these worrisome dysplastic changes early enough to allow prophylactic surgical therapy. The presence of Barrett's metaplasia of the esophagus does not predispose an individual to an increased risk of squamous cell carcinoma (choice A), fungal septicemia (choice B), viral encephalitis (choice C), or esophageal varices (choice E).

660. (E) Nephroblastoma (Wilms' tumor) is a childhood malignant neoplasm composed of primitive renal blastoma. Microscopically, there is usually a mixture of immature tubular, stromal, and glomerular elements. Malignant gland-forming epithelium with glycogen-containing clear cytoplasm and abundant vascularity (choice A) is an accurate description of a renal cell carcinoma. This is an adult neoplasm. An angiosarcoma is composed of malignant endothelial cells forming abortive vascular structures (choice B). Malignant osteoid or cartilage (choice C) would describe an osteosarcoma or a chondrosarcoma, respectively. Malignant adrenal neural crest cells (choice D) would describe a neuroblastoma.

661. (E) Nephroblastoma usually harbors a partial deletion of chromosome 11. A third copy of a chromosome is termed trisomy (choice A). Down syndrome, trisomy 21, is an example of this type of chromosomal abnormality. Trisomy is not routinely seen with Wilms' tumor. Translocations (choice B) may be reciprocal or Robertsonian. Neither type is associated with nephroblastoma. Ring formation (choice C) describes the fusion of the telomeric portions of the chromosome into a ring-shaped structure. It is not usually seen with Wilms' tumor. Inversion (choice D) involves the reordering of gene sequences within the same chromosome. This alteration is not seen with nephroblastoma.

662. (A) With appropriate combined therapy the five-year survival rate for nephroblastoma is about 90%. Lack of therapy, inadequate therapy, and the anaplastic variant of this tumor may imply a negative outcome. The other numerical choices 60% (choice B), 40% (choice C), 20% (choice D), and 5% (choice E) are incorrect.

663. (A) Hemophilia A is a genetic disorder characterized by very low levels of factor VIII, elevated partial thromboplastin time, normal prothrombin time, normal platelet aggregation with ristocetin, and spontaneous hemorrhages into joints, soft tissues, and mucosal surfaces. Hemophilia B (choice B) is a hereditary coagulopathy due to a very low level of factor IX. Von Willebrand's disease (choice C) is characterized by a mild hereditary bleeding diathesis and abnormal platelet aggregation with ristocetin. Christmas disease (choice D) is an alternative term for hemophilia B. Rosenthal's syndrome (choice E) defines a deficiency of factor XI.

664. (A) Hemophilia A is an X-linked recessive disorder. This mode of inheritance means that the disorder is only fully expressed in males and that females may be unaffected carriers of the trait. Hemophilia A is not usually inherited in an X-linked dominant (choice B), autosomal recessive (choice C), autosomal dominant (choice D), or autosomal codominant (choice E) manner.

665. (D) Multiple myeloma is a disease of the elderly classically characterized by numerous lytic bony areas containing atypical plasma cells. The neoplastic plasma cells may secrete a monoclonal paraprotein which can be detected in the patient's serum or urine. The presence of a paraprotein usually results in an elevated total protein and low serum albumin. Metastatic melanoma (choice A) would demonstrate atypical melanocytes on fine needle biopsy, not plasma cells. The total protein is usually low, not elevated. Mononucleosis (choice B) is a viral disorder of young adults characterized by sore throat, lymphadenopathy, and fever. There are no bony lytic lesions with mononucleosis. Metastatic adenocarcinoma (choice C) would display atypical glandular epithelial cells on fine needle biopsy. The total protein is usually low, not elevated. Malignant lymphoma (choice E) would demonstrate atypical lymphoid cells if examined by fine needle aspiration. The total protein is usually decreased.

666. (D) The neoplastic clones of plasma cells usually secrete a monoclonal paraprotein that can be detected by laboratory methods in the serum, urine, or both. Bisalbuminemia (choice A) is a rare hereditary condition characterized by a biclonal albumin band on serum protein electrophoresis. It is a laboratory anomaly in an otherwise healthy individual. The presence of the myeloma paraprotein usually produces hypergammaglobulinemia, rather than hypogammaglobulinemia (choice B). The myeloma paraprotein results in a monoclonal hypergammaglobulinemia, rather than a polyclonal hypergammaglobulinemia (choice C). The alpha fractions (choice E) are usually normal or increased with multiple myeloma.

667. (C) Forty to 50 years ago diethylstilbestrol was actively used to prevent miscarriages. Surviving female fetuses exposed to this agent later demonstrated an increased incidence of vaginal adenosis. The development of vaginal adenosis is not known to be associated with rubella virus (choice A), radiation (choice B), aspirin ingestion (choice D), or administration of methotrexate (choice E).

668. (B) The most serious long-term consequence of vaginal adenosis is the increased risk to develop clear cell adenocarcinoma. Vaginal adenosis does not significantly predispose to the development of endometrial adenocarcinoma (choice A), vaginal sarcoma (choice C), uterine leiomyomas (choice D), or serous papillary carcinoma (choice E).

669. (E) The clinical scenario describes a classic example of Duchenne muscular dystrophy. The weakness is symmetric and most often begins at the pelvic girdle. Fatty pseudohypertrophy with alternating muscle fiber atrophy and hypertrophy typify the histologic changes. Many patients die before their twenties. The other diagnostic options, poliomyelitis (choice A), trichinosis (choice B), cerebral palsy (choice C), and myositis ossificans (choice D), do not fit the given clinical vignette.

670. (A) Muscular dystrophy is a hereditary disorder. In most instances there is a deletion of a portion of the X chromosome which codes for the dystrophin muscle protein. Muscular dystrophy is not caused by viruses (choice B), *Trichinella spiralis* infestation (choice C), a neoplastic process (choice D), or secondary to neonatal trauma (choice E).

671. (A) Healthy skeletal muscle cells contain a number of enzymes which are required for routine physiologic functions. When these cells are damaged, enzymes may leak out into the blood and be used clinically as a marker for muscle cell death. Muscular dystrophy typically displays an elevation of creatine kinase, aldolase, and lactate dehydrogenase. The normal phenotype is present as choice B. Decreases in the muscular enzymes (choice C) would not be expected with muscular dystrophy. Other options (choices D and E) offered only one of the three enzymes elevated. Normally, dying skeletal muscle cells release all three diagnostic enzymes.

672. (E) Right-sided colon cancers typically produce a large ulcerative lesion. Blood loss from the tumor can be detected in the feces as a positive test for occult blood. If sufficient blood is lost, over time the patient will become anemic. The serum CEA is usually elevated as a marker of tumor dedifferentiation back towards a more primitive fetal antigen-synthesizing tissue. A normal CEA, negative occult blood, and normal hemoglobin (choice A) is a triplet of normal laboratory studies. In choice B there is only one item (positive occult blood) of the three that is usually seen with right-sided colon cancers. The elevated hemoglobin in choice C is highly unlikely in this clinical vignette. The other two items are normal. In choice D there is only one item (elevated CEA) of the three that is usually seen with right-sided colonic carcinomas.

673. (E) After metastasizing first to the pericolonic lymph nodes, colonic tumor cells usually are then drained by the mesenteric lymphatics into the blood vessels, the portal vein, and finally, into the liver. The liver is the most common distant site of metastatic right-sided colon carcinoma. The brain (choice A), lung (choice B), adrenal (choice C), and appendix (choice D) are all less likely sites of initial distant tumor spread.

REFERENCES

Chandrasoma P, Taylor CR. *Concise Pathology*, 3rd edition. Appleton and Lange, 1998.

Rubin F, Farber JL. *Pathology*, 2nd edition. JB Lippincott, 1994

Subspecialty List: Pathology

547. Endocrine system
548. Immunopathology
549. Nervous system
550. Inflammation
551. Non-genetic syndromes
552. Immunopathology
553. Genetic or metabolic syndromes
554. Cell injury and response
555. Non-genetic syndromes
556. Endocrine system
557. Non-genetic syndromes
558. Alimentary system
559. Alimentary system
560. Neoplasia
561. Abnormal growth and development
562. Blood and lymphatic system
563. Immunopathology
564. Alimentary system
565. Kidney and urinary system
566. Cardiovascular system
567. Respiratory system
568. Alimentary system
569. Blood and lymphatic system
570. Neoplasia
571. Abnormal growth and development
572. Neoplasia
573. Neoplasia
574. Inflammation
575. Infectious diseases
576. Nervous system
577. Cardiovascular system
578. Breast pathology
579. Alimentary system
580. Abnormal growth and development
581. Neoplasia
582. Respiratory system
583. Alimentary system
584. Genetic or metabolic syndromes
585. Cardiovascular system
586. Cardiovascular system
587. Respiratory system
588. Infectious diseases
589. Inflammation
590. Alimentary system
591. Cardiovascular system
592. Genetic or metabolic syndromes
593. Alimentary system
594. Genital system
595. Breast pathology
596. Cardiovascular pathology
597. Environmental pathology
598. Neoplasia
599. Alimentary system
600. Respiratory system
601. Neoplasia
602. Infectious diseases
603. Cell injury and response
604. Cell injury and response
605. Immunopathology
606. Cell injury and response
607. Endocrine system
608. Blood and lymphatic system
609. Cell injury and response
610. Cardiovascular system
611. Genetic or metabolic syndromes
612. Hemostasis and coagulation
613. Inflammation
614. Neoplasia
615. Genetic or metabolic syndromes
616. Infectious diseases
617. Kidney and urinary system
618. Genetic or metabolic syndromes
619. Environmental pathology
620. Environmental pathology
621. Non-genetic syndromes
622. Non-genetic syndromes

623. Environmental pathology
624. Neoplasia
625. Genital system
626. Genital system
627. Genital system
628. Immunopathology
629. Infectious diseases
630. Genital system
631. Genetic or metabolic syndromes
632. Blood and lymphatic system
633. Breast pathology
634. Respiratory system
635. Miscellaneous
636. Kidney and urinary system
637. Alimentary system
638. Environmental pathology
639. Infectious diseases
640. Genetic or metabolic syndromes
641. Infectious diseases
642. Kidney and urinary system
643. Respiratory system
644. Genital system
645. Infectious diseases
646. Endocrine system
647. Hemostasis and coagulation
648. Hemostasis and coagulation
649. Hemostasis and coagulation
650. Cutaneous pathology
651. Cutaneous pathology
652. Cutaneous pathology
653. Cutaneous pathology
654. Alimentary system
655. Alimentary system
656. Breast pathology
657. Breast pathology
658. Alimentary system
659. Alimentary system
660. Kidney and urinary system
661. Kidney and urinary system
662. Kidney and urinary system
663. Genetic or metabolic syndromes
664. Genetic or metabolic syndromes
665. Blood and lymphatic system
666. Blood and lymphatic system
667. Abnormal growth and development
668. Abnormal growth and development
669. Muscular system
670. Muscular system
671. Muscular system
672. Neoplasia
673. Neoplasia

CHAPTER 6

Pharmacology

Questions

Russell K. Yamazaki, PhD

DIRECTIONS: (Questions 674 through 799): Each of the numbered items or incomplete statements in this section is followed by answers or by completions of the statement. Select the ONE lettered answer or completion that is BEST in each case.

674. The following are pharmacokinetic data for the drug propranolol: clearance, 50 L/hr in a 70 kg adult; effective plasma concentration, 20 ng/ml; oral availability (= 100 × fractional absorption), 25%. Calculate the oral maintenance dosing rate for propranolol in a 70-kg person.

(A) 10 μg/hr
(B) 200 μg/hr
(C) 1 mg/hr
(D) 4 mg/hr
(E) 50 mg/hr

675. In the operating room, a patient has been anesthetized with an inhalational anesthetic and has just been given a single intravenous dose of succinylcholine. Power has now been lost in the operating room, and the surgeon wishes to stop the procedure. What pharmacological treatment will reverse the acute actions of succinylcholine?

(A) pralidoxime
(B) physostigmine
(C) bethanechol
(D) atracurium
(E) none of the above

676. A teenage male patient has been brought to the emergency room in an agitated state. He must be restrained from leaving because he believes that he can fly and wants to jump off the roof. His friend confides that the patient has consumed an extract made from some weeds. The patient appears to have an elevated body temperature but is not perspiring. His pupils are dilated, and his heart rate is elevated. Although the diagnosis is necessarily tentative, the immediate treatment of choice for the patient if his condition appears to be worsening is

(A) methscopolamine
(B) physostigmine
(C) carbachol
(D) neostigmine
(E) ipratropium

677. Circulating levels of norepinephrine correlate with the overall activity of the sympathetic nervous system. For which of the following agents would you expect the circulating levels of norepinephrine to be depressed with administration?

(A) prazosin
(B) phenoxybenzamine
(C) clonidine
(D) phentolamine
(E) amphetamine

Patient A.W. is a 73-year-old female with complaints of mental confusion, exercise fatigue, and breathlessness. Examination reveals swollen ankles, pulmonary rales, and dyspnea upon reclining. This patient is the subject for the next three questions.

678. Treatment of this patient with an ACE inhibitor such as captopril may be beneficial because ACE inhibitors

(A) increase efficiency of oxygen extraction by skeletal and cardiac muscle
(B) decrease both ventricular preload and afterload
(C) produce a positive inotropic effect and negative chronotropic effect
(D) promote ventricular remodeling and compensatory enlargement
(E) increase coronary perfusion

679. If ACE inhibitor treatment alone does not produce the desired therapeutic response, addition of an agent such as hydrochlorothiazide to the regimen may be effective. The primary beneficial action of treatment of such patients with hydrochlorothiazide is a result of

(A) promotion of large artery dilation and subsequent reduction in ventricular afterload
(B) reduction in thirst and subsequent decrease in fluid volume
(C) inhibition of uptake of dietary sodium with subsequent reduction in fluid volume
(D) decrease in cardiac stroke volume with subsequent reduction in ventricular afterload
(E) diuresis with subsequent decrease in sodium and fluid retention

680. Use of a cardiac glycoside such as digoxin in addition to captopril and hydrochlorothiazide may be warranted in this patient. Periodic monitoring of patients being treated with this three-drug combination is necessary because of the serious hazard of primary cardiac arrhythmias caused by

(A) hypocalcemia produced by increased potassium delivery to the distal convoluted tubules
(B) hypokalemia produced by increased sodium delivery to the collecting ducts
(C) toxic accumulation of digoxin, produced by diuretic inhibition of renal excretion of the glycoside
(D) decreased plasma oncotic pressure produced by diuretic-induced proteinuria
(E) desensitization of cardiac beta adrenoceptors produced by decreased bradykinin levels

681. Which of the following descriptions correctly describes the molecular mechanism underlying the therapeutic actions of the statins, such as simvastatin?

(A) inhibition of hepatic VLDL secretion resulting in less production of IDL and LDL
(B) inhibition of hepatic cholesterol synthesis resulting in increased expression of LDL receptor
(C) inhibition of lecithin:cholesterol acyltransferase activity resulting in decreased conversion of IDL to LDL
(D) inhibition of hepatic production of apoCIII resulting in loss of inhibition of lipoprotein lipase activity
(E) increased fecal excretion of bile acid resulting in increased conversion of cholesterol to bile acid

682. Multidrug resistance is a major cause of treatment failure in cancer chemotherapy. One mechanism for multidrug resistance (and therefore a target for pharmacological intervention) to the cancer chemotherapeutic agents doxorubicin, vincristine, paclitaxel (taxol) and dactinomycin (actinomycin D) is produced when tumor cells have

(A) increased activity of DNA repair pathways
(B) decreased doubling time so that a smaller percentage of cells are caught in S phase

(C) increased expression of an outward transport system that removes drug from cells
(D) increased activity of dihydrofolate reductase
(E) reduced activity of deoxycytidine kinase

683. The controlling factor for the time to onset of action of the oral anticoagulant warfarin is

(A) half-life for dissociation of warfarin from plasma protein binding sites
(B) elimination half-life for vitamin K
(C) elimination half-life of warfarin
(D) half-life for circulating antithrombin
(E) half-lives for circulating Gla-containing coagulation factors

684. A 37-year-old African-American male patient with a known allergy to sulfonamides was diagnosed with open-angle glaucoma. After treatment was initiated with topical timolol, he experienced difficulty in breathing and went to the hospital emergency room. He was treated with inhalational albuterol and released. What was the likely mechanism by which timolol caused this episode?

(A) hemolysis caused by hereditary glucose-6-phosphate dehydrogenase deficiency
(B) bronchoconstriction resulting from blockade of β adrenoceptors
(C) drug allergy to timolol
(D) induction of erythrocyte sickling
(E) idiosyncratic response to timolol

• **685.** A patient suffers from partial seizures that have been well controlled by treatment with a carbamazepine regimen. Which of the following new conditions is most likely to cause carbamazepine-induced diplopia and ataxia if the regular regimen is not altered?

(A) hepatitis
(B) coadministration of phenobarbital
(C) initiation of smoking
(D) diuresis with chlorothiazide
(E) coadministration of probenecid

Questions 686 through 688

Figure 6–1 shows plasma concentrations of drug W in a patient following intravenous injection of a single dose of 100 mg of the drug, an agent eliminated from the body by renal excretion. At hour 12, the patient was treated with sodium bicarbonate.

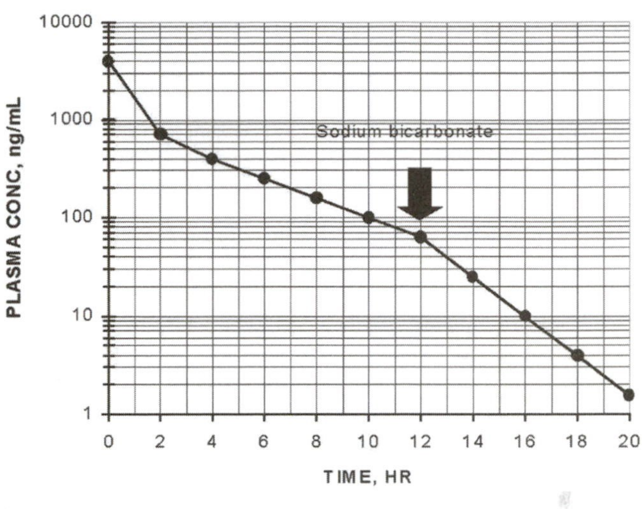

Figure 6–1

686. Using the data before hour 12, the calculated volume of distribution (V_d) for drug W is

(A) 1 liter
(B) 10 liters
(C) 25 liters
(D) 50 liters
(E) 100 liters

687. Using the data before hour 12, the half-life ($t_{1/2}$) for drug W is

(A) 0.5 hr
(B) 1 hr
(C) 3 hr
(D) 7 hr
(E) 10 hr

688. The change in elimination rate after hour 12 when sodium bicarbonate was administered is expected if drug W is which of the following chemical types?

(A) strong base
(B) weak base
(C) non-electrolyte
(D) weak acid
(E) strong acid

689. Patient T.W. has suffered an acute myocardial infarction. After initial treatment, the patient is found to be suffering from pronounced hypotension and reduction of cardiac function with an elevated left ventricular filling pressure. The pharmacological treatment of choice for this condition in this patient is

(A) norepinephrine
(B) epinephrine
(C) atropine
(D) dobutamine
(E) isoproterenol

690. A rational approach for the prevention of prostate cancer would involve the use of which of the following agents?

(A) finasteride
(B) leuprolide
(C) flutamide
(D) ketoconazole
(E) diethylstilbestrol

Questions 691 through 694

Consider a hypothetical synapse which uses the neurotransmitter Q. Q is removed from the synaptic cleft by uptake into the presynaptic terminal. The curve in Figure 6–2 labeled Std shows the relationship between externally applied concentrations of Q (which can enter the synaptic cleft by diffusion) and the biological response.

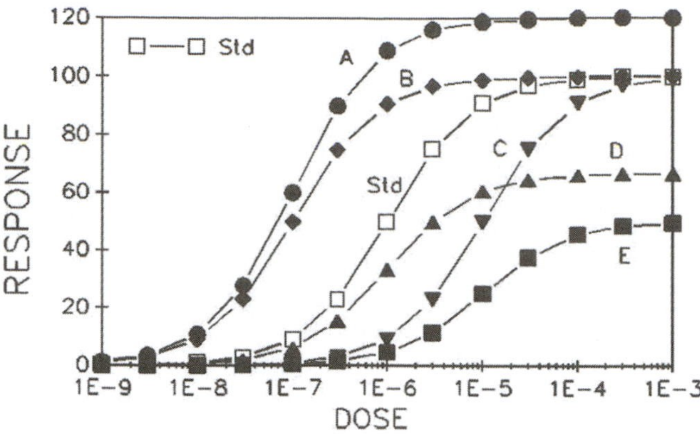

Figure 6–2

691. In this synaptic system, which is the dose-response curve expected for external additions of Q in the presence of a competitive antagonist added at nine times the antagonist's K_i concentration?

(A) curve A
(B) curve B
(C) curve C
(D) curve D
(E) curve E

692. In this synaptic system, which is the dose-response curve expected for external additions of Q in the presence of a pure non-competitive antagonist added at a concentration sufficient to inactivate 33% of the receptors for Q?

(A) curve A
(B) curve B
(C) curve C
(D) curve D
(E) curve E

693. In this synaptic system, which is the dose-response curve expected for external additions of Q in the presence of an inhibitor of the presynaptic uptake of Q?

(A) curve A
(B) curve B
(C) curve C
(D) curve D
(E) curve E

694. In this synaptic system, which is the dose-response curve for additions of R, which is an agonist for the Q receptor with 50% the efficacy of that for Q? Assume that Q is not present.

(A) curve A
(B) curve B
(C) curve C
(D) curve D
(E) curve E

695. A patient who had undergone a liver transplant was found to be suffering from nephrotoxicity without any signs of bone marrow depression. This situation might arise from toxicity from which of the following agents?

(A) cyclosporine
(B) prednisone
(C) muromonab-CD3 monoclonal antibody
(D) azathioprine
(E) cyclophosphamide

696. Cultures from a Caucasian female patient complaining of vaginitis showed the presence of *Trichomonas vaginitis.* Treatment was initiated with this agent. The patient then suffered embarrassment when she became ill and vomited at a wedding reception where champagne was served. This description best fits which agent?

(A) methimazole
(B) metronidazole
(C) mebendazole
(D) primaquine
(E) trimethoprim

697. Patient P.W. suffers from seasonal rhinitis and takes an antihistamine for symptomatic relief. He contracts a systemic fungal infection and is given appropriate treatment. After initiating antifungal therapy, he suffers a serious cardiac arrhythmia that is attributable to the use of terfenadine in conjunction with this antifungal agent.

(A) griseofulvin
(B) amphotericin B
(C) ketoconazole
(D) chloramphenicol
(E) nystatin

698. Because this anti–herpesvirus agent uses viral thymidine kinase as part of its activation pathway, resistance is associated with thymidine-kinase deficient strains of herpesvirus.

(A) foscarnet
(B) zidovudine
(C) amantadine
(D) saquinavir
(E) acyclovir

699. Resistance to this agent used in *Escherichia coli* urinary tract infections can arise through bacterial expression of altered forms of dihydrofolate reductase acquired by spontaneous mutation or plasmid transfer.

(A) methotrexate
(B) trimethoprim
(C) amoxicillin
(D) imipenem
(E) sulfamethoxazole

700. Because this antitubercular agent is an inducer of hepatic cytochrome P450, dosing regimens for oral anticoagulants must be adjusted when it is administered with them.

(A) rifampin
(B) isoniazid
(C) ethambutol
(D) streptomycin
(E) sulfisoxazole

701. A 54-year-old male being treated for hypertension with this agent responded well initially but complained of dizziness upon standing. Subsequently when he was treated for depression with a tricyclic antidepressant, this antihypertensive agent lost its effectiveness.

(A) lisinopril
(B) prazosin
(C) guanethidine
(D) hydralazine
(E) methyldopa

702. A 47-year-old male being treated for hypertension with this agent responded well with minimal adverse effects (dry mouth and some sedation). However, when the patient neglected to take his medication during a vacation, a severe headache and tachycardia led him to seek treatment at a hospital emergency room where he was found to be in hypertensive crisis.

(A) prazosin
(B) captopril
(C) clonidine
(D) hydralazine
(E) chlorothiazide

703. A 44-year-old female being treated for hypertension with this agent complained of arthralgia and myalgia along with skin rashes and fever. The lupus-like syndrome disappeared upon discontinuance of this agent.

(A) hydralazine
(B) captopril
(C) clonidine
(D) propranolol
(E) prazosin

704. A 34-year-old male flutist was treated for hypertension with this agent. Although his blood pressure was reduced, he complained that he was now unable to play his instrument because of a dry cough.

(A) hydralazine
(B) captopril
(C) clonidine
(D) propranolol
(E) prazosin

705. This cancer chemotherapeutic agent requires metabolism by cytochrome P450 for formation of the active alkylating species.

(A) bleomycin
(B) 5-fluorouracil
(C) paclitaxel
(D) cisplatin
(E) cyclophosphamide

706. This agent used in treating testicular cancer requires hydration and diuresis to prevent nephrotoxicity associated with the agent.

(A) bleomycin
(B) 5-fluorouracil
(C) paclitaxel
(D) cisplatin
(E) cyclophosphamide

707. This chemotherapeutic agent's mechanism of action involves inhibition of thymidylate synthase and incorporation into RNA.

(A) bleomycin
(B) 5-fluorouracil
(C) paclitaxel
(D) cisplatin
(E) cyclophosphamide

708. This chemotherapeutic agent's mechanism of action involves inhibition of topoisomerase II, resulting in DNA strand breakage.

(A) bleomycin
(B) 5-fluorouracil
(C) paclitaxel
(D) etoposide
(E) cyclophosphamide

709. When a steady state concentration of drug is present in the systemic circulation and equilibration between the systemic circulation and tissue compartments has been achieved, which of these fluid compartments will have the largest total fluid:blood concentration ratio for the weak acid sulfadiazine (pKa = 6.5).

(A) alkalinized urine at pH 8.0
(B) acidified urine at pH 5.0
(C) breast milk at pH 6.4
(D) jejunum-ileum contents at pH 7.6
(E) stomach contents at pH 2.0

710. When a steady state concentration of drug is present in the systemic circulation and equilibration between the systemic circulation and tissue compartments has been achieved, which of these fluid compartments will have the largest total fluid:blood concentration ratio for the weak base pyrimethamine (pKa = 7.0).

(A) alkalinized urine at pH 8.0
(B) acidified urine at pH 5.0
(C) breast milk at pH 6.4
(D) jejunum-ileum contents at pH 7.6
(E) stomach contents at pH 2.0

711. Which of the following is a correct statement regarding vasopressin (antidiuretic hormone, ADH) and its actions?

(A) Thiazide diuretics are useful in treating nephrogenic (vasopressin-resistant) diabetes insipidus.
(B) Ethanol stimulates vasopressin secretion.
(C) Non-steroidal anti-inflammatory agents (NSAIDs) inhibit the antidiuretic response to vasopressin.
(D) Hyperosmolality inhibits vasopressin secretion.
(E) Vasopressin relaxes vascular smooth muscle.

712. Which of the following matches a drug with its correct action that is used clinically to prevent or relieve anginal pain?

(A) isoproterenol and decreased myocardial contractile force
(B) nitroglycerin and increased cardiac preload
(C) thiosulfate and increased extraction of oxygen from blood
(D) propranolol and decreased heart rate
(E) nifedipine and decreased venous return to the heart

713. Which of the following is a predictable adverse effect of treatment with a phenothiazine such as chlorpromazine?

(A) nausea and vomiting
(B) Tourette's syndrome
(C) excessive salivation
(D) hyperprolactinemia
(E) diarrhea

714. Which of the following is a correct pharmacokinetic generalization?

(A) The intravenous route of administration has more potential for first pass metabolism than the oral route.
(B) After intravenous administration, highly lipid-soluble drugs will distribute to adipose tissue before brain and skeletal muscle.
(C) Stereoisomers of drugs differ in their rates of intestinal absorption.
(D) For drugs highly bound to serum proteins, pharmacological activity correlates best with the total drug rather than the free drug concentration.
(E) A volume of distribution much larger than 1 liter/kg body weight is an indication that the drug will be cleared by hepatic metabolism.

715. Which of the following is a predictable side effect of treatment with a tricyclic antidepressant such as imipramine?

(A) decrease in seizure threshold
(B) weight loss
(C) hyperprolactinemia
(D) excessive salivation
(E) hypertension

716. Which of the following is an agent of choice to treat bronchoconstriction in an acute asthma attack?

(A) aminophylline
(B) terbutaline
(C) ipratropium bromide
(D) cromolyn sodium
(E) propranolol

717. Which of these drugs is used in treatment of gouty arthritis to inhibit the formation of uric acid?

(A) allopurinol
(B) sulfinpyrazone
(C) probenecid
(D) colchicine
(E) indomethacin

718. Which of these drugs is used in treatment of an acute attack of gouty arthritis to inhibit migration and motility of granulocytes?

(A) allopurinol
(B) sulfinpyrazone
(C) probenecid
(D) colchicine
(E) indomethacin

719. H_1 receptor antagonists are used to treat which of the following conditions?

(A) peptic ulcer
(B) allergic rhinitis
(C) narcolepsy
(D) bronchial asthma
(E) diabetes insipidus

720. Following prostate surgery it is discovered that motor nerve damage to the urinary bladder has resulted in a decreased ability to empty the bladder. Which of the following drugs would most effectively promote improved bladder function?

(A) pirenzepine
(B) physostigmine
(C) atropine
(D) bethanechol
(E) phenylephrine

721. The drug labetalol has been useful in some patients with hypertension because it

(A) is a pure α_1-adrenoceptor agonist
(B) blocks α_1 as well as β adrenoceptors
(C) is an α_2-specific adrenoceptor agonist
(D) selectively blocks only the β_2 adrenoceptors of vascular muscle
(E) blocks only the β adrenoceptors of the heart

722. The β-adrenoceptor antagonist atenolol has a pA_2 value of 7.0 for cardiac muscle β adrenoceptors and a pA_2 value of 5.3 for lung β-adrenoceptors. We can therefore conclude that atenolol

(A) is more potent in blocking the heart than lung beta adrenoceptors.
(B) is more potent in the lung than the heart
(C) has a greater efficacy in the heart than the lung
(D) has greater efficacy in the lung than the heart
(E) is equally potent in the heart and lung

723. In a functional transplanted pancreas, which of the following agents would you expect to cause the greatest increase in the secretion of digestive enzymes?

(A) hexamethonium
(B) physostigmine
(C) botulinum toxin type A (Botox)
(D) phenylephrine
(E) pilocarpine

724. Which of the following agents produces vasodilation by increasing nitric oxide synthesis in endothelial cells?

(A) prazosin
(B) isoproterenol
(C) pilocarpine
(D) diphenhydramine
(E) hexamethonium

725. Lidocaine has the property of

(A) being metabolized in the plasma
(B) producing respiratory depression at elevated blood levels
(C) reducing chloride channel conductance
(D) hyperpolarizing neuronal membranes
(E) blocking conduction in A fibers before C fibers in nerve trunks

726. In a patient with possible narrow angle glaucoma who must have a refracted cycloplegic eye examination for prescribing corrective lenses, which of the following would be the safest agent?

(A) phentolamine
(B) phenylephrine
(C) atropine
(D) tropicamide
(E) loratadine

727. Severe renal damage resulting from oxalate formation is characteristic of intoxication by

(A) methanol
(B) ethanol
(C) isopropanol
(D) methylene chloride
(E) ethylene glycol

728. Which of the following statements correctly associates a psychotherapeutic agent with a demonstrated effect on neurotransmitter mechanisms?

(A) fluoxetine—selective inhibition of presynaptic norepinephrine uptake
(B) tranylcypromine—inhibition of O-methylation of catecholamines
(C) trifluoperazine—competitive antagonism of $GABA_A$ receptors
(D) diazepam—facilitation of GABA-stimulated chloride channel opening
(E) pentobarbital—inhibition of NMDA receptors

729. Which of the following agents is associated with numerous drug–drug interactions because of its inhibition of hepatic cytochrome P450 activity?

(A) cromolyn
(B) phenobarbital
(C) atracurium
(D) cimetidine
(E) diazepam

730. Two male patients of similar ages and body composition were treated first with epinephrine and then with ephedrine. What is the best explanation for the observed differences in heart rate response?

	PATIENT A	PATIENT B
Untreated heart rate	72	78
After epinephrine 0.1 mg IV	130	155
After ephedrine 50 mg IV	120	84

(A) Patient B had been pretreated for two weeks with atropine
(B) Patient B had been pretreated for two weeks with tranylcypromine
(C) Patient B had been pretreated for two weeks with propranolol
(D) Patient B had been pretreated for two weeks with prazosin
(E) Patient B had been pretreated for two weeks with imipramine

731. Compared to the parent drug, glucuronide conjugates are more likely to

(A) easily diffuse across the placenta
(B) be poorly reabsorbed into the circulation from the renal tubular urine
(C) have higher oil:water partition coefficients
(D) penetrate the blood–brain barrier
(E) have a longer half-life

732. Propofol has a brief duration of action because it is

(A) very hydrophilic
(B) rapidly distributed from the brain to other tissues
(C) metabolized rapidly in the blood
(D) actively transported out of the choroid plexus
(E) eliminated by active tubular renal secretion

733. Ketamine is characterized by which of the following pharmacologic effects?

(A) depression of blood pressure and heart rate in a dose-dependent fashion
(B) lack of analgesic action unless consciousness is lost
(C) association with disagreeable dreams during and after recovery
(D) production of excellent skeletal muscle relaxation
(E) moderately high risk of bronchospasm

734. The most rapid onset of action of general inhalational anesthetics correlates with the smallest value for the

(A) oil:gas partition coefficient
(B) onset of hepatic metabolism
(C) organ system distribution from the blood
(D) blood:gas partition coefficient
(E) minimum alveolar concentration (MAC)

735. The MAC for which of the following inhalational general anesthetic agents exceeds normal atmospheric pressure?

(A) enflurane
(B) isoflurane
(C) halothane
(D) sevoflurane
(E) nitrous oxide

736. The agent of choice for chronic treatment of simple hypothyroidism (myxedema) is

(A) reverse T_3
(B) desiccated thyroid
(C) levothyroxine (T_4)
(D) liothyronine (T_3)
(E) potassium iodide

737. Which of the following agents is a rational choice for treatment of populations before and during acute exposure to a radioactive iodine release from a nuclear power plant accident to prevent future thyroid cancer?

(A) propylthiouracil
(B) levothyroxine
(C) propranolol
(D) potassium iodide
(E) desiccated thyroid

738. Patient E.W. is a 24-year-old female who presented with hypertension and hypokalemic metabolic alkalosis. Although these symptoms are normally indicative of hyperaldosteronism, this patient's aldosterone levels were found to be undetectable, and no other mineralocorticoid activity was found. A diagnosis of Liddle's syndrome was made on the basis of the signs and symptoms and a family history. Liddle's syndrome is caused by a genetic defect leading to excess accumulation of the "normal" apical sodium channel in the principal cells of the cortical collecting duct. The result is hyperactivity of the apical sodium channel. Which of the following agents would be the best choice for treatment of the hypertension and hypokalemic metabolic alkalosis in this patient?

(A) amiloride
(B) hydrochlorothiazide
(C) spironolactone
(D) lisinopril
(E) fludrocortisone

739. Which of the following correctly describes the mechanism of action for streptokinase?

(A) combines with plasminogen to form an enzymatically active complex
(B) converts plasmin to plasminogen
(C) provides a template for combination of thrombin and antithrombin III
(D) inhibits platelet cyclo-oxygenase activity
(E) competitively blocks binding of plasminogen to fibrin

740. Patient T.R. is a 17-year-old male who has suffered from tonic–clonic seizures. This condition has been well controlled with a regimen of phenytoin. Which of the following signs or symptoms would be indicative of phenytoin toxicity in this patient?

(A) postural hypotension
(B) hyperprolactinemia
(C) rigidity and tremor
(D) gingival hyperplasia
(E) polydipsia and polyuria

741. An antioxidant agent that is effective in cardioprotection because it is accumulated in lipoprotein particles where it can prevent oxidation of LDL is

(A) vitamin A
(B) β-carotene
(C) vitamin C (ascorbic acid)

(D) vitamin D
(E) vitamin E (α-tocopherol)

742. While metabolism of 5-fluorouracil in the gut and liver normally dictates a parenteral route of administration, inhibition of this enzyme allows oral doses of 5-fluorouracil to be effective in treatment of tumors.

(A) thymidylate kinase
(B) cytochrome P4501A12
(C) xanthine oxidase
(D) dihydrofolate reductase
(E) dihydropyridine dehydrogenase

743. Which of the following is a correct statement regarding the treatment of adverse effects of neuroleptic agents such as haloperidol?

(A) Tardive dyskinesia is best treated with levodopa.
(B) Akathisia is best treated by increasing the dosage of the neuroleptic.
(C) Acute dystonic reactions are best treated with clonidine.
(D) Neuroleptic malignant syndrome is first treated by administering a muscarinic agonist such as pilocarpine.
(E) Parkinsonian syndrome is best treated with anticholinergic agents such as benztropine.

744. Patient E.G. has bacterial meningitis and is being treated with a β-lactam antimicrobial agent cleared by both hepatic metabolism and renal excretion of the parent drug. The volume of distribution is 10 L and the half-life for elimination is seven hours in this patient. If the renal contribution to the plasma clearance of the drug is 8.5 mL/min, what percentage of drug elimination can be attributed to the metabolism?

(A) 10%
(B) 25%
(C) 50%
(D) 75%
(E) 90%

745. Normal oral therapeutic doses of nitrendipine are essentially completely absorbed from the digestive tract. However, the drug exhibits a bioavailability of only 10% because of first pass metabolism in the portal circulation. If hepatic blood flow has a value of 1500 mL/min, what is the hepatic clearance for timolol?

(A) 150 mL/min
(B) 375 mL/min
(C) 750 mL/min
(D) 1110 mL/min
(E) 1350 mL/min

746. The target therapeutic plasma steady state concentration for drug Z is 500 μg/mL. When an intravenous loading dose was administered to patient F.P. followed by the "standard" intravenous maintenance dosing rate of 30 mg/hr, a plasma steady state level of 300 μg/mL for drug Z was obtained, too low to provide adequate therapy. Starting at the plasma concentration of 300 μg/mL, which of the following strategies will most rapidly and safely achieve (without exceeding) the target therapeutic steady state plasma concentration, and then maintain a plasma level of 500 μg/mL in this patient?

(A) Give 20% of the loading dose as an IV bolus and then maintain with 80 mg/hr.
(B) Give 30% of the loading dose as an IV bolus and then maintain with 30 mg/hr.
(C) Give 40% of the loading dose as an IV bolus and then maintain with 50 mg/hr.
(D) Give 60% of the loading dose as an IV bolus and then maintain with 30 mg/hr.
(E) Give 40% of the loading dose as an IV bolus and then maintain with 30 mg/hr.

747. The rate of urinary excretion of p-aminohippuric acid, an organic acid, is increased with which of the following treatments?

(A) aspirin in doses used to treat a headache
(B) sodium bicarbonate administration
(C) ammonium chloride administration
(D) probenecid administration
(E) inulin administration

748. Drug X is converted to a single inactive metabolite by a cytochrome P450-catalyzed biotransformation reaction. Cimetidine inhibits this particular P450 isoform. If cimetidine and drug X are administered simultaneously, cimetidine will

(A) shift the dose-response curve of drug X to the right
(B) increase the $t_{1/2}$ for plasma levels of drug X
(C) increase the systemic clearance of drug X
(D) decrease the volume of distribution of drug X
(E) decrease the apparent efficacy of drug X

749. Drug Q has an apparent volume of distribution (V_d) of 400 liters in a 70-kg patient. This suggests that the drug

(A) is extensively bound to plasma proteins
(B) distributes similarly throughout the body
(C) is extensively accumulated or bound at sites outside the circulation
(D) exhibits zero order elimination kinetics
(E) is excreted in the kidney by filtration and secretion without being reabsorbed

750. Which of the following vasoactive drugs exerts its effects through inhibition of cyclic GMP phosphodiesterase?

(A) hydralazine
(B) prazosin
(C) nitroprusside
(D) sildenafil
(E) minoxidil

Questions 750 through 754

Patient P.D. is a 47-year-old obese female with type II (non–insulin-dependent) diabetes mellitus. Because her hyperglycemia was not well controlled with diet and oral hypoglycemic agents, she now is required to self-administer insulin injections. At various times, she has complained of deep, sharp pains, most often occurring at night. She has also complained that her ingested food "sits in my stomach and comes back up and burns." She has now come to her physician's office with a fever and external ear infection from which *Pseudomonas aeruginosa* was cultured. Use this patient case for the next four questions.

751. Which of the following insulin regimens would most closely mimic insulin release from a normally functioning pancreas?

(A) pre-meal injections of an intermediate insulin form plus an injection of regular insulin at bedtime
(B) pre-meal injections of regular insulin plus morning and evening injections of a slow insulin form
(C) post-meal injection of a slow insulin form plus a pre-breakfast injection of a slow insulin form
(D) post-meal injection of an intermediate insulin form
(E) pre-breakfast and pre-dinner injections of a slow insulin form plus a pre-snack injection of regular insulin

752. If aspirin and acetaminophen are not effective in providing relief from the nocturnal sharp pains, which of the following would be the best choice for pain relief?

(A) meperidine
(B) morphine
(C) diphenoxylate
(D) codeine
(E) methadone

753. Which of the following agents would be useful in treating this patient's gastrointestinal problem and is also useful as an antiemetic in cancer chemotherapy?

(A) diphenhydramine
(B) metoclopramide
(C) kaolin
(D) scopolamine
(E) neostigmine

754. Which of the following drugs or drug combinations would be the treatment of choice for the *P. aeruginosa* infection in this patient?

(A) tetracycline
(B) chloramphenicol
(C) nafcillin + kanamycin
(D) sulfamethoxazole + trimethoprim
(E) ticarcillin + tobramycin

755. On the basis of their mechanisms of action, which of the following combinations of drugs would you predict would produce a beneficial additive or synergistic effect in therapy when each agent is present at its effective concentration?

(A) chlortetracycline + amoxicillin
(B) lovastatin + cholestyramine
(C) clomiphene + chorionic gonadotropin
(D) succinylcholine + atracurium
(E) pentazocine + morphine

Figure 6–3 shows the quantal population dose-response curves for the therapeutic effect of drug X and drug Y. Both drugs are agonists at the same receptor to produce the therapeutic response, and the maximum responses obtained with each agent are the same. The toxicity curve in the figure shows the superimposed toxic response curves for drug X and drug Y; they are identical in terms of the concentration dependence.

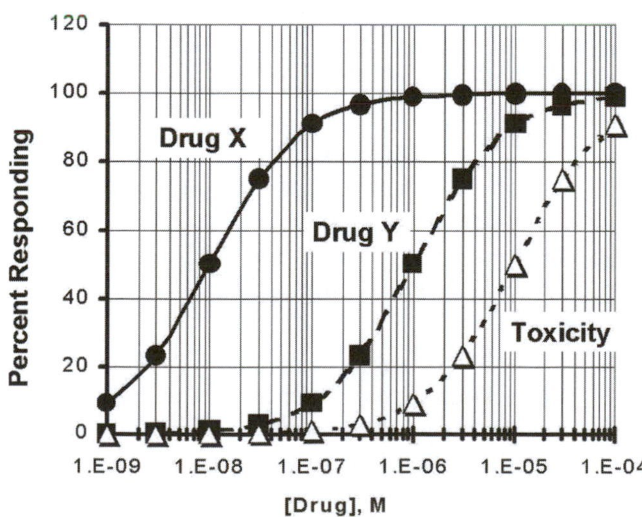

Figure 6–3

756. Which of the following is a correct conclusion that can be deduced from the above data?

(A) Measured in terms of toxicity rather than lethality, drug Y has a larger therapeutic index than drug X.
(B) Toxicity for both drugs is a result of over-stimulation of the same receptor for which they are agonists.
(C) Drug X is more efficacious than drug Y since the midpoint of its response curve lies at a lower concentration value.
(D) Drug X is the better drug to use because, at similar levels of toxicity, a greater response is obtained.
(E) The incidence of adverse effects for both drug X and drug Y should be similar when each is used at its EC_{50} level.

757. Patient B.C. is a 78-year-old male who has been diagnosed with mild hypertension, ankle edema, and mild congestive heart failure. Because of physical problems and lack of suitable transportation, he has great difficulty in making visits to your office. You wish to treat him with a cardiac glycoside and diuresis without hospitalization because he does not have medical insurance. What is the best choice for producing diuresis in this patient?

(A) chlorothiazide
(B) chlorothiazide + ibuprofen
(C) triamterene
(D) hydrochlorothiazide + triamterene
(E) furosemide

758. Figure 6–4 shows an idealized version of measurements of systolic blood pressure (top of bars), mean pressure (filled circle), and diastolic pressure (bottom of bars) in a person. The solid bar at the top of the figure shows the duration for an intravenous infusion of a constant low concentration of drug X. The arrow shows the point at which an intravenous bolus of drug X was administered. Drug X is

(A) phenylephrine
(B) acetylcholine
(C) norepinephrine
(D) amphetamine
(E) epinephrine

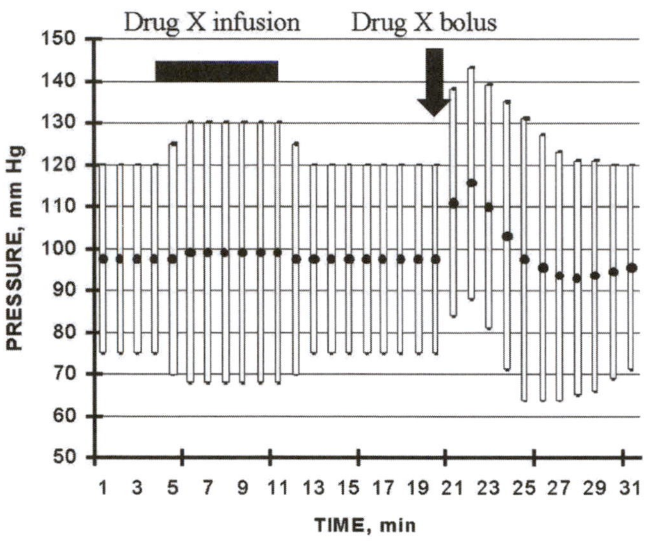

Figure 6–4

759. Patient E.W., an asthmatic 63-year-old female, has been admitted to the hospital suffering from palpitations and syncopal episodes (fainting spells). She is found to be hypotensive and her electrocardiogram indicates the presence of AV nodal re-entrant tachycardia. Which of the following drugs would provide acute treatment of this condition?

(A) digoxin
(B) propranolol
(C) phenylephrine
(D) nitroprusside
(E) norepinephrine

760. Patient H.S. is a 38-year-old male that is being treated for myasthenia gravis with pyridostigmine and propantheline. He is now found to have serious muscle weakness. What is the first course of action in treating this patient?

(A) Administer the daily dose of pyridostigmine on the assumption that he forgot to take his medication.
(B) Administer pralidoxime on the assumption that he inadvertently overdosed himself.
(C) Use the presence or absence of parasympathetic hyperactivity for differential diagnosis.
(D) Administer a test dose of edrophonium.
(E) Administer a test dose of tubocurarine.

761. Assuming the use of equal doses, which of the following routes of drug administration should result in the lowest area under the curve (AUC) for the plasma concentration-time function for the drug diazepam?

(A) oral
(B) intravenous
(C) subcutaneous injection
(D) rectal suppository
(E) sublingual tablet

Questions 762 through 764

PATIENT	BODY WT	V_D	HALF-LIFE	K ELIMINATION
Normal	65 kg	50 L	3.5 hr	0.20/hr
Obese	122 kg	200 L	14 hr	0.05/hr

The above pharmacokinetic data for drug T were determined from analyses of the concentration-time curves for single IV doses of 25 mg in a normal and an obese subject.

762. If the IV loading dose for drug T is 200 mg in the normal subject, what is the IV loading dose that should be used in the obese subject to achieve the same target plasma concentration?

(A) 25 mg
(B) 50 mg

(C) 200 mg
(D) 800 mg
(E) 4000 mg

763. If the IV maintenance infusion rate for the normal patient is 25 mg/hr, what maintenance infusion rate should be used in the obese patient to achieve and maintain the same target plasma concentration?

(A) 25 mg/hr
(B) 50 mg/hr
(C) 200 mg/hr
(D) 800 mg/hr
(E) 4000 mg/hr

764. Based on the pharmacokinetic data given above, which description best fits drug T?

(A) highly polar molecule probably cleared by the kidney
(B) highly polar molecule probably cleared by hepatic metabolism
(C) highly lipophilic molecule probably cleared by the kidney
(D) highly lipophilic molecule probably cleared by hepatic metabolism
(E) negatively charged molecule probably cleared by biliary secretion

765. A patient being continuously infused at 25 mg/min has a plasma steady state level of drug Q (half-life = 6 hr) of 200 mg/mL. Misinterpretation of instructions causes the infusion rate to be increased from 25 mg/min to 50 mg/min. If toxicity usually becomes detectable at a plasma level of 350 mg/mL, how long will it take after the increase in infusion rate for symptoms of toxicity to appear?

(A) 6 hr
(B) 9 hr
(C) 12 hr
(D) 18 hr
(E) 24 hr

766. What is the plasma clearance for a drug that is infused at a rate of 1 mg/min and achieves a steady state plasma concentration of 4 mg/L?

(A) 50 mL/min
(B) 200 mL/min
(C) 250 mL/min
(D) 500 mL/min
(E) 2000 mL/min

767. The neurotoxic actions of botulinum toxin are associated with

(A) nicotinic receptor depolarization blockade
(B) blockade of somatic nerve transmitter exocytosis
(C) inhibition of smooth muscle myosin light chain kinase
(D) irreversible inhibition of cholinesterase
(E) reversal by infusion of heroic doses of choline

768. Which of the following is a rational choice for treatment of open-angle glaucoma, a condition requiring chronic miosis?

(A) scopolamine
(B) pilocarpine
(C) tropicamide
(D) atracurium
(E) hexamethonium

769. Patient C.R. has started taking a medication and now complains about dizziness to the point of almost fainting upon standing up rapidly. This complaint is frequently encountered with therapy using

(A) diazepam
(B) chlorpromazine
(C) lithium carbonate
(D) fluoxetine
(E) chlordiazepoxide

770. Which of the following correctly describes the antiarrhythmic mechanism of action for lidocaine?

(A) blockade of sodium–calcium exchange
(B) blockade of ATP-sensitive potassium channels
(C) blockade of voltage-dependent calcium channels
(D) blockade of β_1 adrenoceptors
(E) blockade of sodium channels

771. Oral anticoagulants such as warfarin exert their anticoagulant effects by

(A) inhibiting calcium binding to coagulation factors
(B) acting as a template for complexing thrombin and antithrombin III
(C) breaking down thrombin
(D) inhibiting hepatic post-translational carboxylation of coagulation factors
(E) forming an active complex with plasminogen

772. Potassium supplementation often is necessary for patients taking

(A) spironolactone
(B) triamterene
(C) furosemide
(D) amiloride
(E) captopril

773. Which of the following disease entities is most likely to respond to the use of the drug ranitidine?

(A) motion sickness
(B) seasonal rhinitis
(C) urticaria
(D) duodenal ulcer
(E) conjunctivitis

774. Which of the following statements is correct regarding therapeutic use of angiotensin-converting enzyme (ACE) inhibitors?

(A) Chronic therapy with ACE inhibitors impairs hemodynamic response to exercise.
(B) Rebound hypertension after abrupt cessation of therapy is a frequent problem.
(C) The use of ACE inhibitors depresses renin activity.
(D) ACE inhibitors are useful in the treatment of essential hypertension.
(E) ACE inhibitors are of little value in therapy of congestive heart failure.

775. Which of the following tricyclic/heterocyclic antidepressants is most selective in blocking reuptake of norepinephrine as compared with serotonin?

(A) doxepin
(B) desipramine
(C) amitriptyline
(D) fluoxetine
(E) trazodone

776. The most common problem associated with use of non-steroidal anti-inflammatory drugs (NSAIDs) such as ibuprofen is

(A) prolonged bleeding time
(B) fluid retention
(C) gastrointestinal complaints
(D) bronchospasm
(E) drowsiness

777. Microcytic hypochromic anemia is best treated with

(A) oral ferric chloride
(B) oral ferrous sulfate
(C) oral vitamin B_{12}
(D) IM vitamin B_{12}
(E) oral folic acid

778. Which of the following insulin preparations is recommended for the provision of basal levels of insulin in multiple dosing regimens because of its long duration of action?

(A) semilente insulin
(B) lente insulin
(C) NPH insulin
(D) regular insulin
(E) ultralente insulin

779. Which of the following items correctly associates the mechanism of action with the corresponding agent used in hyperlipidemia?

(A) nicotinic acid: altered excretion of bile acids
(B) clofibrate: decreased activity of lipoprotein lipase
(C) simvastatin: inhibition of HMG CoA reductase
(D) cholestyramine: increased activity of lipoprotein lipase
(E) gemfibrozil: inhibition of microsomal triglyceride transfer protein

780. Calcium disodium edetate is an antidote for poisoning with

(A) mercury
(B) atropine
(C) arsenic
(D) lead
(E) iron

781. The current drug of choice for treatment of roundworm (*Ascaris*) infections is

(A) mebendazole
(B) ivermectin
(C) praziquantel
(D) niclosamide
(E) diethylcarbamazine

782. Coadministration of which of the following drugs with oral anticoagulants will put the patient at risk for a thromboembolic episode?

(A) rifampin
(B) aspirin
(C) phenylbutazone
(D) cimetidine
(E) ceftriaxone

783. The leukotrienes (LTC_4, LTD_4, and LTE_4)

(A) are long-lasting bronchoconstrictor substances
(B) have their biosynthesis greatly reduced by aspirin
(C) have few cardiovascular effects
(D) are synthesized and stored in platelet granules
(E) are potent chemotactic agents for polymorphonuclear leukocytes

784. Which of the following correctly matches an antiepileptic agent with its mechanism of action?

(A) lamotrigine: activation of potassium channels
(B) carbamazepine: blockade of calcium channels
(C) tiagabine: inhibition of the uptake of gamma-aminobutyric acid
(D) ethosuximide: activation of chloride channels
(E) vigabatrin: competitive blockade of $GABA_A$ receptor

785. The mechanism of action for local anesthetic agents involves

(A) ganglionic blockade
(B) inhibition of pain receptors
(C) inhibition of nerve conduction via blockade of Na^+ channels
(D) inhibition of nerve conduction via blockade of Ca^{2+} channels
(E) hyperpolarization of neurons via enhanced $C1^-$ influx

786. Acute early intoxication with antihistamines (H_1-receptor antagonists) is correctly described as

(A) treatable with histamine therapy
(B) characterized by fever and flushing in adults
(C) causing severe respiratory depression
(D) producing a state similar to atropine poisoning in children
(E) producing joint pain

787. Which of the following describes the mechanism of action for the stimulation of insulin release from pancreatic beta cells by glybenclamide?

(A) inhibition of Na^+-K^+-ATPase
(B) activation of fast sodium channels
(C) inhibition of ATP-sensitive potassium channels
(D) activation of sodium–calcium exchanger
(E) inhibition of voltage-dependent calcium channels

788. Which of the following properties best correlates with the rate of onset of anesthesia for a series of inhalational general anesthetic agents, each administered at its MAC partial pressure?

(A) minimum alveolar concentration for anesthesia (MAC)
(B) blood:oil partition coefficient
(C) anesthetic potency
(D) blood:gas partition coefficient
(E) lipid solubility

789. Which of the following agents is used in thyroid storm because of its ability to inhibit both thyroid iodine organification and peripheral deiodination of thyroxine to triiodothyronine?

(A) reverse T_3
(B) propylthiouracil
(C) radioactive iodine (^{131}I)
(D) propranolol
(E) potassium perchlorate

790. Which of the following drugs is used to promote ovulation through inhibitory actions in the hypothalamus?

(A) flutamide
(B) ethinyl estradiol
(C) norethindrone
(D) clomiphene
(E) diethylstilbestrol

791. A drug with a half-life of 12 hr is administered by continuous intravenous infusion. How long will it take for the drug to reach 94% of its final steady state level?

(A) 18 hr
(B) 24 hr
(C) 30 hr
(D) 40 hr
(E) 48 hr

792. Pharmacologic treatment of severe digitalis intoxication consists of

(A) administration of Fab fragments (digitalis antibodies)
(B) infusion of lidocaine
(C) serum potassium repletion
(D) infusion of atropine
(E) supportive therapy only

793. Which of the following agents may be used as a cardiac stimulant in the treatment of β-blocker overdose?

(A) insulin
(B) glucagon
(C) atrial natriuretic peptide
(D) human growth hormone
(E) epinephrine

794. At a blood alcohol level of 200 mg/dL (0.2%), which of the following correctly describes the systemic elimination process for ethanol?

(A) zero-order elimination via hepatic metabolism
(B) first-order elimination via pulmonary exhalation
(C) first-order elimination via renal excretion
(D) second-order elimination via biliary secretion
(E) constant clearance via liver, kidney, and lungs

795. During the course of an ophthalmological examination, patient W.H. was treated topically with eye drops and later complained that she was blinded by bright light and was unable to read for several days. She probably had been administered

(A) tropicamide
(B) edrophonium
(C) homatropine
(D) phenylephrine
(E) echothiophate

796. The effects of this drug include increased motor activity, loss of appetite, excitement, and, with prolonged administration, stereotyped and psychotic behavior. Frequent repeated use causes a rapid, progressive decline in CNS stimulatory activity. The drug is

(A) amphetamine
(B) cocaine
(C) tetrahydrocannabinol
(D) heroin
(E) ethanol

797. The mechanism of action for the therapeutic effect of saquinavir involves

(A) inhibition of viral reverse transcriptase
(B) incorporation into RNA
(C) inhibition of thymidylate synthase
(D) inhibition of viral DNA polymerase
(E) inhibition of viral protease

798. Patient B.T. is a 58-year-old postmenopausal Caucasian woman (5′10″ tall, 118 lb). She has been diagnosed with osteoporosis after measurements of bone density. She has a strong family history of breast cancer and is concerned about her high risk for this disease. Which of the following agents offers the best single treatment choice in this patient?

(A) parathyroid hormone (PTH)
(B) alendronate
(C) dietary calcium supplementation
(D) conjugated estrogen
(E) raloxifene

799. Which of the following combinations of agents provides the best choice for single, short-term treatment of duodenal ulcer, and that also prevents recurrence of disease?

(A) ranitidine + atropine + omeprazole
(B) cimetidine + colloidal bismuth + magnesium hydroxide
(C) clarithromycin + amoxicillin + omeprazole
(D) misoprostal + ranitidine + sucralfate
(E) ranitidine + colloidal bismuth + diazepam

Answers and Explanations

674. (D) The maintenance dosing rate (D/T) is calculated using the formula (D/T) = (Target) × CL/F where D is the dose administered, T is the time interval between doses, Target is the desired steady state plasma concentration for which we use the effective plasma concentration, CL is the systemic clearance, and F is the fractional absorption. After we multiply the clearance (50 L/hr) times the effective plasma concentration (0.02 mg/L), the resulting product of 1 mg/hr must be divided by the fractional absorption of 0.25, giving a dosing rate of 4 mg/hr. Note that the units for clearance and target concentration must be consistent with respect to volume. The extensive first pass metabolism of propranolol means that we must administer an oral dose four times larger to achieve the same systemic concentration as we would with an intravenous dose.

675. (E) The depolarizing blocking agent succinylcholine acts acutely as a nicotinic receptor agonist at the neuromuscular junction to produce depolarization. Succinylcholine is not hydrolyzed by acetylcholinesterase so that a sustained depolarization that prevents impulse transmission is produced. None of the drugs listed can reverse the acute actions of succinylcholine. Actions of succinylcholine are eventually terminated by diffusion of the drug from the neuromuscular junction and hydrolysis by plasma pseudocholinesterase. With longer exposure (hrs), the characteristics of the blockade with succinylcholine change from depolarization to a situation resembling antagonist blockade where anticholinesterases will alleviate the blockade. Pralidoxime (choice A) is an important agent for reactivation of acetylcholinesterase that has been inhibited by organophosphates, but has no use in this case. The anticholinesterase physostigmine (choice B) will increase acetylcholine concentrations, but will not alleviate the blockade since the junction is already depolarized by the agonist succinylcholine. Bethanechol (choice C) is a muscarinic agonist with negligible action at nicotinic sites. Atracurium (choice D) is a nicotinic receptor antagonist, but will not alleviate the blockade since we simply would be displacing an agonist with an antagonist.

676. (B) The elevated body temperature without perspiration, dilated pupils, and elevated heart rate are indicative of parasympathetic dysfunction such as might occur with atropine intoxication and consequent block of muscarinic receptors. The delusional state indicates central nervous system involvement. Scopolamine and other similar antimuscarinic compounds are found in the seeds and leaves of plants such as Jimson weed (*Datura* species). The treatment consists of inhibition of acetylcholinesterase to increase concentrations of acetylcholine at muscarinic synapses centrally and peripherally. Physostigmine will accomplish this. Methscopolamine (choice A) is a muscarinic antagonist like scopolamine that would exacerbate the toxicity. Carbachol (choice C) is a muscarinic agonist, but does not have central nervous system activity because, as a charged molecule, it does not gain access centrally.

Neostigmine (choice D) is a cholinesterase inhibitor but, unlike physostigmine, it does not readily gain access to the central nervous system because of its charged nature. This difference in distribution between physostigmine and neostigmine is the reason for using neostigmine, but not physostigmine, for treatment of myasthenia gravis where central effects of the drug are undesirable. Ipratropium (choice E) is a muscarinic antagonist administered by inhalation for the acute treatment of asthma.

677. (C) Clonidine, an α_2-adrenoreceptor agonist, acts at the level of the vasopressor centers in the brainstem to decrease sympathetic outflow, thus decreasing norepinephrine release. Prazosin (choice A), an α_1-adrenoreceptor antagonist, lowers blood pressure by direct antagonism of the arteriolar α_1-receptors. The resulting decrease in blood pressure causes a reflex stimulation of the sympathetic nervous system and release of synaptic norepinephrine, some of which escapes neuronal reuptake and elevates circulating levels. Phenoxybenzamine (choice B) is also an α_1-adrenoreceptor antagonist that will increase norepinephrine release. Phentolamine (choice D) is similarly an α_1-adrenoreceptor antagonist that will increase norepinephrine release by the same reflex mechanism. Amphetamine (choice E) is an indirect-acting agent that elevates blood pressure by causing the non-exocytotic release of norepinephrine.

678. (B) The description the patient is indicative of congestive heart failure (CHF). Goals in the treatment of congestive heart failure include decreasing the cardiac workload including preload and afterload, reducing sodium and fluid retention, and increasing myocardial contractility. ACE inhibitors decrease ventricular preload and afterload through multiple actions. These actions originate with the inhibition of angiotensin-converting enzyme (ACE) and the consequent decrease in production of the pressor angiotensin II, along with prolongation of the actions of the vasodilator bradykinin normally degraded by ACE. ACE inhibition also reduces angiotensin II–dependent augmentation of sympathetic nervous system activity. Decreased intrarenal levels of angiotensin II also help correct CHF-induced problems with solute and water resorption in the kidney. Since aldosterone production in the adrenal cortex is also regulated by angiotensin II, the mineralocorticoid actions that promote sodium retention are also lessened. At the level of the heart, the use of ACE inhibitors decreases the local generation of angiotensin II involved in hypertrophy and ventricular remodeling with CHF. All of these factors recommend the use of ACE inhibitors as first line drugs in the treatment of CHF. Choice A is incorrect since efficiency of oxygen extraction by muscle is unaffected by ACE inhibitors. The actions of ACE inhibitors are exerted at the level of hemodynamics. Choice C is incorrect since ACE inhibitors exert no direct effects on inotropicity or chronotropicity. Choice D is incorrect. Use of ACE inhibitors actually prevents ventricular remodeling and compensatory enlargement, making this treatment valuable in CHF. Choice E is incorrect in that ACE inhibitors exert no direct effects on coronary perfusion.

679. (E) The ankle swelling and pulmonary edema seen in the patient are signs of excessive sodium and fluid retention that may be treated with a thiazide diuretic such as hydrochlorothiazide. Diuresis will reduce cardiac workload by reducing the ventricular preload. Diuretic resistance is often encountered when diuretics are used as the sole agents to treat CHF. As alluded to in the previous answer, increases in glomerular filtration fraction in CHF cause increased solute and water resorption in the proximal tubule. Use of ACE inhibitors allows more solute and water to be delivered to the distal convoluted tubules, the site of the electroneutral NaC1 cotransporter that is inhibited by the thiazide diuretics, thereby restoring diuretic sensitivity. Loop diuretics such as furosemide may also be used. Choice A is incorrect because the primary effect of thiazide diuretics is exerted at the level of renal clearance of sodium and thus water. No direct effects of thiazide diuretics on vascular smooth muscle have been observed. Choice B is incorrect since the effects of thiazide diuretics are exerted at the level of the kidney. Choice C is incorrect since the effects of thiazide diuretics are exerted at the level of renal clearance of sodium rather than at the level of intestinal absorption. Choice D is incorrect since thiazide diuretics have no direct effect on cardiac stroke volume. This choice is also incorrect in that a decrease in cardiac stroke volume would result in an increase rather than a reduction of the ventricular afterload.

680. **(B)** Use of loop and thiazide diuretics results in increased sodium and water delivery to the collecting ducts, where exchange of sodium ions with protons and potassium ions will produce a hypokalemic metabolic alkalosis. The cardiac glycosides such as digoxin inhibit Na^+/K^+-ATPase. Inhibition of the sodium pump causes an elevation of intracellular sodium ion concentrations and a resultant decrease in sodium–calcium exchange. The increased intracellular calcium concentration at the contractile machinery produces the therapeutic increase in cardiac contractility needed in CHF. Because potassium ions and cardiac glycosides compete for binding to Na^+/K^+-ATPase, a lowering of serum potassium ion will result in excessive inhibition of the sodium pump. This will result in cardiac toxicities including atrioventricular junctional rhythm, premature ventricular depolarizations, bigeminal rhythm, and second-degree atrioventricular blockade. The use of loop diuretics also brings the potential for magnesium depletion, another risk factor for arrhythmias. Choice A is incorrect since the use of a thiazide diuretic increases delivery of sodium to the distal convoluted tubules, where exchange of sodium for potassium may lead to potassium depletion unless potassium-sparing agents are also used. Thiazide diuretics produce variable effects on calcium excretion, with a slight decrease in renal excretion of calcium ion seen with chronic thiazide treatment. Choice C is incorrect since thiazide diuretics do not inhibit the renal excretion of the glycoside. Choice D is incorrect since diuretics do not induce proteinuria. ACE inhibitors have been reported to produce a slight proteinuria, but this is not a contraindication for their use. Choice E is incorrect on several counts. ACE inhibitors cause an increase in bradykinin levels rather than a decrease. Desensitization of cardiac beta receptors occurs with increased sympathetic drive to the failing heart, but this is attributable to the increased concentration of catecholamines.

681. **(B)** Hepatic intracellular cholesterol levels are tightly controlled through regulation of endocytotic uptake of cholesterol within LDL particles, biosynthesis starting with the enzyme 3-hydroxymethylglutaryl-CoA reductase (HMG CoA reductase), incorporation into VLDL particles, and loss due to conversion to bile acids. Inhibition of cholesterol biosynthesis through statin inhibition of HMG CoA reductase lowers intracellular cholesterol levels. This lowering results in increased transcription of the genes for LDL receptor and HMG CoA reductase, both of which are negatively regulated by oxysterols. Increased expression of hepatic LDL receptors leads to increased endocytic uptake of LDL particles and consequent reduction of circulating levels of LDL cholesterol. This mechanism explains why patients homozygous for defective LDL receptor (familial hypercholesterolemia) have extremely high levels of LDL cholesterol that do not respond to statin treatment. Inhibition of VLDL secretion is the mechanism for lowering of VLDL and LDL by niacin. The loss of inhibition of lipoprotein lipase when the hepatic synthesis of apoCIII is inhibited is the mechanism for lowering of elevated VLDL levels by the fibric acids. Increased fecal excretion of bile acids bound to the bile acid-binding resins such as cholestyramine ultimately leads to increased expression of LDL receptors as is the case with the statins. Also like the statins, patients who are homozygous for defective LDL receptor do not respond to the bile acid-binding resins. Choice A is incorrect since the statins do not affect hepatic VLDL secretion. Inhibition of VLDL secretion does appear to be the mechanism of action for nicotinic acid (niacin) in its ability to lower VLDL and LDL. Choice C is incorrect since the statins do not affect LCAT activity. Choice D is incorrect since the statins do not inhibit the hepatic production of apoCIII. ApoCIII is an inhibitor of lipoprotein lipase. The fibric acids such as clofibrate do inhibit the synthesis of apoCIII. It is currently thought that the loss of apoCIII in VLDL particles contributes to the enhanced clearance of VLDL seen with the fibrates. Choice E is incorrect in that bile acid-binding resins rather than the statins promote increased fecal excretion of bile acids, leading ultimately to increased expression of hepatic LDL receptors.

682. (C) P-glycoprotein, the product of the MDR genes, is an ATP-dependent efflux protein that pumps a number of structurally dissimilar drugs out of cells. The chemotherapeutic agents named in this question have dissimilar mechanisms of action but are all substrates for P-glycoprotein. Doxorubicin and dactinomycin are DNA-intercalating agents and are not cell-cycle specific in their actions. Paclitaxel and vincristine are M-phase specific agents that promote and inhibit microtubule formation, respectively. Increased activity of DNA repair (choice A) is a mechanism for resistance specific to DNA alkylating agents. Decreased doubling time so that a smaller percentage of cells are caught in S phase (choice B) would apply only to S phase-specific agents such as 5-fluorouracil. Increased activity of dihydrofolate reductase (choice D) is a mechanism for resistance to methotrexate. Deletion of deoxycytidine kinase (choice E) is a mechanism for resistance to cytosine arabinoside.

683. (E) Coagulation factors II (prothrombin), VII, IX, and X and proteins C and S are synthesized in the liver and posttranslationally modified by the γ-carboxylation of multiple glutamate residues to yield γ-carboxyglutamate (Gla) residues. The Gla residues within the coagulation proteins provide sites for Ca^{2+} binding necessary for the proteolytic conversion of the zymogen forms to the active forms. The carboxylation reaction requires reduced vitamin K, carbon dioxide, and molecular oxygen. The epoxide form of vitamin K that is generated in the carboxylation reaction must be converted back to the reduced form using NADH. It is this reduction step that is inhibited by the oral anticoagulants, resulting in depletion of reduced vitamin K and inhibition of further carboxylation reactions. The coagulation factors lacking Gla residues are biologically inactive but are still released into the circulation. Although the carboxylation reaction may be rapidly inhibited upon administration of the oral anticoagulants, decreases in coagulation rates are not seen until the levels of the Gla-containing factors are sufficiently depleted. Since the half-lives for the various factors range from six to 50 hrs in the circulation, the full anticoagulant effects of warfarin are not evident for several days after the initial dose was administered. The half-life for dissociation of warfarin from plasma proteins (choice A) plays no role in the time of onset of action since the dissociation is extremely rapid. The elimination half-life for vitamin K (choice B) plays no role in the time to onset of action of warfarin since the drug causes no change in the pharmacokinetics of vitamin K. The elimination of half-life of warfarin (choice C) is a factor that determines the dosing regimen for warfarin, but it does not play a role in the time to onset of action because the loss of active Gla-modified coagulation factors in the circulation is the critical step. Antithrombin (choice D) is an irreversible inhibitor of thrombin, but its half-life plays no role in the time to onset of action of warfarin or the other oral anticoagulants.

684. (B) Open-angle glaucoma is treated by either increasing outflow of aqueous humor through inducing miosis or decreasing production of aqueous humor by the ciliary body. Miosis is produced by muscarinic stimulation through agonists such as pilocarpine or inhibition of acetylcholinesterase by agents such as physostigmine. The carbonic anhydrase inhibitors dorzolamide and acetazolamide decrease production of aqueous humor. Topical beta blockers were found serendipitously to inhibit production of aqueous humor. The mechanism apparently involves β-adrenoceptor stimulation of fluid formation. Topical timolol is a widely used agent for treatment of glaucoma. However, it can undergo systemic absorption from the nasolacrimal system. Use of β blockers may precipitate an asthmatic attack, and their use is contraindicated in known asthmatic patients. Hemolysis (choice A) may produce breathing difficulties, but this condition would not be immediately resolved with inhalational albuterol, a β-adrenoceptor agonist used in asthma attacks. Drug allergy (choice C) might cause angioedema with breathing difficulties, but this condition would not be immediately resolved with inhalational albuterol. Induction of sickling (choice D) may also cause breathing difficulties, but this condition would not be immediately resolved with inhalational albuterol. An idiosyncratic response to timolol (choice E) might also result in breathing difficulties, but the response to albuterol again points to timolol-induced bronchoconstriction.

685. (A) Carbamazepine is a drug of choice for treatment of partial seizures. Its pharmacokinetic profile is complex because a number of other drugs along with the drug itself can induce carbamazepine metabolism. Diplopia and ataxia are indicative of carbamazepine toxicity. Hepatitis will compromise the ability of the liver to metabolize the drug, resulting in a rise in carbamazepine plasma steady state concentrations if the dosing regimen is not adjusted. Phenobarbital (choice B) is an inducer of hepatic drug metabolism and its coadministration would be expected to cause carbamazepine steady state levels to decrease. Smoking (choice C) will induce hepatic drug metabolism and again would be expected to decrease carbamazepine levels. Diuresis (choice D) should have no effect on carbamazepine steady state levels since hepatic metabolism rather than renal excretion is responsible for its clearance. Coadministration of probenecid (choice E), an inhibitor of organic acid active tubular secretion, should have no effect since hepatic metabolism rather than renal excretion controls elimination of the drug.

686. (E) The apparent volume of distribution is a function of the elimination process and is calculated using the equation $V_d = X/C$, where V_d is the volume of distribution, X is the amount of drug present in the body, and C is the plasma (or blood) concentration. We must use time zero for our calculations since this is the only time at which we know the amount of drug in the body because it will immediately be subjected to elimination. The curvature seen in the early data points results from distribution of the drug from blood into tissue compartments. The linear portion of the data reflects the elimination process and must be extrapolated back to time zero to determine the plasma concentration that would have been obtained if distribution had been instantaneous. The administered dose of 100 mg divided by the extrapolated plasma concentration of 1 μg/mL (or 1 mg/L) yields an apparent V_d of 100 L. The volume of distribution is useful in providing a parameter that describes the relationship between the administered dose and the resulting plasma concentration.

687. (C) Using the extrapolated linear portion of the data, the concentration at time zero is 1 μg/mL. By definition, the elimination half-life is the time interval for 50% reduction in concentration for single-dose drug disappearance under conditions when the drug disappearance is controlled by the elimination process. The plasma concentration of 0.5 μg/mL is achieved after 3 hrs. The elimination half-life provides information necessary for calculation of dosing regimens to achieve and maintain the plasma concentration at a specified concentration to provide effective therapy without producing toxicity. In many cases, the pharmacokinetic information for a given drug is supplied as the clearance. Clearance is the product $[V_d * \ln 2/t_{1/2}]$.

688. (D) By inspection of the graph, it is observed that administration of sodium bicarbonate increases the rate of renal elimination of the drug. Sodium bicarbonate produces alkalinization of urinary pH. This alkalinization will cause increased ionization of weak acids and accelerate their urinary excretion since the anions cannot be reabsorbed through the tubular epithelium, whereas the uncharged form of many weak acids may undergo reabsorption. Urinary alkalinization is a therapeutic strategy used to hasten the excretion of weak acids such as aspirin in overdose situations. A strong base (choice A) will be protonated at all attainable urinary pH values so that alteration of urinary pH will have no effect on its excretion. Excretion of a weak base (choice B) will be slowed by alkalinization of urinary pH since the uncharged form of the base that is readily reabsorbed from the tubular urine will predominate. Excretion of a non-electrolyte (choice C) will be unaffected by changes in urinary pH since the polarity of non-electrolytes is not sensitive to pH. A strong acid (choice E) will be unprotonated at all attainable urinary pH values so that alteration of urinary pH will have no effect on its excretion.

689. **(D)** The description of shock with reduced cardiac function and elevated left ventricular filling pressure indicates cardiogenic shock. In cardiogenic shock, an agent that increases myocardial contractility without increasing heart rate and peripheral resistance is required. Particularly in cardiogenic shock resulting from acute myocardial infarction, it is important to select an agent that does not increase the cardiac workload and further extend myocardial damage. Dobutamine, a selective β_1-adrenoceptor agonist, will increase myocardial contractility without producing increases in heart rate or peripheral resistance. Norepinephrine (choice A) will increase myocardial contractility but will also greatly increase peripheral resistance. The latter effect will increase the cardiac workload, a situation that is to be avoided in cardiogenic shock. Epinephrine (choice B) can also increase myocardial contractility but also will increase heart rate and, at doses that produce increased contractility, will also increase peripheral resistance. Atropine (choice C), a muscarinic antagonist, may produce an increase of myocardial contractility under conditions when vagal tone is high, but is not useful in cardiogenic shock where direct stimulation of the myocardium is needed. Isoproterenol (choice E), a non-selective β-adrenoreceptor agonist, again will increase contractility but will also produce tachycardia, thus increasing the cardiac workload.

690. **(A)** In a prostatic cancer chemoprevention program, an agent that acts to decrease androgenic actions at the prostate level without producing major systemic changes in testosterone levels is needed. Finasteride is an inhibitor of the 5α-reductase that converts testosterone to dihydrotestosterone in the prostate. Since continuous conversion of testosterone to dihydrotestosterone is essential for the androgenic effects in the prostate, inhibition of the 5α-reductase will decrease the stimulation of the prostate. Use of finasteride will produce fewer systemic side effects than use of androgen receptor antagonists or gonadotropin-releasing hormone (GnRH) receptor agonists. Finasteride is used for the treatment of prostatic hyperplasia because it produces a consistent decrease in prostatic size. Leuprolide (choice B) is a GnRH agonist that suppresses plasma testosterone levels to the level of pharmacological castration. It is used in the treatment of prostatic cancer. Flutamide (choice C) is a nonsteroidal antiandrogen that is used in the treatment of prostatic cancer. Ketoconazole (choice D) in an antifungal agent that has the property of inhibiting the cytochrome P450 isoforms of steroid biosynthesis. It is also used in the treatment of prostatic cancer. Diethylstilbestrol (choice E) is a non-steroidal synthetic estrogen that is used in the treatment of prostatic cancer. Use of this agent in a noncancerous patient would produce undesirable feminization.

691. **(C)** Curve C shows a dose-response curve in which the efficacy or maximum effect of the agonist is unchanged, but the apparent potency, the inverse of the concentration for half-maximal effect, has been decreased. A competitive antagonist, by occupying the receptor site for the agonist, causes the dose-response curve for the agonist to retain the same shape but to be shifted to the right. Curve A (choice A) is not a possible curve for antagonism since both the apparent efficacy and potency of the agonist are increased. Antagonists must decrease either or both of these properties since antagonists by definition interfere with receptor function. Curve B (choice B) is also not a possible curve since the apparent potency has been increased. Curve D (choice D) shows a diminution of the apparent efficacy of the agonist, a property of a non-competitive antagonist. By definition, the effects of a competitive antagonist may be overcome or competed away by using larger concentrations of the agonist. This overcoming of the competition will result in a decrease in the apparent potency for the agonist but the maximum effect will be unchanged. Curve E (choice E) is an example of the dose-response curve expected for an antagonist that has both competitive and non-competitive properties, thus resulting in both a decrease in the apparent potency and apparent efficacy of the agonist.

692. (D) The effect of a noncompetitive antagonist is to reduce the apparent efficacy or maximal response of the agonist. This may be accomplished by direct receptor inactivation or through interference with postreceptor steps leading to the biological response. Inactivation of 33% of the receptors would leave 67% of the receptors available to produce the response. If we assume that space receptors are not present, this should lead to a decrease in the apparent efficacy to the 67% level. Increasing the agonist concentration does not yield any greater response. Curve A (choice A) is not a possible curve for antagonism since both the apparent efficacy and apparent potency of the agonist are increased. Antagonists must decrease either or both of these properties since antagonists by definition interfere with receptor function. Curve B (choice B) is also not a possible curve since the apparent potency has been increased. Curve C (choice C) shows the properties of competitive antagonism as discussed in the preceding question. Curve E (choice E) is an example of the dose-response curve expected for an antagonist that has both competitive and non-competitive properties, thus resulting in both a decrease in the apparent potency and apparent efficacy of the agonist.

693. (B) An inhibitor of the presynaptic uptake of drug Q would be expected to increase the synaptic concentrations of Q since the synaptic concentration is determined by the balance between the appearance of the neurotransmitter (whether by synaptic release under physiological conditions or diffusion from the external medium in this experimental system) and the disappearance due to the uptake system. Inhibition of the uptake system will allow concentrations of Q in the medium to yield larger synaptic concentrations of Q than would be the case without inhibition of the uptake. This results in a shift of the dose-response curve to lower concentrations. The maximum response is unaffected. In the case of synaptic norepinephrine (NE), approximately 70% of the disappearance of NE is attributable to the amine pump responsible for the presynaptic uptake system. Inhibition of the NE and other biogenic amine uptake systems by agents such as cocaine or fluoxetine underlies the mechanistic basis of action for the clinical actions of such agents. Curve A (choice A) is not a possible choice since the apparent efficacy of the agonist Q has been increased. Increases in the maximum response are possible with agents that act as allosteric receptor activators or that act downstream of the receptor, but an inhibitor of the presynaptic uptake as described in this question would exert its effects upstream of the receptor. Curve C (choice C) is not a possible choice since an inhibitor of presynaptic uptake would lead to higher, rather than lower, synaptic concentrations of Q. Curve C might arise if the uptake inhibitor was also a competitive antagonist at the Q receptor, but there is no reason to assume this is the case. Curve D (choice D) is not a possible choice for the same reasons as indicated for curve C above. Curve D might arise if the inhibitor was a non-competitive receptor inhibitor, but again there is no reason to assume this to be the case. Curve E (choice E) is not a possible choice as indicated above. Curve E might arise if the inhibitor showed both competitive and non-competitive antagonism, but again there is no reason to assume this.

694. (D) If the drug R has 50% of the efficacy of Q, the maximum response expected is 50% of that for Q. Curve A (choice A) is not a possible answer since the apparent efficacy is greater than that for Q. Curve B (choice B) is not a possible answer since the efficacy is the same as that for Q. Curve C (choice C) is not a possible answer since the efficacy is the same as that for Q. Curve E (choice E) is not a possible answer since the efficacy shown is lower than 50% of that for Q.

695. (A) Cyclosporine is a major agent used for immunosuppression in organ transplantation. Use of this agent along with tacrolimus is responsible for the remarkable progress in the prevention and treatment of organ rejection. Cyclosporine acts by blocking the activation of T cells through formation of complexes with the cyclophilin family of protein. These cyclosporine-cyclophilin complexes inhibit function of the protein complex calcineurin, preventing the transcriptional activation necessary for lymphokine expression. Cyclosporine produces nephrotoxicity in a majority of patients, but exhibits no bone marrow depression. Prednisone (choice B) is used in transplantation because it reduces circulating levels of lymphocytes and inhibits T-cell proliferation. Toxicity is that expected of glucocorticoids (ulcers, hyperglycemia, and osteoporosis) and includes neither nephrotoxicity nor bone marrow depression. Muromonab-CD3 monoclonal antibody (choice C) is a mouse monoclonal antibody whose T-cell epitope is in close proximity to the antigen recognition complex. Binding to T cells prevents antigen binding to the antigen recognition complex and activates cytokine release. This ultimately results in the appearance of T cells with CD3 and antigen recognition complex being absent, resulting in the immunosuppressive actions. Toxicities include cytokine release syndrome, anaphylactoid reactions, and central nervous system effects, but do not include nephrotoxicity or bone marrow depression. Azathioprine (choice D) is a purine antimetabolite that prevents the clonal expansion of B and T lymphocytes, thus producing immunosuppressive actions. Because it is a cytotoxic agent, it produces bone marrow depression along with toxicity to gastrointestinal cells. Cyclophosphamide (choice E) is an alkylating agent used in immunosuppression as well as in cancer chemotherapy. Toxicities include bone marrow depression along with hemorrhagic cystitis and cardiotoxicity.

696. (B) Metronidazole is the agent of choice for the treatment of trichomoniasis. It produces a selective toxicity to anaerobic organisms by initiating redox cycling in these organisms. Because metronidazole produces a disulfiram-like action, patients should be cautioned to avoid alcohol consumption when taking the drug. Methimazole (choice A) is an antithyroid agent that inhibits formation of thyroid hormone. Mebendazole (choice C) is an antihelminthic agent used to treat roundworm infections such as ascariasis, pinworms, or whipworm. Primaquine (choice D) is used to treat relapsing malarias caused by *Plasmodium vivax* and *P. ovale.* Trimethoprim (choice E), in combination with sulfamethoxazole, is used prophylactically in antiparasitic treatments to prevent *Pneumocystis carinii* infections in immune-deficient patients, as well as being used to treat bacterial urinary tract infections.

697. (C) Ketoconazole is an inhibitor of the cytochrome P450 isoforms involved in sterol and steroid biosynthesis in fungal cells as well as host cells. The inhibition of sterol synthesis compromises the fungal cell membrane function. The inhibition of steroid biosynthesis may be used advantageously to reduce corticosteroid or testosterone biosynthesis in adrenal hyperplasia or prostate cancer, respectively. Ketoconazole will also inhibit the P450-mediated metabolism of a number of other drugs including terfenadine, astemizole, warfarin, and cyclosporine. In this case, raising circulating terfenadine levels leads to depressed cardiac conduction, a situation that may result in fatal torsades de pointes. Griseofulvin (choice A) exerts its antifungal activity by disrupting the fungal mitotic spindle, and is an inducer rather than an inhibitor of hepatic drug metabolism. Amphotericin B (choice B) is a polyene macrolide that binds to fungal sterols and forms channels in the fungal cell membrane. Amphotericin B does not produce any significant alterations in hepatic metabolism of other drugs. Chloramphenicol (choice D) is an antibacterial agent that inhibits eukaryotic protein synthesis by binding to the bacterial 50S ribosomal subunit. It is not effective in the treatment of fungal infections. Chloramphenicol is an irreversible inhibitor of cytochrome P450 isoforms and will decrease the hepatic clearance of a wide variety of drugs. Nystatin (choice E) is similar in structure and mechanism of action to amphotericin B, but, because of its greater toxicity, it is not used systemically. It is a useful topical antifungal agent.

698. **(E)** Acyclovir is an anti–herpesvirus agent that acts by terminating DNA polymerization in a manner that results in suicide inactivation of the DNA polymerase. Acyclovir is an acylic guanine nucleoside analog that undergoes phosphorylation by herpesviral thymidine kinase in the pathway to formation of the acyclovir triphosphate form that is involved in DNA chain termination. Resistance involves deletion or reduction, along with altered catalytic activity of herpesvirus thymidine kinase. Foscarnet (choice A) is a pyrophosphate analog that inhibits herpesvirus nucleic acid synthesis at the level of the viral DNA polymerase. Resistance involves point mutations in the viral DNA polymerase. Zidovudine (choice B) is an antiretroviral thymidine analog. The triphosphate is a competitive inhibitor of reverse transcriptase and a DNA chain terminator. The monophosphate is a competitive inhibitor of thymidine kinase. Resistance involves point mutations in reverse transcriptase. Amantadine (choice C) is a tricyclic amine that inhibits uncoating of influenza A virus. It is used for the prevention and treatment of influenza A virus. It also is used in the treatment of parkinsonism. Saquinavir (choice D) is an HIV protease inhibitor. Resistance involves point mutations in the protease.

699. **(B)** Trimethoprim is an inhibitor of dihydrofolate reductase that exhibits great specificity for binding to the bacterial form as opposed to the human form (10^5 higher concentrations are required for inhibition of host dihydrofolate reductase). Trimethoprim is combined with sulfamethoxazole to provide inhibition of sequential steps in bacterial tetrahydrofolate synthesis. Resistance may arise by mutation of bacterial dihydrofolate reductase, although acquisition of a plasmid encoding altered dihydrofolate reductase is more common for gram-negative bacteria. Methotrexate (choice A) is an inhibitor of dihydrofolate reductase but this drug, unlike trimethoprim, shows no specificity for bacterial forms as opposed to host cell forms. This lack of specificity makes it unsuitable for antibacterial therapy. Methotrexate and similar antifolates such as trimetrexate and 5,10-dideazatetrahydrofolate are used in cancer chemotherapy. Methotrexate is also used in rheumatoid arthritis. Amoxicillin (choice C) is a β-lactamase sensitive penicillin whose spectrum of activity includes the gram-negative bacteria. Because amoxicillin achieves high concentrations in the urine, it is useful for *E. coli* urinary tract infections, although resistance is increasingly a problem. Its mechanism of action involves osmotic lysis of the bacteria secondary to inhibition of cell wall synthesis. Imipenem (choice D) is a β-lactam antibiotic whose structure is distinct from the penicillins and cephalosporins. It exhibits good activity against a wide variety of bacteria. It is resistant to hydrolysis by bacterial β-lactamases and kills susceptible organisms by inhibiting cell wall synthesis leading to osmotic lysis. Imipenem is combined with cilastatin, an inhibitor of dipeptidases, to improve its half-life in the body. Sulfamethoxazole (choice E) is a sulfonamide that shares the property of inhibiting incorporation of p-aminobenzoic acid into folate in bacteria. It is often combined with trimethoprim to provide sequential inhibition of reduced folate synthesis as indicated above.

700. **(A)** Rifampin selectively inhibits bacterial DNA-dependent RNA polymerase. It is highly useful in treating mycobacterial infections since it can penetrate cells and kill intracellular mycobacteria. It is a potent and notorious inducer of cytochrome P450, leading to increased hepatic clearance of many other drugs including the oral anticoagulants, cyclosporine, propranolol, digitoxin, corticosteroids, and oral contraceptives. Isoniazid (choice B) is the most widely used antitubercular agent worldwide. It functions by inhibiting mycolic acid biosynthesis. Isoniazid is cleared by metabolism via N-acetylase and hydrolytic activity. Early population studies of isoniazid metabolism provided clear evidence of genetic heterogeneity in rates of acetylation and led to the classifications of fast and slow acetylators. Ethambutol (choice C) is often combined with isoniazid in antitubercular regimens. Clearance is primarily via renal excretion. Streptomycin (choice D) was the first effective drug for the treatment of tuberculosis, but, because of its ototoxicity and nephrotoxicity and the development of less toxic agents, use of streptomycin is limited to the severe forms of the disease. Sulfisoxazole (choice E) may be used in antitubercular regimens in combination with other drugs. Clearance is primarily via glomerular filtration.

701. (C) Orthostatic hypotension is associated more frequently with antihypertensive agents working peripherally than those acting centrally. Loss of efficacy with administration of a tricyclic antidepressant indicates either a hastening of the clearance of the antihypertensive agent or a loss of activity at the site of action. Tricyclic antidepressants are cleared by hepatic metabolism, but there is no evidence to indicate that they induce their own metabolism or that of other drugs. The interference by a tricyclic antidepressant points to guanethidine. This agent appears to work within the sympathetic nerve terminal by depleting vesicular catecholamine stores as well as preventing exocytotic vesicle fusion with the plasma membrane. Guanethidine requires entry into the terminal via the catecholamine transporter that is inhibited by tricyclic antidepressants. Even without this drug–drug interaction, the use of tricyclic antidepressants with antihypertensive agents that produce orthostatic hypotension is unwise since the tricyclics also block α_1-adrenoceptors and cause orthostatic hypotension. A serotonin-reuptake inhibitor such as fluoxetine might be a better choice for treating depression in this patient since these agents have fewer and less severe cardiovascular side effects. Lisinopril (choice A) is an ACE inhibitor used in antihypertensive therapy. Orthostatic hypotension is not a problem with lisinopril. ACE inhibitors are cleared both by renal excretion and metabolism to glucuronide and cysteine conjugates. The clearance of an ACE inhibitor should not be affected by a tricyclic antidepressant. Tricyclic antidepressants should have no effect on ACE inhibitor activity. Prazosin (choice B) is an α_1-adrenoceptor antagonist. Because it acts by blocking arteriolar smooth muscle α_1-receptors, orthostatic hypotension is a significant side effect. Coadministration of a tricyclic antidepressant with α_1-blocking actions with prazosin should intensify the antihypertensive actions and the orthostatic hypotension. Hydralazine (choice D) is an arteriolar smooth muscle relaxing agent. Because its actions are selective for arteriolar smooth muscle, postural hypotension is not a problem. Hydralazine is cleared by hepatic acetylation as well as formation of oxo-acid hydrazones. Methyldopa (choice E) is metabolized by the normal enzymes of catecholamine biosynthesis to α-methylnorepinephrine, an α_2 agonist that acts at the level of the vasopressor centers in the brainstem to decrease sympathetic outflow to the periphery. Methyldopa enters neurons via the amino acid uptake system, and its entry is not inhibited by the tricyclic antidepressants.

702. (C) Clonidine, an α_2-selective agonist, acts at the vasopressor centers in the brainstem to decrease sympathetic outflow to the periphery. Sedation and xerostomia occur in many patients; these side effects usually abate after a few weeks of treatment although the persistence of these and other adverse effects may force cessation of clonidine treatment. Abrupt cessation of clonidine, especially in high-dose regimens, may precipitate a withdrawal syndrome with headache, tremors, sweating, and tachycardia. This condition may be treated with the usual dose of clonidine (the effect may take several hours) or with a vasodilator such as sodium nitroprusside if a more rapid reduction in pressure is needed. Although it is not included in the list here, the β-receptor blockers such as propranolol also show a rebound hypertension with abrupt withdrawal in antihypertensive regimens. Prazosin (choice A) is associated with a first-dose phenomenon in which profound orthostatic hypotension occurs after the first dose. Patients should be warned to take the first dose at night before going to bed. Although tolerance develops to this, some degree of orthostatic hypotension is seen with chronic use. No significant rebound hypertension is seen with abrupt withdrawal of prazosin. Captopril (choice B) is an ACE inhibitor. Serious side effects of ACE inhibitors are rare. No significant rebound hypertension is seen with abrupt withdrawal. Hydralazine (choice D) is an arteriolar smooth muscle relaxing agent. The side effects with this agent are those associated with hypotension including headache, palpitations, dizziness, and tachycardia along with production of a lupus-like syndrome. No significant rebound hypertension is associated with abrupt withdrawal of this agent. Chlorothiazide (choice E) is a thiazide diuretic that is used to reduce body sodium and fluid volume. No rebound hypertension is seen with abrupt withdrawal.

703. (A) Hydralazine is an arteriolar smooth muscle relaxing agent. In addition to producing side effects associated with hypotension, hydralazine may produce immunological reactions, the most common being a lupus-like syndrome. The incidence is four times higher in women than in men. Studies of the effect of acetylator genotype with the syndrome indicate that slow acetylators develop positive antinuclear antibodies more rapidly. This suggests that the parent compound rather than the acetylated metabolite is responsible. The syndrome usually disappears upon cessation of hydralazine treatment. The ACE inhibitor captopril (choice B) may cause a skin rash in some patients but does not produce a lupus-like syndrome. Clonidine (choice C), the centrally acting α_2-receptor agonist, does not produce an immunological reaction. The β-blocker propranolol (choice D) does not produce an immunological reaction. The α_1-receptor antagonist prazosin (choice E) does not elicit an immunological reaction.

704. (B) Captopril and other ACE inhibitors cause a dry cough in 5 to 20% of patients. This may be due to accumulation of bradykinin in the lungs as a result of ACE inhibition since bradykinin is also metabolized by ACE. The cough will disappear with cessation of ACE inhibitor treatment. The arteriolar smooth muscle relaxing agent hydralazine (choice A) produces troublesome side effects attendant with hypotension along with a lupus-like syndrome, but does not cause a cough. Clonidine (choice C), the centrally acting α_2-receptor agonist, produces sedation and xerostomia but no cough. The β-blocker propranolol (choice D) may produce a variety of side effects including precipitating heart failure and asthma in susceptible patients. It does not cause a cough. Propranolol has been used by musicians to control palpitations associated with stage fright. The α_1-receptor antagonist prazosin (choice E) produces postural hypotension but not cough.

705. (E) Cyclophosphamide is metabolized by the cytochrome P450 CYP2A isoform to species that eventually lead to phosphoramide mustard, an alkylating agent, and acrolein, a chemical irritant that causes hemorrhagic cystitis, to be generated. The natural product bleomycin (choice A) binds to DNA and forms an iron complex that is capable of generating active oxygen species in the presence of a reducing agent. The reactive oxygen species then generate single- and double-strand breaks, leading to cytotoxicity. Bleomycin has a serious toxicity-involved production of pulmonary fibrosis. The pyrimidine analog 5-fluorouracil (choice B) is metabolized by ribosylation and phosphorylation to the nucleotide level. F-UMP is further metabolized to F-dUMP, an inhibitor of thymidylate synthase. Cells then become starved for TTP and incorporate F-dUTP and dUTP in its place in DNA. Fluorouracil also becomes incorporated in RNA, leading to inhibition of RNA processing. Paclitaxel (choice C) is a natural product isolated from the bark of the Western yew tree. Paclitaxel is a mitotic inhibitor by promoting microtubule formation. Cisplatin (choice D), an inorganic platinum-containing complex, becomes hydrated and binds to DNA where it forms intra- and interstrand crosslinks.

706. (D) Cisplatin, an inorganic platinum-containing complex, becomes hydrated and binds to DNA where it forms intra- and interstrand crosslinks. Cisplatin is particularly effective in testicular and ovarian cancers in combination with other antitumor agents. Cisplatin exerts a renal toxicity that may be prevented by the infusion of one to two liters of saline prior to administration. Ototoxicity involving high-frequency hearing loss is an effect that is not prevented by hydration. The natural product bleomycin (choice A) binds to DNA and forms an iron complex that is capable of generating active oxygen species in the presence of a reducing agent. The reactive oxygen species then generate single- and double-strand breaks, leading to cytotoxicity. The drug is particularly useful against germ cell tumors of the testes and ovary. Bleomycin has a serious toxicity that involves production of pulmonary fibrosis. The pyrimidine analog 5-fluorouracil (5-FU) (choice B) is metabolized by ribosylation and phosphorylation to the nucleotide level. F-UMP is further metabolized to F-dUMP, an inhibitor of thymidylate synthase. Cells then become starved for TTP and incorporate F-dUFP and dUTP in its place in DNA. 5-FU also becomes incorporated in RNA, leading to inhibition of RNA processing. 5-FU is used to treat a wide variety of carcinomas. Toxicity from 5-FU is expressed as GI disturbances (anorexia, nausea, stomatitis, and diarrhea) and myelosuppression. Paclitaxel (choice C) is a natural product isolated from the bark of the Western yew tree. Paclitaxel is a mitotic inhibitor by promoting microtubule formation. This drug is particularly useful in treating metastatic breast and ovarian cancer. The primary toxicity of paclitaxel is bone marrow suppression. Cyclophosphamide (choice E) is metabolized by the cytochrome P450 CYP2A isoform to the phosphoramide mustard that acts as the alkylating agent. This agent is widely used in combination regimens. Nausea and vomiting are the most common toxicities. Hemorrhagic cystitis attributable to the acrolein also produced from cyclophosphamide metabolites may be minimized by hydration and frequent voiding of the bladder. Note that this toxicity is not at the level of the kidney.

707. (B) The pyrimidine analog 5-fluorouracil (5-FU) is metabolized by ribosylation and phosphorylation to the nucleotide level. F-UMP is further metabolized to F-dUMP, an inhibitor of thymidylate synthase. Cells then become starved for TTP and incorporate F-dUTP and dUTP in its place in DNA. 5-FU also becomes incorporated in RNA, leading to inhibition of RNA processing. 5-FU is used to treat a wide variety of carcinomas. Toxicity from 5-FU is expressed as GI disturbances (anorexia, nausea, stomatitis, and diarrhea) and myelosuppression. The natural product bleomycin (choice A) binds to DNA and forms an iron complex that is capable of generating active oxygen species in the presence of a reducing agent. The reactive oxygen species then generate single- and double-strand breaks, leading to cytotoxicity. The drug is particularly useful against germ cell tumors of the testes and ovary. Bleomycin has a serious toxicity that involves production of pulmonary fibrosis. Paclitaxel (choice C) is a natural product isolated from the bark of the Western yew tree. Paclitaxel is a mitotic inhibitor by promoting microtubule formation. This drug is particularly useful in treating metastatic breast and ovarian cancer. The primary toxicity of paclitaxel is bone marrow suppression. Cisplatin (choice D), an inorganic platinum-containing complex, becomes hydrated and binds to DNA where it forms intra- and interstrand crosslinks. Cisplatin is particularly effective in testicular and ovarian cancers in combination with other antitumor agents. Cisplatin exerts a renal toxicity that may be prevented by the infusion of one to two liters of saline prior to administration. Ototoxicity involving high-frequency hearing loss is an effect that is not prevented by hydration. Cyclophosphamide (choice E) is metabolized by the cytochrome P450 CYP2A isoform to the phosphoramide mustard that acts as the alkylating agent. This agent is widely used in combination regimens. Nausea and vomiting are the most common toxicities. Hemorrhagic cystitis attributable to the acrolein also produced from cyclophosphamide metabolites may be minimized by hydration and frequent voiding of the bladder.

708. **(D)** Etoposide is a semisynthetic derivative of podophyllotoxin, a constituent of the mandrake plant. Etoposide is an inhibitor of topoisomerase II, an enzyme that relaxes DNA supercoiling by breaking one strand and passing the second strand through the break before closing the break. Etoposide inhibits the closure step and results in an accumulation of DNA strand breaks, leading to cell death. Etoposide is used to treat testicular tumors and small cell carcinoma of the lung in combination with cisplatin. Leukopenia is the dose-limiting toxicity seen with this drug. The natural product bleomycin (choice A) binds to DNA and forms an iron complex that is capable of generating active oxygen species in the presence of a reducing agent. The reactive oxygen species then generate single- and double-strand breaks, leading to cytotoxicity. The drug is particularly useful against germ cell tumors of the testes and ovary. Bleomycin has a serious toxicity that involves production of pulmonary fibrosis. The pyrimidine analog 5-fluorouracil (5-FU) (choice B) is metabolized by ribosylation and phosphorylation to the nucleotide level. F-UMP is further metabolized to F-dUMP, an inhibitor of thymidylate synthase. Cells then become starved for TTP and incorporate F-dUTP and dUTP in its place in DNA. 5-FU also becomes incorporated in RNA, leading to inhibition of RNA processing. 5-FU is used to treat a wide variety of carcinomas. Toxicity from 5-FU is expressed as GI disturbances (anorexia, nausea, stomatitis, and diarrhea) and myelosuppression. Paclitaxel (choice C) is a natural product isolated from the bark of the Western yew tree. Paclitaxel is a mitotic inhibitor by promoting microtubule formation. This drug is particularly useful in treating metastatic breast and ovarian cancer. The primary toxicity of paclitaxel is bone marrow suppression. Cyclophosphamide (choice E) is metabolized by the cytochrome P450 CYP2A isoform to the phosphoramide mustard that acts as the alkylating agent. This agent is widely used in combination regimens. Nausea and vomiting are the most common toxicities. Hemorrhagic cystitis attributable to the acrolein also produced from cyclophosphamide metabolites may be minimized by hydration and frequent voiding of the bladder.

709. **(A)** Sulfadiazine is stated to be a weak acid with a pKa value of 6.5. The protonated form will be uncharged and will be the permeant species that crosses biological membranes. At equilibrium the concentration of the permeant species will be the same on both sides of the membrane, but the total amount (protonated form + anion) present in each compartment will depend on the pH of the compartment. For a weak acid, the total amount will be the highest in the most alkaline compartment. This is because higher pH values will cause dissociation of the acid to the anion that becomes trapped in the compartment since the charged anion cannot cross the membrane. The higher the pH value for the compartment, the greater will be the total amount present. Alkalinized urine at pH 8.0 has the highest pH value. The value for the total amount may be calculated using the Henderson–Hasselbalch equation [pH = pKa + log (unprotonated form/protonated form)].

710. **(E)** Pyrimethamine is a weak base with a pKa value of 7.0. The unprotonated form (or the "free base") will be unchanged and will be the permeant species that crosses biological membranes. At equilibrium the concentration of the permeant species will be the same on both sides of the membrane, but the total amount (base + protonated form) present in each compartment will depend on the pH of the compartment. For a weak base, the total amount will be the highest in the most acidic compartment. This is because lower pH values will cause protonation of the base to the protonated form that becomes trapped in the compartment since the charged protonated base cannot cross the membrane. The lower the pH value for the compartment, the greater will be the total amount present. Stomach contents at pH 2.0 has the lowest pH value. The value for the total amount at any pH may be calculated using the Henderson–Hasselbalch equation [pH = pKa + log (unprotonated form/protonated form)].

711. (A) Vasopressin is a peptide hormone synthesized in the supraoptic and paraventricular nuclei of the hypothalamus and transported to the posterior lobe of the neurohypophyseal system. Osmoreceptors in the hypothalamus, close to the nuclei that synthesize and secrete ADH, are stimulated to cause release of vasopressin by an increase in plasma osmolality. Vasopressin acts through G protein-linked receptors on vascular smooth muscle (V_1 receptors) to mediate vasoconstriction and on V_2 receptors in the collecting ducts to increase permeability to water, thus aiding in the formation of hypertonic urine. Diabetes insipidus is a disease characterized by formation of large quantities of dilute urine. This can be due to either inadequate vasopressin secretion (pituitary diabetes insipidus) or inadequate renal response to vasopressin (nephrogenic diabetes insipidus). In a seemingly paradoxical manner, vasopressin-resistant diabetes insipidus can be treated with thiazide diuretics which act by decreasing plasma volume and decreasing fluid delivery to the collecting ducts. Desmopressin is used as an intranasal spray for the treatment of pituitary diabetes insipidus. This derivative is less susceptible to peptidase breakdown, and the intranasal route avoids GI tract peptidases. Other uses of vasopressin include treatment of bleeding esophageal varices since the vasoconstrictor effects of vasopressin appear to be marked in splanchnic circulation. Ethanol (choice B) inhibits vasopressin secretion, resulting in the well-known alcohol-induced diuresis. NSAIDs (choice C) enhance the antidiuretic response to vasopressin by inhibiting the formation of prostaglandins which decrease the antidiuretic response. Hyperosmolality (choice D) is the primary physiological stimulus for vasopressin secretion. The osmoreceptive complex, a series of structures of the central nervous system, sense osmolality and regulate vasopressin secretion. Vasopressin (choice E) acting on V_1 G protein-linked receptors in vascular smooth muscle, causes formation of IP_3 which increases intracellular calcium ion concentrations and promotes contraction.

712. (D) Propranolol is used prophylactically to prevent the onset of anginal attacks because of its β-blocking action in decreasing heart rate and preventing increases in heart rate with exertion. This effect decreases the myocardial oxygen demand and prevents the ischemic episodes that trigger the anginal pain. Isoproterenol (choice A) is a β-receptor agonist that will increase heart rate and contractile force, precipitating an anginal attack or even myocardial infarction in a patient with compromised coronary blood flow. Nitroglycerin (choice B) is used to terminate anginal attacks. Its vasodilating actions cause venous pooling of blood and a decrease in peripheral resistance, thereby reducing the cardiac preload and afterload. This results in a diminution of the cardiac workload and a consequent decrease in myocardial oxygen demand. Nitroglycerin and other organic nitrates also appear to increase blood flow to ischemic areas in the myocardium, but the primary action is considered to be the decrease in cardiac workload and reduction of myocardial oxygen demand. Thiosulfate (choice C) is an agent used to treat cyanide toxicity. The mitochondrial enzyme rhodanese will combine cyanide and thiosulfate to form thiocyanate, which is excreted by the kidney. Nifedipine (choice E) is a dihydropyridine calcium channel blocker that is beneficially combined with propranolol to treat angina. Nifedipine selectively dilates arterial resistance vessels with little effect on venous pooling. The decrease in arterial pressure will result in tachycardia and increased force of contraction, effects that will be attenuated by combination of nifedipine with a β blocker such as propranolol. The decreased peripheral resistance causes a decrease in cardiac workload. Because nifedipine does not alter venous tone, venous return to the heart is relatively unaltered.

713. (D) The phenothiazines and neuroleptic agents in general have been characterized as being antagonists of dopamine D_2 receptors in the limbic system. More recent data casts some doubt on this as being the total explanation for the antipsychotic actions, since the atypical antipsychotic agents such as clozapine have a low affinity for D_2 receptors. Most of the adverse effects of the neuroleptics involving dopamine receptors are attributable to blockade of D_2 receptors. Because prolactin secretion from the anterior pituitary is under negative regulation by dopamine, blockade of D_2 receptors by chlorpromazine will stimulate prolactin secretion. This may result in breast engorgement and galactorrhea in females. Nausea and vomiting (choice A) are not seen with chlorpromazine since this and other neuroleptics exert an antiemetic effect at the chemoreceptor trigger zone. Tourette's syndrome (choice B) involves tics and other involuntary movements and obscene vocalizations. The neuroleptic agent haloperidol is the current drug of choice for the treatment of this disease. Excessive salivation (choice C) is not correct since the phenothiazines, by virtue of their antimuscarinic effects, produce dry mouth and other signs of blockade of parasympathetic nervous system action. Diarrhea (choice E) is not correct since the antimuscarinic effects of chlorpromazine will result in constipation.

714. (E) A volume of distribution much larger than 1 liter/kg body weight for a drug indicates in general that the drug is highly lipid-soluble and is able to move from plasma through capillary membranes and cell membranes. Such highly lipid-soluble drugs are usually cleared from the body by metabolism since the hepatic drug metabolizing system works on highly lipid-soluble compounds. It is, of course, possible for a drug to have a large volume of distribution and to be relatively lipid-insoluble if it can pass through fenestrations and becomes tightly bound to a structural component such as bone matrix or extracellular matrix. As a general rule, however, a large volume of distribution indicates high lipid solubility and clearance by hepatic metabolism. Note that the converse is not necessarily true as evidenced by the observation that the lipid-soluble anxiolytic agent chlordiazepoxide has a volume of distribution of 0.30 liter/kg body weight because it is highly bound to plasma protein. Choice A is incorrect since the definition of first-pass metabolism involves oral administration with the drug having to pass first through the portal circulation where it may be extensively metabolized prior to reaching the systemic circulation. The intravenous route will bypass this first pass through the liver. Choice B is incorrect as evidenced by the kinetics of distribution of thiopental as used in induction of anesthesia. When administered intravenously, the highly lipid-soluble thiopental distributes first to the brain because of the large percentage of cardiac output that the brain receives. The drug will then redistribute to skeletal muscle and, only slowly, to adipose tissue. The tissue distribution is dependent on the tissue perfusion rate. Since adipose tissue is relatively poorly perfused, the drug is only slowly distributed to it. Stereoisomers (choice C) usually show no differences in their rates of intestinal absorption since the process of passive diffusion by which most drugs are absorbed shows no stereoselectivity. Choice D is incorrect since pharmacological activity correlates with free drug. It is the free drug that interacts with receptors to produce the biological response.

715. (A) Tricyclic antidepressants produce an increased risk of tonic–clonic seizures. Accidental and deliberate overdoses in children carry a high risk of death. Weight gain rather than weight loss (choice B) is a common side effect of tricyclics. Hyperprolactinemia (choice C) is a side effect of neuroleptics because of their D_2-receptor blocking activity. Dopamine is inhibitory to prolactin release; blockade of dopamine receptors elevates serum prolactin levels. Although the phenothiazines and tricyclic antidepressants share many side effects such as α_1-receptor and muscarinic receptor blocking activities, tricyclics do not block dopamine receptors and so do not affect prolactin levels. Inhibition of salivation rather than excessive salivation (choice D) is expected since the tricyclic antidepressants exert pronounced antimuscarinic actions. Postural hypotension rather than hypertension (choice E) is expected since the tricyclics have α_1-receptor blocking actions.

716. (B) Inhalational terbutaline (or other β_2-selective receptor agonists including albuterol, pirbuterol, bitolterol) are the agents of choice for treating bronchoconstriction in an acute asthma attack. The β_2-selective agonists produce bronchial relaxation by stimulating cyclic AMP formation in bronchiolar smooth muscle. β_2-selective agonists may be combined with ipratropium to enhance the bronchiolar relaxation. The use of aminophylline (choice A) and other methylxanthines in asthma has declined with the advent of better and safer drugs. Use of methylxanthines is prophylactic in that the drug must be used regularly to prevent acute episodes. The methylxanthines are not effective in terminating acute bronchoconstriction. Inhalational ipratropium (choice C) produces bronchial relaxation more slowly than the β_2 agonists and should not be the sole agent used to treat acute exacerbations. It may be combined with a β_2 agonist beneficially. Cromolyn sodium (choice D) is an agent that must be used prophylactically to prevent acute episodes. It is not a smooth muscle relaxing agent. Rather it appears to prevent release of histamine and other mediators of inflammation from mast cells. The β-blocker propranolol (choice E) would precipitate rather than relieve an acute episode in an asthmatic patient since bronchiolar relaxing activity is important in preventing and terminating acute episodes.

717. (A) Allopurinol and its metabolite alloxanthine inhibit xanthine oxidase, thus preventing conversion of xanthine and hypoxanthine to uric acid. Deposition of uric acid crystals in joints leads to acute gout attacks. By slowing the formation of uric acid, allopurinol prevents deposition of uric acid crystals in joints. Allopurinol is not useful in an acute gout attack; it must be used prophylactically. Sulfinpyrazone (choice B) is a uricosuric agent. Renal uric acid excretion is determined by the balance between the amount filtered plus that actively secreted and the amount undergoing passive and active reabsorption. At low doses, sulfinpyrazone inhibits active secretion and thus promotes retention of uric acid. At higher doses, both active secretion and active reabsorption are inhibited, with the result that excretion is enhanced. The decreased plasma level of uric acid prevents deposition of uric acid crystals or tophi. Combined use with probenecid will lower plasma uric acid levels to such an extent that uric acid tophi already present will shrink and disappear. Probenecid (choice C) is a uricosuric agent with an action similar to sulfinpyrazone. However, the combination of the two uricosuric agents is additive, allowing their combined use to greatly increase uric acid excretion. Probenecid was originally designed to inhibit active tubular secretion of penicillin and prolong the half-life of the antibiotic when that drug was in short supply, and it still finds use in this capacity today. Colchicine (choice D) is an inhibitor of microtubule function that brings relief in an acute gout attack by inhibiting the motility of granulocytes and preventing the formation of mediators of inflammation by leukocytes. Indomethacin (choice E) is a non-steroidal anti-inflammatory drug (NSAID) that, by inhibiting cyclo-oxygenase, prevents formation of prostaglandins and eicosanoids involved in the inflammatory process and pain perception in an acute episode of gouty arthritis.

718. (D) Colchicine is an inhibitor of microtubule function that brings relief in an acute gout attack by inhibiting the motility of granulocytes and preventing the formation of mediators of inflammation by leukocytes. Allopurinol (choice A) and its metabolite alloxanthine inhibit xanthine oxidase, thus preventing conversion of xanthine and hypoxanthine to uric acid. Deposition of uric acid crystals in joints leads to acute gout attacks. By slowing the formation of uric acid, allopurinol prevents deposition of uric acid crystals in joints. Allopurinol is not useful in an acute gout attack; it must be used prophylactically. Sulfinpyrazone (choice B) is a uricosuric agent. Renal uric acid excretion is determined by the balance between the amount of filtered plus that actively secreted and the amount undergoing passive and active reabsorption. At low doses, sulfinpyrazone inhibits active secretion and thus promotes retention of uric acid. At higher doses, both active secretion and active reabsorption are inhibited, with the result that excretion is enhanced. The decreased plasma level of uric acid prevents deposition of uric acid crystals or tophi. Combined use with probenecid will lower plasma uric acid levels to such an extent that uric acid tophi already present will shrink and disappear. Probenecid (choice C) is a uricosuric agent with an action similar to sulfinpyrazone. However, the combination of the two uricosuric agents is additive, allowing their combined use to greatly increase uric acid excretion. Probenecid was originally designed to inhibit active tubular secretion of penicillin and prolong the half-life of the antibiotic when that drug was in short supply, and it still finds use in this capacity today. Indomethacin (choice E) is a nonsteroidal anti-inflammatory drug (NSAID) that, by inhibiting cyclooxygenase, prevents formation of prostaglandins and eicosanoids involved in the inflammatory process and pain perception in an acute episode of gouty arthritis.

719. (B) One of the primary uses of H_1-receptor antagonists (antihistamines) is the symptomatic treatment of allergic rhinitis (hay fever). The older antihistamines have pronounced sedative actions (making them useful as OTC sleeping pills) and anticholinergic actions that may aid in reducing secretions but are otherwise usually annoying. The newer agents such as loratadine and astemizole are largely devoid of the sedative and anticholinergic activities. Treatment of peptic ulcer (choice A) is a property of the H_2-receptor antagonists such as cimetidine and ranitidine. Narcolepsy (choice C) is sleep disorder in which the affected individual falls asleep at inappropriate times during the day. It may arise from sleep apnea or other disorders that prevent restful sleep during the night. With their tendency to produce sedation, antihistamines would tend to exacerbate this condition. Although asthma involves activated mast cells that secrete histamine, H_1-receptor antagonists have only limited efficacy in the treatment of asthma (choice D). Rather the treatment of asthma involves bronchodilation or prevention of bronchoconstriction. Diabetes insipidus (choice E) is characterized by production of large quantities of dilute urine and may arise from inadequate secretion of vasopressin from the pituitary or an inadequate response to vasopressin at the kidney. Antihistamines have no effect in this disease.

720. (D) In a normally innervated bladder, parasympathetic activity will stimulate the detrusor muscle and relax the trigone and sphincter muscles, allowing emptying of the bladder. Sympathetic activity inhibits bladder control by producing opposing effects on the same muscles. The muscarinic agonist bethanechol will stimulate the urinary bladder. Bethanechol is preferred over carbachol and methacholine because it possesses less nicotinic activity at the ganglion level, thus reducing side effects. Pirenzipine (choice A) is an agent with antimuscarinic activity selective for the M_1-receptor subtype. It is used primarily as a research tool to identify muscarinic receptor subtype specificity when characterizing either receptors or their biological responses. Since there is no nerve releasing acetylcholine, pirenzipine should have no effect. Physostigmine (choice B) is a tertiary ammonium cholinesterase inhibitor. Inhibition of acetylcholinesterase will increase synaptic concentrations of acetylcholine previously released. Because it penetrates the blood–brain barrier, physostigmine finds use in counteracting the central as well as peripheral antimuscarinic actions of atropine and tricyclic antidepressant intoxication. Physostigmine has no effect in this patient, however, since there is no functional nerve to release acetylcholine. Atropine (choice C), the muscarinic receptor antagonist, would normally cause a decreased ability to void, but will be without effect in this patient in the absence of other drugs and without a nerve to release ACh. Atropine preadministration will block the actions of bethanechol in promoting voiding. Phenylephrine (choice E) is an α-receptor agonist that will cause contraction of the trigone and sphincter muscles and relax the detrusor muscle of the bladder, effects detrimental to emptying of the bladder.

721. (B) Labetolol blocks α_1-adrenoceptors as well as β_1- and β_2-adrenoceptors. The molecule contains two chiral centers and the clinically utilized preparations contain approximately equal amounts of the four enantiomers, each of which exhibits somewhat different receptor actions. The mixture provides α_1-selective antagonism, antagonism of β_1- and β_2-adrenoceptors and partial agonism at β_2-adrenoceptors, as well as inhibition of the presynaptic catecholamine transporter. Overall the β blockade is five- to tenfold greater than the α blockade. The blockade of α adrenoceptors as well as activation of vascular smooth muscle β_2-adrenoceptors in skeletal muscle decreases peripheral resistance, lowering arterial pressure, and the β-blocking actions prevent the reflex response of the heart.

722. (A) The pA_2 value is the negative logarithm of the concentration of a competitive antagonist required to cause an apparent doubling of the effective concentration at 50% response for the receptor agonist. This is a method for determination of the receptor affinity for the antagonist in terms of how the dose-response relationship for the agonist is altered by the presence of antagonist. It was extensively used before ligand-binding techniques were available. Assuming a 1:1 relationship between receptor occupancy and the response (i.e., no spare receptors), the pA_2 value should be equivalent to the negative logarithm of the dissociation constant for the inhibitor-receptor complex. Thus cardiac β adrenoceptors show a dissociation constant of 10^{-7} M whereas lung β adrenoceptors show a dissociation constant of 5×10^{-6} M for atenolol. This indicates that atenolol is more potent in blocking cardiac β adrenoceptors than lung β adrenoceptors. Choices B and E are incorrect as indicated above. Choices C and D are incorrect since they refer to efficacy. Efficacy is a property of agonists in defining the maximum response obtained. Antagonists do not have efficacies since they do not produce a response by themselves. They only alter the response to an agonist.

723. (E) In normally innervated pancreatic acini, parasympathetic activity will stimulate secretion and sympathetic activity will decrease secretion of digestive enzymes. The alkaloid pilocarpine has pronounced muscarinic agonist properties at exocrine glands. Hexamethonium (choice A) is a nicotinic blocking agent at ganglionic nicotinic sites. Ganglionic blocking agents were once used in the treatment of hypertension, but have been replaced by agents without the many side effects, such as bladder and gastrointestinal atony, cycloplegia, absence of sweating, and others, that ganglionic blockade entails. Hexamethonium will not affect secretion in the non-innervated pancreas. Physostigmine (choice B) is an anticholinesterase that stimulates pancreatic secretion in the presence of a functional parasympathetic nerve by preventing the breakdown of ACh released from the nerve. Without a functional nerve, physostigmine will have no effect. Botox (choice C) is a preparation from botulinum toxin that enters cholinergic nerve terminals and causes proteolysis of proteins necessary for exocytotic release of ACh. The result is an inhibition of acetylcholine release. This is the basis of the toxicity of botulinum toxin. Clinically Botox is used by local injection to provide temporary (weeks to months) relief from involuntary tics and to provide cosmetic treatment of facial frown lines. Botox would have no effect on this pancreas since there is no nerve releasing acetylcholine. Phenylephrine (choice D) is an α-adrenoceptor agonist that would be expected to inhibit release of digestive enzymes from the pancreas.

724. (C) Although there is no cholinergic innervation of most blood vessels, the endothelial cells have muscarinic receptors of the M_3

subtype. Activation of these receptors results in stimulated synthesis of nitric oxide (NO) that diffuses to vascular smooth muscle cells and promotes relaxation by raising cyclic GMP levels through activation of NO-stimulated guanylyl cyclase activity. The alkaloid pilocarpine is a muscarinic agonist that produces a large fall in blood pressure when given intravenously. Prazosin (choice A) is an α blocker that produces vasodilation through inhibition of the actions of norepinephrine at arteriolar α_1-adrenoceptors. Actions of NO are not involved. Isoproterenol (choice B) produces vasodilation by its agonistic actions on β_2-adrenoceptors in the vascular beds of skeletal muscle. Actions of NO are not involved. Diphenhydramine (choice D) is an H_1-receptor antagonist that blocks histamine-induced smooth muscle vasoconstriction and histamine-induced vasodilation produced by histamine stimulation of endothelial cells. Hexamethonium (choice E) is a nicotinic ganglionic blocker that will produce vasodilation by decreasing sympathetic tone to arteriolar smooth muscle. Actions of NO are not involved.

725. **(B)** The local anesthetic lidocaine will produce CNS depression, respiratory depression, seizures, and coma as plasma levels increase to toxic levels. Lidocaine is an amide class local anesthetic that is cleared by hepatic metabolism through cytochrome P450 oxidation and amidase activities rather than plasma metabolism (choice A). Memory device for local anesthetic classes and prototypes: L for *L*idocaine and *L*iver (metabolism); P for *P*rocaine and *P*lasma (metabolism), Pseudocholin*ester*ase (ester type). Choice C is incorrect in that lidocaine does not alter chloride channel conductance. It blocks fast sodium channels and prevents propagation of action potentials. Lidocaine does not cause hyperpolarization of neuronal membranes (choice D). It does not alter resting membrane potential; rather it prevents depolarization by blocking fast sodium channels. Lidocaine blocks conduction in the smaller unmyelinated C fibers before affecting the larger myelinated A fibers in nerve trunks rather than the reverse (choice E).

726. **(D)** To carry out such an examination, an agent that produces both cycloplegia (paralysis of the ciliary muscle) and mydriasis (pupillary dilation) is needed. Parasympathetic activity causes contraction of the ciliary muscle to allow focusing on near objects and contraction of the sphincter muscle of the iris to cause pupillary constriction or miosis. Sympathetic activity causes contraction of the radial muscle to produce pupillary dilation or mydriasis. Use of muscarinic antagonists to block parasympathetic tone causes both cycloplegia and mydriasis. Mydriasis may cause a mechanical obstruction of the outflow of aqueous humor and raise intraocular pressure, a danger in a patient with possible glaucoma. Both tropicamide and atropine (choice C) are muscarinic antagonists, but tropicamide has a shorter duration of action (hours versus days) so it is the preferred agent for use. Phentolamine (choice A) is an α-adrenoceptor antagonist that would produce miosis without cycloplegia. Phenylephrine (choice B) is an α-adrenoceptor agonist that would produce mydriasis without cycloplegia. Loratadine (choice E) is an H_1-receptor antagonist and is not useful in a refracted cycloplegic eye examination.

727. **(E)** Ethylene glycol, commonly used as antifreeze in cars, is metabolized to glycoaldehyde by alcohol dehydrogenase and then to glycolic (hydroxyacetic) acid by aldehyde dehydrogenase. Glycolic acid is further metabolized by α-hydroxyacid oxidase to glyoxylic acid. Glyoxylic acid can then be metabolized by lactate dehydrogenase to oxalic acid. Ethylene glycol is a CNS depressant. Its relatively low molecular weight means that ingestion of small amounts will generate high concentrations of metabolites, thus producing a profound metabolic acidosis. Treatment consists of sodium bicarbonate for the metabolic acidosis and measures to inhibit further metabolism. This may include ethanol as a competitive substrate for alcohol dehydrogenase or 4-methylpyrazole as an inhibitor. Hemodialysis may be useful. Methanol (choice A) follows a similar path of metabolism, with the toxic metabolites being formaldehyde and formic acid. Ethanol (choice B) is metabolized to acetaldehyde and acetic acid. Isopropanol (choice C) is slowly metabolized to acetone. Methylene chloride (choice D) is metabolized by cytochrome P450 to carbon monoxide.

728. **(D)** The benzodiazepine anxiolytic agents including diazepam appear to potentiate the actions of the inhibitory neurotransmitter GABA acting upon $GABA_A$ receptors in the opening of choride ion channels. Fluoxetine (choice A) is a selective inhibitor of serotonin uptake. Tranylcypromine (choice B) is an inhibitor of monoamine oxidase (MAO) rather than catechol-O-methyltransferase (COMT). Trifluoperazine (choice C) is a phenothiazine that is an antagonist for dopamine receptors. Pentobarbital (choice E) is a modulator of the GABA-sensitive chloride channel.

729. **(D)** The H_2-receptor antagonist cimetidine has been notorious for producing many drug–drug interactions at the level of cytochrome P450 inhibition by cimetidine and consequent increases in plasma concentrations of other P450 substrate drugs. Cimetidine was widely used to decrease gastric acid secretion in peptic ulcer disease. Because other H_2-receptor antagonists such as ranitidine and famotidine with little or no inhibition of P450 are now available, use of cimetidine has declined. Newer antibiotic regimens to eradicate *Helicobacter pylori,* a causative agent for peptic ulcers, have also contributed to a decline in use of H_2 blockers. Cromolyn sodium (choice A) is used in prophylaxis of asthma because of its ability to inhibit the release of histamine and other mediators of inflammation from mast cells. It is not a substrate or inhibitor of cytochrome P450. The drug is excreted unchanged in the urine and bile. Phenobarbital (choice B) produces many drug interactions because of its ability to induce (rather than inhibit) cytochrome P450 activity. Phenobarbital was widely used as a sedative-hypnotic and antiepileptic agent, but its use today is limited because of respiratory depression and drug interaction properties. Atracurium (choice C) is a competitive antagonist for nicotinic receptors at the neuromuscular junction. It is used to produce skeletal muscle relaxation during surgery. It is eliminated by a spontaneous chemical reaction and by plasma cholinesterases and is not a substrate or inhibitor of cytochrome P450. Diazepam (choice E) is used to treat anxiety and muscle spastic states by virtue of its ability to facilitate inhibitory actions exerted by the $GABA_A$ receptor at chloride channels. It is eliminated by cytochrome P450 metabolism but is not an inducer of activity. Although it may compete with other P450 substrates for metabolism, inhibition of metabolism of other drugs is not a major effect of diazepam or other benzodiazepines.

730. **(E)** Since the answer choices all involve alterations in Patient B, we assume that Patient A is the control. Without treatment, the heart rate for Patient B is slightly higher. This observation is consistent with block of parasympathetic tone by atropine (choice A). Pretreatment with the nonspecific monoamine oxidase (MAO) inhibitor tranylcypromine (choice B) will cause an accumulation of norepinephrine in synaptic vesicles. MAO inhibitors may, through effects on ganglionic transmission, reduce arterial blood pressure. Heart rate might then be slightly elevated. Pretreatment with the β-blocker propranolol (choice C) is not consistent since we would expect decreased heart rate with β blockade. Pretreatment with the α_1-blocker prazosin (choice D) might increase heart rate through a reflex response to decreased arterial pressure. The combination of atropine block and catecholamine transporter block by imipramine would be expected to cause a slight increase in heart rate.

When epinephrine is administered, the heart rate increases in the control Patient A. A larger increase in rate is seen in Patient B. The greater rate is consistent with atropine pretreatment since muscarinic blockade would prevent the reflex slowing following the rise in arterial pressure with the α-adrenoceptor effects of epinephrine. Pretreatment with tranylcypromine would not be expected to intensify the increase in heart rate with epinephrine treatment since MAO activity is not a controlling factor for circulating levels of catecholamines. Propranolol pretreatment is again ruled out since propranolol should block the increase in heart rate. Pretreatment with prazosin is consistent since the α-blockade of prazosin will allow the β-positive chronotropic actions of epinephrine to be unopposed by reflex slowing. The higher heart rate in Patient B is also consistent with pretreatment by imipramine since the tricyclic antidepressant, by blocking the catecholamine transporter uptake of epinephrine, will induce a greater stimulation of heart rate, in addition to having the reflex slowing blocked by the antimuscarinic effects.

Ephedrine is a non-catecholamine compound that has both indirect and direct agonistic properties. Its primary actions are produced when it enters sympathetic nerve terminals via the catecholamine transporter and displaces endogenous norepinephrine, thus producing the actions of norepinephrine released from nerve terminals. It also is a weak direct agonist for α- and β-adrenoceptors. Ephedrine treatment in the control produced a rise in heart rate nearly equal to that seen with epinephrine. In Patient B, we see only a slight increase in heart rate. This is not consistent with atropine pretreatment since we would expect the heart rate response to be similar to or greater than that seen with epinephrine. The response seen is also not consistent with tranylcypromine pretreatment because ephedrine should elicit a very large increase in heart rate (and arterial pressure) since the synaptic stores of norepinephrine are increased after MAO pretreatment. Propranolol pretreatment has already been ruled out above. The response seen is not consistent with prazosin pretreatment since this α blocker should not affect the ability of ephedrine to displace norepinephrine and increase heart rate. The response to ephedrine is consistent with imipramine pretreatment since the tricyclic will block the entry of ephedrine into sympathetic nerve terminals and prevent the displacement of norepinephrine. We would expect to see only the weak agonistic properties of ephedrine on chronotropicity. We are thus left with pretreatment with imipramine as the correct explanation.

731. (B) Addition of the glucuronic acid moiety to a drug will impart a negative charge, making the metabolite more polar and thus less able to be reabsorbed from the tubular urine back into the systemic circulation. Attachment of the glucuronic acid group may also turn the metabolite into a substrate for active tubular secretion by the organic acid secretion system. Diffusion across the placenta (choice A) is decreased because of the more polar nature of the glucuronide conjugate. Formation of the glucuronide will decrease rather than increase the oil:water partition coefficient (choice C), a measure of the lipid solubility of the compound. Formation of a glucuronide will decrease the ability of the drug to penetrate the blood–brain barrier (choice D) since penetration normally depends on high lipid solubility. In general, glucuronide conjugates have a shorter half-life (choice E) as compared with the parent compound because of the active tubular secretion and decreased reabsorption in the kidney.

732. (B) The intravenous anesthetic propofol shares the properties of rapid induction of anesthesia and brief duration of action with thiopental because both agents are highly lipid-soluble and are rapidly distributed to the brain via the relatively large percentage of cardiac output it receives. The drugs are redistributed from the brain to the skeletal muscle and eventually to adipose tissue as determined by the relative rates of perfusion for these tissues. Propofol is rapidly metabolized in the liver by glucuronide conjugation, but the controlling factor for the duration of action is the redistribution from brain to other tissues. Propofol is widely used for induction of anesthesia because of its rapidity of onset and rate of recovery, which is more rapid than that from thiopental. Propofol is devoid of major side effects and may be used for maintenance of anesthesia as well. Propofol is very hydrophobic as opposed to being hydrophilic (choice A). Propofol is metabolized primarily in the liver rather than in the blood (choice C). Propofol is not actively transported out of the choroid plexus (choice

D) and does not undergo active tubular secretion (choice E).

733. (C) Use of the dissociative anesthetic agent ketamine is associated with disagreeable dreams during and after recovery. Ketamine produces a feeling of being dissociated from the environment, and it is related chemically to the veterinary anesthetic phencylidine, a drug discontinued for human use because of the high frequency of hallucinations and psychological problems. Recovery from ketamine may take hours and may involve disturbing dreams and hallucinations that may recur for weeks. Coadministration of midazolam or another benzodiazepine lessens this occurrence. The frequency of these effects is lower in children. Ketamine is unusual among anesthetic agents in that it stimulates sympathetic nervous system activity rather than depressing it (choice A). Heart rate may increase by 25%. This property is considered useful for patients in shock. Ketamine exerts good amnesia and analgesia effects, even when consciousness is maintained (choice B). Its use is associated with increased muscle tone, making it a poor agent for production of skeletal muscle relaxation (choice D). Ketamine abolishes bronchospasm rather than causing it (choice E).

734. (D) The blood:gas partition coefficient is a measure of the solubility of the inhalation anesthetic in the blood. Blood provides the means of delivery to the brain. The solubility of the agent in blood determines how rapidly the partial pressure will rise in the blood. Agents with high solubility (large blood gas partition coefficients) require large amounts of the anesthetic to be put into the blood before the partial pressure in the blood will increase enough to effectively deliver the agent to the brain. Thus agents with lower blood solubilities (small blood:gas partition coefficients) will have more rapid rates of onset of anesthesia. Desirable properties for inhalation anesthetic agents include high potency and low blood solubility. The halogenated hydrocarbons such as desflurane and sevoflurane fit these criteria and are used extensively. The oil:gas partition coefficient (choice A) is a measure of the lipid solubility of the anesthetic agent. This correlates with the potency as measured by the MAC, the minimum alveolar concentration required for anesthesia. Hepatic metabolism (choice B) plays no role in onset of action, but may be important in terms of possible liver and kidney damage resulting from the production of toxic metabolites from some of the halogenated inhalational anesthetic agents. The organ system distribution from the blood (choice C) does not play a role in the rate of onset for inhalational general anesthetic agents, unlike the situation with thiopental and propofol, where high lipid solubility and relative tissue perfusion rates cause distribution and redistribution to be primary determinants of rates of onset and recovery. The MAC value (choice E) is a measure of the potency of the agent, but does not give an indication of the rate of onset for an agent.

735. (E) The MAC value for nitrous oxide is 105% (atmospheric partial pressure) meaning that for nitrous oxide to be used as the sole anesthetic agent, hyperbaric conditions must be used to deliver both the nitrous oxide for anesthesia and oxygen for life. The other commonly used inhalational agents, including enflurane, isoflurane, halothane, and sevoflurane (choices A–D) have MAC values of 6% or less. Although these data might be interpreted to imply that nitrous oxide is not useful in anesthesia, it is highly valued because of its pronounced analgesic actions at subanesthetic levels. It is usefully combined with other inhalational agents that possess less analgesic activity.

736. (C) The agent of choice in treating simple hypothyroidism is levothyroxine (T_4). Administered thyroxine is bound in plasma in the same way and metabolized to triiodothyronine in the same manner as native thyroxine. Although T_3 is more active as a thyroid hormone, its shorter half-life of one day as compared with the T_4 half-life of six to seven days means that thyroxine has a longer duration of action. The use of synthetic forms of thyroxine also allows more precise dosages to be administered. T_4 (3,5,3′,5′-tetraiodothyronine) is converted by deiodinases to the active T_3 (3,5,3′-triiodothyronine) and the inactive reverse T_3 (3,3′,5′-triiodothyronine) in equal amounts (choice A). Desiccated thyroid (choice B) from animal sources was once used in the treatment of hypothyroidism. That practice is now abandoned because the thyroid hormone content of such preparations was highly variable from batch to batch. T_3 (choice D) is utilized under special circumstances when immediate actions of thyroid hormone are desired, but it is not generally used to treat hypothyroidism because of its higher cost and shorter duration of action relative to levothyroxine. At high concentrations, iodide in the form of potassium (choice E) or other salts is an inhibitor of thyroid gland function. Iodide inhibits its own uptake into thyroid cells and inhibits the release of thyroxine and triiodothyronine from the gland. Escape from iodide inhibitions occurs so that iodide cannot be used to treat chronic hyperthyroidism. Iodide treatment is useful in preparation for surgical thyroidectomy since the gland becomes firmer and vascularity is reduced. In the event of a nuclear accident, administration of 100 mg of potassium iodide to children in an exposure area to prevent uptake of radioactive iodine will decrease the later risk of thyroid cancer.

737. **(D)** The iodine radioisotopes ^{131}I and ^{125}I are generated in nuclear reactions. These radioisotopes gain entry into the body by direct exposure and ingestion of liquids and foods from sources that have been exposed (e.g., drinking milk from exposed cows). When these isotopes gain entry into the body, they will accumulate in the thyroid gland where their decay generates ionizing radiation that is genotoxic and may ultimately lead to thyroid cancer. Prevention of exposure is the best strategy, but this may not be possible with a large-scale radioactive release near a densely populated region. The therapeutic strategy is to administer iodide before and during acute exposure. This results in a dilution of the radioactive iodide, but more importantly, high concentrations of iodide have the effect of inhibiting iodide uptake by the thyroid gland. The usefulness of this strategy was shown in European areas downwind of Chernobyl after the 1986 release of radioisotopes, when pre-exposure administration of potassium iodide to children resulted in many fewer cases of thyroid cancer than might otherwise have occurred. Propylthiouracil (choice A) is a thiourylene antithyroid agent that inhibits the peroxidase reactions of organification and coupling involved in thyroid hormone synthesis. It is useful in the treatment of hyperthyroidism prior to partial surgical removal or radioiodine ablation of the thyroid gland or in anticipation of spontaneous remission of Graves' disease. Levothyroxine (choice B) is the synthetic version of thyroxine and is the agent of choice for thyroid hormone replacement in simple hypothyroidism. The β-blocker propranolol (choice C) is used in treatment of thyroid storm to decrease the elevated heart rate that arises with the hyperactivity of the sympathetic nervous system with thyroid hormone excess. It serves no useful purpose in preventing thyroid cancer. Dessicated thyroid (choice E) is a preparation from animal thyroid glands that was used to treat hypothyroidism before the advent of levothyroxine. Use of this form is to be avoided since the available content of thyroid hormone may be highly variable.

738. **(A)** Liddle's syndrome is an autosomal dominant disease in which there is hyperactivity of the apical sodium channel in the principal cells in the cortical collecting duct due to mutations in the β subunit. These mutations cause the ubiquitin-dependent proteolytic turnover of the sodium channel protein to become reduced, with a resulting excess in activity. Treatment consists of direct inhibition of the sodium channel by either amiloride or triamterene, both of which are classified as potassium-sparing diuretics. Hydrochlorothiazide (choice B), a thiazide diuretic, would exacerbate the problem since inhibition of the Na^+-$C1^-$-symporter in the distal convoluted tubule would result in delivery of more sodium to the cortical collecting duct, where the hyperactivity of the sodium channel and resulting potassium extrusion along with increased proton exchange from type A intercalated cells would result in greater hypokalemia and alkalosis. Spironolactone (choice C) is a synthetic steroid that acts as an antagonist at the aldosterone receptor. It is used as a potassium-sparing diuretic. In the case of Liddle's disease, spironolactone has no utility since aldosterone does not play a primary role and its levels are depressed. Lisinopril (choice D) is an ACE inhibitor that is used in the treatment of essential hypertension. Since the problem in Liddle's disease is specific to sodium channel hyperactivity within the principal cells in the cortical collecting duct, use of an ACE inhibitor would not correct the pathophysiology underlying the hypokalemia and metabolic alkalosis. Fludrocortisone (choice E) is a synthetic mineralocorticoid used for replacement therapy of hypoaldosteronism. Although aldosterone levels are reduced in this patient, administration of a mineralocorticoid will exacerbate rather than relieve the hypertension and hypokalemic metabolic alkalosis.

739. **(A)** Streptokinase is a protein produced by β-hemolytic streptococci. It has no intrinsic enzymatic activity, but instead forms a stable complex with plasminogen that is enzymatically active in cleaving free plasminogen to plasmin. The streptokinase-plasminogen complex is not inhibited by antiplasmin. The other thrombolytic agents, tissue plasminogen activator (tPA) and urokinase, are enzymatically active by themselves. Conversion of plasmin to plasminogen (choice B) is an incorrect choice since it is plasminogen that is converted to plasmin in the thrombolytic actions. Heparin exerts its anticoagulant actions by providing a template for the combination of thrombin and antithrombin III (choice C). Inhibition of cyclo-oxygenase activity (choice D) is a property of the non-steroidal anti-inflammatory drugs (NSAIDs) that contributes to prevention of platelet aggregation and thrombosis. Competitive blocking of binding of plasminogen to fibrin (choice E) is a property of aminocaproic acid (AMICAR), a lysine analog used to inhibit fibrinolysis, and apolipoprotein A, a variant form of LDL that produces a procoagulant state by preventing the interaction of plasminogen with fibrin.

740. **(D)** Gingival hyperplasia is seen in 20% of patients receiving chronic phenytoin. It is the most common symptom of phenytoin toxicity in children and adolescents. Other manifestations of toxicity include ataxia, diplopia, nystagmus, and vertigo. Metabolic effects that phenytoin may produce include hyperglycemia (by inhibiting insulin release from the pancreas), and osteomalacia (loss of bone mineralization), by altering vitamin D metabolism and increasing the metabolism of vitamin K, a factor necessary for production of bone proteins and four coagulation factors. Postural hypotension (choice A) is not an adverse effect of phenytoin. Postural hypotension can be produced by antihypertensive agents that work peripherally rather than centrally, as well as antipsychotic agents such as the phenothiazines that have α_1-adrenoceptor blocking actions. Hyperprolactinemia (choice B) is an adverse effect of antipsychotic agents such as the phenothiazines, which are antagonists at dopamine receptors, since dopamine exerts negative control of prolactin secretion at the anterior pituitary. It is not an effect of phenytoin toxicity. Rigidity and tremor (choice C) are symptoms of parkinsonism. These symptoms may be produced by dopamine antagonists such as antipsychotic agents, but are not associated with phenytoin toxicity. Polydipsia and polyuria (choice E) are symptoms of diabetes insipidus. These symptoms may be produced by lithium toxicity during treatment of bipolar depression. They are not associated with phenytoin toxicity.

741. **(E)** α-Tocopherol, the most active of the natural tocopherols, becomes associated with lipoprotein particles after dietary absorption. Because it is lipophilic and is associated with lipoprotein particles, it can function effectively as an antioxidant to prevent peroxidation of unsaturated fatty acids, a process leading to production of modified forms of LDL that undergo endocytosis by the scavenger receptors of macrophages. These events are currently thought to be involved in the initial stages of atherogenesis. In the limited studies to date, supplementation of the diet with α-tocopherol appears to provide cardioprotection. Although vitamin A (choice A) is lipid-soluble and has antioxidant properties, the more important physiological roles for the various forms of vitamin A seem to lie in control of cell differentiation and proliferation (retinoic acid) and vision (retinal). In vitro studies of β-carotene (choice B) have demonstrated antioxidant properties for this precursor of vitamin A, but clinical trials of β-carotene have not demonstrated efficacy in cardioprotection and have implicated β-carotene in increasing the risk of lung cancer. Vitamin C or ascorbic acid (choice C) is water-soluble and functions as an antioxidant in the aqueous phase of cells, and as a cofactor for many hydroxylation biosynthetic reactions. Vitamin D (choice D) is a positive regulator of calcium homeostasis in the body. It does not possess antioxidant activity.

742. **(E)** Dihydropyridine dehydrogenase activity is present in the intestinal mucosa and liver. This enzyme converts 5-fluorouracil (5-FU) to a fluoro-dihydrouracil form that is subsequently converted to fluoro-alanine. Patients with an inherited deficiency of this enzyme were found to be highly sensitive to 5-FU. Inhibition of this enzyme by coadministration of compounds such as eniluracil allows oral 5-FU to be used effectively for treatment of a variety of cancers. Thymidylate kinase (choice A) is an enzyme involved in the eventual conversion of the antiretroviral agent zidovudine to its deoxynucleotide triphosphate, the form active in inhibiting reverse transcriptase. Zidovudine monophosphate acts as a competitive inhibitor of thymidylate kinase with resulting reduction in levels of TTP. This effect contributes to the antiviral activity. The cytochrome P4501A12 system is involved with the oxidation of certain drugs, such as acetaminophen, by the liver. It does not actively participate in the metabolism of 5-fluorouracil. Xanthine oxidase (choice C) is the enzyme responsible for converting hypoxanthine and xanthine to uric acid. Inhibition of xanthine oxidase by allopurinol is used as a strategy in gout for preventing formation of uric acid tophi, and in ischemic injury to reduce the formation of pathogenic reactive oxygen species. Dihydrofolate reductase (choice D) is the enzyme that converts dihydrofolate to tetrahydrofolate, a step necessary for one-carbon metabolism in the synthesis of purines and pyrimidines. This enzyme is a target for inhibition by the antibacterial agent trimethoprim and the antitumor/antiarthritic agent methotrexate.

743. **(E)** Parkinsonian syndrome is a common adverse effect whose occurrence is predictable from the dopaminergic blocking actions of the neuroleptics. The syndrome, which is characterized by akinesia and rigidity, particularly in the facial muscles, can be treated with a centrally acting muscarinic antagonist such as benztropine. Tardive dyskinesia (choice A) is a late-occurring syndrome that is most frequently seen in elderly female patients with chronic treatment. The syndrome is characterized by choreoathetoid movements that appear to arise as a consequence of dopamine supersensitivity in the basal ganglia. Because there is no satisfactory treatment of the condition, prevention is crucial. Akathisia (choice B) or motor restlessness is an early occurring adverse effect that is treated by reduction of the dose or changing the neuroleptic. It must be differentiated from agitation, since the latter would be treated by increasing the dose of neuroleptic. Acute dystonic reactions (choice C) are the earliest-occurring adverse effects of neuroleptic treatment. They are characterized by spasms of the muscles of the face, tongue, neck, and back. The dystonia may be treated with a centrally acting antihistamine such as diphenhydramine. Clonidine, an α_2-adrenoceptor agonist, has no role in the treatment of these adverse effects of neuroleptic agents, since the control of fine motor function involves dopamine and acetylcholine as neurotransmitters. Neuroleptic malignant syndrome (choice D) is a rare condition that presents a medical emergency because there is a 10% fatality rate. It is characterized by catatonia and fluctuations in blood pressure and heart rate. The first step in the treatment is to stop administration of the neuroleptic.

Muscle relaxants such as benzodiazepines or dantrolene may help. Bromocriptine may also be useful. Muscarinic agonists such as pilocarpine would exacerbate the situation, since the pathophysiology in the basal ganglia arises from dopamine receptor blockade with resulting excess cholinergic activity.

744. (C) The total plasma clearance of the drug is the product of the volume of distribution times the elimination rate constant ($CL_{TOTAL} = V_d \times k_e$). The elimination rate constant k_e is found by using the relationship $k_e = \ln(2)/t_{1/2}$ where ln(2) is the natural logarithm of 2 (or approximately 0.7) and $t_{1/2}$ is the half-life (seven hours in this case). The value for k_e is therefore (10 liters × 0.1 per hr) or 1 liter/hr. This is equivalent to 1000 mL/60 min or about 17 mL/min. Since we are given that the renal clearance value is 8.5 mL/min, hepatic metabolism must account for the remaining 8.5 mL/min. Thus, hepatic metabolism accounts for 50% of the total drug elimination.

745. (E) Clearance is defined as the apparent volume of blood or plasma per unit time that is completely emptied of drug. Although the actual mechanisms involved do not function in such a manner, clearance is a theoretical construct that is highly useful in pharmacokinetics. If nitrendipine is completely absorbed but shows only 10% bioavailability, 90% of the drug must have been cleared in the first pass through the liver. Since hepatic blood flow is 1500 mL/min, the hepatic clearance must be 90% of that value or 1350 mL/min.

746. (C) The plasma level is already at 60% of the target concentration. To achieve 100% of the target of 500 mg/mL quickly, we must administer 40% of the loading dose, since a loading dose is defined as that amount given in one dose that will achieve 100% of the target plasma concentration. To maintain the patient at this new steady state level, the maintenance dosing regimen must be 50 mg/hr. There is a direct relationship between the maintenance dosing regimen and the steady state plasma level. If the steady state level must be increased by 67% (from 300 µg/mL to 500 µg/mL), the maintenance dose must also increase proportionally by 67% (from 30 mg/hr to 50 mg/hr).

747. (B) The urinary excretion of organic acids is increased by alkalinization of urine with sodium bicarbonate administration. This is because higher urinary pH values favor the formation of the charged, anionic form over the uncharged protonated form of organic acids. The charged, anionic form is prevented from being reabsorbed from the tubular urine by its polar nature and is thus "pH-trapped" in alkaline urine, causing increased urinary excretion. This strategy of alkalizing the urine to promote renal excretion is used for overdoses of organic acids such as salicylic acid and phenobarbital, but is only effective in producing large scale increases in excretion when the pKa of the acid lies within the normal limits of urinary pH values of 5 to 8. The presence of aspirin (choice A) at doses used to treat a headache will inhibit the renal excretion of organic acids, since aspirin at low doses will compete for the active tubular secretion system for organic acids. Administration of ammonium chloride (choice C) is a strategy used in drug intoxication to hasten the urinary excretion of organic bases. Through a series of biochemical steps involving synthesis of glutamine in the liver and deamination in the kidney to cause renal excretion of ammonia and a proton, ammonium chloride produces an acidification of urine. This will cause pH-trapping of organic bases in the urine and promote their excretion. Urinary acidification will slow the excretion of an organic acid, since more of the acid will be in the protonated or uncharged form that is more easily reabsorbed from tubular urine. Probenecid (choice D) is an organic acid that will compete with other organic acids at the level of the active tubular secretion system for organic acids, thus inhibiting their renal excretion. Probenecid is used in this way to inhibit the renal excretion of penicillins, thereby prolonging their duration of action. Probenecid used at high doses is also effective in promoting renal excretion of uric acid through inhibition of the active uptake system that normally allows uric acid to be reabsorbed from tubular urine. Inulin (choice E) is an organic molecule that undergoes filtration without reabsorption in the kidney. It is used to measure glomerular filtration rates, and its presence in the kidney will not affect the excretion of organic acids.

748. (B) By inhibiting the metabolism of drug X, cimetidine will cause an increase in its plasma half-life. Because it inhibits the P450-dependent metabolism of a wide variety of drugs, cimetidine has achieved a notoriety of sorts in terms of producing drug interaction problems. The newer H_2 antagonists such as ranitidine and famotidine do not share this P450-inhibitory activity. A shift in the dose-response curve to the right (choice A) is incorrect. Coadministration of cimetidine will cause the dose-response curve to be shifted to the left since the administered doses of drug X will have a greater average plasma concentration. This effect would be particularly evident if drug X normally exhibits extensive first-pass metabolism. The systemic clearance of drug X (choice C) will be decreased rather than increased by the addition of cimetidine since the metabolism of drug X will be decreased. The volume of distribution of drug X (choice D) should not change with coadministration of cimetidine. This statement must be tempered somewhat since the volume of distribution is a calculated value whose determination depends on the slope of the elimination curve. It is possible for a change in half-life to cause a change in the calculated volume of distribution. It is not possible to predict a priori what the effect will be. Clearly answer B is the most obvious correct choice. The efficacy of drug X (choice E) is a measure of the maximum response that the drug will produce. Changes in the elimination rate will have no effect on the maximum response, although decreased metabolism will decrease the concentration of drug X needed to achieve the maximum response.

749. (C) The volume of distribution is calculated by dividing the amount present in the body by the plasma concentration. If a drug is highly lipophilic, it will partition out of the blood and into tissues such as brain and fat. This results in a very low concentration measured in the plasma and may yield an impossibly large value for the volume of distribution. In such a case, the calculated volume is an apparent rather than real volume. Other mechanisms such as active uptake by tissues or tight binding to structural components such as bone or extracellular matrix may also result in very large calculated volumes of distribution. Extensive binding to plasma proteins (choice A) results in a very low calculated volume of distribution since much of the total drug is trapped in the plasma. A similar distribution throughout the body (choice B) is incorrect since the drug must distribute differently between blood and other tissues for the volume of distribution to exceed total body water. Zero-order kinetics (choice D) is incorrect since the calculation of the volume of distribution assumes that first order kinetics apply, allowing the low (concentration) versus time curve to be extrapolated in a linear fashion to time zero. Excretion in the kidney without reabsorption (choice E) is incorrect since most drugs with large volumes of distribution are highly lipophilic molecules that must be cleared by hepatic metabolism since they undergo extensive reabsorption in the kidney.

750. (D) One mechanism for the production of vasodilation involves an increase in cyclic GMP (cGMP) levels in vascular smooth muscle cells, causing relaxation. The organic nitrates and nitroprusside (nitrovasodilators) increase cGMP levels by generating nitric oxide (NO) that subsequently activates a soluble form of guanylyl cyclase. Activation of muscarinic receptors on vascular endothelial cells results in formation of NO (earlier identified as endothelial-derived relaxing factor) that diffuses to smooth muscle cells and relaxes them through increased cGMP levels. Erection of the penis involves neuronally regulated formation of NO, increased cGMP levels in the corpus cavernosum, and relaxation of vascular smooth muscle to increase local blood flow in erectile tissue. Rather than acting at the level of guanylyl cyclase, sildenafil (Viagra) acts as a selective inhibitor of cGMP phosphodiesterase type 5 to enhance the actions of NO-stimulated cGMP levels. The fact that sildenafil acts downstream of NO stimulation of guanylyl cyclase accounts for the toxic interactions between nitrovasodilators and sildenafil. The mechanism for relaxation of vascular smooth muscle by hydralazine (choice A) is unknown although it does not involve NO or prostaglandin I_2. Speculations have included interference with calcium entry and activation of transcription of unknown factors to cause an increase in cGMP levels. Prazosin (choice B) produces vasodilation by inhibiting α_1 adrenoceptors on arteriolar smooth muscle to block sympathetic nervous system activation of vasoconstriction. Nitroprusside (choice C) is a nitrovasodilator as described above. Its metabolism generates NO by a mechanism distinct from that used by the organic nitrates. Minoxidil (choice E) is metabolized to minoxidil-O-sulfate which activates an ATP-sensitive potassium channel in smooth muscle. The outflow of potassium produces hyperpolarization and subsequent relaxation of smooth muscle cells.

751. (B) A normally functioning endocrine pancreas will provide a low basal level of circulating insulin and spikes of insulin release triggered by the ingestion of food. Use of morning and evening injections of a slow insulin form (ultralente) will provide a basal level of circulating insulin attributable to the slow release properties of this insulin preparation. The pre-meal injections of regular insulin will provide the spikes of circulating insulin needed to deal with the dietary glucose load. Regular insulin is needed here because the release kinetics from either the intermediate or slow forms do not provide a sufficiently high circulating level of insulin to control the blood glucose level nor to provide adequate control of the enzymes of glucose homeostasis after a meal.

752. (D) Diabetic neuropathy may result in deep severe pain sensations. Extreme pain usually subsides after a period of months to a few years. Treatment of the pain presents a therapeutic dilemma since opioid analgesics may be needed but addiction is a strong possibility. Analgesia along with the addictive properties is associated with μ-type opioid receptors. Of the analgesics listed, codeine is a weak agonist at μ receptors, whereas the other opioid analgesics are full agonists. Therefore codeine is less efficacious but also has the lowest addiction and abuse liability and would be the agent of choice within this list. Meperidine (choice A) is a synthetic μ opioid receptor agonist with high addictive liability. Morphine (choice B) is the prototype μ opioid receptor agonist and possesses high addictive liability. Diphenoxylate (choice C) is a congener of meperidine that is used to control gastrointestinal hypermotility. At its therapeutic dose levels, no morphine-like effects are observed. Methadone (choice E) is a μ opioid receptor agonist with good oral efficacy and a long plasma half-life (15 to 40 hr). It is used in treatment of heroin addicts.

753. (B) Metoclopramide has dopamine receptor antagonistic properties that include blocking emesis induced by apomorphine and producing hyperprolactinemia. It does not possess useful antipsychotic activity, but high doses may produce extrapyramidal symptoms that are controlled with antimuscarinic agents such as diphenhydramine and benztropine. Metoclopramide is effective against severe chemotherapy-induced emesis. The complaint of the patient indicates that she is suffering from gastroparesis and esophageal reflux as a result of diabetic peripheral neuropathy. Metoclopramide increases the motility of smooth muscle from the esophagus to small bowel and would therefore be effective in treating this patient. Diphenhydramine (choice A) is an antihistamine (H_1 blocker) with antimuscarinic activity that is useful in treating extrapyramidal symptoms of dopamine receptor blockers as indicated above. Diphenhydramine itself possesses weak antiemetic activity, but may be used effectively in combination with other agents such as metoclopramide to reduce the dosage, and therefore the adverse effects, of the other agent. In the gastrointestinal tract, diphenhydramine would produce hypomotility because of its antimuscarinic activity. Kaolin (choice C) is an adsorbent agent widely used as an antidiarrheal, although agents such as diphenoxylate and loperamide are more effective. It does not possess antiemetic activity. Scopolamine (choice D) is a muscarinic receptor antagonist with weak antiemetic properties. It would produce hypomotility of the gastrointestinal tract. Neostigmine (choice E) is a reversible inhibitor of cholinesterases. It would stimulate motility in the gastrointestinal tract but would produce no antiemetic effect.

754. (E) *Pseudomonas aeruginosa* is an aerobic gram-negative bacterium that is frequently the causative agent in diabetic malignant external otitis. Increased susceptibility to infection in diabetes probably arises through impairment of leukocyte function with poor glycemic control. Such *P. aeruginosa* infections are best treated with a broad-spectrum β-lactam cell wall synthesis inhibitor such as ticarcillin in combination with a broad-spectrum aminoglycoside such as tobramycin. Tetracycline (choice A) is a bacteriostatic protein synthesis inhibitor. When first introduced, tetracycline was effective in treating *Pseudomonas*, but now all strains are resistant. Chloramphenicol (choice B) is a bacteriostatic protein synthesis inhibitor. *P. aeruginosa* is resistant to chloramphenicol. Nafcillin + kanamycin (choice C) is a combination of a penicillinase-resistant penicillin plus a limited spectrum aminoglycoside. Nafcillin is useful in treating penicillinase-producing staphylococcal infections, but does not possess a broad enough antibacterial spectrum to treat *P. aeruginosa.* Kanamycin is not effective against *P. aeruginosa.* Sulfamethoxazole + trimethoprim (choice D) is a combination of folate synthesis inhibitor plus dihydrofolate reductase inhibitor that is effective in treating urinary tract infections. *P. aeruginosa* is resistant to this combination.

755. (B) The hydroxymethylglutaryl-CoA (HMG CoA) reductase inhibitor lovastatin and the bile acid-binding resin cholestyramine both exert their effects through lowering the intrahepatocytic concentration of cholesterol, but by different mechanisms. Inhibition of HMG CoA reductase by the statins prevents hepatocytes from synthesizing cholesterol from HMG CoA. Bile acid binding in the intestinal lumen produces a depletion of intracellular bile acid and consequent increased conversion of cholesterol to bile acid. In both cases, the lowering of intracellular cholesterol levels results in a loss of oxysterol repression of the transcription of the genes for LDL receptor and HMG CoA reductase. The increased expression and activity of LDL receptor lowers circulating LDL-cholesterol levels through increased endocytosis of the lipoprotein particles. Because the two agents lower intracellular cholesterol by different mechanisms, along with the ability of the statin to inhibit increased HMG CoA reductase activity, the effects of the combination in lowering LDL-cholesterol levels are additive or synergistic. The combination of chlortetracycline and amoxicillin (choice A) would provide an antagonism of antibacterial action. The β-lactam cell wall synthesis inhibitors such as the penicillins and cephalosporins are bactericidal, but are effective only when the bacteria are rapidly proliferating. Tetracyclines are bacteriostatic agents that slow or inhibit the growth of bacterial cells by inhibiting protein synthesis. The combination of clomiphene and chorionic gonadotropin (choice C) would not produce any beneficial additive action. Both agents are used to treat female infertility. Clomiphene is an estrogen receptor antagonist that functions at the level of the hypothalamus to stimulate release of gonadotropin-releasing hormone (GnRH). The increased release of GnRH results in increased release of the gonadotropins LH and FSH from the anterior pituitary. This results in stimulation of ovulation. Administration of chorionic gonadotropin also stimulates ovulation. Since both preparations function through increases in gonadotropin levels and both are present at their effective concentrations, there would not be a beneficial additive effect. Succinylcholine and atracurium (choice D) are both skeletal muscle-relaxing agents that block muscle contraction at the neuromuscular junction. Succinylcholine is a depolarizing blocker that acts as a long-lasting agonist at the nicotinic receptor. Atracurium is a competitive antagonist at the same receptor. Since both are blocking function at the same receptor and are present at their effective concentrations, there would not be any beneficial additive effect. The combination of pentazocine and morphine (choice E) would not produce a beneficial interaction. Pentazocine exerts its pain-relieving activity by being a weak agonist at μ opioid receptors. Morphine is a full agonist at the same receptors. When the two analgesic agents are combined, pentazocine acts as an antagonist for morphine at μ receptors. The result is precipitation of withdrawal in addicted patients and dysphoria and loss of morphine analgesia in nonaddicted patients.

756. (D) If we choose a toxic response value of about 2% (this occurs at a concentration of about 3×10^{-7} M), we can see that drug X provides a therapeutic response in about 98% of the population whereas drug Y provides a response in about 23% of the population. Thus by using doses that yield this concentration, we can provide effective therapy in 98% of the population and expect only 2% of the population to show signs of toxicity. A more conservative approach might be to use doses yielding concentrations effective in 90% of the population, where we expect less than 1% occurrence of toxicity. Clearly by this criterion, drug X is the better drug to use. Drug Y has a smaller, rather than larger, therapeutic index than drug X (choice A). The therapeutic index is calculated as the ratio of LC_{50}/EC_{50} where LC refers to lethal concentration and EC refers to the effective concentration. The subscript numbers refer to the percent of the population responding. In this case, we are defining the therapeutic index in terms of TC_{50}/EC_{50} where TC refers to the toxic concentration. The EC_{50} (found at the midpoint) for drug X is 1×10^{-8} M. The EC_{50} for drug Y is 1×10^{-6} M. The TC_{50} for both is 1×10^{-5} M. Thus the therapeutic indexes for drug X and drug Y are 10^3 and 10, respectively. Drug X has the larger therapeutic index, and by this criterion, is the safer drug. Toxicity for both drugs is unlikely to be the result of over-stimulation of the same receptor for which they are agonists (choice B) because mass action considerations would predict that the toxicity curve for each drug should be displaced the same distance from its respective effective curve. In the graph, we see that the toxic response curves are superimposed. It is more likely that toxicity is expressed through a receptor or site of action distinct from that producing the therapeutic response. Drug X is not more efficacious than drug Y (choice C). We are told that both agonists produce the same maximum response, indicating that they have the same efficacy. Potency rather than efficacy is determined by the relative position of the midpoint of the response curve. Choice E is incorrect since, at their respective EC_{50} levels, drug X should produce toxicity in 0% of the population, whereas drug Y should produce toxicity in about 8% of the population.

757. (D) Use of hydrochlorothiazide will provide mild diuresis to reduce sodium and water retention in this patient. The thiazide diuretics inhibit the Na^+-$C1^-$-symporter in the distal convoluted tubule. This results in less sodium and water resorption in this region of the kidney. The increased delivery of sodium to the cortical collecting duct will lead to increased potassium exchange and subsequent K^+ excretion in the urine. Hypokalemia increases the risk of adverse reactions with the cardiac glycosides since they function through inhibition of Na^+/K^+-ATPase. A decrease in serum potassium ion allows toxic levels of the cardiac glycosides to bind to the ATPase. The concurrent administration of a potassium-sparing diuretic such as triamterene will prevent thiazide-induced hypokalemia. Chlorothiazide alone (choice A) will provide diuresis, but brings the risk of cardiac glycoside toxicity as indicated above. Chlorothiazide plus ibuprofen (choice B) presents a problem since non-steroidal anti-inflammatory drugs (NSAIDs) such as ibuprofen, by inhibiting cyclo-oxygenase and the production of prostaglandins, cause resistance to diuretic actions. Triamterene (choice C) is a potassium-sparing diuretic as detailed above. Its diuretic actions alone are not sufficient to treat the patient. Furosemide (choice

E) is a high ceiling or loop diuretic that inhibits the Na^+-K^+-$2Cl^-$-symporter in the thick ascending limb of the loop of Henle. Its use produces a profound sodium diuresis with attendant high risk of hypokalemia. Furosemide is effective as a single diuretic in the treatment of advanced congestive heart failure, but, because of its great efficacy, patients need to be closely monitored for electrolyte and fluid balance. Because the patient described is being treated as an outpatient with close monitoring not practical, a less efficacious diuretic is indicated.

758. (E) With constant infusion of drug X, we observe an increase in systolic pressure indicative of an increase in cardiac output. Increased cardiac output indicates an increase in cardiac function that might result from an agent exhibiting positive inotropicity. Epinephrine acts on cardiac β_1 adrenoceptors to stimulate inotropicity. The decrease in diastolic pressure indicates that peripheral resistance has decreased. Epinephrine acts on β_2 adrenoceptors in skeletal muscle to relax vascular smooth muscle. Since skeletal muscle constitutes a large percentage of the body mass, total peripheral resistance will decrease even though epinephrine also acts on α_1 adrenoceptors in arterioles throughout the body to produce vasoconstriction. Note that this effect of reducing total peripheral resistance is dependent on the concentration of epinephrine. At higher epinephrine concentrations, an increase in total peripheral resistance would be observed. This concentration dependence of action is attributable to the differences in affinity of the α_1 and β_2 adrenoceptors for epinephrine, with β_2 receptors having a higher affinity and therefore responding at lower epinephrine concentrations. The large pulse pressure (the difference between systolic and diastolic) and small effect on mean pressure are characteristic of epinephrine. With the bolus injection, epinephrine initially produces increases in both systolic and diastolic pressures. As the plasma epinephrine concentration declines with time, the systolic pressure rapidly decreases toward the baseline value whereas diastolic pressure remains depressed for a longer period due to the higher affinity of the β_2 adrenoceptors for epinephrine. Phenylephrine (choice A) is an α_1-adrenoceptor agonist. It would increase diastolic pressure by increasing total peripheral resistance. It should have little direct effect on the heart, but the increase in diastolic pressure will cause a reflex bradycardia and negative inotropicity. Acetylcholine (choice B) will decrease total peripheral resistance through activation of vascular muscarinic receptors (present in spite of the lack of cholinergic innervation), and cause relaxation of vascular smooth muscle mediated through formation of nitric oxide and a rise in smooth muscle intracellular cyclic GMP levels. Acetylcholine will directly depress cardiac function, but reflex activation of the sympathetic nervous system will attenuate these effects. Generally, high concentrations of acetylcholine are needed to elicit any response, because acetylcholine is hydrolyzed very rapidly by plasma cholinesterase activity. Norepinephrine (choice C) will stimulate the heart to cause an increase in systolic pressure, but it also produces a large increase in total peripheral resistance, thereby raising diastolic pressure. Norepinephrine is bound by β_2 receptors with poor affinity so that β_2 effects are not evident in its actions. Amphetamine (choice D), because it displaces norepinephrine from adrenergic nerve terminals, produces similar responses to those of norepinephrine. Amphetamine does not exhibit direct β actions.

759. (C) Cautious intravenous administration of the α_1-adrenoceptor agonist phenylephrine will activate constriction of arteriolar smooth muscle, thereby raising total peripheral resistance in this hypotensive patient. The resulting rise in blood pressure will increase vagal tone, causing release of acetylcholine at the heart to terminate the arrhythmia. Carotid sinus pressure is sometimes used in combination with phenylephrine. Digoxin (choice A) may be used chronically to treat atrial tachycardia, but it is not a drug of choice in an acute situation because of the slow onset of action. Propranolol (choice B) may be used to treat AV nodal reentrant tachycardia, but it is contraindicated in this asthmatic patient. Nitroprusside (choice D) is a vasodilator that would exacerbate the hypotension and thus increase sympathetic drive to the heart and further contribute to the tachyarrhythmia. Norepinephrine (choice E) would raise the blood pressure and increase vagal tone. However, the direct β_1 effects of norepinephrine would produce tachycardia.

760. (D) Myasthenia gravis is an autoimmune disease of muscle weakness attributable to an impairment of nicotinic receptor function at the neuromuscular junction by antireceptor antibodies. Treatment consists of increasing the junctional concentration of acetylcholine with a reversible anticholinesterase such as pyridostigmine. In this patient, the problem is to distinguish whether the muscle weakness is attributable to myasthenic crisis (too little medication) or cholinergic crisis (too much medication) since both conditions cause muscle weakness. The safest definitive method is to administer a small dose of the short-acting anticholinesterase edrophonium. If the patient is in myasthenic crisis, an immediate improvement in muscle function should be evident. If the patient is in cholinergic crisis, the patient's condition may worsen, but because the duration of action for edrophonium is five minutes, this test provides less risk than other alternatives. Atropine should be available to treat excess parasympathetic activity. Administration of pyridostigmine (choice A) is unwise since a patient in cholinergic crisis is put at risk of exacerbation and extension of the toxic episode for a significant period of time. Administration of pralidoxime (choice B) is incorrect since pralidoxime is useful for reactivation of cholinesterase only in the case of organophosphate intoxication of recent origin. Symptoms of parasympathetic hyperactivity (choice C) would normally be evident in cholinergic crisis, except that this patient is being treated with the muscarinic antagonist propantheline. Administration of a test dose of tubocurarine (choice E) to elicit muscle weakness is a provocative test that is dangerous and does not provide definitive evidence for diagnosis.

761. (A) The anxiolytic agent diazepam, like most CNS active drugs, gains access to the CNS by virtue of possessing high lipid solubility. Hepatic metabolism is the usual elimination fate of drugs with high lipid solubility. Because the blood flow from the GI tract first passes through the liver, orally administered diazepam will undergo extensive first pass hepatic metabolism, decreasing the amount reaching the systemic circulation and thus reducing the area under the curve (AUC) for the concentration-time function. The AUC is a measurement of the amount of the administered dose reaching the systemic circulation. The intravenous route (choice B) should have the largest AUC since all of the administered dose is in the systemic circulation. Subcutaneous injection (choice C) should eventually deliver all of the administered dose to the systemic circulation, so that route should have an AUC similar to the intravenous route. Absorption from rectal suppositories (choice D) bypasses much of the first pass hepatic circulation so the AUC for this route should be larger than that for the oral route. Sublingual tablets (choice E) also avoid first pass metabolism so the AUC should be larger than the oral route. Administration of nitroglycerin for anginal pain utilizes this route because the drug is essentially completely destroyed by first pass metabolism when taken orally.

762. (D) The loading dose is the amount of drug given in a single bolus that will achieve the target or desired steady-state plasma level. The loading dose is equal to the steady-state plasma concentration times the apparent volume of distribution. Since the apparent volume of distribution is four times larger in the obese patient, the loading dose must be four times larger to achieve the same plasma concentration.

763. (A) Comparison of the clearances (calculated from the product of $V_d \times k_{elimination}$) indicates the clearances are the same in both patients. Since the target plasma concentrations are the same, the maintenance infusion rates must be the same.

764. (D) The relatively large volume of distribution of 50 L in the normal and 200 L in the obese patient indicates high lipid solubility as evidenced by distribution out of the blood and the increase in V_d with obesity. Drugs with high lipid solubility (high lipophilicity) are usually cleared by hepatic metabolism. A highly polar molecule (choice A) would be cleared by renal excretion and would be expected to have a volume of distribution smaller than that of total body water since polar molecules do not easily pass through lipid membranes. Highly polar molecules (choice B) are usually cleared by renal excretion rather than hepatic metabolism, since polar molecules are not well reabsorbed after filtration and do not gain access to the metabolizing enzymes within the membranes of the endoplasmic reticulum in the liver. Highly lipophilic molecules (choice C) are not cleared by renal excretion since they are readily reabsorbed from the tubular urine. The purpose of the hepatic drug metabolizing system is the conversion of lipophilic molecules to polar molecules that can be excreted by the kidney. A negatively charged molecule (choice E) would by definition be polar and would be expected to have a small volume of distribution.

765. (C) When the infusion rate is increased by a factor of two while clearance remains constant, the plasma concentration will approach a new steady state level of 400 mg/mL (two times the original). In one half-life (6 hr), the plasma level will be at 300 mg/mL, 50% of the distance to the new steady state. In two half-lives (12 hr), the plasma level will be at 350 mg/mL or 75% of the way to the new steady state.

766. (C) Clearance equals the input rate divided by the plasma steady state concentration. Thus the clearance is (1 mg/min)/(4 mg/L) or 250 mL/min.

767. (B) Botulinum toxin has an intrinsic zinc protease activity, which enters the presynaptic motor nerve terminal and cleaves proteins involved in neurotransmitter exocytosis. The resulting loss of exocytosis causes muscle weakness and paralysis. Preparations of the toxin (Botox) are used therapeutically for severe muscle spasms and tics. Botox is also used cosmetically to reduce or obliterate facial frown lines. Nicotinic receptor depolarization blockade (choice A) is the mechanism for skeletal muscle relaxation by succinylcholine. Inhibition of smooth muscle myosin light chain kinase (choice C) would produce smooth muscle relaxation. It is not clear whether this is a mechanism for any vasodilators at this time. Irreversible inhibition of cholinesterase (choice D) as seen in organophosphate intoxication results in exaggerated muscarinic actions and muscle paralysis attributable to depolarization blockade at the neuromuscular junction. Because the problem in botulism toxicity is at the level of loss of exocytosis, choline administration (choice E) would have no effect.

768. (B) The muscarinic agonist pilocarpine will cause contraction of the sphincter muscle of the iris, thereby producing miosis and reducing intraocular pressure by facilitating outflow of aqueous humor through the canal of Schlemm. The muscarinic antagonist scopolamine (choice A) will exacerbate glaucoma since it is a mydriatic agent that will impede the outflow of aqueous humor by exerting pressure on the canal of Schlemm. Tropicamide (choice C) is a short-acting muscarinic antagonist that will exacerbate glaucoma. Atracurium (choice D) is a skeletal muscle-relaxing agent that is a competitive inhibitor at the neuromuscular junction nicotinic receptor. It has no utility in the treatment of glaucoma. Hexamethonium (choice E) is a nicotinic receptor antagonist at ganglia. It would provide no direct benefit. Ganglionic blocking agents are rarely used because of the wide range of adverse effects associated with loss of sympathetic and parasympathetic function.

769. (B) Orthostatic hypotension, manifested as dizziness upon standing and attributable to α_1-adrenergic blocking effects, is frequently observed with therapy using phenothiazine antipsychotic agents. Chlorpromazine may cause orthostatic hypotension and reflex tachycardia because of the combination of α-adrenergic blockade and central actions of the drug. The anxiolytic agent diazepam (choice A) is not associated with orthostatic hypotension. It does not affect α-adrenoceptors or sympathetic nervous system activity. Sedation is the most frequent adverse effect. Lithium carbonate (choice C) is used in the treatment of bipolar depression. It does not affect sympathetic nervous system function. Adverse effects of lithium include polydipsia, polyuria, sedation, tremor, and mental confusion. Fluoxetine (choice D) is a selective serotonin uptake inhibitor used in the treatment of depression. It is free of anticholinergic and antiadrenergic adverse reactions. Adverse effects include nausea and loss of libido. Chlordiazepoxide (choice E) is a benzodiazepine anxiolytic agent that does not affect sympathetic function.

770. (E) Lidocaine, a class IB antiarrhythmic agent, exerts its effects through blocking both active and inactive sodium channels. By adding to depolarization-induced blockade or inactivation of sodium channels, lidocaine will selectively suppress electrical activity in depolarized arrhythmogenic tissue. Blockade of the sodium–calcium exchanger (choice A) is not a mechanism of drug action. Blockade of hyperpolarizing ATP-sensitive potassium channels (choice B) is the mechanism of action for the sulfonylurea-induced stimulation of insulin release from pancreatic β-cells but is not a mechanism for antiarrhythmic therapy. Blockade of voltage-dependent calcium channels (choice C) is the mechanism for the Class IV antiarrhythmic actions of the calcium channel blockers but not for lidocaine. Blockade of B_1 adrenoceptors (choice D) is the mechanism for the Class II antiarrhythmic agents such as propranolol.

771. (D) The oral anticoagulants such as warfarin block the vitamin K–dependent step in the synthesis of coagulation factors VII, IX, X, and prothrombin. Carboxylation of descarboxyprothrombin to form prothrombin containing γ-carboxyglutamate residues requires the reduced form of vitamin K as a cofactor. Vitamin K epoxide is formed as a product. KH_2 must be regenerated by an NADH-dependent epoxide reductase for the next round of carboxylation. It is the epoxide reductase step that is blocked by oral anticoagulants. The oral anticoagulants do not inhibit calcium binding to coagulation factors (choice A), but calcium binding is reduced because of the absence of γ-carboxyglutamate residues within the sequences of the coagulation factors VII, IX, X, and prothrombin. Heparin exerts its anticoagulant actions by acting as a template for combining thrombin and antithrombin III (choice B). Warfarin exerts its anticoagulant effect by inhibiting the synthesis of prothrombin. Warfarin has no degradative actions (choice C) against the thrombin molecule. The thrombolytic agent streptokinase becomes active in fibrinolysis by forming an active complex with plasminogen (choice E).

772. (C) The loop diuretic furosemide, because of its inhibition of the Na^+-K^+-$2Cl^-$-symporter in the ascending limb of the loop of Henle, promotes sodium–potassium exchange in the cortical convoluted tubule and subsequent potassium loss. The use of loop diuretics often requires concomitant supplemental potassium administration or use of a potassium-sparing diuretic. Spironolactone (choice A) is a synthetic steroid that acts as a competitive antagonist of aldosterone. Aldosterone increases activity of sodium–potassium and sodium–proton exchange in the distal convoluted tubule to conserve body sodium. Loss of the exchange activity leads to potassium-sparing diuresis, and therefore may cause hyperkalemia if potassium supplements are also administered. Triamterene (choice B) and amiloride (choice D) are potassium-sparing diuretics that inhibit the epithelial sodium channel in the late distal tubule and the principal cells of the collecting duct. Inhibition of this sodium channel prevents the outflow of potassium ion and thereby inhibits the sodium–potassium exchange process. Potassium supplementation would lead to hyperkalemia in combination with these agents. Captopril (choice E) is an ACE inhibitor whose use, because it indirectly inhibits aldosterone formation by preventing formation of angiotensin II, can cause hyperkalemia with potassium supplementation. This is rarely a problem in the absence of potassium supplementation or the use of potassium-sparing diuretics.

773. (D) Ranitidine is an H_2-receptor antagonist. H_2 receptors have been identified in numerous sites, including the stomach, uterus, ileum, and bronchial musculature. Gastric acid secretion involves activation of H_2 receptors, and disorders of acid secretion such as duodenal ulcer respond to treatment with H_2-receptor antagonists. Treatment of this condition is beginning to focus on eradication of *Helicobacter pylori* since this bacterium appears to be the causative agent for duodenal ulcers. Motion sickness (choice A), seasonal rhinitis (choice B), urticaria (choice C), and conjunctivitis (choice E) are all conditions that respond to conventional antihistamines (H_1 antagonists) but not to H_2 antagonists.

774. (D) ACE inhibitors such as captopril and enalapril are effective agents in the treatment of systemic hypertension. By inhibiting ACE, these drugs impair conversion of angiotensin I to angiotensin II while also prolonging the half-life of bradykinin, a vasodilator that normally is partially degraded by ACE. Unlike β blockers, ACE inhibitors do not interfere with reflex sympathetic activity, and thus the response to exercise is unimpaired (choice A). Unlike centrally acting agents such as clonidine, there is no indication of rebound hypertension after abrupt cessation of therapy (choice B). Renin levels (choice C) will rise as feedback inhibition via production of angiotensin II is removed. ACE inhibitors are highly useful in the treatment of congestive heart failure (choice E). The drugs decrease cardiac preload and afterload and prevent ventricular remodeling.

775. (B) Tricyclic/heterocyclic antidepressants block reuptake of biogenic amine neurotransmitters into the presynaptic nerve terminals. Although increased synaptic concentrations of neurotransmitter should, according to the classical biogenic amine-deficient model of depression result in a cure, clinical improvement seems to correlate better temporally with down-regulation of receptors. These agents are relatively selective for certain neurotransmitters. Desipramine is the most selective agent for blocking uptake of norepinephrine. Although these agents show selectivity in their inhibition of amine uptake, the differences do not seem to correlate with clinical efficacy. The selective serotonin uptake inhibitors do offer the advantage that they do not produce autonomic side effects, in contrast to the tricyclic/heterocyclic antidepressants. Doxepin (choice A) shows some selectivity for serotonin over norepinephrine. Amitriptyline (choice C) is relatively selective for serotonin. Fluoxetine (choice D) is highly selective for serotonin. Trazodone (choice E) is relatively selective for serotonin.

776. (C) The most common side effect of NSAIDs is gastrointestinal complaints including gastric upset, gastritis, and peptic ulceration. Prostaglandins PGI_2 and PGE_2 are cytoprotective agents important in inhibiting acid secretion by the stomach and promoting formation of mucus in the intestine. Inhibition of cyclo-oxygenase by the NSAIDs prevents synthesis of prostaglandins and removes the protective barrier. NSAIDs may also allow back diffusion of secreted protons. Prolongation of bleeding time (choice A) is attributable to inhibition of cyclooxygenase in platelets. This leads to less production of thromboxane A_2, a platelet-aggregating agent. Thus platelet function in coagulation is inhibited. Fluid retention (choice B) is produced by loss of prostaglandin function in the kidney. This is not a problem in normal individuals, but becomes evident in patients with congestive heart failure, hepatic cirrhosis, or renal disease. Bronchospasm (choice D) may be produced by NSAIDs in intolerant patients. The mechanism is unclear but the occurrence seems to correlate with inhibition of cyclo-oxygenase, suggesting either a loss of prostaglandin function or shunting of arachidonic acid to the lipoxygenase pathway with subsequent formation of bronchoconstrictor leukotrienes in the etiology. Drowsiness (choice E) is not a common adverse effect of NSAIDs.

777. (B) Microcytic hypochromic anemia is an indication of iron deficiency. Inadequate dietary intake is rare these days in industrialized countries with the fortification of flour and the widespread use of iron supplements. A more common cause of iron deficiency is blood loss from gastrointestinal bleeding or menstruation. The cause of iron loss must be investigated since it may be a sign of a bleeding ulcer or gastrointestinal cancer. Iron deficiency must be adequately treated since iron is needed for the functioning of many enzymes including cytochromes and other hemoproteins. Oral iron preparations in the form of ferrous salts (sulfate, fumarate, and gluconate) are the preferred and most inexpensive treatments for microcytic hypochromic (iron-deficiency) anemia. The bioavailability of various oral ferrous salts is relatively similar. Ferrous sulfate is less expensive than the other forms, however, and should be considered the treatment of choice. Ferric salts such as ferric chloride (choice A) show poorer absorption than the ferrous forms of iron. Macrocytic megaloblastic anemias arise from derangements in DNA metabolism and are symptoms of either vitamin B_{12} (choices C and D) or folate deficiency (choice E). Diagnosis of the underlying cause of the anemia must precede the treatment, since folate administration will correct the anemia, but allow undetected neurological damage associated with B_{12}-deficiency to progress.

778. (E) The duration of action of various insulin preparations is related to the rate of absorption from the subcutaneous injection site. Formation of complexes with various compounds such as protamine and zinc results in slower absorption of insulin. Ultralente insulin, an extended insulin zinc suspension, will provide stable low levels of insulin for a particularly long duration of action (approximately 36 hr) and is thus well suited to use in maintaining basal levels of insulin in a multiple dosing regimen. Semilente insulin (choice A), a prompt insulin zinc suspension, has a duration of action of 12 to 16 hr. Lente insulin (choice B), an intermediate insulin zinc suspension, has a duration of action of 18 to 24 hr. NPH insulin (choice C) is a complex of insulin, zinc, and protamine in phosphate buffer and has a duration of action of 18 to 24 hr. Regular insulin (choice D) has a duration of action of 5 to 8 hr and, because of its rapid onset and short duration of action, is the form taken before meals in most multiple dosing regimens.

779. (C) Simvastatin is one of the statin inhibitors of HMG CoA reductase, the rate-limiting enzyme in cholesterol biosynthesis within the liver. The statins are the most efficacious agents in the treatment of elevated LDL-cholesterol levels. Inhibition of HMG-CoA reductase prevents hepatocytes from synthesizing cholesterol from HMG-CoA. The lowering of intracellular cholesterol levels results in a loss of oxysterol repression of the transcription of the genes for LDL receptor and HMG CoA reductase. The increased expression and activity of LDL receptor lowers circulating LDL-cholesterol levels through increased endocytosis of the lipoprotein particles. Niacin or nicotinic acid (choice A), through unknown mechanisms decreases the production of VLDL particles, which in turn leads to less conversion to LDL particles. Clofibrate (choice B) and the other fibric acid derivatives including gemfibrozil (choice E) reduce plasma triglyceride levels by decreasing the VLDL content of apoprotein CIII which acts as an inhibitor of lipoprotein lipase activity. The resulting increased lipoprotein lipase activity allows more rapid catabolism of VLDL particles in skeletal muscle and adipose tissue vascular beds. Gemfibrozil causes a beneficial increase in HDL cholesterol levels through unknown mechanisms. The mechanism indicated in choice E, inhibition of microsomal triglyceride transfer protein, is not associated with any current drugs, but is an area of intense research that may result in highly efficacious cholesterol-lowering agents in the future. Bile acid-binding resins including cholestyramine (choice D) and colestipol are somewhat less efficacious and more bothersome to take orally (gritty fluid suspensions or chewable bars). By sequestering the bile acids in the intestinal lumen, the bile acid-binding resins decrease negative feedback regulation of the conversion of cholesterol to bile acids within the liver. The resulting lower LDL cholesterol level allows increased expression and activity of hepatic LDL receptors that mediate endocytosis of LDL particles. Bile acid-binding resins produce less lowering of LDL-cholesterol levels than the statins because HMG-CoA reductase activity is also increased with both treatments, but this activity is inhibited only by the statins.

780. (D) Recognition of lead as an environmental toxin of industrialization has resulted in lower population exposure through the use of nonleaded gasoline and the removal of lead from paints. Lead still remains a concern, however, because of its ubiquitous nature. Chronic lead poisoning results in a condition known as lead encephalopathy. This condition is more common in children than adults. Its symptoms range from ataxia to lowering of IQ and even convulsions. Lead at low concentrations inhibits the synthesis of heme and causes accumulation of porphyrins and increased activity of the enzyme δ-aminolevulinic acid synthase, two biochemical events that may aid diagnosis. When blood lead levels exceed 50 μg/dL, chelation treatment is indicated. The calcium ion in calcium disodium edetate is readily displaced by lead, forming a lead chelate that is excreted in the urine. Calcium disodium EDTA will bind any available divalent or trivalent metal that has a greater affinity for EDTA than calcium. Mercury (choice A) is not chelated by EDTA. Inorganic mercury poisoning is treated by using chelation therapy with dimercaprol or penicillamine. Organic mercury poisoning is more difficult to treat because of the lipophilic nature of the organomercury compounds. Methylmercury poisoning has been treated successfully with the introduction into the intestine of an insoluble polythiol resin that binds methylmercury, since this compound undergoes extensive enterohepatic circulation. Atropine (choice B) is a lipophilic muscarinic receptor antagonist that will block parasympathetic functions and produce hallucinations and psychosis. Treatment of atropine intoxication consists of administration of the lipid-soluble anticholinesterase physostigmine. Arsenic (choice C) exists naturally in both inorganic and organic forms with various valence states. Arsenate can substitute for phosphate in oxidative phosphorylation to form an unstable ATP analog that spontaneously hydrolyzes, thus essentially uncoupling oxidative phosphorylation. The trivalent forms readily react with sulfhydryl compounds including enzymes and lipoic acid. Pyruvate dehydrogenase is particularly sensitive to this inhibition. Arsenic poisoning is treated with chelation therapy using dimercaprol, succimer (2,3-dimercaptosuccinic acid), and penicillamine. Toxicity from iron (choice E) may arise from ingestion of iron supplements (as with children swallowing adult preparations) or diseases such as thalassemia. Treatment consists of the use of the iron chelating agent deferoxamine.

781. (A) Mebendazole is a broad-spectrum anthelmintic that is effective against a variety of nematodes including hookworm (*Necator, Ancylostoma*), whipworm (*Thichuris*), threadworm (*Stronglyloides*), and pinworm (*Enterobius*). Adverse effects are rare. Ivermectin (choice B) is used to treat *Onchocerca volvulus,* the agent responsible for river blindness in west and central Africa. Praziquantel (choice C) is the agent of choice for the treatment of beef tapeworm (*Taenia saginata*), pork tapeworm (*Taenia solium*), and dwarf tapeworm (*Hymenolepis nana*). It is also effective in treating flukes (*Schistosoma haematobium, Schistosoma mansoni, Fasciola hepatica* and others). Niclosamide (choice D) shows an anthelmintic spectrum similar to praziquantal and is considered a second-choice drug for many of the same indications. It should not be used, however, in the treatment of *Taenia solium,* since it does not kill ova that will be liberated following digestion of dead adult segments. Diethylcarbamazine (choice E) was developed during World War II in a search for a treatment for filariasis. Because of adverse effects that include nausea, vomiting, headache, leukocytosis, and proteinuria, its use today has been largely supplanted by other antifilarial agents, except in the case of *Loa loa,* where it remains the drug of choice.

782. (A) Rifampin is an efficacious inducer of hepatic cytochrome P450 activity. One or more of the rifampin-induced P450 isoforms metabolizes the coumarin anticoagulants so that hepatic clearance of the anticoagulants is increased. This will result in a reduction of anticoagulant activity, putting the patient at risk for thrombosis and embolism. Aspirin (choice B), phenylbutazone (choice C), and other NSAID cyclo-oxygenase inhibitors will increase the risk of hemorrhage with oral anticoagulants by inhibiting platelet function and promoting gastric ulceration. Displacement of coumarin anticoagulants from serum protein-binding sites by these compounds will also contribute acutely to increased anticoagulant activity. The H_2-blocker cimetidine (choice D) will increase anticoagulant activity by inhibiting the hepatic metabolism of the coumarins. This places the patient at risk for hemorrhage. Ceftriaxone (choice E) is a third-generation cephalosporin that is the agent of choice in the treatment of gonorrhea. The cephalosporins increase the risk of hemorrhage with the oral anticoagulants in two ways: (a) they decrease the intestinal flora, an important source of vitamin K, and (b) the cephalosporins such as ceftriaxone with heterocyclic side chains inhibit the same vitamin K epoxide reductase that the oral anticoagulants inhibit.

783. (A) The leukotrienes LTC_4, LTD_4, and LTE_4 are cysteine-linked 5′-lipoxygenase metabolites of arachidonic acid. When lung tissue is challenged with antigen in sensitive individuals, LTC_4 is formed and is subsequently metabolized to LTD_4 and LTE_4. These leukotrienes produce bronchoconstriction, increased capillary permeability, and increased mucus formation for an extended duration because of their slow tissue clearance. A prominent role for the leukotrienes in asthmatic bronchoconstriction is indicated by the observation that zafirlukast, an antagonist at LTC_4, LTD_4, and LTE_4 receptors, provides significant relief from asthmatic symptoms with chronic use. This drug is not a bronchodilator and is not effective in acute episodes. Because the first step in synthesis of leukotrienes from arachidonic acid is 5′-lipoxygenase rather than cyclo-oxygenase, aspirin (choice B) does not inhibit their biosynthesis. An increased formation of leukotrienes with cyclo-oxygenase inhibition and shunting of arachidonate to the lipoxygenase pathway has been postulated. The leukotrienes possess significant cardiovascular effects (choice C). The cysteinyl-leukotrienes produce hypotension by decreasing intravascular volume and reducing cardiac contractility by constricting coronary vessels, thus reducing coronary blood flow. They also increase capillary permeability to cause fluid exudation. Platelets do not contain 5′-lipoxygenase (although they do contain 12′-lipoxygenase), and leukotrienes are not stored in platelet granules (choice D). The cyclooxygenase product of arachidonic acid, TXA_2, is critical in platelet physiology, and acetylation of this enzyme by aspirin accounts for the effect of this drug in inhibiting platelet function. LTB_4 is a potent chemotactic agent for polymorphonuclear leukocytes (choice E), but the cysteine-linked leukotrienes LTC_4, LTD_4, and LTE_4 do not share this property.

784. (C) Recent advances in unraveling the mechanisms for control of neuronal firing have led to an understanding of the actions of older antiepileptic agents and the design of new ones. The mechanisms of action for the agents that are effective in treating partial and secondarily generalized tonic–clonic seizures fall into two primary areas: (a) promoting the inactive state of voltage-dependent sodium channels to inhibit sustained repetitive neuronal firing and (b) enhancing gamma-amino butyrate (GABA) inhibition of synaptic transmission. The mechanism of action for agents effective against absence seizures involves limiting the activation of T-type voltage-dependent calcium channels. GABA is the most abundant inhibitory neurotransmitter in the brain. Tiagabine was designed as an inhibitor of uptake of GABA, thereby enhancing its actions in inhibiting synaptic function. It is effective against both partial and generalized tonic–clonic seizures. Its adverse effects include dizziness, tremor, and nervousness. Lamotrigine (choice A), like phenytoin and carbamazepine, inhibits sodium channel function to inhibit high-frequency repetitive neuronal firing. Lamotrigine does this by promoting the voltage- and use-dependent inactivation of the sodium channel. Lamotrigine is effective alone against partial seizures as well as absence and generalized seizures. Adverse effects include dizziness, ataxia, double vision, nausea and vomiting. Carbamazepine (choice B) slows the rate of recovery of inactivated sodium channels. It is a primary drug for the treatment of partial and tonic–clonic seizures. Carbamazepine is cleared by hepatic metabolism and induces its own metabolism. Adverse effects include drowsiness, vertigo, ataxia, and double vision. Ethosuximide (choice D) inhibits T-type calcium channels that are involved in the thalamic 3 Hz spike rhythm of absence seizures. Adverse effects include nausea, vomiting, drowsiness, dizziness, and headache. Vigabatrin (choice E) is an irreversible inhibitor of GABA aminotransferase, the enzyme responsible for metabolic inactivation of GABA. It is effective against partial seizures. Adverse effects include drowsiness, dizziness, and weight gain.

785. (C) Local anesthetic agents inhibit sensory nerve conduction through blockade of voltage-dependent fast sodium channels. As a result, the threshold of excitability of the nerve is increased, and the ability of the nerve to propagate an action potential is decreased. Ultimately, transmission of sensory stimuli to the CNS is suppressed, and motor function involving small fibers in the vicinity of the injection is also lost. Ganglionic blockade (choice A) inhibits the functioning of the sympathetic and parasympathetic nervous systems, but has no effect on pain perception or motor nerve function. Inhibition of pain receptors (choice B) is not a current mechanism for analgesic agents although antagonists at the neurokinin receptors involved in nociception (pain perception) are an area of intense research. Inhibition of nerve conduction via blockade of Ca^{2+} channels (choice D) is not a mechanism for local anesthetic agents. Inhibition of T-type calcium channels to inhibit synaptic transmission in the thalamus is the mechanism for the antiepileptic agent ethosuximide. Hyperpolarization of neurons via enhanced Cl^- influx (choice E) is not a mechanism for local anesthetic agents, but is the mechanism for inhibition of repetitive neuronal firing by the benzodiazepines, barbiturates, and GABA-mimetic and enhancing agents that act by modulating or activating the $GABA_A$ receptor-chloride channel of neurons.

786. (D) In an individual severely intoxicated by antihistamines, the combination of central excitatory and depressive effects causes the greatest danger. In a child, the dominant effect is excitation, and hallucinations, ataxia, incoordination, and convulsions may occur. Symptoms such as fixed and dilated pupils, a flushed face, and fever are common and markedly resemble those of atropine intoxication. There is no specific therapy for antihistamine intoxication; treatment is usually supportive. Histamine administration (choice A), in addition to being dangerous because of the potential for anaphylactic reactions, would not be useful because the primary problems involve the CNS, where histamine does not gain access. Fever and flushing generally are not manifestations of antihistamine intoxication in adults (choice B). Deepening coma and cardiorespiratory collapse (choice C) characterize the late or terminal phases of the intoxication. Joint pain (choice E) is not associated with acute early antihistamine intoxication.

787. (C) Pancreatic beta cells are electrically active and exhibit a slow rate of Phase IV spontaneous depolarization. Depolarization causes entry of calcium and activation of insulin exocytosis. Under conditions of low glucose, the tendency to depolarize is counteracted by the activity of an ATP-sensitive hyperpolarizing potassium channel. When glucose levels are high, glucose enters beta cells via an insulin-independent transporter and is metabolized to yield ATP. The increased ATP (or other unknown compound) levels inhibit the potassium channel, allowing the cell to depolarize and secrete insulin. Sulfonylureas such as glybenclamide bind to a cell surface protein to cause inhibition of the hyperpolarizing potassium channel, thereby allowing the beta cell to spontaneously depolarize and secrete insulin. Na^+-K^+-ATPase (choice A) is unaffected by the oral hypoglycemic agents, but is the target for the digitalis glycosides. Fast sodium channels (choice B) are unaffected by oral hypoglycemic agents. Inhibition of fast sodium channels in pancreatic beta cells by agents such as local anesthetics or tetrodotoxin will inhibit insulin release by preventing rapid depolarization. Activation of a sodium-calcium exchanger (choice D) is not a mechanism for oral hypoglycemic agents. Inhibition of Na^+-K^+-ATPase by cardiac glycosides will result in increased sodium–calcium exchange in the heart to raise intracellular calcium levels and produce an inotropic response. Inhibition of voltage-dependent calcium channels (choice E) is not associated with oral hypoglycemic agents, but is the mechanism for the treatment of absence seizures by agents such as ethosuximide and reduction of blood pressure and reduced arrhythmogenesis by the calcium channel blockers such as nifedipine.

788. (D) The blood:gas partition coefficient determines the rate of onset of anesthesia. Blood provides the means of delivery to the brain. The blood solubility of the agent determines how rapidly the partial pressure rises in the blood. Agents with high solubility (large blood:gas partition coefficients) require large amounts of the anesthetic to be put into the blood before the partial pressure in the blood will increase enough to effectively deliver the agent to the brain. The MAC value (choice A) and the other properties listed [blood:oil partition coefficient (choice B); anesthetic potency (choice C); lipid solubility (choice E)], are all measures of the potency, which is a measure of the amount or partial pressure of the agent needed in the brain to produce anesthesia. Potency and rate of onset are independent properties of anesthetic agents. Desirable properties for inhalation anesthetic agents include high potency and low blood solubility. The halogenated hydrocarbons such as desflurane and isoflurane fit these criteria and are extensively used. Analgesia is also desirable. Nitrous oxide, which has a MAC value exceeding normal atmospheric pressure, is used in combination with other general anesthetic agents to provide analgesia.

789. (B) Thyroid storm, a malignant manifestation of thyrotoxicosis, involves an exaggeration of the features of thyrotoxicosis including fever, tachycardia, vomiting, and agitation. The thioamide propylthiouracil exerts its primary antithyroid actions by inhibiting the thyroid peroxidase, which carries out iodine organification, and coupling of iodotyrosines. The ability of propylthiouracil to block the peripheral deiodination of thyroxine to triiodothyronine adds to the treatment of thyroid storm. Reverse T_3 (choice A) or 3,3′,5′-triiodothyronine is formed from thyroxine by the selenocysteine 5′-deiodinase in almost equimolar amounts with normal triiodothyronine (3,5,3′-triiodothyronine). Reverse T_3 is metabolically inactive. Radioactive iodine (^{131}I) (choice C) is used in ablation of hyperactive thyroid tissue in Graves' disease. The preparation is administered orally and rapidly accumulates in the thyroid gland where the ionizing radiation destroys the tissue. Propranolol (choice D) is a nonselective β_2-adrenoceptor antagonist that is used to treat the tachycardia of thyrotoxicosis and thyroid storm. Potassium perchlorate (choice E) is an agent that will inhibit the uptake of iodide by the thyroid gland. It must be used cautiously since excessive doses can produce fatal aplastic anemia.

790. (D) Clomiphene is a weak partial agonist at estrogen receptors. When clomiphene is bound, it acts as a competitive antagonist of endogenous estrogen. Clomiphene blocks estrogen feedback inhibition of gonadotropin releasing hormone secretion from the hypothalamus. This allows levels of gonadotropin releasing hormone and the gonadotropins to increase, stimulating ovulation. Flutamide (choice A) is an antiandrogen used in the palliative treatment of prostate cancer. Ethinyl estradiol (choice B), a synthetic estrogen, and norethindrone (choice C), a synthetic progestin, are commonly used separately for replacement therapy or combined for oral contraception. The non-steroidal synthetic compound diethylstilbestrol (choice E) is used as a postcoital contraceptive.

791. **(E)** The kinetics for the approach to the steady state concentration are controlled by the elimination half-life. If we think of the difference between the starting concentration (zero in this case) and the final steady state concentration as a distance that must be traversed, the concentration will traverse half of the remaining distance in each half-life. In this case, after 12 hr or one half-life, the concentration will be 50% of the steady state level. After 24 hr or two half-lives, the concentration will be at 75% of steady state. After 48 hr or four half-lives, the concentration will be at 93.75% of the steady-state level. Mathematically, the steady state asymptote is only achieved after an infinite amount of time, but the normal rule of thumb is to use 4 × half-life as a measure of the time to essentially achieve the steady state level.

792. **(A)** In severe digitalis intoxication, serum potassium is elevated and automaticity is depressed. Treatment usually consists of insertion of a temporary cardiac pacemaker catheter and the use of purified Fab fragments from ovine anti-digoxin antisera. The cross-reacting properties also allow digoxin intoxication to be treated. Many cases of severe intoxication have turned out to be deliberate attempts at suicide. Immunotherapy is expensive ($2000 to $3000). Infusion of lidocaine (choice B) or other antiarrhythmics and cardioversion to control arrhythmias are contraindicated since these procedures may lead to cardiac arrest. Serum potassium repletion (choice C) is not needed since serum potassium is already elevated due to the inhibition of Na^+-K^+-ATPase and subsequent loss of intracellular potassium from cells. Much of the excess serum potassium comes from skeletal muscle, since this tissue represents a large percentage of the total body mass. Infusion of atropine (choice D) is contraindicated since it may lead to cardiac arrest. Supportive therapy only (choice E) is not sufficient since continued massive inhibition of Na^+-K^+-ATPase will result in cessation of cellular functions.

793. **(B)** The cardiac manifestations of β-blocker intoxication depend on the specific agent and its selectivity of action at various adrenoceptors. Hypotension and bradycardia are common. The heart has glucagon receptors linked to stimulation of adenylyl cyclase independent of the β_1 adrenoceptor. Glucagon plays a primary role in raising blood glucose levels through activation of glycogenolysis and gluconeogenesis, but also exerts inotropic and chronotropic effects in the heart. Insulin (choice A) activates entry of glucose into sensitive tissues such as skeletal muscle and promotes glycogen and triglyceride storage. It has no direct effects on cardiac function. Atrial natriuretic peptide (choice C) is released from atria and stimulates vasodilation through activation of membrane-bound guanylyl cyclase in arteriolar smooth muscle, and sodium excretion in the urine through an increase in glomerular filtration rate and consequent increase in filtration fraction. Human growth hormone (choice D) is a peptide hormone produced by the anterior pituitary. It stimulates growth at open epiphyses through production of the insulin-like growth factors (IGFs). It has no direct effect on cardiac function. Epinephrine (choice E) will be relatively ineffective in the presence of profound β-adrenoceptor blockade.

794. **(A)** At a blood alcohol level of 200 mg/dL, most individuals are grossly inebriated; a level of 100 mg/dL (0.1%) is considered the threshold for legal intoxication in most states. Ethanol is metabolized by alcohol dehydrogenase (and to a lesser extent by the microsomal ethanol oxidizing system) to acetaldehyde, primarily in the liver. When ethanol concentrations are very high relative to normal cellular metabolites, the metabolizing system becomes rate-limited at the level of the reoxidation of NADH since the cellular redox state becomes very reduced. As a result, zero-order kinetics are observed. A typical adult will show a constant elimination rate that translates as a decline in blood level of 22 mg/dL/hr. As blood alcohol levels drop below about 100 mg/dL, elimination has characteristics intermediate between zero and first order. Only at concentrations below 1 mg/dL is the elimination truly first order. At the high levels of ethanol where zero-order kinetics apply, clearance is not constant since constant clearance implies first-order elimination. Pulmonary exhalation (choice B) of ethanol accounts for only a minor component of elimination. Exhalation of ethanol is used to estimate the level of intoxication in drivers suspected of driving under the influence of alcohol. Renal excretion (choice C) also accounts for only a minor component of systemic elimination of alcohol. Because of the lipophilic nature of ethanol, most of the alcohol undergoing filtration at the glomerulus is reabsorbed. Biliary secretion (choice D) is generally important only for large molecules. This route is not significant in ethanol elimination. Biliary secretion is an active transport system and typically exhibits first-order kinetics. At a concentration of 200 mg/dL blood alcohol is eliminated at zero-order kinetics via hepatic alcoholic dehydrogenase. The clearance via kidney and lung (choice E) is minimal.

795. (C) For a complete refractive eye examination, both mydriasis (pupillary dilation) and cycloplegia (paralysis of accommodation) are needed. Muscarinic cholinoceptor antagonists produce both of these effects. The description of this patient best fits homatropine because it produces mydriasis and cycloplegia for several days. Tropicamide (choice A), a muscarinic receptor antagonist, is routinely used for cycloplegic refractive ophthalmologic examinations because its actions have a shorter duration of action (6 hr) as compared with two days for homatropine and one week for atropine. Edrophonium (choice B) is a short-acting anticholinesterase that is used to diagnose myasthenia gravis. Anticholinesterase activity in the eye will produce contraction of the ciliary body (miosis), thus facilitating outflow of aqueous humor and reducing intraocular pressure in glaucoma. In treatment of glaucoma, muscarinic agonists such as pilocarpine or long-acting anticholinesterases such as physostigmine or echothiophate are used. Phenylephrine (choice D) will produce mydriasis without cycloplegia. Echothiophate (choice E) is a stable organophosphate anticholinesterase that is used topically for glaucoma. Because of its high polarity, systemic effects are not seen due to lack of absorption, in contrast to other organophosphate anticholinesterases.

796. (A) The description indicates a CNS stimulant such as amphetamine or cocaine. The rapid loss of CNS activity with frequent repeated use is indicative of amphetamine for which tolerance rapidly develops (tachyphylaxis). This may arise in part from depletion of cytoplasmic biogenic amine stores caused by amphetamine displacement. Cocaine (choice B), by virtue of its actions in inhibiting synaptic reuptake of biogenic amines, is also a stimulant. Cocaine exhibits a shorter duration of action and has a lower tendency to produce stereotyped behavior than does amphetamine. Rapidly developing tolerance to the stimulating actions is not seen with cocaine. Tetrahydrocannabinol (choice C) use produces a "high" that is different from that produced by the stimulants. Appetite is stimulated and psychotic behavior may occur, but is uncommon. Tachyphylaxis is not observed with tetrahydrocannabinol. Heroin (choice D) or diacetylmorphine, along with its metabolite monoacetylmorphine, gain rapid access to the CNS because of their high lipid solubility. Tolerance is observed with heroin and other opioids, but opioid tolerance is not rapid in development as compared with tachyphylaxis, which occurs over a period of hours. Ethanol (choice E) is categorized as a CNS depressant rather than a stimulant, although certain behaviors may appear to be excitatory as a result of loss of inhibitory influences. Tachyphylaxis is not seen with ethanol.

797. (E) Saquinavir is an HIV protease inhibitor. Viral protease cleavage of a polyprotein is necessary for production of the viral coat protein. The HIV protease inhibitors were designed as specific inhibitors of this activity. The current HIV protease inhibitors are not sufficient for monotherapy because of the rapid emergence of resistance due to mutations in the HIV protease sequence. Combination therapy using saquinavir with two of the reverse transcriptase inhibitors such as zidovudine, lamivudine, or didanosine is currently effective in making patients virus-free. The HIV protease inhibitors are expensive and generally unavailable in underdeveloped countries. Inhibition of viral reverse transcriptase (choice A) is a property of the nucleosides zidovudine (AZT), didanosine (ddI), lamivudine (3TC), and zalcitabine (ddC). These nucleosides are metabolized to the triphosphate forms that competitively inhibit reverse transcriptase. Combinations of agents are utilized since resistance arising through mutations in the reverse transcriptase sequence frequently arises with monotherapy. Incorporation into RNA (choice B) is part of the mechanism of action for the antitumor agent 5-fluorouracil (5-FU). 5-FU may be converted to 5-fluorouridine and incorporated into RNA, where it affects both processing and function of RNA. Inhibition of thymidylate synthase (choice C) is another part of the mechanism of action for the antitumor agent 5-FU. 5-FU is converted to 5-FdUMP, a potent inhibitor of thymidylate synthase. This inhibition leads to loss of production of TTP necessary for DNA synthesis. Inhibition of viral DNA polymerase (choice D) is a mechanism of action for the antiherpesvirus nucleosides acyclovir, valacyclovir, famciclovir, and ganciclovir. These agents are metabolized to their nucleotide triphosphate forms that competitively inhibit the herpesvirus DNA polymerase. Acyclovir and valacyclovir also cause DNA chain termination.

798. (E) Osteoporosis is one of the leading public health considerations in aging women. It arises when the rate of bone resorption exceeds the rate of bone formation. Loss of estrogen after menopause increases the rate of bone resorption. Other risk factors for osteoporosis include being of Asian or Caucasian descent, slender body build, smoking, alcohol consumption, low calcium diet, sedentary life style, and a family history of the disease. Postmenopausal estrogen replacement therapy is satisfactory for treatment of osteoporosis in many women. It is not recommended in women with a high risk of breast cancer because of the potential for carcinogenesis and stimulation of tumor growth. Raloxifene, a selective estrogen receptor modulator, offers the best choice in this patient because it produces an estrogen-like effect in decreasing bone resorption, while giving antiestrogenic activity in breast tissue to provide chemoprotection against breast cancer. Parathyroid hormone (PTH) (choice A) appears to work at the level of bone to stimulate bone resorption through inhibition of osteoblasts and recruitment of osteoclast precursor cells into bone remodeling units. Intermittent administration of PTH in combination with estrogen has shown efficacy in increasing bone mineralization. This combination is experimental and, because of the estrogen component, would not be advised in this patient. Alendronate (choice B) is a bisphosphonate inhibitor of bone resorption. The bisphosphonates are analogs of pyrophosphate and appear to be incorporated into bone matrix, where they are ingested and inhibit osteoclast function. Alendronate is useful in treating osteoporosis and Paget's disease. It and other second generation bisphosphonates do not inhibit bone mineralization, an adverse effect of the first generation bisphosphonate etidronate. Although effective in treating osteoporosis alone, alendronate would not offer protection against breast cancer in this patient. Dietary calcium supplementation (choice C) using milk or calcium salts (such as in calcium antacid tablets) will prevent bone loss and even increase bone mass in some patients. This treatment will not offer protection against breast cancer. Conjugated estrogen (choice D) and other estrogen preparations as discussed above will reduce or prevent osteoporosis, but are contraindicated in this patient.

799. (C) Recent studies indicated that 90% of duodenal ulcers are caused by the presence of *Helicobacter pylori.* Treatment is aimed at reducing the gastric acid irritation of the ulcer and eradicating the bacterium. A 10-day course of clarithromycin, amoxicillin, and omeprazole has been shown to be 75 to 90% effective in healing duodenal ulcer and eradicating *H. pylori.* Clarithromycin, an erythromycin analog that is acid-stable, is a protein synthesis inhibitor that exhibits the same general antimicrobial spectrum as erythromycin. It is an effective oral agent against gram-positive organisms including *H. pylori,* and certain gram-negative organisms. Amoxicillin is an orally active extended spectrum penicillin. Omeprazole is an irreversible inhibitor of the gastric parietal cell proton pump. A single daily oral dose produces complete inhibition of gastric acid secretion. The combination is well tolerated. Adverse effects include diarrhea, strange taste, and headache.

Ranitidine + atropine + omeprazole (choice A) will abolish gastric acid secretion and allow healing of duodenal ulcer but, because the causative agent is still present, will allow recurrence. Ranitidine is an H_2-receptor antagonist that indirectly reduces gastric acid secretion. Atropine is a muscarinic receptor antagonist that was formerly used to provide some inhibition of gastric acid secretion. Omeprazole is an inhibitor of the parietal cell proton pump as indicated above.

Cimetidine + colloidal bismuth + magnesium hydroxide (choice B) will provide some relief from duodenal ulcer but will not provide long-term prevention of recurrence. Cimetidine is an H_2-receptor antagonist that will indirectly reduce gastric acid secretion. Colloidal bismuth provides a coating that will prevent gastric acid and pepsin irritation of duodenal ulcer. Magnesium hydroxide is a common ingredient in antacid preparations.

Misoprostal + ranitidine + sucralfate (choice D) is not a rational combination. Misoprostal, a PGE_1 analog, provides cytoprotection against ulcers generated by NSAID-induced inhibition of formation of prostaglandins. It inhibits gastric acid secretion and promotes mucus formation. Misoprostal use is not indicated except for ulceration attributable to NSAID use. Sucralfate is a sulfated disaccharide that polymerizes under acidic conditions to form a barrier that protects ulcer tissue from acid and pepsin. Because the polymerization requires acid pH, it should not be administered with omeprazole, antacids, or an H_2-receptor antagonist such as ranitidine.

Ranitidine + colloidal bismuth + diazepam (choice E) may give temporary relief but does not prevent recurrence and is not to be recommended. The actions of ranitidine and colloidal bismuth are discussed above. Anxiolytic sedative agents such as diazepam were used before either development of H_2 blockers or recognition of *H. pylori* as a causative agent for duodenal ulcers. The agents were administered under the theory that individuals experiencing chronic high stress are hypersecretors of gastric acid, and administration of a sedative agent will calm the individual and decrease acid secretion. While this may or may not be the case, chronic use of a sedative agent brings definite risks of impairment of cognitive function and habituation or addiction.

REFERENCES

Katzung BG. *Basic & Clinical Pharmacology,* 7th edition. Stamford, CT: Appleton & Lange, 1998

Hardman JG, Limbird LE, Molinoff PB, et al. *Goodman & Gilman's The Pharmacological Basis of Therapeutics,* 9th edition. New York: McGraw-Hill, 1996

Fauci AS, Braunwald E, Isselbacher KJ, et al. *Harrison's Principles of Internal Medicine,* 14th edition. New York: McGraw-Hill, 1998

Lewis WH, Elvin-Lewis MPF. *Medical Botany.* New York: John Wiley & Sons, 1977

Subspecialty List: Pharmacology

Question Number and Subspecialty

674. General principles
675. Neuromuscular system
676. Nervous system
677. Nervous system
678. Cardiovascular system
679. Cardiovascular system
680. Cardiovascular system
681. Lipid-lowering agents
682. Antineoplastics
683. Anticoagulants
684. Adverse side effects
685. Antiepileptics
686. General principles
687. General principles
688. General principles
689. Cardiovascular system
690. Antiandrogen therapy
691. General principles
692. General principles
693. General principles
694. General principles
695. Immunosuppression
696. Drug interactions
697. Drug interactions
698. Antivirals
699. Antimicrobials
700. Drug interactions
701. Drug interactions
702. Adverse side effects
703. Adverse side effects
704. Adverse side effects
705. Antineoplastics
706. Antineoplastics
707. Antineoplastics
708. Antineoplastics
709. General principles
710. General principles
711. Hormones
712. Cardiovascular system
713. Neuroleptics
714. General principles
715. Antidepressants
716. Asthma medicines
717. Gout
718. Gout
719. Antihistamines
720. Autonomic system—bladder
721. Antihypertensives
722. General principles
723. Autonomic system—pancreas
724. Cardiovascular
725. Anesthetic agents
726. Eye
727. Ethylene glycol poisoning
728. Nervous system
729. Drug interactions
730. Cardiovascular
731. General principles
732. Anesthetic agents
733. Anesthetic agents
734. Anesthetic agents
735. Anesthetic agents
736. Hormones
737. Miscellaneous
738. Kidney
739. Thrombolysis
740. Nervous system
741. Vitamins
742. Antineoplastics
743. Nervous system
744. General principles
745. General principles
746. General principles
747. General principles

748. General principles
749. General principles
750. Vascular system
751. Hormones
752. Analgesia
753. Miscellaneous
754. Antimicrobials
755. Drug interactions
756. General principles
757. Cardiovascular
758. Cardiovascular
759. Cardiovascular
760. Neuromuscular system
761. General principles
762. General principles
763. General principles
764. General principles
765. General principles
766. General principles
767. Neuromuscular system
768. Eye
769. Cardiovascular
770. Cardiovascular
771. Anticoagulants
772. Kidney
773. Antihistamines
774. Cardiovascular
775. Antidepressants
776. Adverse side effects
777. Miscellaneous
778. Hormones
779. Lipid-lowering agents
780. Lead poisoning
781. Antiparasitics
782. Drug interactions
783. Leukotrienes
784. Antiepileptics
785. Anesthetic agents
786. Antihistamines
787. Hormones
788. Anesthetic agents
789. Hormones
790. Hormones
791. General principles
792. Treatment of overdosage
793. Treatment of overdosage
794. Ethanol elimination
795. Eye
796. Nervous system
797. Antivirals
798. Osteoporosis
799. Antiulcer therapy

CHAPTER 7

Behavioral Sciences

Questions

Hoyle Leigh, MD

DIRECTIONS: (Questions 800 through 899): Each of the numbered items or incomplete statements in this section is followed by answers or by completions of the statement. Select the ONE lettered answer or completion that is BEST in each case.

800. A patient who had a painful bee sting is now afraid of flies and birds. This is an example of

(A) shaping
(B) classical conditioning
(C) flooding
(D) operant conditioning
(E) stimulus generalization

801. Which of the following is a superego function?

(A) psychological defense mechanisms
(B) reality testing
(C) conscience
(D) perception
(E) cognition

802. The multiaxial diagnostic system in psychiatric disorders implies that

(A) psychiatric disorders are complex
(B) psychiatric disorders and other diseases can coexist
(C) all psychiatric disorders are personality disorders
(D) all medical diseases have psychiatric symptoms
(E) all of the above

803. A most characteristic element of a health maintenance organization (HMO) is

(A) it provides specialized care
(B) it emphasizes prevention and health promotion
(C) it is fee for service
(D) physicians may be salaried
(E) it is a form of managed care

804. According to projections for the United States for the year 2000 as of 1992, which of the following statements is true?

(A) There will be an overall shortage of physicians.
(B) There will be an overall shortage of surgical specialists.
(C) There will be a shortage of family practitioners.
(D) There will be a shortage of pediatricians.
(E) There will be an overall increase in primary care physicians.

805. Which of the following statements is true concerning infant mortality in the United States?

(A) Infant mortality in the United States is high compared to other developed nations.
(B) The leading cause of infant mortality in the United States is the acquired immune deficiency syndrome (AIDS).
(C) Prenatal care, disappointingly, has not been shown to reduce infant mortality.
(D) The mortality rate for white infants is greater than that of black infants.
(E) Very few Asian Americans receive prenatal care as compared to African Americans or Hispanic Americans.

806. Binge drinking is characteristic of which type of alcoholism?

(A) alpha
(B) epsilon
(C) crash
(D) blackouts
(E) gamma

807. The most significant contraindication to electroconvulsive therapy (ECT) is

(A) recent cerebrovascular accident
(B) history of fracture
(C) advanced age
(D) cachexia
(E) history of seizure disorder

808. A patient is convinced that an IV injection she received has made her immortal. This is an example of

(A) reality testing
(B) illusion
(C) hallucination
(D) delusion
(E) delirium

809. The latest to develop during infancy is

(A) the smiling response
(B) sense of body image
(C) reality testing
(D) attachment behavior
(E) sense of gender

810. A 32-year-old male presented himself to a sex therapy clinic with the chief complaint of premature ejaculation. Which of the following procedures may be appropriate?

(A) stop–start technique
(B) psychotherapy
(C) physical examination
(D) CBC
(E) all of the above

811. Which of the following is a normal sexual function?

(A) anorgasmia
(B) premature ejaculation
(C) masturbation
(D) dyspareunia
(E) all of the above

812. A 45-year-old woman came to a sexual dysfunction clinic because of an inability to achieve orgasm. If she had never achieved orgasm in the past, the diagnosis would be

(A) vaginismus
(B) primary orgasmic dysfunction
(C) dyspareunia
(D) psychogenic frigidity
(E) Turner's syndrome

813. A 40-year-old woman who has enjoyed sex and was orgasmic in the past loses sexual desire. She is also apathetic to other activities that used to be pleasurable, and develops insomnia. The most likely diagnosis is

(A) Turner's syndrome
(B) primary orgasmic dysfunction
(C) major depression
(D) marital problem
(E) hypothyroidism

814. Which of the following is the most common dementing disease of the elderly?

(A) Alzheimer's disease
(B) Pick's disease
(C) multiinfarct dementia
(D) Creutzfeld–Jakob disease
(E) secondary dementia

815. A 76-year-old man was brought to the clinic because of increasing confusion and episodes of dizziness. Upon examination, the patient shows upgoing toes on the left side, and his blood pressure is found to be 178/115 mm Hg. The most likely diagnosis is

(A) Alzheimer's disease
(B) Pick's disease
(C) multi-infarct dementia
(D) Creutzfeld–Jakob disease
(E) secondary dementia

816. All patients who have trisomy of autosome 21 who survive to adulthood develop what condition?

(A) Down syndrome
(B) Pick's disease
(C) multiinfarct dementia
(D) Creutzfeld–Jakob disease
(E) secondary dementia

817. Which form of dementia is often reversible with treatment with tricyclics such as imipramine or serotonin reuptake inhibitors such as fluoxetine?

(A) Alzheimer's disease
(B) Pick's disease
(C) multiinfarct dementia
(D) Creutzfeld–Jakob disease
(E) pseudodementia

818. The most common type of substance dependency in the United States is

(A) alcohol
(B) tobacco
(C) cannabis
(D) heroin
(E) barbiturates

819. The incidence of addiction to what drug in physicians is estimated to be 30 to 100 times greater than that of the general population?

(A) alcohol
(B) tobacco
(C) opiates
(D) cocaine
(E) cannabis

820. The abstinence syndrome to this drug is triphasic. During the second phase, protracted dysphoria occurs with decreased activity, amotivation, and intense boredom and anhedonia.

(A) cannabis
(B) cocaine
(C) opiates
(D) barbiturates
(E) alcohol

821. One sensitive laboratory indicator of heavy use of alcohol is

(A) elevated serum gamma-glutamyl transpeptidase (GGT)
(B) decreased serum alkaline phosphatase
(C) elevated serum indirect bilirubin
(D) decreased mean corpuscular volume (MCV)
(E) elevated serum creatinine

822. The activity of which structure in the pons is suppressed by opioids, clonidine, and gamma-aminobutyric acid (GABA), and produces most of the noradrenergic input to the brain?

(A) nucleus pulposus
(B) mammillary bodies
(C) nucleus solitarius
(D) locus ceruleus
(E) substantia nigra

823. Unmyelinated C fibers are thought to carry which types of pain sensation?

(A) pricking pain
(B) excruciating pain
(C) sharp pain
(D) pulsating pain
(E) burning pain

824. Which theory concerning pain postulates that nonpain sensations such as vibration or pressure may affect the transmission and perception of pain sensation?

(A) specificity theory
(B) pattern theory
(C) gate control theory
(D) chemical transmission theory
(E) electrical transmission theory

Questions 825 through 827

A man complaining of severe back pain was given an injection of saline. The pain seems to have subsided considerably.

825. The most likely reason for the pain relief is

(A) hypnotic suggestion
(B) secondary gain was achieved
(C) the pain of injection caused counterirritation
(D) the saline injection induced endorphins
(E) the saline injection induced GABA

826. This phenomenon indicates that placebos can be effectively used

(A) as a research tool
(B) as a differential diagnostic tool between psychogenic and organic pain
(C) as an opiate substitute
(D) as a muscle relaxant
(E) all of the above

827. If an injection of naloxone had preceded the injection of saline

(A) the back pain would be even more alleviated
(B) the back pain would be worse
(C) the back pain would be better, but the patient would be drowsy
(D) the pain would be more localized
(E) the pain would be better, but the patient would be more anxious

828. The most characteristic aspect of the Oedipus complex is

(A) penis envy
(B) grandiosity
(C) intense love for parent of the opposite sex
(D) intense hate for the parent of the opposite sex
(E) all of the above

829. Harry Harlow's experiments with young monkeys separated from their mothers demonstrated that

(A) they had normal sexual development
(B) they became docile and domesticated
(C) they all died of dehydration
(D) they tended to adjust to stress rapidly
(E) they chose terrycloth as a mother substitute

830. Susan was tending the goose eggs when they hatched. The young goslings started following Susan, even when the mother was calling them. This is an example of

(A) maternal bonding
(B) imprinting
(C) instinctual behavior
(D) operant conditioning
(E) classical conditioning

831. "Executive monkeys" as described by Brady tended to develop bleeding ulcers. They were

(A) alpha monkeys that have the highest level of testosterone in the colony
(B) humans with weak egos and many decisions to make
(C) monkeys that had to keep pressing bars to avoid shock

(D) male monkeys that had too many available females
(E) monkeys that had to press a bar to get a pellet of food

832. James is three years old and he will not part with his filthy terrycloth blanket. Whenever it's taken away from him, he throws a temper tantrum to get it back. He holds it, sucks on it, and seems content when he has it. This is an example of

(A) childhood fetishism
(B) castration anxiety
(C) codependence
(D) transitional object
(E) displacement

Questions 833 through 835

Sara is eight years old.

833. Usually at this age one expects her to spend a lot of time playing with

(A) adults
(B) boys
(C) girls
(D) furry toys
(E) guns

834. According to Piaget, children of this age typically engage in

(A) concrete operations
(B) abstract thinking
(C) circular reactions
(D) preoperational activities
(E) repetitive learning

835. During this period, according to Erikson, a major developmental task for the child is

(A) developing intimate relationships
(B) developing a sense of integrity
(C) learning basic skills such as reading and arithmetic
(D) learning to be independent
(E) developing a clear identity

836. According to psychoanalytic theory, which of the following is a function of the id?

(A) curiosity
(B) sexual urge
(C) music appreciation
(D) movement
(E) perception

Questions 837 through 841

A 70-year-old man is brought to the clinic by the family because he is exhibiting confusion.

837. Upon mental status examination, the patient demonstrates fluctuating levels of awareness. For example, he seems lucid one minute, then becomes somnolent or stuporous the next. The patient most likely has

(A) Alzheimer's disease
(B) Pick's disease
(C) dementia praecox
(D) secondary dementia
(E) delirium

838. The family informs you that the patient was found walking aimlessly in the fields in hot weather for several hours before being brought to the clinic. The most useful lab test would be

(A) electroencephalogram
(B) urinalysis
(C) serum electrolytes
(D) electrocardiogram
(E) HIV test

839. This patient's EEG shows general slowing with occasional delta waves. This confirms the diagnosis of

(A) Alzheimer's disease
(B) Pick's disease
(C) delirium
(D) secondary dementia
(E) seizure disorder

840. Upon further inquiry, the family reports that the patient's mental status has been deteriorating for the past several years, and extensive work-up has not shown any diagnosable medical disease underlying the mental status change. The most likely cause of this gradual deterioration of mental status is

(A) old age
(B) vitamin deficiency
(C) Alzheimer's disease
(D) multiinfarct dementia
(E) Korsakoff's syndrome

841. If, upon further observation, this patient shows urinary incontinence and ataxia, a therapeutic procedure that may be considered is

(A) electroconvulsive therapy
(B) ventriculoperitoneal shunt
(C) megavitamin therapy
(D) benzodiazepines
(E) urocholine

Questions 842 through 844

A 23-year-old female complains of depression and anxiety. While describing her symptoms, she looks dazed. A minute later, she looks around the room slowly, and says, in a heavily accented voice with a different tone, "Where am I?"

842. This presentation is suggestive of

(A) schizophrenia
(B) major depression
(C) catatonia
(D) dissociative identity disorder
(E) adjustment disorder

843. A careful history is likely to reveal

(A) physical or sexual abuse in childhood
(B) history of criminal behavior during childhood
(C) an excellent school record
(D) setting of fires in childhood
(E) all of the above

844. This disorder shares a general classification with

(A) schizophrenia
(B) depersonalization disorder
(C) major depression
(D) dependent personality disorder
(E) multiinfarct dementia

Questions 845 through 849

A 50-year-old man is brought to the emergency room by the police because he was on the street screaming that the water supply was poisoned.

845. The man is very agitated, and requires restraint by the attendants. As you, the on-call physician, try to interview him, he tries to hit you and screams at you. A reasonable first approach would be

(A) reason with him that the water is not poisoned
(B) do a physical examination
(C) give him an injection of naloxone
(D) give him an injection of haloperidol
(E) give him amobarbital by mouth

846. If an injection of naloxone results in dramatic improvement of the patient's behavior, this may indicate

(A) the patient had a toxic psychosis secondary to heroin
(B) the patient is a placebo responder
(C) the patient had a psilocybin-induced psychosis
(D) the patient is a drug seeker
(E) the patient has schizophrenia

847. The mechanism of action of haloperidol seems to be

(A) blockade of serotonin reuptake
(B) facilitation of cholinergic transmission
(C) postsynaptic blockade of dopamine receptors
(D) presynaptic blockade of norepinephrine receptors
(E) generalized CNS depressant effect

848. It is learned that the patient suddenly developed the idea that the water supply in the city was poisoned about a week ago. In considering the diagnosis of schizophrenia, a crucial piece of information would be

(A) the patient has no history of psychotic episodes in the past
(B) the patient is a toxicologist
(C) the patient has a history of substance abuse
(D) the patient does not smoke
(E) the patient is single

849. If, on further evaluation, you find that the patient's parents were both schizophrenic, the probability that any of the patient's siblings would be schizophrenic is

(A) 1%
(B) 12%
(C) 15%
(D) 20%
(E) 50%

Questions 850 through 852

A 25-year-old man was admitted to the hospital when he complained of vomiting blood. All tests were negative, and he was observed stealing a test tube of blood from the lab technician's cart.

850. Which of the following is a likely diagnosis?

(A) hypochondriasis
(B) malingering
(C) body dysmorphic disorder
(D) conversion disorder
(E) factitious disorder

851. This condition may be considered to be

(A) a learned behavior
(B) a form of psychosis
(C) an integral part of antisocial personality
(D) a sick-role addiction
(E) all of the above

852. If the physician learns that the patient would have been incarcerated for a criminal offense if he had not been hospitalized, which of the following diagnoses becomes most likely?

(A) antisocial personality disorder
(B) borderline personality disorder
(C) sick-role addiction
(D) malingering
(E) Munchausen's syndrome

Questions 853 and 854

Concerning "sick-role" as described by Talcott Parsons,

853. One of the rights of the sick individual is to be

(A) hospitalized
(B) provided low-cost medical care
(C) exempted from normal obligations
(D) provided outpatient care
(E) exempted from income tax during the period of illness

854. One of the obligations of the sick individual is to

(A) have a consultation by a physician
(B) consider being ill an undesirable state
(C) pay for medical care received
(D) participate in health-promotion activities
(E) attempt to get better by "pulling oneself together"

Questions 855 through 859

A 48-year-old woman came to the doctor complaining of vague pains in the legs and thighs.

855. On physical examination, the only positive findings were varicose veins of 20 years' duration. The patient, upon being told of this, insists on being operated on for the varicose veins immediately. Underlying this wish for immediate surgery is likely to be

(A) anxiety
(B) drug dependence
(C) psychosis
(D) depression
(E) all of the above

856. If the patient, instead of requesting surgery, told the doctor, "In spite of what you say, doctor, I know that I have a serious illness, probably cancer" the next step should be

(A) ask why she thinks she has cancer
(B) tell her that she does not have cancer
(C) tell her that she has anxiety
(D) tell her that she has depression
(E) tell her to see a psychiatrist

857. The patient further confides in you that she has been losing weight with loss of appetite, has been unable to concentrate, and has had difficulty sleeping through the night. You should suspect

(A) generalized anxiety disorder
(B) schizophrenia
(C) mood disorder
(D) factitious disorder
(E) hypochondriasis

858. In obtaining further history, you find that the patient has a very strong family history of cancer. You decide to do further medical work-up to rule out cancer. Which malignancy is most likely in this patient?

(A) glioblastoma
(B) carcinoma of the lung
(C) carcinoma of the stomach
(D) carcinoma of the pancreas
(E) Kaposi's sarcoma

859. If cancer is ruled out in this patient, you are likely to use which of the following drugs to treat this patient?

(A) diazepam
(B) sertraline
(C) dextroamphetamine
(D) olanzapine
(E) valproic acid

860. Which of the following statements is true concerning medical care of persons of lower socioeconomic status?

(A) They sense that doctors do not expect them to ask questions.
(B) There is a problem of language that results from their unfamiliarity with physicians.
(C) They often regard physicians with a sense of awe.
(D) They feel socially distant from physicians.
(E) all of the above

861. One advantage of technical language is

(A) specificity
(B) ease of communication
(C) ease of visualization
(D) familiarity
(E) all of the above

862. One of the social expectations of the doctor is

(A) the doctor will treat the patient without the cost in mind
(B) the doctor will be competent in what he or she does
(C) the doctor will share all information
(D) the doctor will treat all pathology he or she discovers
(E) all of the above

863. Affective neutrality expected of a doctor means

(A) the doctor should always have a stone face
(B) the doctor should treat patients equally, whether or not he or she likes the patient
(C) the doctor should suppress all feelings about patients
(D) all countertransference should be analyzed
(E) all of the above

Questions 864 through 868

A young man presents to the physician with the chief complaint of palpitations.

864. He also complains of feelings that he is going to die, with feelings of dizziness. Possible diagnosis is

(A) panic attack
(B) acute anxiety attack
(C) cardiac arrhythmia
(D) substance-induced anxiety
(E) all of the above

865. If further evaluation reveals that the patient had used a substance heavily, but stopped about three days prior to experiencing symptoms, the most likely substance used is

(A) cocaine
(B) dextroamphetamine
(C) alprazolam
(D) heroin
(E) cannabis

866. If further evaluation reveals that the patient had not used any substances recently, but that he has been curtailing going outside, especially in open spaces, because he was afraid that he might have one of those attacks and become immobilized, which of the following diagnoses becomes more likely?

(A) acute anxiety attack
(B) agoraphobia with panic attack
(C) cocaine withdrawal
(D) agoraphobia without panic attack
(E) anxiety secondary to a medical condition

867. If the patient turns out to have a panic disorder, a useful drug for treatment would be

(A) olanzapine
(B) paroxetine
(C) bupropion
(D) phenobarbital
(E) valproic acid

868. If further evaluation based on laboratory tests determines that the patient has a general medical condition that underlies the symptoms, it is likely to be

(A) hyperthyroidism
(B) hypothyroidism
(C) hyperparathyroidism
(D) cancer of the pancreas
(E) Addison's disease

869. Concerning emotion

(A) it may be dysregulated
(B) it is often used synonymously with affect
(C) it involves a neurophysiologic discharge
(D) sadness is an example of emotion
(E) all of the above are correct

Questions 870 through 874

A 21-year-old female college student came to the doctor complaining of lightheadedness, palpitation, and tingling of the fingers and toes. She was terrified by this experience and is afraid that she may have a serious disease.

870. If you were the physician, your first approach would be to

(A) reassure her that she does not have a serious medical disease
(B) prescribe her a small dose of diazepam
(C) do a physical examination
(D) ask about any stressors
(E) all of the above

871. Upon further evaluation, there is no evidence of a serious medical condition. The patient, however, has major stress related to her boyfriend. A likely diagnosis is

(A) hyperventilation syndrome
(B) psychogenic syncope
(C) generalized anxiety disorder
(D) panic disorder
(E) agoraphobia

872. Blood lab work on this patient is likely to reveal

(A) reduced P_{CO_2}
(B) increased P_{CO_2}
(C) decreased hemoglobin
(D) increased hemoglobin
(E) increased MCV

873. The tingling of fingers and toes may be due to

(A) hypoxia
(B) peripheral neuropathy
(C) hypocalcemia
(D) thiamine deficiency
(E) niacin deficiency

874. An effective treatment for the acute symptoms of this patient is

(A) Trendelenburg position
(B) rotating tourniquets
(C) intravenous injection of benztropine
(D) ice packs
(E) paperbag rebreathing

Questions 875 through 879

A 50-year-old man developed confusion and difficulty with memory and concentration over a period of several months.

875. This presentation is atypical for Alzheimer's disease because

(A) confusion is not likely in Alzheimer's disease
(B) the age of onset and progression are atypical
(C) the gender of the patient is atypical
(D) difficulty in concentration indicates delirium rather than dementia
(E) all of the above

876. The most effective test to confirm the diagnosis of Alzheimer's disease would be

(A) brain biopsy
(B) blood test for abnormal proteins
(C) serum aluminum level
(D) urine test for homocysteine
(E) DNA mapping

877. If a physical examination reveals that the patient has right hemiparesis, the most likely diagnosis is

(A) Alzheimer's disease
(B) Pick's disease
(C) vascular dementia
(D) dementia secondary to general medical condition
(E) alcoholic dementia

878. If further evaluation reveals that the patient also has myoclonus, ataxia, and seizures, the most likely diagnosis is

(A) Alzheimer's disease
(B) vascular dementia
(C) Creutzfeldt–Jakob disease
(D) Pick's disease
(E) dementia secondary to general medical condition

879. If this patient had Creutzfeld–Jakob disease, a characteristic finding on autopsy would be

(A) senile plaques
(B) aluminum deposits in the brain
(C) punctate hemorrhage in the hippocampus
(D) spongiform encephalopathy
(E) multiple ischemic degeneration

Questions 880 through 884

Sean is eight years old. He was referred to you by his school because he is habitually disruptive in class.

880. A useful area to explore at this point would be

(A) his criminal record
(B) history of enuresis
(C) history of cruelty to animals
(D) his attention span
(E) his relationship with his mother

881. If further evaluation reveals that Sean has been unable to sleep at night for at least three months out of fear that his parents may divorce, an important diagnostic possibility would be

(A) conduct disorder
(B) generalized anxiety disorder
(C) separation anxiety disorder
(D) anaclitic depression
(E) attention-deficit disorder

882. If further evaluation reveals that Sean has had inattention, hyperactivity, and impulsivity since the age of five, the likely diagnosis is

(A) attention-deficit disorder
(B) generalized anxiety disorder
(C) anaclitic depression
(D) separation anxiety disorder
(E) conduct disorder

883. For the most likely diagnosis in question 882, the drug of choice would be

(A) paroxetine
(B) buspirone
(C) nefazodone
(D) clomipramine
(E) dextroamphetamine

884. If further evaluation shows that Sean has had marked impairment in social interaction, and developed restricted, repetitive patterns of behavior and activities, including mannerisms, then the diagnosis that should be considered is

(A) schizophrenia
(B) Asperger's disorder
(C) Rett's disorder
(D) attention-deficit hyperactivity disorder
(E) Munchausen's syndrome

Questions 885 through 889

A 30-year-old woman complains of insomnia.

885. The differential diagnosis should include

(A) mania
(B) depression
(C) alcohol withdrawal
(D) hypothyroidism
(E) all of the above

886. Which of the following neurotransmitters is considered to be most involved in slow-wave sleep?

(A) norepinephrine
(B) dopamine
(C) phenylalanine
(D) serotonin
(E) endorphin

887. If the patient states that one of the reasons she wakes up from sleep is that she has very vivid nightmares, which of the following drugs might provide most effective temporary relief?

(A) aspirin
(B) tranylcypromine
(C) trazodone
(D) zolpidem
(E) chloral hydrate

888. If she also states that in addition to the vivid nightmares, she has attacks of intense anxiety during sleep, such as feeling crushed, and wakes up with a blood-curdling scream, but cannot remember any specific dream, this is most likely a case of

(A) hysteria
(B) flashback
(C) night terror
(D) factitious disorder
(E) non-REM dream

889. For the condition defined in question 888, an effective treatment likely to show short-term results would be

(A) psychoanalysis
(B) hypnosis
(C) benzodiazepines
(D) tranylcypromine
(E) behavior therapy

890. The hospital system is characterized by

(A) democracy
(B) extreme division of labor
(C) ease of mobility
(D) lack of hierarchy
(E) all of the above

Questions 891 and 892

Concerning intensive or coronary care units (ICUs and CCUs)

891. The environment is often characterized by

(A) rigid and predictable schedule
(B) structured activity
(C) chaotic activity
(D) sensory deprivation and overload
(E) loud noise

892. This environment may lead to

(A) panic disorder
(B) obsessive-compulsive disorder
(C) ICU psychosis
(D) delusional disorder
(E) major depression

893. A 53-year-old male executive underwent an emergency appendectomy. Three days after surgery, he became tremulous and diaphoretic, and started having frightening visual hallucinations. At this point, the most likely diagnosis is

(A) alcohol withdrawal
(B) schizophrenia
(C) bipolar disorder
(D) ICU psychosis
(E) panic disorder

894. If the patient in question 893 turns out to have none of the above diagnosed disorders, the most likely diagnosis is

(A) thyrotoxicosis
(B) schizoaffective disorder
(C) drug-induced psychosis
(D) Cushing's syndrome
(E) Capgras' syndrome

895. If the patient turns out to have had a recent psychiatric procedure, it is likely to have been

(A) psychoanalysis
(B) electroconvulsive therapy
(C) sodium amytal interview
(D) hypnosis
(E) psychosurgery

896. During the course of the interview, the patient says that he is very happy to see you again. You know that this is the first time you are seeing him. Nevertheless, he tells you that he enjoyed the dinner he had with you and your family. The most likely diagnosis is

(A) schizophrenia
(B) acute mania
(C) delusional disorder
(D) Ganser syndrome
(E) Korsakoff's syndrome

897. If the patient has an amnestic syndrome due to thiamine deficiency, the lesions are most likely to be in the

(A) frontal lobe
(B) parietal lobe
(C) occipital lobe
(D) limbic system
(E) cerebellum

898. Further history reveals that the patient has been hospitalized recently because of confusion, difficulty with walking, and inability to move his eyeballs. The diagnosis at that time was probably

(A) cerebral hemorrhage
(B) cerebral ischemia
(C) Wernicke's syndrome
(D) vitamin B_6 deficiency
(E) pellagra

899. Concerning the use of hypnosis

(A) hypnosis utilizes animal magnetism
(B) under hypnosis, the subject is completely under the power of the hypnotist
(C) memories recovered under hypnosis are tantamount to facts
(D) hypnosis can cure warts
(E) all of the above are true

Answers and Explanations

800. (E) Stimulus generalization is a process through which a conditioned response is transferred from one stimulus to another stimulus that, in some sense, resembles the conditioned stimulus. In this case, the patient generalized the conditioned stimulus from bees to other flying objects—flies and birds. All the other terms (choices A, B, C, and D) refer to other aspects of learning.

801. (C) The superego is the collection of psychological functions having to do with conscience: moral/ethical attitudes and standards. The ego functions to mediate between the personality system on one hand and the demands of external reality and the superego on the other hand. Thus, psychological defense mechanisms, reality testing, perception, and cognition are all ego functions (choices A, B, D, and E).

802. (B) Axis I of the multiaxial system is for clinical psychiatric disorders such as schizophrenia and mood disorders. Axis II is for personality disorders and mental retardation. Axis III is for general medical conditions (such as myocardial infarction). Axis IV is for psychosocial and environmental problems, and Axis V is for global assessment of functioning. This classificatory system clearly indicates that psychiatric disorders (Axis I) and general medical disorders (Axis III) often do coexist and may influence each other. Choices A, C, D, and E are not part of the multiaxial system.

803. (E) The HMO is a form of managed care providing services in all specialties. Members enroll in a plan and prepay a premium (or a capitation fee paid by the employer or government agency) to cover all health care services for a fixed period of time. The emphasis of an HMO is to reduce health care costs through prevention, health promotion, and reduction of unnecessary health care costs. The physicians may contract with an HMO as a group through an individual practice association (IPA) or may be salaried. Choices A, B, and D are somewhat true, but not always. Choice C is, by definition, in contradistinction to an HMO.

804. (E) It is estimated that there will be more than 650,000 physicians in the United States by the year 2000. There will be an oversupply of physicians in surgery, ophthalmology, internal medicine, obstetrics and gynecology, and neurosurgery; therefore, choices A and B are incorrect. It is expected that the supply will equal the demand in dermatology, family practice, otolaryngology, and pediatrics; therefore, choices C and D are incorrect. There is a trend toward increasing the number of primary care physicians to approximately 50% of all physicians, especially with the advent of managed care and certain legal initiatives.

805. (A) The infant mortality rate in the United States is 8.9 deaths per 1000 live births as of 1989, which ranks the United States behind 11 other developed countries. The leading causes of infant death are congenital anomalies, respiratory distress syndrome, and sudden infant death syndrome; therefore, choice B is incorrect. Choices C, D, and E are incorrect because prenatal care does reduce infant mortality, but only 80% of Caucasian women receive prenatal care, followed by 75% of Asian American women, 65% of African American women, and 60% of Native American women. The infant mortality rate for black infants is greater than that of white infants (choice D).

806. **(B)** Jellinek labeled the types of alcoholism as alpha through epsilon. Alpha alcoholics (choice A) drink to deal with discomfort, and have not yet lost control. Epsilon alcoholics (choice B) are characterized by periodic or binge drinking. Gamma alcoholics (choice E) conform closely to the popular notion of alcoholism, with loss of control, tolerance, physical dependence, and withdrawal symptoms. Blackouts (choice D) are also common in this category, but not in epsilon alcoholics. Crash (choice C) is the first phase of cocaine abstinence, characterized by a crash of mood and energy immediately following the cessation of a binge.

807. **(A)** Electroconvulsive therapy is a safe and painless procedure performed with muscle relaxation and general anesthesia (choices B, C, D, and E are not significant contraindications). The only serious contraindication is increased intracranial pressure, as in cases of recent cerebrovascular accident, because of the danger of herniation due to transient further increase in intracranial pressure during the procedure.

808. **(D)** Delusion (choice D) is a fixed idea or belief that does not correspond to reality. Reality testing (choice A) refers to a person's ability to determine what percepts are real. Illusion and hallucination (choices B and C) are examples of impaired reality testing. In illusion, a stimulus is misperceived. Hallucination is perception without stimulus. Delirium (choice E) involves an alteration of the sensorium, with confusion and disorientation.

809. **(E)** Sense of gender or gender identity is usually established during the second year of life. The smiling response (choice A) develops at about three months of age. A sense of body image (choice B) develops after the first three months of life, which leads to reality testing (choice C). Attachment behavior (choice D) is manifest in infancy, including smiling, clinging, and the development of stranger anxiety.

810. **(E)** In evaluating sexual dysfunction, it is appropriate to perform a complete physical examination (choice C) and laboratory tests (choice D) to rule out a medical condition that may underlie the condition. Psychotherapy (choice B) is often indicated if there is major anxiety or conflict associated with the dysfunction. Stop–start technique (choice A) is a specific behavioral technique used to treat premature ejaculation. During manual stimulation of the penis by the partner, as soon as the patient feels a premonitory urge to ejaculate, he signals the partner to stop. The urge then disappears, and stimulation is begun again. Ejaculation is permitted in the fourth sequence.

811. **(C)** Masturbation is virtually universal among men and women of all cultures. It is common among married as well as single people. Many sex therapists recommend self-stimulation as an auxiliary treatment technique for a variety of sexual dysfunctions. Choices A, B, and D are sexual dysfunctions.

812. **(B)** Orgasmic phase dysfunctions include anorgasmia (frigidity), premature ejaculation, and erectile dysfunction (impotence), as well as delayed ejaculation. In this case, as she has never experienced orgasm, primary as opposed to secondary orgasmic dysfunction is the correct diagnosis. As we do not know the cause yet, psychogenic frigidity cannot be assumed (choice D). Dyspareunia is pain on intercourse (choice C), and vaginismus (choice A) is contraction of the muscles surrounding the vagina. While Turner's syndrome (choice E) may underlie some sexual dysfunctions, there is no evidence at this point of that disorder.

813. **(C)** Anhedonia, including lack of sexual desire and interest, is part of the symptomatology of depression. Depression is an important diagnosis to consider whenever a sexual complaint is the presenting problem. While Turner's syndrome, primary orgasmic dysfunction, marital problems, or hypothyroidism (choices A, B, D, and E) may underlie depression, one cannot at this point make those diagnoses.

814. (A) Alzheimer's disease is the most common primary dementia in the elderly. About 50% of brains of demented patients show evidence of Alzheimer's disease. Pick's disease is a rare cause of cortical dementia. The presence of unilateral cortical atrophy in Pick's disease contrasts with the bilateral atrophy evident in Alzheimer's disease. Microscopically, Pick bodies composed of densely packed neurofilaments are seen within diseased neurons. Multi-infarct dementia (choice C) is secondary to repeated cerebrovascular accidents in patients with underlying atherosclerosis or hypertension. It is more common among men than women. Creutzfeldt–Jakob (choice D) disease and kuru are slow-virus infections that show clinical and histological features similar to Alzheimer's disease. Secondary dementia (choice E) constitutes less than 10% of dementias in the elderly, but is important because the treatment of the underlying disease may reverse or retard the progression of dementia.

815. (C) As the patient shows signs of an old cerebrovascular accident (upgoing toes) and possible transient episodes of cerebral ischemia (episodes of dizziness) with hypertension, the most likely diagnosis is multiinfarct dementia. Multi-infarct dementia is a result of repeated CVAs, and successful treatment of the cardiovascular condition, including hypertension, may retard the progression of the dementia. Choices A, B, D, and E are therefore less likely.

816. (A) Down syndrome is a congenital mental retardation associated with trisomy of autosome 21. All patients with Down syndrome who survive into adulthood develop the brain pathologies of Alzheimer's disease, rendering support to the notion that at least one form of Alzheimer's disease may be associated with an autosome 21 abnormality. Choices B, C, D, and E are not associated with trisomy of autosome 21.

817. (E) Major depression may cause difficulty with concentration, memory, and mental acuity indistinguishable from dementia. Careful examination, however, usually reveals symptoms and signs of depression, such as depressed mood, anhedonia, loss of appetite, and sleep disturbance. Antidepressants are often effective for this type of syndrome called pseudodementia. Choices A, B, C, and D are not reversible with antidepressants.

818. (B) Tobacco addiction is the most common type of drug dependency in the United States. Nicotine is extremely addictive. Since the Surgeon General's report in 1964 that identified the health risks of tobacco smoking, there has been an encouraging trend in the United States. Approximately 42% of the U.S. adult population smoked cigarettes in 1965. The rate was 37% in 1975 and 30% in 1985. The reduction rate of smoking has been more pronounced in males than in females. Choices A, C, D, and E are therefore incorrect.

819. (C) Because of easy drug availability and their high stress occupation, physicians are at high risk for narcotic drug addiction, the incidence estimated to be 30 to 100 times greater than that of the general population. Choices A, B, D, and E are therefore incorrect.

820. (B) The abstinence syndrome to cocaine is triphasic. Phase 1 is called "crash," Phase 2 is a withdrawal phase with protracted dysphoria, and Phase 3 is an "extinction" phase that follows the resolution of withdrawal anhedonia. Choices A, C, D, and E do not show this type of triphasic syndrome.

821. (A) An elevated gamma-glutamyl transpeptidase (GGT) level may be the only laboratory abnormality in an alcohol abuse patient. At least 70% of persons with a high GGT (over 30 units) are persistent heavy drinkers. Heavy drinkers may also have increased mean corpuscular volume (MCV), but this is not as sensitive as GGT (choice D). Choices B, C, and E are incorrect.

822. (D) The locus ceruleus, located in the pons, produces most of the noradrenergic input to the brain, and has receptors for opioids and autoreceptors for norepinephrine (alpha 2) as well as GABA. The locus ceruleus seems to be involved in alertness and anxiety response. Choices A, B, C, and E refer to structures elsewhere.

823. (E) It is now believed that specific pain receptors (free nerve endings) are stimulated mainly by chemicals such as bradykinin, and that two types of pain sensations ("pricking pain" and "burning pain") are transmitted by different types of nerves. The burning pain sensation is transmitted by small C-fibers, while the pricking pain sensation is transmitted by larger, myelinated A delta fibers. The pain fibers eventually terminate in the thalamus in a somatotopical fashion. Therefore, choices A, B, C, and D are incorrect.

824. (C) The theories involving pain perception are: (1) the specificity theory (choice A), postulating that there are specific pain receptors transmitting specific pain signals through specific neurons to specific areas of the brain; (2) the pattern theory (choice B), postulating the existence of "reverberating circuits" to explain phantom pain; and (3) the gate control theory (choice C), postulating an interaction between pain sensation and other sensations competing for transmission at the spinal cord level. Choices D and E do not postulate the interaction with non-pain sensations.

825. (D) Placebo-induced analgesia has been shown to be reversed with naloxone, indicating an endorphinergic mechanism. Therefore, choices A, B, C, and E are incorrect.

826. (A) Placebos are inconsistently effective, but they are far from being inert. Placebos should never be used as a differential diagnostic tool between psychogenic and organic pain, as they may be equally effective in both. The best current use of placebo is as a research tool in double-blind, placebo-controlled studies. Therefore, choices B, C, D, and E are incorrect.

827. (B) As placebo-induced analgesia is blocked by naloxone, the pain would be likely to worsen, because the naloxone would also block whatever endorphin there was alleviating pain before the saline injection. Further, if the patient were habituated to opiates, there could be withdrawal symptoms, including heightened anxiety. Choices A, C, D, and E are therefore incorrect.

828. (C) Between the ages of approximately three and five years, a child develops a so-called Oedipus complex, an intense love toward the parent of the opposite sex with a wish to have an exclusive relationship with him or her. As marrying and having a sexual relationship with a parent is socially unacceptable (the development of superego), the child eventually veers away from this intense love and turns his or her attention to schoolwork and peers of the same sex, while identifying with the parent of the same sex. This period (approximately 6 years of age until adolescence) is called the latency period. Choice A may be a part of the Oedipus complex but is not the central theme, choice B is not characteristic of the complex, and choice D, if it occurs, is secondary to it.

829. (E) During infancy, the presence of a mothering figure and close contact with her (or even a suitable substitute, such as a "terrycloth mother") provides a basic sense of security. Choices A, B, and D are incorrect; if anything, the opposite effects were observed. Death from dehydration (choice C) did not occur.

830. (B) Imprinting is an ethological term that indicates a critical period in a newborn animal's life. For example, if goslings are exposed to humans rather than geese shortly after hatching, they will follow humans rather than their own mother.

831. (C) Monkeys that were placed in a highly complex operant conditioning program to avoid electric shock developed bleeding gastric ulcers, while yoked controls who received the same amount of shock, but did not have to perform the complex task, did not. The lack of a confirmatory feedback (such as a safe light or food to indicate a shock-free interval) seems to be especially ulcerogenic in Brady's "executive monkeys." Choices A, B, D, and E are therefore incorrect.

832. **(D)** Transitional objects are "mother substitutes" such as a blanket or a soft toy, to which a child may become attached and which she or he may carry around all the time. This is a normal developmental phenomenon and not a sign of pathology. Choices A, B, C, and E do not refer to this phenomenon.

833. **(C)** During latency (approximately seven years of age until puberty), the child relinquishes the intense sexual interest which characterized the Oedipal period, and tends play with peers of the same sex. Therefore, choices A, B, D, and E are incorrect.

834. **(A)** According to Piaget, at about age seven, the child develops the notion of conservation of volume or weight, and a clear concept of hierarchical classifications, especially of concrete objects. This is called the phase of concrete operations, which is followed by the phase of abstract operations in adolescence. Choices B, C, D, and E refer to other concepts and phases.

835. **(C)** Erikson identified the major tasks of the period paralleling Freudian latency to be industry versus inferiority. The child learns to win recognition by learning and producing things. Children receive systematic instruction in basic skills during this period. Unsuccessful completion of this stage results in a sense of inadequacy and inferiority. Choice A is developed in young adulthood, choice B is developed in older age, and choices D and E are developed in adolescence.

836. **(B)** The id is the collection of functions having to do with basic instinctual drives, such as sexual drive. Ego is the collection of functions that mediate relations between the demands of the id and the constraints of social reality and conscience. All the rest of the responses to this question (choices A, C, D, and E) are therefore ego functions.

837. **(E)** Fluctuating levels of awareness are characteristic of delirium, which is indicative of an encephalopathy due to metabolic derangement of the brain, such as anoxia, electrolyte imbalance, or hypoglycemia. While delirium may be superimposed on dementia, at this point there is no evidence that the patient has the more stable cognitive deficits characteristic of dementia (choices A, B, C, and D).

838. **(C)** An elderly man who was exposed to hot sunlight for hours may be dehydrated, and testing serum electrolytes may confirm this suspicion. While the other tests (choices A, B, D, and E) may be indicated at some point, they are not the most urgent tests in this case.

839. **(C)** Generalized slowing of the EEG is characteristic of delirium or metabolic encephalopathy. While some slowing of the EEG may be present in dementia (choices A, B, and D), often this test is normal. Seizure disorder (choice E) is characterized by spikes and sharp waves rather than generalized slowing.

840. **(C)** Alzheimer's disease is the most common primary dementia in the elderly. Multi-infarct dementia (choice D) is caused by repeated CVA, and there should be evidence of cardiovascular disease, such as hypertension. Old age (choice A), by itself is no cause for dementia. Korsakoff's syndrome (choice E), characterized by confabulation, is associated with alcohol withdrawal and thiamine deficiency (choice B). There is no evidence of either in this case.

841. **(B)** Normal pressure hydrocephalus is associated with the symptoms of dementia, ataxia, and urinary incontinence. On brain imaging, the ventricles are often enlarged, but CSF pressure is normal. A ventriculoperitoneal shunt is often therapeutic for this condition. Choices A, C, D, and E are inappropriate.

842. (D) Dissociative identity disorder (multiple personality disorder) is often associated with memory disturbance, and an alternate personality who may have a different speech tone, accent, or voice. Schizophrenia (choice A) is unlikely as there is no sign of psychosis, major depression (choice B) is unlikely as there is no sign of depression, catatonia (choice C) refers to muscle rigidity and mutism, and adjustment disorder (choice E) is a broad diagnostic category that does not include this presentation.

843. (A) Dissociative identity disorder (multiple personality disorder) is often associated with a history of severe emotional, physical, or sexual abuse in childhood. The dissociation may serve an adaptive function enabling the patient to tolerate an intolerable situation. The patient's school record is often poor due to memory disturbance associated with the disorder. Choices B and C are associated with antisocial personality, and choice C is unlikely as dissociation often causes inattention and poor school grades.

844. (B) Dissociative disorders include dissociative amnesia; dissociative fugue; dissociative identity disorder; depersonalization disorder; and dissociative disorder, not otherwise specified. Many dissociative disorders show symptoms and history similar to those seen in posttraumatic stress disorder and borderline personality disorder. Choices A, C, D, and E are inappropriate.

845. (D) The management of acute psychosis involves use of parenteral antipsychotic drugs, such as haloperidol. Reasoning with a delusional patient (choice A) is usually futile, and an agitated and uncooperative patient is unlikely to permit a physical examination (choice B) or take an oral medication (choice E). Unless you know that the patient is intoxicated with opiates, naloxone (choice C) is unlikely to be of benefit.

846. (A) Naloxone is an opiate antagonist, and would be effective in toxic psychosis due to heroin. The placebo analgesic effect seems to be endorphin-mediated, and naloxone would block it. The other choices (choices B, C, D, and E) do not deal with naloxone's specific antiopioid activity.

847. (C) The mechanism of action of haloperidol is believed to be the blockade of dopaminergic receptors, particularly in the mesolimbic system. Many of the more recently marketed antidepressants are serotonin reuptake blockers. Therefore, choices A, B, D, and E are incorrect.

848. (A) While all the other items (choices B, C, D, and E) may be of significance, one cannot make a diagnosis of schizophrenia if the patient has never had an episode of psychotic symptoms lasting for at least six months.

849. (E) The risk of developing schizophrenia in the general population is about 1%, while the prevalence for parents of children who are schizophrenic is 12%. The morbidity risk for schizophrenia for full siblings of schizophrenic patients is 13 to 14%. The risk for children of one schizophrenic parent is about 8 to 18%. The risk for children with both parents who are schizophrenic is about 50%. Therefore, choices A, B, C, and D are incorrect.

850. (E) Factitious disorder's essential feature is the intentional production of physical signs or symptoms in the absence of an external incentive as a motivation. If the latter is present, then malingering is diagnosed (choice B). Hypochondriasis (choice A) is incorrect because it is characterized by preoccupation with fears of having a serious disease based on a misinterpretation of bodily signs or symptoms. If the preoccupation is with a physical defect, either slight or imagined, then body dysmorphic disorder (dysmorphophobia) is diagnosed (choice C). Conversion disorder (choice D) is incorrect because it involves symptoms or deficits involving voluntary motor or sensory function as a result of a psychological conflict.

851. **(D)** The caring environment of hospitalization and exemption from normal responsibilities accompanying the sick role may be the unconscious motivation for many patients with factitious disorders to undergo very uncomfortable and often painful procedures or self-inflicted injuries to become a patient. There is no clear-cut learning, psychosis, or personality disorder that accompanies this condition, so choices A, B, C, and E are incorrect.

852. **(D)** When there is an external incentive for causing the symptom or injury, malingering is more likely than factitious disorder (Munchausen's syndrome), the motivation of which is often quite unclear. While there may be concomitant personality disorders, malingering is not diagnostic of any specific personality disorder. Choices A, B, C, and E are less likely as there seems to be an obvious and conscious motivation in this case.

853. **(C)** According to Parsons, a sick person is exempted from normal role expectations, such as going to school and work. A sick person is expected to be cared for, but this does not include any specific rights such as medical care, hospitalization, outpatient care, or legal obligations such as paying taxes (choices A, B, D, and E).

854. **(B)** With the obligation to consider being ill an undesirable state comes the obligation to seek competent help, but the help need not be by consultation with a physician (choice A). The sick role expectation also involves the notion that being ill is not one's own fault, and that the patient cannot be expected to get better by oneself (choice E) without help. While participating in health-promotion activities (choice D) is laudable, it is not part of the original sick-role expectations formulated by Parsons, and neither is paying for medical care (choice C).

855. **(A)** Anxiety or concomitant stress is a common trigger for help-seeking behavior, especially if the symptom or sign is of long duration. While depression (choice D) can cause vague discomfort and precipitate help-seeking, insisting on an operation immediately seems to indicate anxiety rather than depression, which is more likely to cause indecision or inaction. A drug-dependent person (choice B) is more likely to insist on drugs. There is no evidence of psychosis (choice C).

856. **(A)** When a patient presents with a conviction that she has a serious illness, it is important to find out more about why the patient has the notion, because in the process the doctor may be able to diagnose emotional distress in the form of anxiety, depression, or simple misperception, as well as hypochondriasis. All the other choices (B, C, D, and E) bring about a premature closure.

857. **(C)** Depression, which is a major part of mood disorder, is often accompanied by vague physical symptoms. When a depressed patient presents herself to a primary physician, it is important that the presence of depression be ascertained by careful history, as depressed patients are often suicidal, and about 70% of successful suicides have seen their physician in the previous month. Choices A, B, D, and E are not supported by the signs presented in this question.

858. **(D)** Carcinoma of the tail of the pancreas often presents with symptoms of depression. While other carcinomas and neoplasms (choices A, B, C, and E) may also cause depression, pancreatic cancer has to be ruled out first in a patient with severe depression.

859. **(B)** Sertraline is a selective serotonin reuptake inhibitor (SSRI), an antidepressant, and would be the drug used in treating this patient's depression. Diazepam (choice A) is an antianxiety agent, dextroamphetamine (choice C) is a CNS stimulant, olanzapine (choice D) is a new atypical antipsychotic, and valproic acid (choice E) is an anticonvulsant drug used to treat bipolar disorder.

860. **(E)** In spite of all the barriers listed here, the general desire for medical knowledge, regardless of social status of the individual, is the same. Therefore, the seeming lack of interest should not deter the physician from providing appropriate information to all patients.

861. (A) Technical language can be quite specific and precise. It suffers, however, from being unfamiliar to lay persons, and often impedes rather than facilitates communication between physician and patient. For choices B, C, and D, the opposite is true, especially when technical language is spoken to a lay person.

862. (B) In addition to technical competence, Talcott Parsons listed universalism, functional specificity, affective neutrality, and collectivity orientation as being part of doctor-role expectations. While it may be desirable for doctors to share all information (choice C) and treat patients without cost in mind (choice A), these are not general social expectations of the doctor. Requiring a doctor to treat all pathology (choice D) is counter to the functional specificity expectation that the doctor will treat only conditions for which he or she has competence.

863. (B) Affective neutrality implies that the physician will not become emotionally involved with patients or act on emotions generated by the patient. This includes not becoming intimate with a patient, or becoming emotionally aroused (either erotically or aggressively). Choices A, C, and D, are incorrect and impractical.

864. (E) The anxiety symptoms presented so far could be a part of any of the conditions listed, and only further history and evaluation will lead to a diagnosis.

865. (C) Benzodiazepine withdrawal is often associated with anxiety symptoms. Cocaine (choice A) may cause a "crash" with anxiety soon after cessation of use, but by day three there is more likely to be dysphoria than anxiety. While withdrawal from other substances (choices B, D, and E) can cause similar anxiety, benzodiazepine withdrawal is the most common cause of this type of symptomatology.

866. (B) The symptoms of panic associated with fear and avoidance of being in places where escape may be difficult or embarrassing call for the consideration of agoraphobia with panic attack. Choices A, C, D, and E are not associated with the characteristic phenomenon described here.

867. (B) In addition to selective serotonin reuptake blockers such as paroxetine and fluoxetine, tricyclic antidepressants, MAO inhibitors, and high-potency benzodiazepines such as alprazolam and clonazepam may be effective in panic disorder. Choice A (olanzapine) is an atypical antipsychotic and has not been shown to be effective in panic disorder. Neither are choices C, D, and E (bupropion, an antidepressant; phenobarbital, a CNS depressant; and valproic acid, an anticonvulsant and antimanic drug).

868. (A) Hyperthyroidism is often associated with anxiety and panic symptoms. While these symptoms may also occur in any of the other medical conditions, depression and slowed mentation are more common in hypothyroidism, hyperparathyroidism, and Addison's disease; cancer of the pancreas is often associated with severe depression.

869. (E) Emotions, or affects, include three main components—a subjective feeling tone, a neurophysiologic discharge, and perception of the bodily sensations caused by the motor discharge, e.g., palpitation. Dysregulation of emotion results in anxiety or mood disorders.

870. (D) Although the known symptoms are indicative of an anxiety disorder, one needs more information to proceed. As stressors are important in anxiety symptoms, asking about them would be the first approach. Choices A, B, and C bring about premature closure.

871. (A) Lightheadedness, palpitation, and tingling in the fingers and toes are characteristic of hyperventilation syndrome. Choice B is incorrect because there is no syncope, and choices C, D, and E need further evidence and are not supported by known symptoms.

872. (A) In hyperventilation syndrome, there is respiratory alkalosis due to CO_2 loss. This may in turn lead to decreased ionization of calcium. Choices B, C, D, and E are incorrect as there is no reason for such changes.

873. (C) In hyperventilation syndrome, there is often hypocalcemia associated with respiratory alkalosis. Choices A, B, D, and E are not supported by the evidence found so far.

874. (E) Paperbag rebreathing restores P_{CO_2}, and normalizes the blood pH and calcium. This technique and education about hyperventilation, as well as appropriate coping with stressors, can prevent and control hyperventilation syndrome. Choices A, B, C, and D may be appropriate for other conditions.

875. (B) While some types of Alzheimer's disease have a rapid progression and younger age of onset, it is primarily a disease of the elderly with relatively slow progression (years). Confusion and difficulty with concentration are quite common in Alzheimer's, which affects both sexes, although females may be at slightly higher risk. Therefore, choices A, C, and D are less appropriate than B.

876. (A) Even though it is not practical in most cases, microscopic examination of the brain is most accurately diagnostic of the pathology of Alzheimer's disease, consisting of neurofibrillary tangles, senile plaques, and granulovacuolar bodies. Choices B, C, D, and E have not been shown to confirm the diagnosis of Alzheimer's.

877. (C) Evidence of CVA, such as hemiparesis, increases the likelihood that the dementia is due to repeated vascular events in the brain (multiinfarct dementia). Evidence of CVA is not present in the other disorders (choices A, B, D, and E).

878. (C) Creutzfeldt–Jakob disease, caused by protein fragments called "prions," is characterized by relatively rapid onset of dementia, myoclonus, seizures, and ataxia. Choices A, B, D, and E are not associated with these severe neurologic signs.

879. (D) Creutzfeldt–Jakob disease is a spongiform encephalopathy similar to kuru and "mad cow disease." Unlike Alzheimer's disease (choice A), senile plaques or neurofibrillary tangles are usually absent in the brains of patients with Creutzfeld–Jakob disease. Punctate hemorrhage (choice C) in the hippocampus is seen in Wernicke's disease, and multiple ischemic degeneration (choice E) is more likely in vascular dementia. Choice B (aluminum deposits) were suspected in Alzheimer's, but not in Creutzfeld–Jakob disease.

880. (D) A common cause of disruptiveness in a child is attention-deficit hyperactivity disorder, characterized by inattention and hyperactivity. Enuresis (choice B), cruelty to animals (choice C), and trouble with the law (choice A) are often found in the childhoods of those who are eventually diagnosed as having an antisocial personality, but disruptiveness in class is more indicative of hyperactivity. Exploring choice E may be useful, but not as much so as D.

881. (C) Separation anxiety disorder involves excessive anxiety concerning separation from the home or someone to whom the child is attached. The disturbance must continue for more than four weeks, with onset before age 18. Choices A, B, D, and E are not particularly indicated by the new information in this question.

882. (A) The diagnostic criteria for attention-deficit disorder include inattention, hyperactivity, and impulsivity in various areas, and the symptoms must have been present before the age of seven. The specific history of inattention and hyperactivity tend to rule out choices B, C, D, and E, although there may be some elements of conduct disorder.

883. (E) Dextroamphetamine and methylphenidate are effective in treating attention-deficit hyperactivity disorder. Paroxetine (choice A) and nefazodone (choice C) are antidepressants, clomipramine (choice D) is a tricyclic that has special use in obsessive-compulsive disorders, and buspirone (choice B) is an antianxiety agent.

884. (B) Asperger's disorder and Rett's disorder are forms of pervasive developmental disorder. In Rett's disorder (choice C), there is the development of multiple specific deficits following a period of normal functioning after birth. In Asperger's disorder, there is severe and sustained impairment in social interaction and restricted, repetitive patterns of behavior, interests, and activities. There is no evidence of schizophrenia or factitious disorder (choices A and E). If attention-deficit hyperactivity symptoms exist (choice D) in addition to symptoms of pervasive developmental disorder, the latter is diagnosed.

885. (E) Insomnia is seen in depression, sedative withdrawal including alcohol, hypothyroidism, and mania, although in mania the patient may not feel the need to sleep or complain about the lack of sleep.

886. (D) Non-REM or slow-wave sleep is an active phenomenon probably brought about by the activation of the serotonergic neurons of the pontine raphe system. Noradrenergic (choice A) and possibly cholinergic systems are involved in REM sleep, and dopamine (choice B) seems more involved in attention and reward mechanisms. Phenylalanine (choice C) is an amino acid, and endorphins (choice E) are neuromodulators that may contribute to modulation of sleep.

887. (B) Vivid dreams usually occur during rapid eye movement (REM) sleep. Many drugs suppress REM, but monoamine oxidase inhibitors, such as tranylcypromine, are most potent in this effect. The other drugs listed (choices A, C, D, and E) have little effect on REM sleep.

888. (C) This is a typical description of night terrors, which, unlike nightmares, occur during the NREM delta-wave sleep. Hysteria and flashback (choices A and B) are not sleep disorders, and non-REM dreams (choice E) are usually not terrifying as in night terrors. While in factitious disorder (choice D), the patient may give a manufactured account of what happened, the case fits the description of night terror the best.

889. (C) As night terror is an NREM, particularly stage 4, sleep phenomenon, benzodiazepines that suppress stage 4 sleep such as diazepam can be effective. There is no evidence that psychotherapy, including psychoanalysis, hypnosis, or behavioral therapy (choices A, B, and E) are effective in the short term for this condition. Tranylcypromine (choice D), a monoamine oxidase inhibitor, suppresses REM but not NREM sleep.

890. (B) The professional, administrative, and nonprofessional staffs in a hospital have clearly distinguishable and separate tasks, orientations, and loyalties. The clerk does not operate, and the doctor does not collect bills. A hospital is a hierarchy, and there is often blocked mobility—a nurse cannot be a doctor without first changing his or her career, and vice versa. Therefore, choices A, C, and D are incorrect.

891. (D) Various activities occur simultaneously in the ICU and CCU, and structured activity is often impossible due to the urgent nature of medical care needed. Noise is usually suppressed, and while there are a variety of activities, they are not chaotic, but instead are medically ordered. Sensory deprivation and overload both may occur due to the suppression of sound and lighting, contrasted with the constant beep of the monitors and the clamor of cardiac resuscitation. Therefore, choices A, B, C, and E are incorrect.

892. (C) Sensory deprivation and overload superimposed on physiologic aberrations such as electrolyte imbalance or narcotic analgesics may cause a psychotic syndrome characterized by hallucinations and delusions called ICU psychosis. While panic disorder (choice A) is possible, all the other disorders listed (choices B, D, and E) are primary psychiatric disorders that can be diagnosed only after ruling out ICU psychosis.

893. **(A)** Emergency surgery results in unexpected withdrawal from habituated drugs, including alcohol. The symptoms are characteristic of delirium tremens. Schizophrenia (choice B) is unlikely because the psychosis is sudden, and the hallucinations are primarily visual (in schizophrenia, they are more likely to be auditory). ICU psychosis (choice D) is not impossible, but most likely by the third postsurgical day, the patient is out of the ICU. Being tremulous and diaphoretic are not typical features of bipolar disorder (choice C), and hallucinations do not occur in panic disorder (choice E).

894. **(C)** Next to sedative drug withdrawal, visual hallucinations during the postoperative period should raise the index of suspicion for drug-induced psychosis, especially due to narcotic analgesics. While all the other listed disorders (choices A, B, D, and E) could produce a psychotic syndrome, the acute course in this patient suggests delirium.

895. **(B)** ECT often causes memory disturbance, especially of short-term memory. Psychoanalysis, amytal interview, and hypnosis (choices A, C, and D) may be used to attempt to recover certain types of memory, but are unlikely to be causes of this disturbance. Modern psychosurgery (choice E) is often very localized and unlikely to involve memory loss.

896. **(E)** Korsakoff's syndrome, caused by thiamine deficiency in alcoholics, is characterized by confabulation as in this case. Ganser syndrome (choice D) is associated with approximate but inaccurate answers, and schizophrenia and acute mania (choices A and B) are usually associated with their characteristic symptoms, although confabulation may occasionally occur. Delusional disorder (choice C) is possible, but the patient presented with memory problems, which are in delusional disorder.

897. **(D)** The amnestic syndrome is associated with lesions in the limbic system, including the hippocampus, fornix, and mammillary bodies. Therefore, choices A, B, C, and E are incorrect.

898. **(C)** Wernicke's syndrome is characterized by ophthalmoplegia, ataxia, and delirium. Wernicke's syndrome may progress to Wernicke–Korsakoff syndrome, with amnesia, nystagmus, and ataxia. Peripheral neuropathy is usually present. While all the other disorders (choices A, B, D, and E) could produce neurologic symptoms and confusion, the presenting symptoms are characteristic of Wernicke's encephalopathy. Furthermore, the patient's current condition (Korsakoff's syndrome) must be a progression of the recent Wernicke's syndrome.

899. **(D)** Hypnotic suggestion can make warts disappear by reducing blood flow to their base. Hypnosis, however, is not an all-powerful tool to control others (choice B), but rather a method of enhancing the concentration and attention of the subject. Historically, Anton Mesmer proposed that the hypnotic phenomenon was based on animal magnetism (choice A), but the association between hypnosis and magnetism was disproved by the famous French Royal Commission Report. Memory retrieved under hypnosis (choice C) is no more accurate than non-hypnotic recall (in fact, it is less reliable).

REFERENCES

Elkin GD. *Introduction to Clinical Psychiatry.* Stamford, CT: Appleton & Lange, 1998

Kaplan HI, Sadock BJ. *Comprehensive Textbook of Psychiatry/VI CD-ROM.* Teton Data Systems, Jackson, Wyoming, Baltimore: Williams & Wilkins, 1998

Kaplan HI, Sadock BJ. *Kaplan and Sadock's Synopsis of Psychiatry,* 8th edition. Baltimore: Williams & Wilkins, 1998

Leigh H, Reiser MF. *The Patient: Biological, Psychological, and Social Dimensions of Medical Practice,* 3rd edition. New York: Plenum Press, 1992

Subspecialty List: Behavioral Sciences

Question Number and Subspecialty

800. Psychological and social factors
801. Psychoanalytical theory
802. Miscellaneous
803. Medical ethics
804. Future trends in medicine
805. Infant mortality
806. Substance abuse
807. Miscellaneous
808. Psychotic disorders
809. Life cycle
810. Human sexuality
811. Human sexuality
812. Human sexuality
813. Mood disorders
814. Dementia
815. Dementia
816. Miscellaneous
817. Dementia
818. Substance abuse
819. Substance abuse
820. Substance abuse
821. Substance abuse
822. Psychologic correlates of behavior
823. Pain sensation
824. Pain sensation
825. Metabolic correlates
826. Placebo effect
827. Metabolic correlates
828. Life cycle
829. Life cycle
830. Animal and human behavior
831. Animal and human behavior
832. Life cycle
833. Life cycle
834. Life cycle
835. Life cycle
836. Psychoanalytical theory
837. Delirium
838. Delirium
839. Delirium
840. Dementia
841. Miscellaneous
842. Dissociative identity disorders
843. Dissociative identity disorders
844. Dissociative identity disorders
845. Psychotic disorders
846. Psychotic disorders
847. Pharmacology
848. Psychotic disorders
849. Psychotic disorders
850. Personality disorders
851. Personality disorders
852. Personality disorders
853. Psychological and social factors
854. Psychological and social factors
855. Anxiety disorders
856. Anxiety disorders
857. Mood disorders
858. Mood disorders
859. Mood disorders
860. Medical ethics
861. Medical ethics
862. Medical ethics
863. Medical ethics
864. Anxiety disorders
865. Substance abuse
866. Anxiety disorders
867. Anxiety disorders
868. Anxiety disorders
869. Emotions
870. Anxiety disorders
871. Anxiety disorders
872. Metabolic correlates
873. Metabolic correlates

874. Anxiety disorders
875. Organic dementia
876. Organic dementia
877. Organic dementia
878. Organic dementia
879. Organic dementia
880. Attention-deficit disorder
881. Separation anxiety disorder
882. Attention-deficit disorder
883. Attention-deficit disorder
884. Developmental disorder
885. Sleep
886. Sleep
887. Sleep
888. Sleep
889. Sleep
890. Medical ethics
891. Psychological and social factors
892. Psychological and social factors
893. Substance abuse
894. Psychotic disorders
895. Organic correlates
896. Organic correlates
897. Organic correlates
898. Organic correlates
899. Hypnosis

CHAPTER 8

Practice Tests

Carefully read the following instructions before taking the Practice Tests.

1. This examination consists of questions divided into two testing periods. Each test contains 150 questions. You are allowed two hours to complete each batch of 150 questions. At this pace you need to answer a question about every 50 seconds.
2. The tests simulate the USMLE. You should not carry any extra time from one test over to the other. Any remaining time from either test should be used to review your answers in that test only. You should take a break of 1 or 2 hours between the two tests.
3. Be sure you have an adequate number of pencils and erasers, a clock, and a comfortable setting, and an adequate amount of undisturbed, distraction-free time to complete each test.
4. Be sure to fill out the answer sheet properly. The answer sheets are at the end of the book.
5. After you have completed a test, check your responses against the answers that appear on the pages directly following each exam.
6. Good luck on these Practice Tests and on the USMLE.

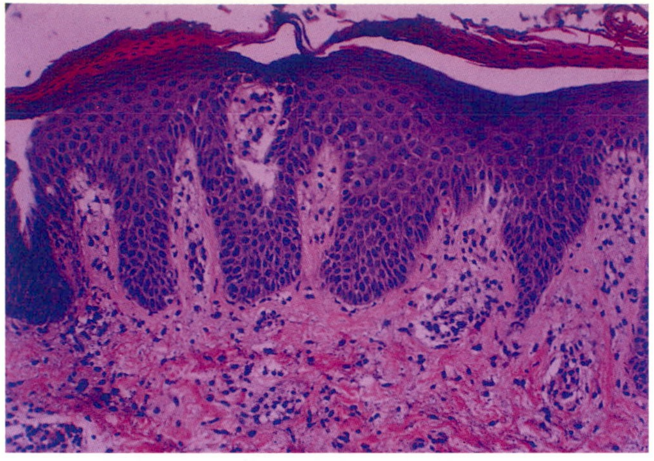

Figure 8–3 (Question 21)

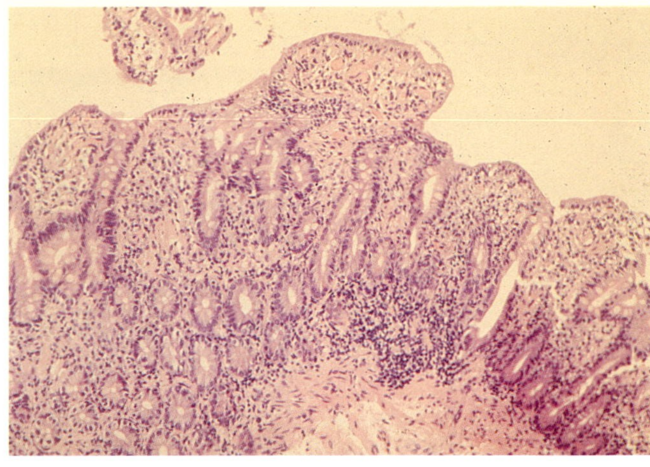

Figure 8–4 (Question 28)

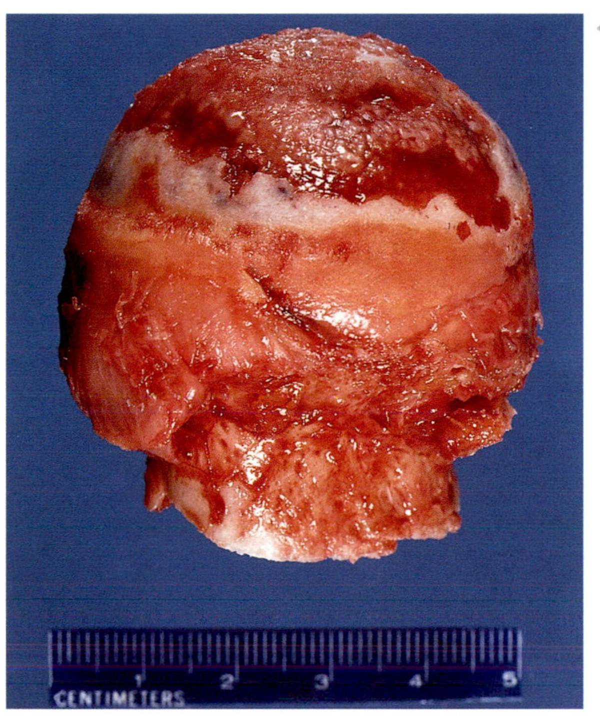

Figure 8–6 (Question 38)

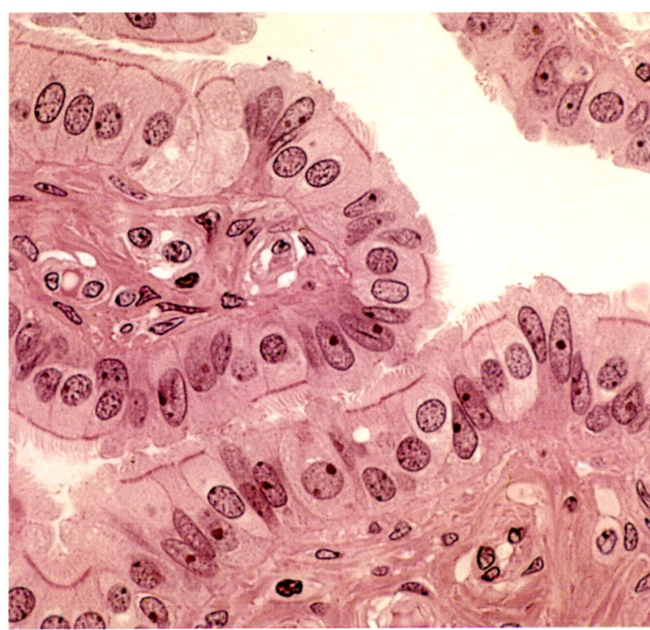

Figure 8–7 (Question 57)

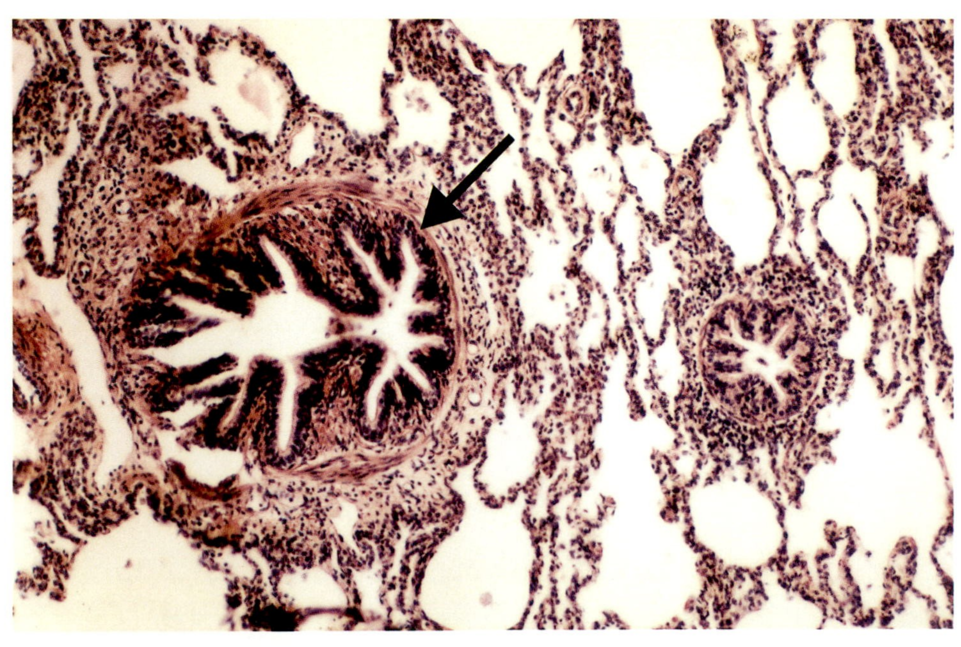

Figure 8–9 (Question 63)

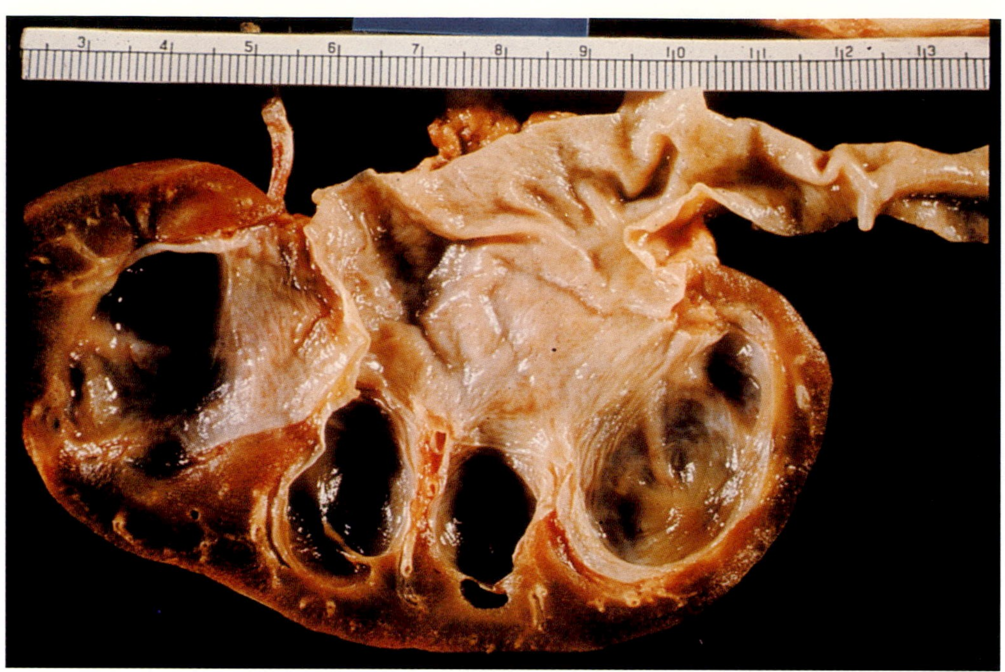

Figure 8–10 (Question 66)

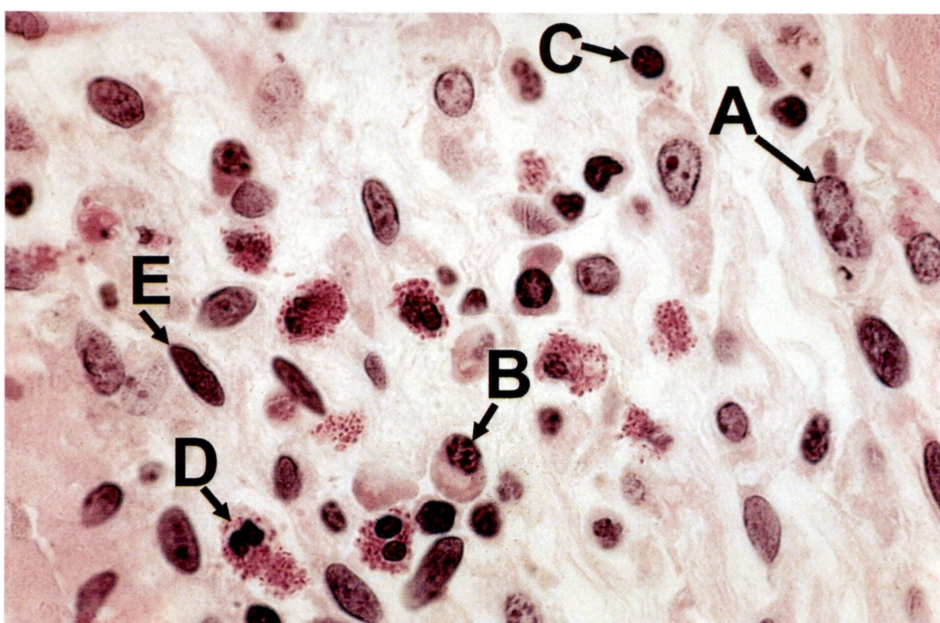

Figure 8–11 (Question 80)

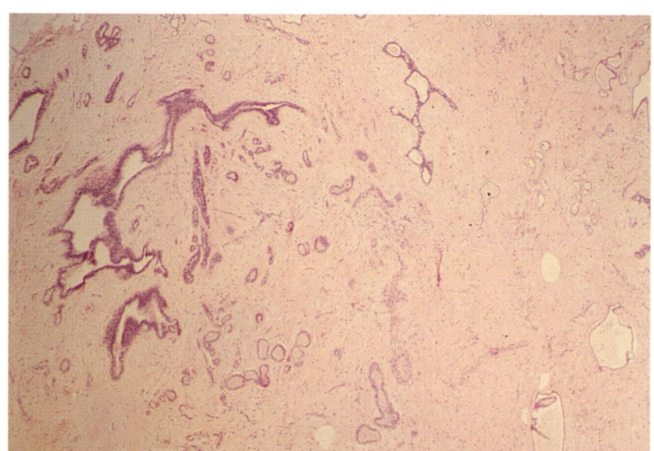

Figure 8–13 (Question 88)

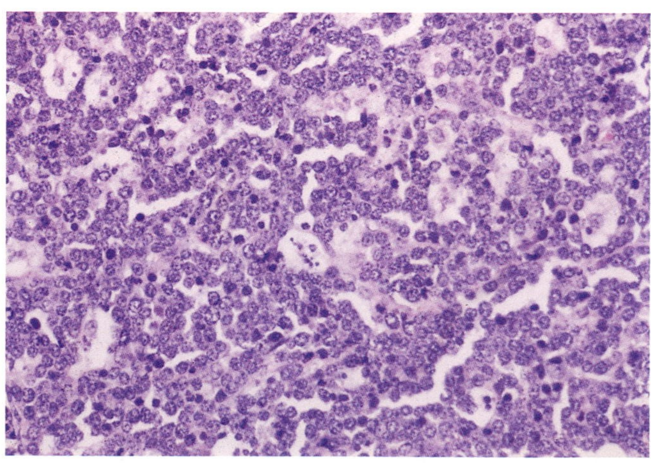

Figure 8–14 (Questions 95 and 96)

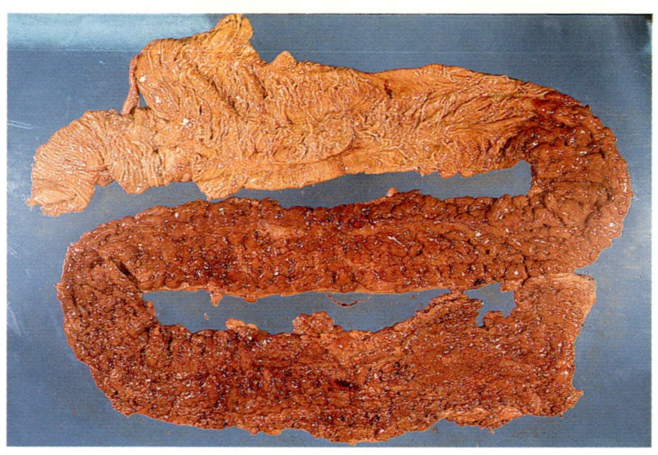

Figure 8–17 (Question 122)

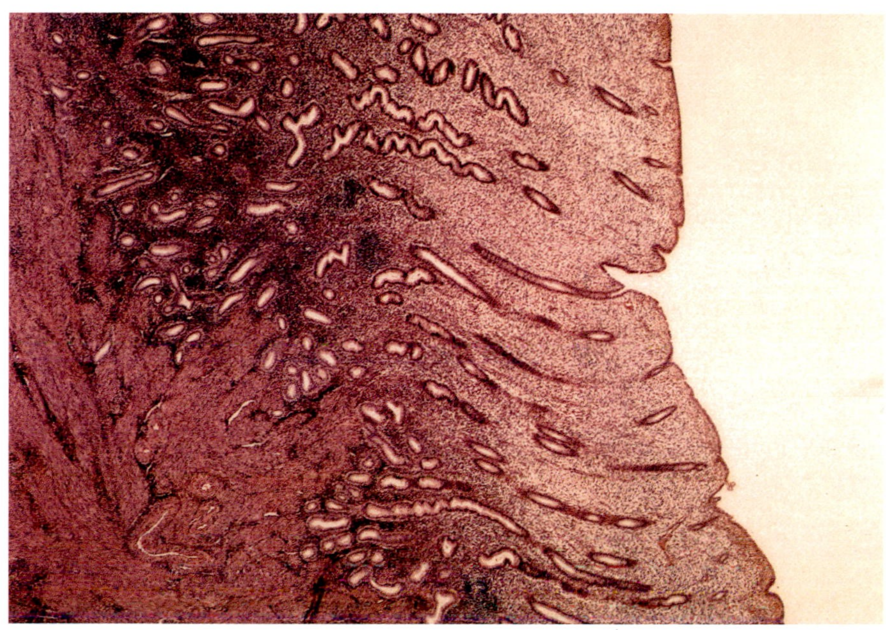

Figure 8–18 (Question 133)

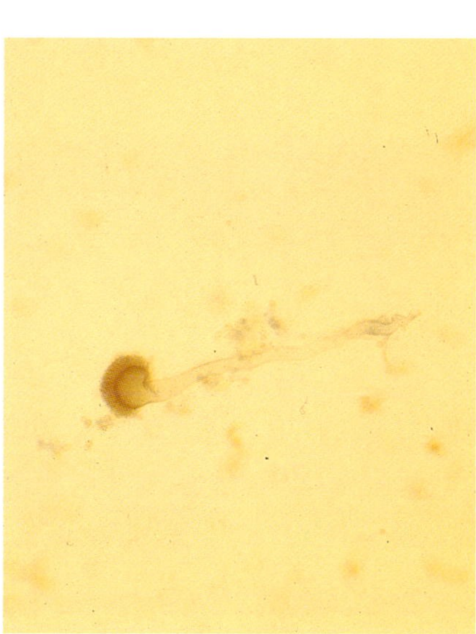

Figure 9–1 (Question 2)

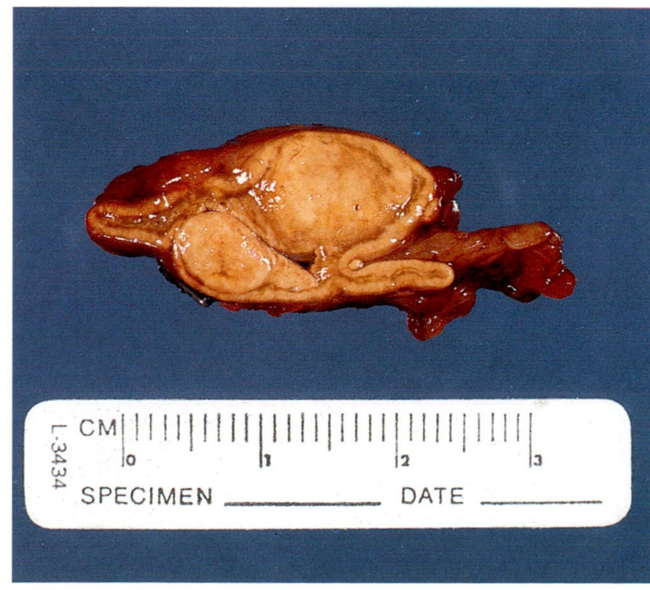

Figure 9–4 (Question 14)

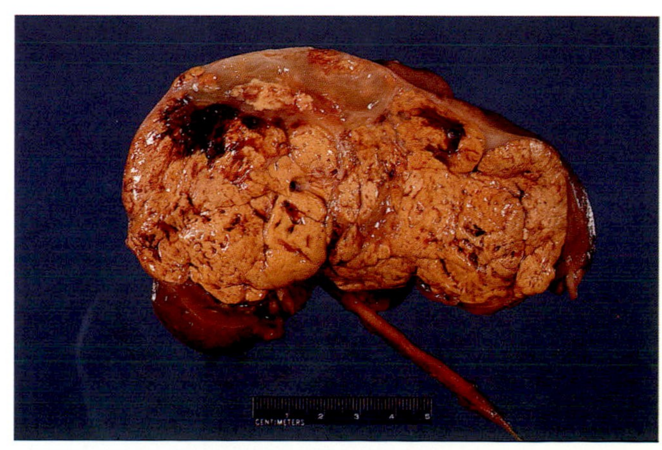

Figure 9–7 (Question 33)

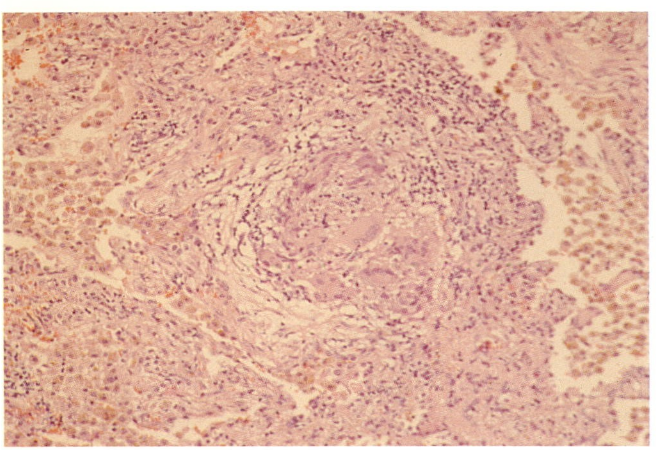

Figure 9–9 (Question 48)

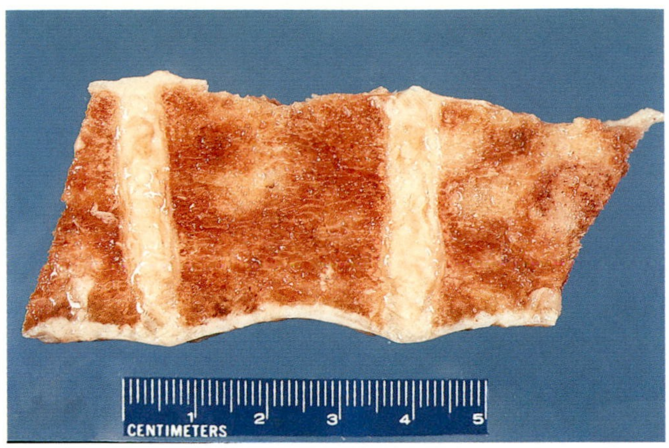

Figure 9–10 (Question 62)

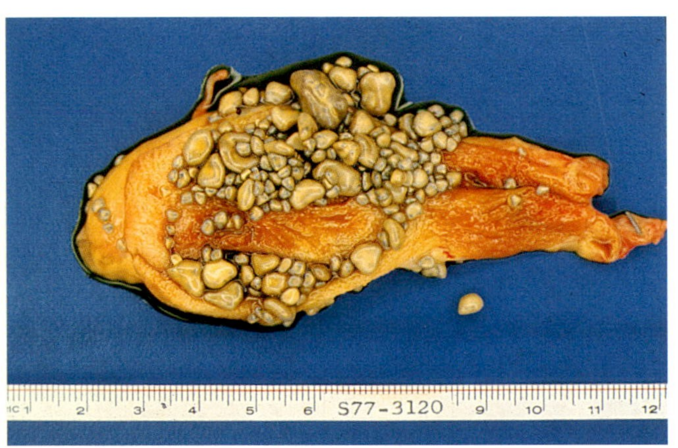

Figure 9–13 (Question 91)

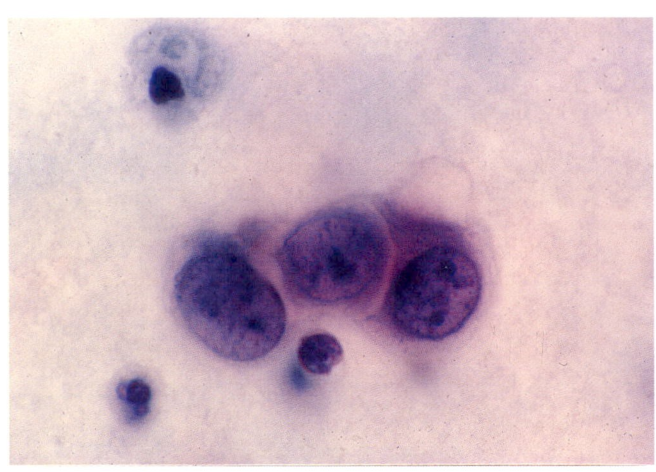

Figure 9–19 (Question 128)

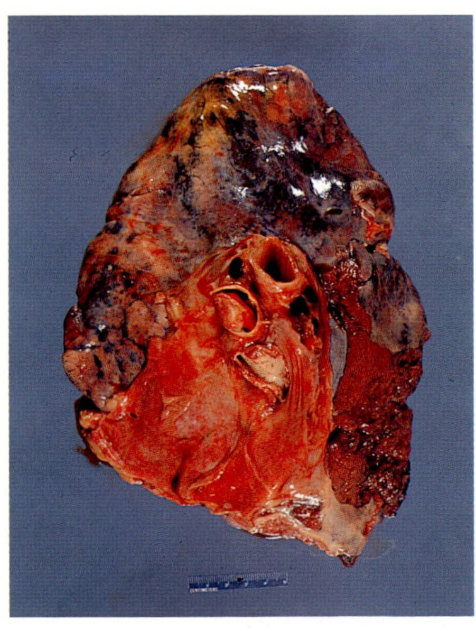

Figure 9–20 (Question 137)

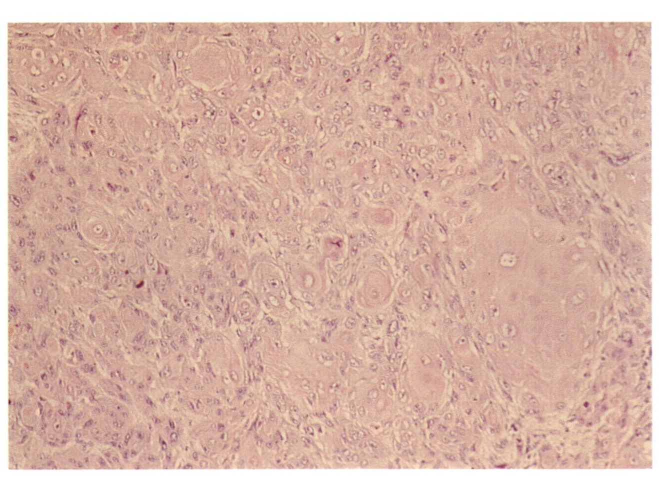

Figure 9–22 (Question 149)

Practice Test I
Questions

DIRECTIONS: (Questions 1 through 150: Each of the numbered items or incomplete statements in this section is followed by answers or by completions of the statement. Select the ONE lettered answer or completion that is BEST in each case.

1. Which of the following fatty acids can be the precursor of prostaglandins in humans?

(A) oleic
(B) palmitic
(C) stearic
(D) arachidonic
(E) palmitoleic

2. You determine that your young patient has an enlarged right side of the heart due to significant shunting of blood from the left to the right atrium. You suspect that this interatrial septal defect is due to an abnormally large foramen ovale resulting from incomplete development of the

(A) septum primum
(B) septum secundum
(C) muscular interventricular septum
(D) ostium primum
(E) ostium secundum

Use Figure 8–1 for questions 3 and 4.

3. Drug L, when administered as a single-bolus IV dose of 30 mg to a 70-kg (154-lb) patient, yields the plasma values shown in Figure 8–1 as a function of time after injection. The apparent volume of distribution is

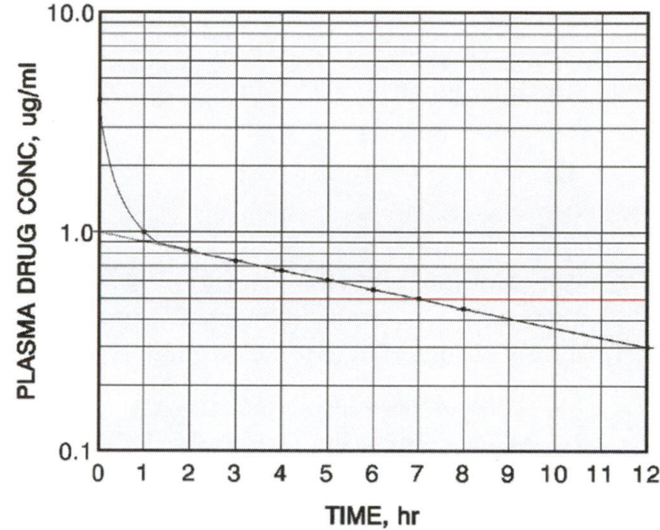

Figure 8–1

(A) 0.25 L
(B) 4.0 L
(C) 14 L
(D) 30 L
(E) 100 L

4. In Figure 8–1, the elimination half-life for drug L is

(A) 0.25 hr
(B) 1.0 hr
(C) 7.0 hr
(D) 12.0 hr
(E) 28.0 hr

5. When a person thinks about biting into a sour apple, he or she may have increased salivation. This phenomenon is probably an example of

(A) classical conditioning
(B) cognitive learning
(C) operant conditioning
(D) shaping
(E) imprinting

6. Mutations of the p53 gene are associated with

(A) carcinogenesis
(B) micrognathia
(C) cystic fibrosis
(D) pulmonary fibrosis
(E) essential hypertension

7. Which of the following symptoms is attributable to the vitamin deficiency most commonly observed in chronic alcoholics?

(A) corneal vascularization
(B) weakening of the rectus muscles of the eye
(C) dark, scaling skin lesions of the mouth
(D) severe eye itch and burning
(E) periosteal hemorrhaging

Questions 8 through 10

8. A 24-year-old male model has a mononucleosis-like illness, characterized by apathy, slow responsiveness, fever, generalized enlargement of lymph nodes, leukopenia, and a maculopapular rash. Cultivation of lymphocytes obtained from this patient resulted in the isolation of the virus responsible for his illness. The virus had an envelope, two molecules of simple-stranded, positive-polarity RNA, and a reverse transcriptase. The most likely diagnosis is

(A) mumps
(B) infectious hepatitis
(C) lymphocyte choriomeningitis
(D) acquired immune deficiency syndrome
(E) pleurodynia

9. The key pathogenic event for this patient is

(A) infection of meninges
(B) invasion of spinal fluid
(C) invasion of bone marrow
(D) reduction of plasma cells
(E) destruction of cells bearing the CD4 molecule

10. The most notable opportunistic neoplasia associated with the illness of this patient is

(A) Kaposi's sarcoma
(B) herpes simplex type 1 lymphoma
(C) Burkitt's lymphoma
(D) Rous sarcoma
(E) herpes simplex type 2 carcinoma

11. In the illustration in Figure 8–2 a patient receives a continuous infusion of gastrin. The production of gastric acid and pancreatic bicarbonate secretion is monitored before and after administration of peptide x (at arrow). Which of the following hormones is most likely to produce the changes observed?

(A) motilin
(B) angiotensin II
(C) cholecystokinin (CCK)
(D) somatostatin
(E) secretin

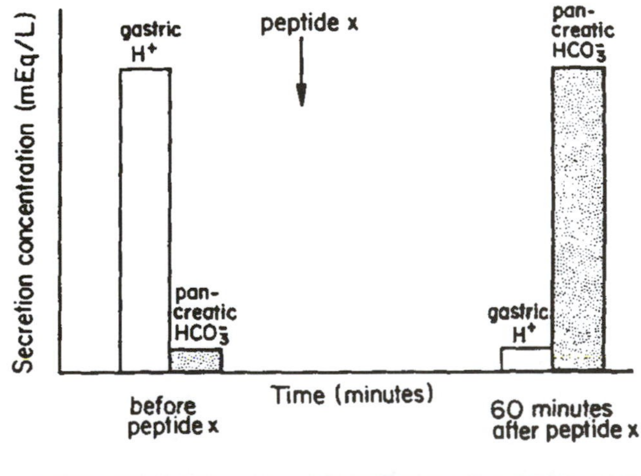

Figure 8–2

12. Based on the part of the brain it supplies, an occlusion of which of the following vessels would produce a visual field deficit?

(A) lenticulostriate artery
(B) calcarine artery
(C) PICA
(D) A_2
(E) medial striate artery

13. Which of the following is true concerning tobacco?

(A) It is the most common type of drug dependency in the United States.
(B) Nicotine is associated with psychological dependence but no physical withdrawal symptoms.
(C) Tobacco dependence usually begins in childhood.
(D) The relapse rate of most smoking cessation programs is 30%.
(E) Physical complications of chronic tobacco use usually begin to appear in 40 pack-years.

14. The second law of thermodynamics states that

(A) reactions that are spontaneous proceed as written because the products of the reaction possess a minimal energy content
(B) the natural tendency of molecules is to increase their state of disorder
(C) the total energy of a molecule is equal to the sum of all internal energies of all the bonds within that molecule
(D) the total energy of the universe cannot increase or decrease
(E) energy cannot change form

15. Which of the following is a mechanism for resistance to trimethoprim by *Escherichia coli*?

(A) expression of β-lactamase activity
(B) acquisition of altered forms of dihydrofolate reductase through plasmid transfer
(C) thickening of the bacterial cell wall
(D) expression of altered forms of the transpeptidase involved in cell wall synthesis
(E) mutating ribosomal subunits to reduce drug binding

16. A 27-year-old recent Asian immigrant is hospitalized because of cyclic severe fevers occurring about every 72 hours due to infection by *Plasmodium malariae.* What is the pathogenic mechanism responsible for the recurrent quartan fever?

(A) central hypothalamic fever due to cerebral malaria
(B) hepatocyte infestation with cyclic lysis
(C) immune mediated destruction of organisms by cytotoxic antimalarial antibodies
(D) red cell lysis upon release of proliferating merozoites
(E) cell-mediated cytokines invoke pyrogen production

17. A 71-year-old male is admitted for TEA (thromboendarterectomy) because of an 85% stenosis of his left common carotid artery documented by Doppler echography. As part of this procedure a brief occlusion of the carotid artery is unavoidable. During this occlusion the anesthesiologist would expect

(A) an increase in the number of impulses from the carotid sinus nerve
(B) vasodilatation throughout the peripheral circulation
(C) a decrease in heart rate
(D) an increase in arterial pressure
(E) an increase in venous capacity

18. Binding of O_2 to hemoglobin

(A) results in a release of the heme from the interior to the exterior of the β subunits leading to an increase in O_2 affinity of the α subunits
(B) causes a large shift of the surrounding secondary structures leading to decreased affinity of the deoxy subunits for CO_2
(C) is cooperative, meaning that after the first O_2 binds, the other subunits are more readily oxygenated
(D) occurs with equal affinity at all four subunits
(E) results in a release of the heme from the interior to the exterior of the α subunits leading to an increase in O_2 affinity of the β subunits

19. You are about to remove a small lesion from the mucosa of the laryngeal vestibule and want to anesthetize the nerve that supplies general sensation to the mucous membrane of that area. The nerve you are interested in is the

(A) pharyngeal plexus
(B) glossopharyngeal nerve
(C) internal laryngeal nerve
(D) external laryngeal nerve
(E) inferior laryngeal nerve

20. On routine examination, a 35-year-old male is found to have a blood pressure of 145/89 mm Hg. Thorough workup excludes an immediate cause of his hypertension and a diagnosis of essential hypertension is made. Long-term regulation of arterial blood pressure in this patient is primarily a function of

(A) total peripheral vascular resistance
(B) peripheral baroreceptors
(C) the autonomic nervous system
(D) urine output and fluid intake
(E) the CNS

21. An adult male has recurrent skin lesions which first appeared over his elbows and knees as well-defined pink papules covered by a micaceous silvery scale. A skin biopsy microphotograph is displayed from one of his lesions in Figure 8–3. The diagnosis is

(A) basal cell carcinoma
(B) malignant melanoma
(C) squamous cell carcinoma
(D) pemphigus vulgaris
(E) psoriasis

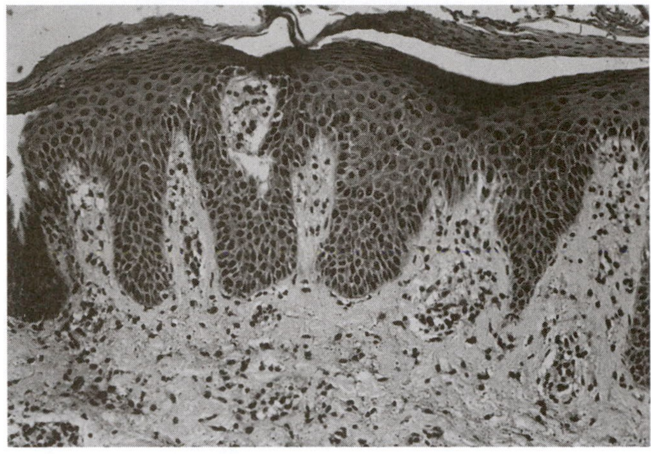

Figure 8–3 (see also Color Insert)

22. Which of the following drugs may produce tachycardia as an adverse effect?

(A) clonidine
(B) nifedipine
(C) propranolol
(D) digoxin
(E) pyridostigmine

23. Which of the following is associated with the use of benzodiazepines?

(A) muscle relaxant effects
(B) agitation in the elderly
(C) addictive effects
(D) non-impairment of conditioned avoidance learning
(E) all of the above

24. The major amino acid precursor for gluconeogenesis is

(A) alanine
(B) aspartate

(C) cysteine
(D) glutamate
(E) serine

25. During the course of a neurological exam you notice that your patient exhibits a loss of all somatosensation on the right side of the body, accompanied by obvious weakness and hyperreflexia in the arm and leg on that side. When protruded, the patient's tongue also deviates to the right. Occlusion of which of the following vessels would account for these deficits?

(A) anterior spinal artery on left
(B) lenticulostriate arteries on left
(C) paramedian branches of basilar bifurcation on right
(D) lenticulostriate arteries on right
(E) posterior spinal artery on right

26. The occurrence of malignant mesothelioma has been correlated with industrial exposure to

(A) beryllium
(B) silica
(C) coal dust
(D) asbestos
(E) nitrogen dioxide

27. A tetraplegic patient has a complete spinal transection between the cervical and thoracic levels. Which of the following statements applies to this patient?

(A) Vital capacity is only slightly compromised.
(B) The maximal inspiratory pressures are more compromised than the expiratory ones.
(C) Functional residual capacity equals residual volume.
(D) The inspiratory reserve volume is greatly reduced (less than 10% of normal).
(E) The ventilatory response to limb exercise is characterized by an increase in tidal volume contributed by the expiratory reserve volume.

28. A six-year-old child presents with diarrhea, malabsorption, and steatorrhea. A microphotograph from a small intestinal mucosal biopsy is displayed in Figure 8–4. An appropriate treatment would be

(A) antineoplastic drugs
(B) β-interferon therapy
(C) a diet free of gluten
(D) surgical resection of a segment of small bowel
(E) a referral to hospice for supportive care

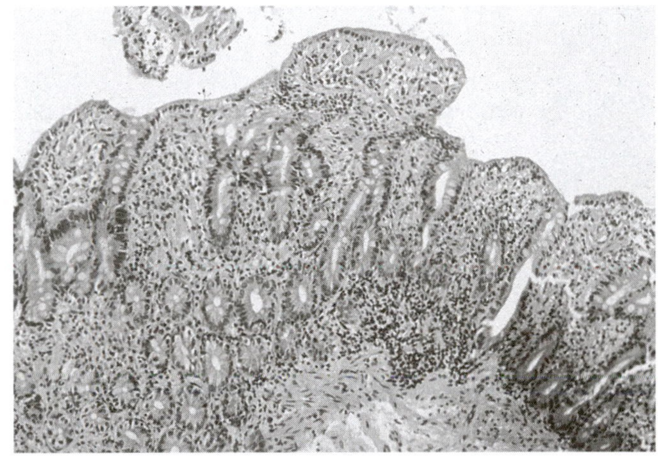

Figure 8–4 (see also Color Insert)

29. Which of the following affects the duration of anesthesia with thiopental?

(A) serum elimination half-life
(B) urinary pH
(C) tissue redistribution
(D) hepatic blood flow
(E) induction of hepatic drug metabolism

30. Hepatic pyruvate kinase is inhibited by which of the following?

(A) phosphofructokinase-2–mediated phosphorylation
(B) cAMP-dependent protein kinase–mediated phosphorylation
(C) oxaloacetate acting allosterically
(D) citrate-mediated polymerization
(E) proteolytic cleavage by chymotrypsin

31. Your patient has a pituitary tumor that has encroached on the cavernous sinus, compressing the internal carotid artery and the adjacent abducens nerve. Interruption of the abducens nerve in the cavernous sinus is most likely to result in

(A) a loss of visual accommodation
(B) ptosis of the upper eyelid
(C) medial deviation of the pupil (internal strabismus)
(D) lateral deviation of the pupil (external strabismus)
(E) dilatation of the pupil

32. Which of the following statements concerning neuroleptic antipsychotic drugs is true?

(A) most are serotonin receptor blockers
(B) most are ineffective against negative symptoms of schizophrenia
(C) most decrease serum prolactin levels
(D) combined use with anticholinergic agents is contraindicated
(E) most of them are non-sedating

33. A 52-year-old male with a history of fainting episodes is admitted for cardiac monitoring. A representative section of his ECG is shown in Figure 8–5. Which of the following statements best describes the pathophysiologic condition of this patient?

(A) The ECG of this patient shows a life-threatening condition and requires immediate application of strong electric current to place the entire myocardium in refractory period.
(B) A drug such as quinidine, which acts in part by prolonging the effective refractory period of conducting tissue, is useful therapy.
(C) The P waves on the ECG recordings are normal in this patient.
(D) The interval between QRS complexes remains constant in this patient.
(E) Since the atria contribute little to ventricular function, the pulse of this patient is expected to be extremely regular in spite of the abnormality.

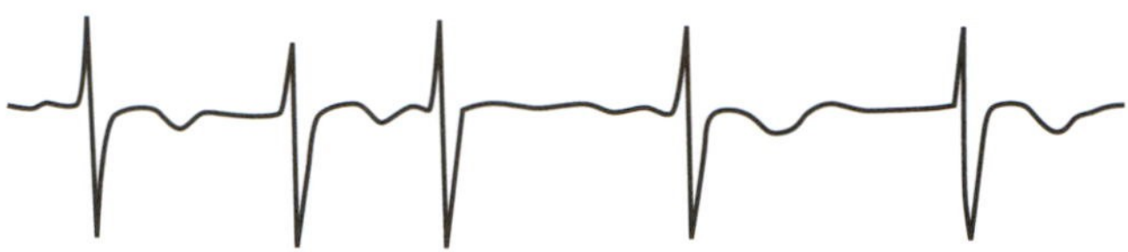

Figure 8–5

34. The inclusion body seen in cells infected with rabies virus is called a(n)

(A) Negri body
(B) Guarnieri's body
(C) reticulate body
(D) elementary body
(E) Ammon's body

35. Which of the following amino acids is purely ketogenic?

(A) cysteine
(B) serine
(C) glycine
(D) leucine
(E) alanine

36. A temporary increase in the number of circulating reticulocytes will most predictably result when an individual

(A) has a bacterial infection
(B) receives a vaccination against measles
(C) has a viral infection
(D) moves from sea level to a high altitude
(E) experiences an allergic reaction to ragweed pollen

37. The production of edema during an acute inflammatory reaction is primarily due to

(A) interleukin-5 secretion by T cells
(B) widening of capillary and venous endothelial pores
(C) reversible swelling of endoplasmic reticulum
(D) pinocytosis
(E) margination of neutrophils

38. A 66-year-old female has complained of hip pain for about three years. A prosthetic hip replacement is recommended. A photograph of her diseased femoral head is displayed in Figure 8–6. What is the likely cause of this abnormality?

(A) degenerative process
(B) benign neoplastic process
(C) infection
(D) malignant neoplastic process
(E) coagulopathy

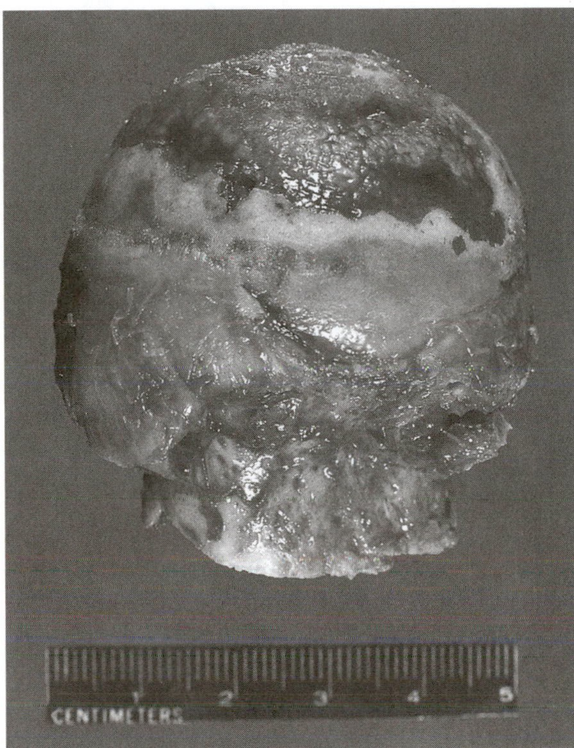

Figure 8–6 (see also Color Insert)

39. An activator of the alternate complement pathway is

(A) interleukin-1 (IL-1)
(B) β interferon
(C) lipoproteins
(D) endotoxin
(E) complement component C1

40. Which of the following is a pharmacologic effect associated with opiate use?

(A) pupillary constriction
(B) intestinal hypermotility
(C) respiratory stimulation
(D) relaxation of the lower end of the common bile duct
(E) stimulation of the cough reflex

41. Phosphofructokinase-2 can best be characterized as

(A) one of the enzymes whose activity is required in the TCA cycle
(B) an enzyme regulated by phosphorylation, an event that increases the rate at which the enzyme phosphorylates its substrate
(C) an enzyme that has fructose-1,6-bisphosphate as a substrate
(D) a bifunctional enzyme that can function as a kinase or as a phosphatase
(E) an allosteric activator of phosphofructokinase-1

42. Observing the protruded tongue tests the competence of the innervation to the muscles of the tongue. A deviation of the protruded tongue to the right indicates damage to the

(A) right hypoglossal nerve
(B) left hypoglossal nerve
(C) right lingual nerve
(D) left lingual nerve
(E) right glossopharyngeal nerve

43. Which of the following is most likely to cause depression?

(A) cancer of the pancreas
(B) cancer of the cervix
(C) cancer of the stomach
(D) cancer of the skin
(E) cancer of the lung

44. A 56-year-old male is slowly losing vision in his right eye. The ophthalmologist notes that the conjunctiva, sclera, and lens are normal on examination. The intraocular pressure, however, is markedly elevated and there is pressure atrophy of the optic disk. What is the likely diagnosis?

(A) glaucoma
(B) cataract
(C) retrolental fibroplasia
(D) arcus senilis
(E) pinguecula

45. During a snowboarding accident a 19-year-old male suffers a complete transection of the upper lumbar spinal cord. During the first 12 hours after this accident you would expect a(n)

(A) exaggerated knee stretch reflex
(B) normal knee stretch reflex
(C) diminished bladder reflex
(D) normal bladder reflex
(E) normal sense of vibration in the legs

46. A worker in a nuclear power plant is exposed to 17 cGy. What acute clinical symptoms are likely to be observed?

(A) none
(B) acute radiation syndrome
(C) hematopoietic syndrome
(D) gastrointestinal syndrome
(E) cerebral syndrome

47. The conversion of fibrinogen to fibrin is catalyzed by

(A) prothrombin
(B) thrombin
(C) antithrombin III
(D) plasmin
(E) heparin

48. A 13-year-old girl has leukemia and needs a bone marrow transplant. Using this girl's leukocytes and irradiated leukocytes from her relatives in mixed leukocyte cultures, the following results were obtained:

SOURCE OF LEUKOCYTES	COUNTS/MIN OF TRITIATED THYMIDINE INCORPORATED
Sister	540
Brother	2000
Mother	280
Grandmother	650
Grandfather	980

The best bone marrow donor for this 13-year-old girl is

(A) sister
(B) brother
(C) mother
(D) grandmother
(E) grandfather

49. A 20-week-old infant suffers from hypothermia, jaundice, and muscular hypotonia. A diagnosis of cretinism is made. What is the proper therapy?

(A) vitamin D
(B) thyroxine
(C) thiamine
(D) antibiotics
(E) growth hormone

50. The thrombolytic mechanism of action of tissue plasminogen activator (tPA) involves

(A) direct conversion of plasminogen to plasmin
(B) proteolytic breakdown of fibrin
(C) depletion of α_2 antiplasmin
(D) formation of an active complex with plasminogen
(E) proteolytic activation of fibrinogen

51. Bipolar cells are located in the

(A) spinal cord
(B) retina
(C) dorsal root ganglion
(D) pyramidal neuron
(E) semilunar ganglia

52. Concerning human immunodeficiency virus (HIV) infection

(A) affected individuals should not engage in vaginal or anal intercourse under any circumstances
(B) affected individuals should not donate blood unless under triple therapy
(C) affected individuals may manifest a cortical but not subcortical dementia
(D) affected individuals can engage in kissing
(E) affected individuals may not safely masturbate

53. Phosphofructokinase-1 can best be characterized by which of the following statements?

(A) The enzyme is activated as the concentration of AMP rises.
(B) The enzyme is negatively regulated by fructose-1,6-bisphosphate.
(C) The enzyme is positively regulated by fructose-1,6-bisphosphatase.
(D) The enzyme is activated when the concentration of NADH is rising.
(E) The enzyme uses AMP in a substrate level phosphorylation to yield ATP.

54. You are called for consultation on a patient who has been comatose for several days. To determine the oxygen consumption of the brain the following measurements are made:

Carotid artery oxygen concentration: 20 ml/O_2 per 100 mL

Jugular vein oxygen concentration: 15 ml/O_2 per 100 mL

Blood flow through brain: 500 mL/min

Oxygen consumption of the brain is

(A) 2.5 mL O_2/min
(B) 5 mL O_2/min
(C) 10 mL O_2/min
(D) 15 mL O_2/min
(E) 25 mL O_2/min

55. A 30-year-old man has a viral infection characterized by fever, myalgia, headache, and a dry, nonproductive cough which lasts for three days. The virus responsible for this infection is an orthomyxovirus and undergoes frequent antigenic changes. It is reasonable to assume that this virus

(A) lacks H antigen
(B) lacks N antigen
(C) has a segmented RNA genome
(D) is a non-enveloped virus
(E) is a bullet-shaped virus

56. An abnormal accumulation of sphingomyelin within reticuloendothelial cells is the primary pathologic alteration seen with

(A) Tay–Sachs disease
(B) Lesch–Nyhan syndrome
(C) Niemann–Pick disease
(D) Pompe's disease
(E) Fabry's disease

57. The section shown in the photomicrograph in Figure 8–7 is typical of the mucosa from the

(A) small intestine
(B) trachea
(C) oviduct
(D) epididymal duct
(E) oropharynx

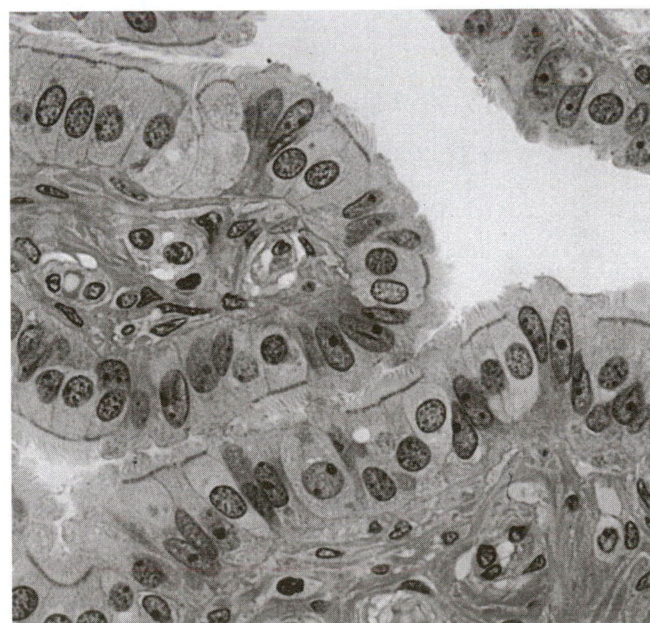

Figure 8–7 (see also Color Insert)

58. Which of the following sets of drugs and description or mechanism of action pairs a drug with its correct description or mechanism?

(A) pralidoxime: reversible cholinesterase inhibitor
(B) isoflurophate: used in treatment of myasthenia gravis
(C) physostigmine: irreversible cholinesterase inhibitor
(D) neostigmine: cholinesterase inhibitor specific for muscarinic synapses
(E) edrophonium: short-acting cholinesterase inhibitor

59. Down syndrome is characterized by the karyotype

(A) trisomy 13
(B) trisomy 18
(C) trisomy 21
(D) XO
(E) XXY

60. The graph in Figure 8–8 shows loss of vision (shaded areas) in the visual field of a patient.

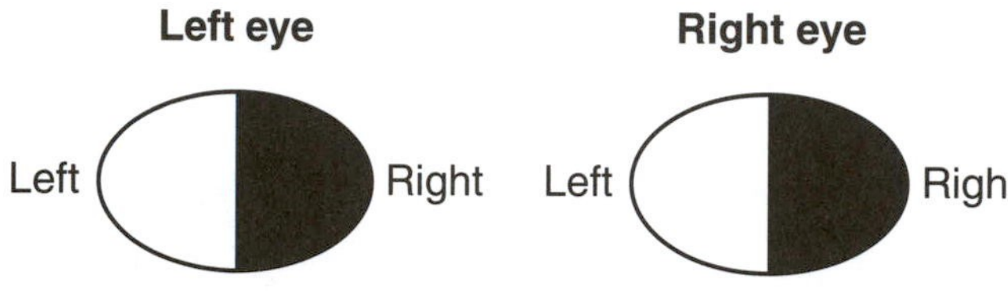

Figure 8–8

This patient has most likely a lesion in the

(A) left optical nerve
(B) right optical nerve
(C) left optical tract
(D) right optical tract
(E) optic chiasm

61. Ethanol consumption inhibits the delivery of glucose to the blood primarily as a consequence of the activity of alcohol dehydrogenase. The effect of this reaction is to reduce the level of NAD^+ which in turn

(A) activates glycolysis by increasing the rate of ATP utilization, signaling a need to oxidize more carbohydrate within hepatocytes
(B) activates the glycolytic reaction catalyzed by glyceraldehyde-3-phosphate dehydrogenase, thereby inhibiting the rate of gluconeogenesis
(C) inhibits the ability of the cell to deliver gluconeogenic substrates in the form of phosphoenol pyruvate as a result of a shift in the equilibrium of the malate dehydrogenase catalyzed reaction
(D) inhibits the gluconeogenic reaction catalyzed by glyceraldehyde-3-phosphate dehydrogenase which requires NAD^+ as a substrate
(E) signals a reduced level of hepatocyte ATP which results in an activation of phosphofructokinase-1

62. Degeneration of the substantia nigra results in

(A) "cogwheel" rigidity
(B) intention tremor
(C) hyperkinesia
(D) chorea
(E) athetosis

63. The arrow in the photomicrograph in Figure 8–9 indicates

(A) the trachea
(B) a bronchus
(C) a bronchiole
(D) an alveolar duct
(E) an arteriole

64. An antihyperlipidemic agent whose actions in lowering LDL cholesterol depend on the expression of functional LDL receptors in the liver is

(A) gemfibrozil
(B) probucol
(C) niacin
(D) etretinate
(E) colestipol

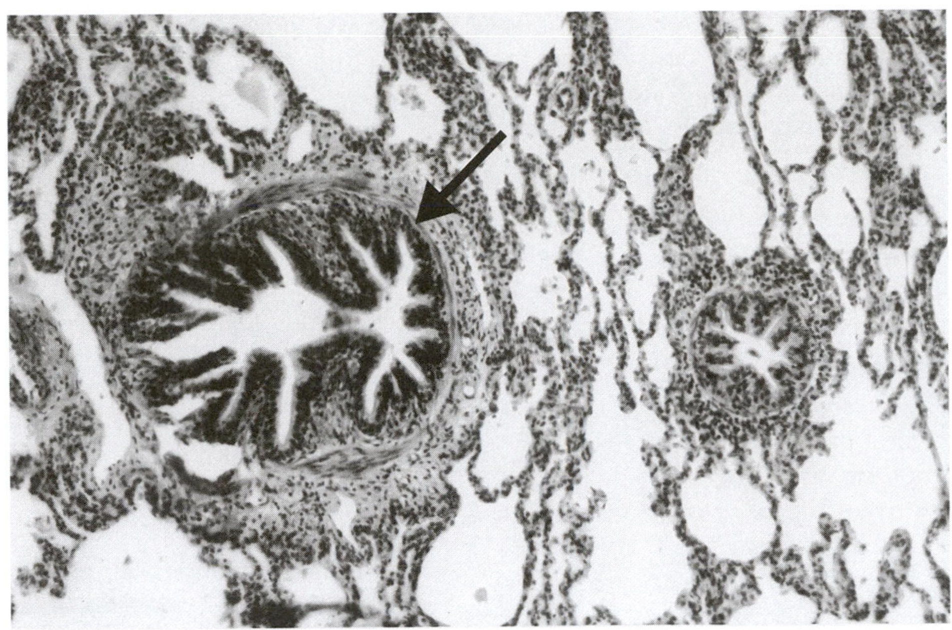

Figure 8–9 (see also Color Insert)

65. The antibody residues that predominantly make up the antigen-combining site as the "contact" amino acids are located within the

(A) constant domains
(B) heavy chains
(C) hypervariable regions
(D) disulfide bonds
(E) framework regions

66. The changes seen in the kidney shown in the photograph in Figure 8–10 may be produced by

(A) postrenal obstruction
(B) renal infarct
(C) hypertension
(D) renal cell carcinoma
(E) abuse of analgesics

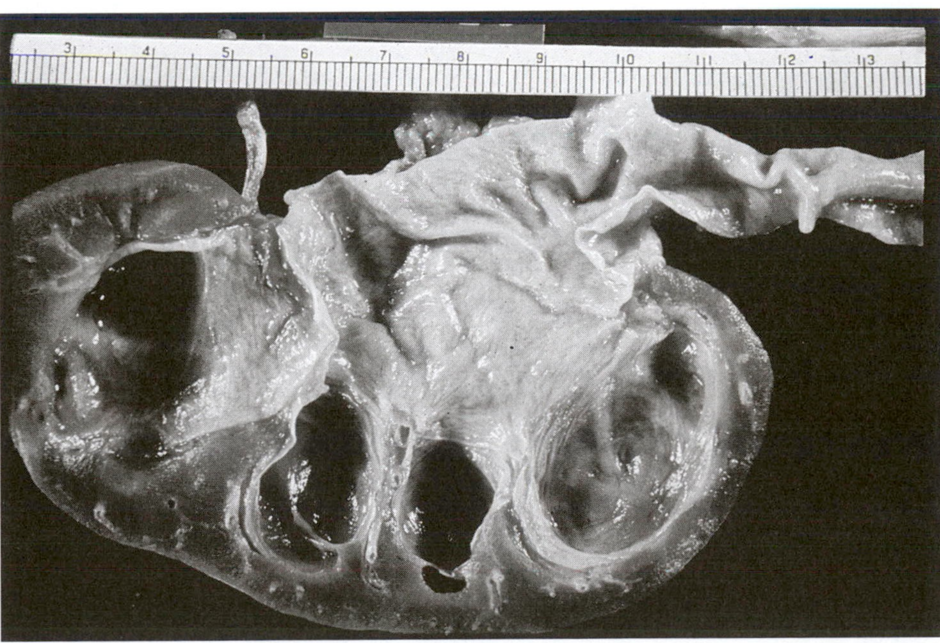

Figure 8–10 (see also Color Insert)

67. The stimulation in salivary gland acini results in a loss of intracellular and a rise in extracellular potassium ions. The efflux of potassium ions is believed to be primarily due to the action of

(A) an Na^+-K^+ exchange mechanism
(B) voltage-dependent non-specific cation channels
(C) calcium-activated K^+ channels
(D) Na^+-K^+-$C1^-$ cotransport
(E) an ouabain-sensitive pump

68. Herniation of the uncal region of the temporal lobe over the free edge of the tentorium and through the tentorial notch compresses the ipsilateral crus cerebri and nearby structures such as the oculomotor nerve. Which of the following combination of signs might be seen in such a case?

(A) contralateral hemiplegia—paralysis of ipsilateral lower facial expression
(B) contralateral hemiplegia—paralysis of the ipsilateral medial rectus muscle
(C) contralateral hemiplegia—contralateral upper facial expression paralysis
(D) ipsilateral hemiplegia—deviation of the tongue toward the side opposite the lesion
(E) ipsilateral hemiplegia—paralysis of the ipsilateral medial rectus muscle

69. Which of the following is present only in the intrinsic pathway of clotting?

(A) fibrinogen (factor I)
(B) accelerin (factor V)
(C) prothrombin (factor II)
(D) antihemophilic factor (factor VIII)
(E) Stuart factor (factor X)

Questions 70 through 75

A 30-year-old woman complains of fatigue, insomnia, and depression.

70. If the patient had weight loss in spite of increased appetite, which of the following tests would be most useful?

(A) dexamethasone suppression test
(B) Rorschach test
(C) thyroid function test
(D) serum calcium level
(E) trail-making test

71. If the patient seems unable to sit still, bursts out crying repeatedly, and is literally wringing her hands, this phenomonon is called

(A) hysteria
(B) psychomotor retardation
(C) pseudobulbar palsy
(D) psychomotor agitation
(E) restless leg syndrome

72. If the patient described in question 71 says that she intends to kill herself by taking an overdose, you should

(A) hospitalize her
(B) prescribe amitriptyline 50 mg at night for 30 days
(C) prescribe fluoxetine 20 mg every day for 14 days
(D) provide supportive psychotherapy
(E) provide explorative psychotherapy

73. If further history reveals that she had attempted suicide several times in the past, which of the following statements would be most useful?

(A) The patient is probably a habitual slasher.
(B) The risk of successful suicide is increased.
(C) The risk of successful suicide is decreased.
(D) The patient's current statement about suicide is probably not serious.
(E) The patient probably has a personality disorder.

74. Which additional information would be most useful in treating this patient at this point?

(A) family history of dysthymia
(B) family history of somatization disorder
(C) family history of bipolar disorder
(D) family history of suicide
(E) family history of schizophrenia

75. If this patient turns out to have unipolar depression, the pharmacologic agent most likely to help the patient's symptomatology is

(A) fluoxetine
(B) nefazodone
(C) tranylcypromine
(D) buspirone
(E) risperidone

76. In the condition known as Bell's palsy, injury to the facial nerve may result in

(A) a loss of sensory innervation to the cornea and conjunctiva
(B) reduced secretion of the parotid gland
(C) an inability to blink
(D) warm and dry skin on the face
(E) chronic constriction of the pupil

77. The blood protein thrombin is known to

(A) have an enzymatic specificity similar to trypsin
(B) form clots by complexing with fibrin
(C) be an oligomeric protein
(D) require vitamin K in its activated form
(E) contain γ-carboxyglutamate residues

78. Which of these agents finds use in the acute treatment of cardiogenic shock because of its ability to increase cardiac inotropicity without producing large increases in chronotropicity?

(A) epinephrine
(B) dobutamine
(C) propranolol
(D) digoxin
(E) atropine

79. A patient's laboratory analysis of arterial plasma showed a pH of 7.44, bicarbonate 15 mEq/L, PO_2 = 80 mm Hg, and PCO_2 = 25 mm Hg. This patient probably

(A) has severe chronic lung disease
(B) is a lowlander who has been vacationing at high altitude for two weeks
(C) is an emergency room patient with severely depressed respiration as a result of a heroin overdose
(D) is an adult psychiatric patient who swallowed an overdose of aspirin
(E) is a subject in a clinical research experiment who has been breathing a gas mixture of 10% oxygen and 90% nitrogen for a few minutes

80. Which letter indicates a macrophage in the photomicrograph of a section of the lamina propria of the cervix in Figure 8–11?

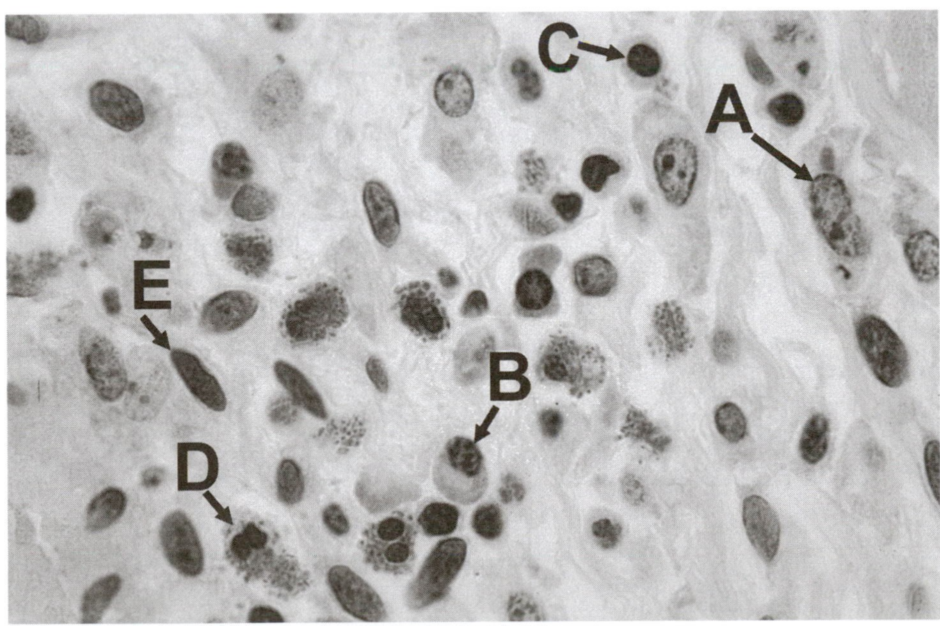

Figure 8–11 (see also Color Insert)

81. A baseball player has pain in his stomach which is relieved by food intake. If gastritis due to *Helicobacter pylori* is suspected, the most useful and rapid diagnostic test to be employed is

(A) determination of IgE
(B) in vivo, or in vitro tests for urease
(C) carbohydrate utilization tests
(D) Gram's stain of the gastric contents
(E) culture of gastric contents on blood agar containing metronidazole and bismuth salts

82. A clinically apparent accumulation of fluid in the peritoneal cavity is termed

(A) empyema
(B) varicosity
(C) urticaria
(D) acantholysis
(E) ascites

83. The number of moles of ATP produced by complete mitochondrial oxidation of 1 mol of pyruvate to CO_2 and water is

(A) 1
(B) 6
(C) 12
(D) 15
(E) 24

84. Figure 8–12 represents filtration through the glomerular membrane and shows the locations of the Starling forces. In which of the following is there a positive ultrafiltration pressure ($P_{uf} > 0$) for formation of glomerular filtrate? (Numbers in mm Hg)

	P_{GC}	P_{BS}	Π_{GC}	Π_{BS}
(A)	40	20	30	10
(B)	40	15	25	0
(C)	40	10	20	0
(D)	50	20	30	0
(E)	55	25	40	5

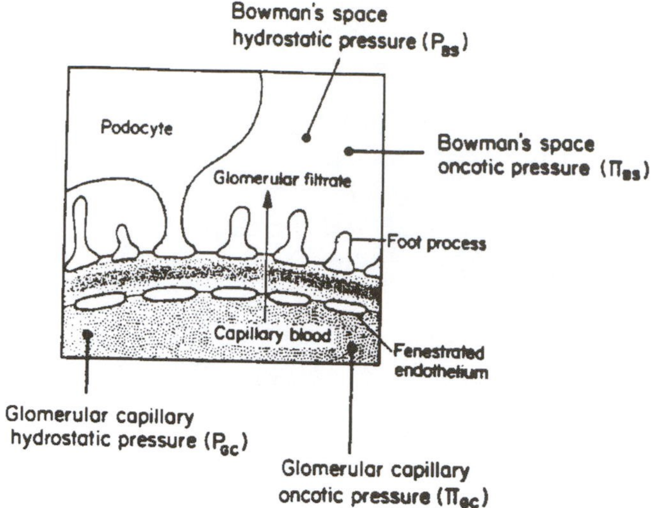

Figure 8–12

85. A 3-year-old child has a temperature of 101°F. On examination, discrete vesiculoulcerative lesions (Koplik's spots) are noted on the mucous membranes of the mouth. The most probable diagnosis is

(A) rubella
(B) herpangina
(C) measles
(D) thrush
(E) scarlet fever

86. Which of the following descriptions best fits the time course for blockade of the motor end plate by a single dose of succinylcholine?

(A) reversible by edrophonium at all times until recovery
(B) reversible early by edrophonium—later not reversed by edrophonium
(C) not reversed early by edrophonium—later reversed by edrophonium
(D) not reversed by edrophonium at all times until recovery
(E) reversible by pralidoxime at all times

87. Histological examination of a lymph node reveals the presence of germinal centers but an absence of the deep cortical (paracortical) zone. This finding is consistent with a condition of

(A) agammaglobulinemia
(B) thymic hypoplasia
(C) combined immunodeficiency
(D) an acute bacterial infection
(E) thrombocytopenia

88. A 35-year-old woman has noticed a slowly growing mass in her left breast over the past four months. At surgery, the mass is found to be predominantly solid, tan-white, rubbery, well circumscribed, and measuring about 3 × 3 × 3 cm. A representative photomicrograph of the lesion is displayed in Figure 8–13. What is the diagnosis?

(A) medullary carcinoma
(B) fibroadenoma
(C) Paget's disease
(D) intraductal carcinoma
(E) scirrhous carcinoma

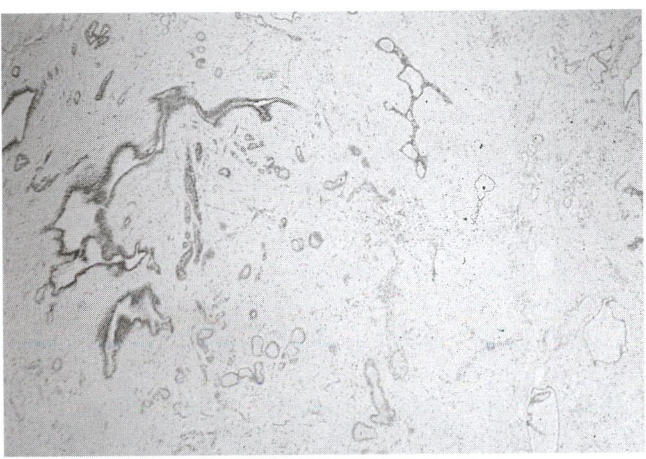

Figure 8–13 (see also Color Insert)

89. Most blood vessels dilate under ischemic conditions. In which arterial region does hypoxia cause vasoconstriction?

(A) coronary arteries
(B) pulmonary arteries
(C) renal arteries
(D) gastrointestinal arteries
(E) skeletal muscle arteries

90. Which of the following reflects the most accurate effects of the increased cAMP that results in hepatocytes in response to glucagon?

(A) an increased activity of pyruvate kinase
(B) an increased activity of phosphofructokinase-1
(C) an increase in the kinase activity of phosphofructokinase-2
(D) an increase in the phosphatase activity of phosphofructokinase-2
(E) an increased activity in phosphoprotein phosphatases

91. Irrigation of the seated patient's right ear with warm water should produce

(A) slow conjugate horizontal eye movement to the right
(B) fast conjugate horizontal eye movement to the left
(C) slow conjugate horizontal eye movement to the left
(D) slow horizontal movement of right eye and fast movement of left eye
(E) no horizontal eye movements

92. Concerning human immunodeficiency virus (HIV) infection, which of the following statements is correct?

(A) The sex ratio between infected males and females is about the same.
(B) The number of infected men is growing at a higher rate than infected women.
(C) The percentage of total cases among gay and bisexual men has declined in the United States.
(D) The percentage of heterosexual men with HIV is decreasing.
(E) Most women acquire HIV infection through IV drugs.

93. A drug has a V_d of 30 L and a total systemic clearance rate of 20 L/hr, with 80% being eliminated by the liver and 20% eliminated by the kidney. The maintenance infusion rate for a normal patient is 20 mg/hr. Which of the following infusion rates should be used to maintain the same steady state plasma concentration in a patient with 50% renal function?

(A) 4 mg/hr
(B) 10 mg/hr
(C) 15 mg/hr
(D) 18 mg/hr
(E) 20 mg/hr

94. The DiGeorge syndrome is characterized by

(A) a depletion of lymph node lymphocytes in both T- and B-dependent areas
(B) defective development of the third and fourth pharyngeal pouches
(C) an absence of isohemagglutinins
(D) a defect in neutrophil chemotaxis
(E) a depletion of B-dependent areas in lymph nodes

Questions 95 and 96

A 12-year-old African male has developed a large facial tumor. The histology of the lesion obtained during a fine needle biopsy is displayed in Figure 8–14.

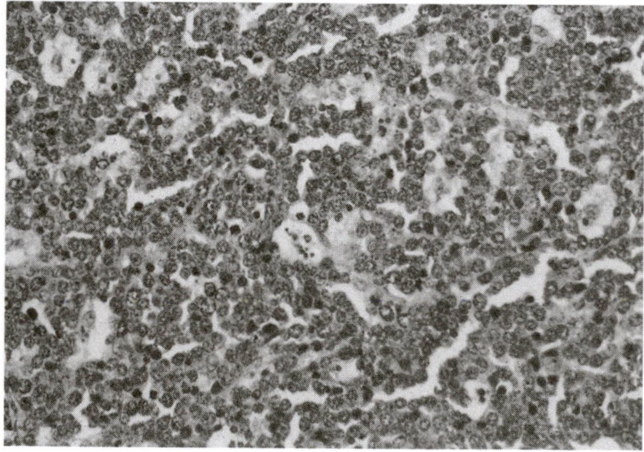

Figure 8–14 (see also Color Insert)

95. What is the diagnosis?

(A) parasitic lymphadenitis
(B) Burkitt's lymphoma
(C) salivary gland lymphoepithelioma
(D) chronic lymphocytic leukemia–lymphoma
(E) adenocarcinoma

96. The development of this lesion is associated with

(A) infection with *Wuchereria bancrofti*
(B) Sjögren syndrome
(C) aflatoxin exposure
(D) deficiency of an essential dietary nutrient
(E) infection with Epstein–Barr virus

97. When lactate is used as a source of carbon atoms for gluconeogenesis, the NADH required for the glyceraldehyde-3-phosphate dehydrogenase reaction comes from the action of which enzyme?

(A) glucose-6-phosphate dehydrogenase
(B) glycerol-3-phosphate dehydrogenase
(C) malate dehydrogenase
(D) lactate dehydrogenase
(E) phosphoenol pyruvate carboxykinase

98. The characteristic pathologic lesion of sarcoid is

(A) fibroblastic proliferation
(B) non-caseating granuloma
(C) pyogenic abscess
(D) mucoid cyst
(E) hyaline membrane formation

99. You ask your patient to look medially and then down. Which muscle is he using when he looks down?

(A) superior rectus
(B) inferior rectus
(C) medial rectus
(D) inferior oblique
(E) superior oblique

100. Which of the following agents has good antipyretic activity but poor anti-inflammatory activity?

(A) indomethacin
(B) aspirin
(C) acetaminophen
(D) nabumetone
(E) tolmetin

101. A research assistant is involved in the production of anthrax vaccine. He must destroy all vegetative cells and spores of *Bacillus anthracis* that have contaminated the glassware he used. This can best be accomplished by

(A) boiling
(B) use of ethyl alcohol
(C) use of anionic detergents
(D) use of oxidizing agents
(E) autoclaving

102. In normal adult men, the major source of circulating estradiol is provided by

(A) secretion from the Leydig cells in the testes
(B) secretion from the Sertoli cells in the testes
(C) the action of aromatase on circulating androgens
(D) release from the inner layers of the adrenal cortex
(E) the action of aromatase on circulating estrone

103. During pregnancy the smooth muscle cells of the uterus reversibly increase in size but do not add any additional new cells within the myometrium. What term best defines this alteration?

(A) hypoxia
(B) hyperplasia
(C) hypertrophy
(D) metaplasia
(E) dysplasia

104. Symptoms of von Gierke's disease include massive enlargement of the liver, severe hypoglycemia, ketosis, hyperlipemia, and hyperuricemia. Biopsy of the tissues of an affected person would show that the liver had a specific deficiency of the enzyme

(A) glucokinase
(B) hexokinase
(C) glucose 6-phosphatase
(D) phosphofructokinase-1
(E) α-1,4-glucosidase

105. Figure 8–15 shows a cardiac pacemaker potential (bold line = normal). Which of the curves best represents the effect of sympathetic stimulation on the pacemaker potential?

(A) curve A
(B) curve B
(C) curve C
(D) curve D
(E) sympathetic stimulation does not alter the pacemaker potential

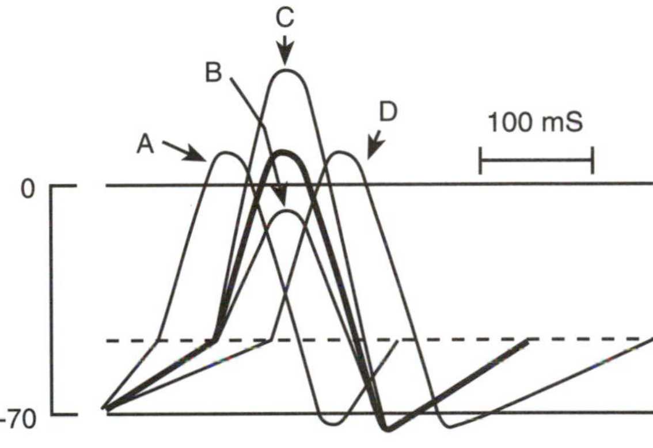

Figure 8–15

106. An indication for HIV testing would be

(A) homosexuality
(B) patients who request testing
(C) psychiatric hospitalization
(D) medical students
(E) induction into the military

107. Which of the following statements can be correctly applied to spasticity?

(A) Spasticity is usually associated with hypotonia.
(B) Lesions involving lower motor neurons are typically associated with spasticity.
(C) Spasticity involves an increase in the resistance to passive movement.
(D) A C8 spinal cord hemisection would lead to spasticity in the contralateral lower extremity.
(E) Clinically, spasticity and rigidity are similar entities and reflect injury to the same brain systems.

108. Methimazole is useful in the treatment of

(A) Hashimoto's thyroiditis
(B) hyperthyroidism
(C) thyrotoxicosis factitia
(D) hypoparathyroidism
(E) hypothyroidism

109. In a positive viral hemagglutination inhibition test, hemagglutination is inhibited by which one of the following substances in the serum?

(A) antiviral antibody
(B) latex agglutinins
(C) Rh antibody
(D) hemolysin
(E) virus

110. Which of the following clinical situations is most likely associated with an increase in predominantly conjugated ("direct") bilirubin?

(A) Gilbert's syndrome
(B) physiological jaundice of the neonate
(C) kernicterus following rhesus incompatibility
(D) pancreatic head tumor
(E) colon tumor

111. Figure 8–16 demonstrates enzyme kinetics of

(A) a competitively inhibited enzyme
(B) a noncompetitively inhibited enzyme
(C) an allosteric enzyme with and without effector
(D) two enzymes, each with a different V_{max}
(E) an irreversibly inhibited enzyme

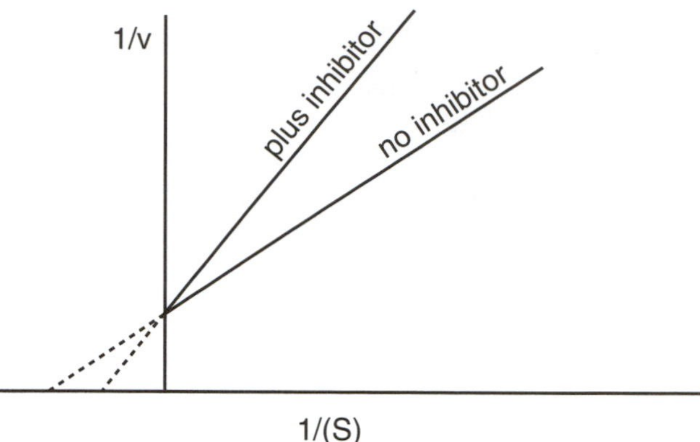

Figure 8–16

112. A 28-year-old male with a history of paroxysmal hypertensive episodes due to a benign pheochromocytoma undergoes a bilateral adrenalectomy. In the absence of hormone replacement therapy, this procedure could result in death within a few days. Most likely the cause of death in this patient would be due to loss of adrenal production of

(A) cortisol
(B) corticosterone
(C) aldosterone
(D) dehydroepiandrosterone
(E) catecholamines

113. A serious adverse effect that may occur with a single therapeutic dose of one aspirin tablet is

(A) infertility
(B) hepatotoxicity
(C) nephrotoxicity
(D) bronchoconstriction
(E) hemolytic anemia

114. In an influenza virus complement-fixation procedure, the indicator system consists of complement, sheep RBCs, plus

(A) ^{51}Cr-labeled sheep RBCs
(B) antibody to influenza virus

(C) fluorescent-tagged virus
(D) antibody to sheep RBCs
(E) neuraminidase

115. A 67-year-old man has a primary well-differentiated adenocarcinoma of the sigmoid colon that invades into, but not through, the muscularis propria. Eleven lymph nodes in the sigmoid resection specimen are examined pathologically and two are found to contain metastatic carcinoma. During surgery there was no evidence of distant metastases to the liver. How would you stage this cancer?

(A) T1 N0 M0
(B) T2 N0 M1
(C) T2 N1 M0
(D) T3 N0 M1
(E) T4 N0 M1

116. A patient with unexplained episodes of hypoglycemia is admitted for evaluation of a possible pancreatic islet tumor. Glucagon secretion from α cells of the pancreatic islets normally is

(A) inhibited by elevated cAMP levels
(B) inhibited by elevated amino acid concentrations in plasma
(C) stimulated by elevated plasma glucose
(D) stimulated by insulin
(E) enhanced by sympathetic stimulation

117. A 36-year-old avid hiker has a four-week history of migratory arthritis and malaise. Her serum contains IgM and IgG antibodies against *Borrelia burgdorferi.* What is the likely diagnosis?

(A) rheumatoid arthritis
(B) Lyme disease
(C) achondroplasia
(D) osteoarthritis
(E) ochronosis

118. The appearance of high levels of phenylpyruvate and phenyllactate in the urine is indicative of which disorder?

(A) Hartnup disease
(B) phenylketonuria
(C) maple syrup urine disease
(D) alcaptonuria
(E) hepatorenal tyrosinemia

119. The microscopic manifestation of highly condensed, transcriptionally inactive DNA is

(A) euchromatin
(B) heterochromatin
(C) nucleolus
(D) nuclear pore
(E) rough endoplasmic reticulum (rER)

120. Patient A.S. is an 82-year-old Caucasian male with a heart murmur. He has been placed on a regimen of an oral anticoagulant. An increased anticoagulant response would be expected with the co-administration of

(A) phenobarbital
(B) rifampin
(C) cefotaxime
(D) cholestyramine
(E) ranitidine

121. A graft-versus-host reaction may occur

(A) because the graft is contaminated with gram-negative microorganisms
(B) only when tumor tissues are grafted
(C) when immunocompetent lymphoid cells are present in the graft and the recipient is immunosuppressed
(D) because the graft has histocompatibility antigens not found in the recipient
(E) when a histocompatible graft is irradiated before use

Questions 122 and 123

A 28-year-old male has a long history of intermittent bloody diarrhea.

122. The colon is surgically removed and displayed in Figure 8–17. What is the likely diagnosis?

(A) pseudomembranous colitis
(B) amebic colitis
(C) ulcerative colitis
(D) collagenous colitis
(E) gangrenous colitis

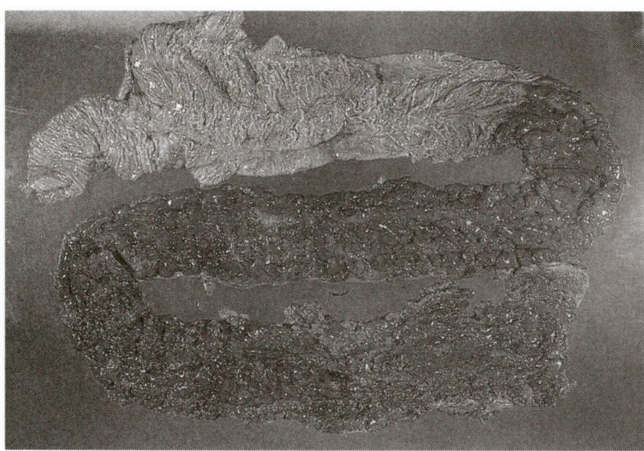

Figure 8–17 (see also Color Insert)

123. The rationale for a colonic surgical resection relates to an increased risk of developing

(A) melanoma
(B) liver abscess
(C) amyloidosis
(D) stricture
(E) carcinoma

124. Endothelin contracts vascular smooth muscle cells by

(A) increasing cellular cAMP
(B) increasing cellular cGMP
(C) activation of tyrosine kinase
(D) increasing cellular inositol-tris-phosphate
(E) regulation of gene expression

125. Introns are correctly described as

(A) noncoding intervening sequences splitting genes for a single protein
(B) noncoding intervening sequences separating genes for different proteins
(C) all noncoding sequences of DNA
(D) untranslated regions of mature mRNA that separate different protein messages
(E) untranslated regions of mature mRNA that intervene in the message for a single protein

126. The muscles of the pharynx have a common innervation except for the stylopharyngeus muscle, which receives its innervation from the

(A) pharyngeal plexus
(B) vagus nerve
(C) glossopharyngeal nerve
(D) facial nerve
(E) mandibular nerve

127. Propranolol is beneficial in the treatment of angina because it

(A) dilates capacitance vessels
(B) increases coronary blood flow
(C) increases oxygen delivery
(D) inhibits renin release
(E) reduces oxygen demand

128. A 30-year-old patient with cystic fibrosis has fever and is coughing sputum, which when grown on nutrient agar produces gram-negative, motile rods that elaborate a blue-green color. This microorganism most likely is

(A) *Pseudomonas aeruginosa*
(B) *Legionella pneumophila*
(C) *Mycoplasma pneumoniae*
(D) *Staphylococcus aureus*
(E) *Staphylococcus epidermidis*

129. The term "personality" may be best defined as a

(A) person's defensive armamentarium
(B) person's ego

(C) person's characteristic patterns of thought, behavior, and feelings
(D) combination of the person's ego and superego
(E) person's characteristic means of relating with reality

130. A 17-year-old male is admitted with a gunshot wound to his left temporal cortex. Damage to Wernicke's area of the cerebral cortex is associated with

(A) impaired vocalization
(B) impaired comprehension of speech
(C) impaired recognition of visual forms
(D) dyslexia
(E) loss of short-term memory

131. Rh_o-specific immune globulin (RhoGAM) therapeutic preparations are correctly described as composed of

(A) anti-inflammatory agents
(B) blocking antibodies
(C) antilymphocyte antibodies
(D) antiallergen antibodies
(E) enhancing antibodies

132. Which glycosaminoglycan is a major component of mast cells lining the blood vessels?

(A) hyaluronate
(B) chondroitin sulfate
(C) dermatan sulfate
(D) keratan sulfate
(E) heparin

133. The photomicrograph in Figure 8–18 illustrates the appearance of the endometrium at what approximate day of a nominal 28-day menstrual cycle?

(A) 2
(B) 9
(C) 16
(D) 21
(E) 26

134. In persons suffering from severe anaphylactic shock, the drug of choice for restoring circulation and relieving angioedema is

(A) epinephrine
(B) norepinephrine
(C) isoproterenol
(D) phenylephrine
(E) dopamine

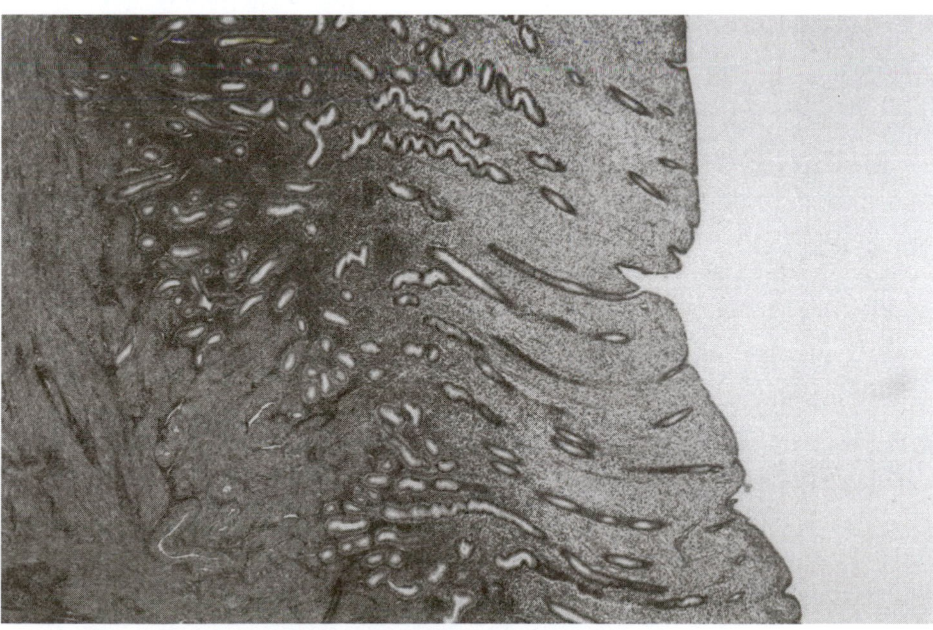

Figure 8–18 (see also Color Insert)

135. In testicular feminization syndrome the karyotype is

(A) 46,XY
(B) 46,XX
(C) 45,XO
(D) 47,XXY
(E) 47,XXX

136. A medical student has been immunized with hepatitis B virus (HBV) recombinant vaccine. The curve in Figure 8–19 represents the production of protective antibodies to the viral component present in the recombinant vaccine. This viral component most likely is

(A) RNA genome of HBV
(B) nucleocapsid proteins of HBV
(C) viral core antigen (HBcAg)
(D) viral surface antigen (HBsAg)
(E) viral e antigen (HBeAg)

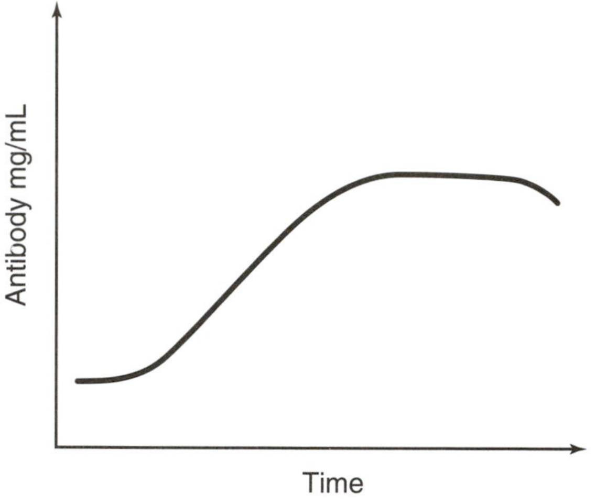

Figure 8–19

137. The central processes of muscle (spindle) afferents from the upper extremity terminate within the

(A) dorsal horn from C3 to C5
(B) nucleus dorsalis from C5 to T1
(C) ipsilateral lateral (accessory) cuneate nucleus
(D) contralateral cuneate nucleus
(E) ipsilateral nucleus gracilis

138. Patient E.W. is a 67-year-old Caucasian female who follows a vegetarian diet. She complains of weakness and "pins and needles" sensations throughout her body. The woman's daughter confides that her mother has undergone a personality change with periods of irritability and confusion. Examination of a blood sample showed the presence of macrocytic megaloblastic anemia. This patient will probably require administration of

(A) folic acid
(B) vitamin B_{12}
(C) ferrous sulfate
(D) intrinsic factor
(E) thiamine

139. The reaction order for $A + B \rightarrow P$ is

(A) first order
(B) second order
(C) third order
(D) pseudo-first order
(E) zero order

140. The illustration in Figure 8–20 displays the organism that may cause

(A) phycomycosis
(B) tinea barbae
(C) tinea corporis
(D) tinea pedis
(E) aspergillosis

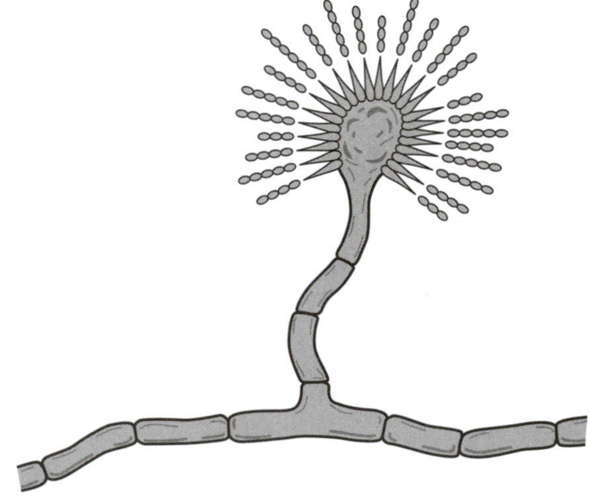

Figure 8–20

141. Some clinical improvement in a limited number of Alzheimer's disease patients has been noted with the chronic use of

(A) atropine
(B) cimetidine
(C) tacrine
(D) atracurium
(E) ipratropium

142. A patient is suffering from eruptions and multiple draining sinuses with copious suppuration. The lesions are located in the cervicofacial region. Microscopic examination of material taken from the lesions reveals small sulfur granules. This patient is most likely suffering from

(A) amebiasis
(B) mucormycosis
(C) histoplasmosis
(D) candidiasis
(E) actinomycosis

143. You are attending a patient with a long-standing history of angina pectoris. Left coronary blood flow normally is greatest

(A) in early systole
(B) at the peak aortic systolic
(C) near the end of systole
(D) in early diastole
(E) near the end of diastole

144. Which statement concerning the processing of precise tactile localization on the face is correct?

(A) Signals from the right side of the face reach the ipsilateral chief sensory nucleus.
(B) Signals from the right side of the face reach the ipsilateral spinal trigeminal nucleus.
(C) Pain sensation from the upper (maxillary) teeth is carried in the contralateral spinal trigeminal tract.
(D) The ventral posterior medial nucleus of the thalamus receives information from the ipsilateral side of the face.
(E) The ventral trigeminothalamic tract terminates in the chief sensory trigeminal nucleus.

145. A 35-year-old apparently healthy black male undergoes a medical examination in application for purchasing life insurance. He is not anemic. His hemoglobin electrophoresis is reported as Hb A, 62%; Hb S, 35%; Hb F, 1%; Hb A2, 1%; no variant C, D, G, or H bands detected. What is the likely diagnosis?

(A) thalassemia minor
(B) thalassemia major
(C) sickle trait
(D) sickle cell disease
(E) sickle thalassemia minor

146. The family of diseases termed "mucopolysaccharidoses" are the result of the

(A) inability of neuronal cells to synthesize the glycoprotein portion of their myelin sheaths
(B) excess synthesis of glycosaminoglycans in hepatocytes
(C) excess synthesis of proteoglycans in nerve cells
(D) loss of lysosomal enzymes necessary for the degradation of glycosaminoglycans
(E) loss of enzymes necessary for the synthesis of lysosomal glycosaminoglycans

147. In the Figure 8–21, the curve labeled STANDARD shows the response generated with increasing concentrations of a standard agonist. Which of the lettered curves shows the response expected with increasing concentrations of the standard agonist in the presence of a concentration of a competitive antagonist at a concentration of ninefold excess over its dissociation constant?

(A) curve A
(B) curve B
(C) curve C
(D) curve D
(E) curve E

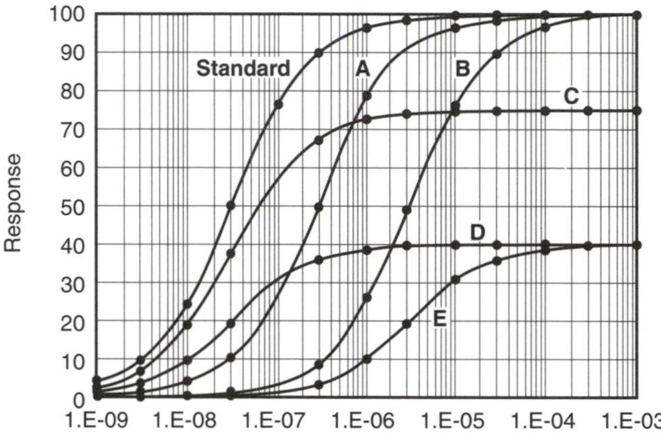

Figure 8–21

148. A banker has been told by his physician that the rash on his arm is due to delayed-type hypersensitivity. If this is actually the case, which one of the following statements is accurate?

(A) This type of allergy usually occurs after inhalation of grass pollens.
(B) This allergy is due to IgE absorbed on mast cells.
(C) This allergy does not cause tissue damage.
(D) Delayed-type hypersensitivity is suppressed by antihistaminic drugs.
(E) Delayed-type hypersensitivity can be transferred passively to volunteers by sensitized lymphocytes.

149. Average hemoglobin levels are 16 g/dL for males and 14 g/dL for females. What is the main reason for the low hemoglobin level in females?

(A) shorter erythrocyte half-life time
(B) smaller number of bone marrow stem cells
(C) decreased responsiveness of bone marrow stem cells to erythropoietin
(D) low testosterone levels in the female
(E) blood loss during menstruation

150. The following are pharmacokinetic data for the drug kanamycin: clearance, 6 L/hr in a 70-kg adult; effective plasma concentration, 5 μg/mL. Calculate the intravenous maintenance infusion rate for kanamycin in a 70-kg person.

(A) 6 mg/hr
(B) 30 mg/hr
(C) 120 mg/hr
(D) 350 mg/hr
(E) 420 mg/hr

Answers and Explanations

1. **(D)** Except for arachidonic, all of the fatty acids listed (choices A, B, C, and E) in the question are non-essential and cannot be precursors for the synthesis of essential fatty acids in humans. Prostaglandins are synthesized from arachidonic acid (cis-5,8,11,14-eicosatetraenoic acid) or other 20-carbon fatty acids that have at least three double bonds. Prostaglandins are 20-carbon fatty acids that contain a 5-carbon ring. They are hormonelike in their action, but unlike hormones, they often directly modulate the activities of the cells in which they are synthesized.

2. **(B)** The septum secundum is a crescent-shaped wedge of tissue that incompletely partitions the developing atria leaving a defect called the foramen ovale near the floor of the right atrium. The septum primum (choice A) is the first partition of the atria and would result in complete partitioning except for the timely development of the ostium secundum. The muscular interventricular septum (choice C) arises from the inferior part of the bulboventricular sulcus to incompletely partition the developing ventricles. The defect in the interventricular septum is closed by growth of the endocardial cushions creating the membranous interventricular septum. The ostium primum (choice D) is the opening between the right and left sides of the developing atrium that is gradually closed by the developing septum primum. The ostium secundum (choice E) is formed by the resorption of the superior part of the septum primum before it completely partitions the ventricles.

3. **(D)** The apparent volume of distribution is a function of the elimination process and is calculated from the formula $V_d = X/C$, where V_d is the volume of distribution, X is the amount of drug present in the body, and C is the plasma (or blood) concentration. We must use time zero for our calculations since this is the only time at which we know the amount in the body, because the drug will immediately be subjected to elimination. The curvature seen in the early data points results from distribution of the drug from blood into tissue compartments. The linear portion of the data reflects the elimination process and must be extrapolated back to time zero to determine the plasma concentration, which would have been obtained if distribution had been instantaneous. The administered amount X of 30 mg divided by the extrapolated plasma concentration of 1 μg/ml yields an apparent V_d of 30 L.

4. **(C)** Using the linear portion of the data (including the dashed extrapolation), the concentration at time zero is 1 mg/mL. By definition, the half-life is the time interval for 50% reduction in concentration for single-dose drug disappearance. The plasma concentration of 0.5 mg/mL is reached after 7 hrs. The half-life will predict the approach to plateau for any situation in which first order kinetics apply. Single-dose disappearance kinetics can be thought of as the approach to a plateau of zero.

5. **(A)** By repeated exposure to the pairing of a stimulus (thinking of an apple) to another stimulus (sour taste) that produces a re-

sponse (salivation), simply thinking of a sour apple produces salivation. This type of learning is called classical (Pavlovian) conditioning. Choice B is incorrect because it refers to learning by thinking. The person in this case probably learned the association between sourness and salivation through experience first, not by thinking about it. Operant conditioning (choice C) refers to learning by rewarding desired behavior. It is unlikely that salivation was rewarded. Shaping (choice D) is a form of operant conditioning. Choice E, imprinting, involves learning during a critical period, as in the case of goslings that follow a human if exposed to a human just after birth.

6. **(A)** The p53 gene is a negative regulator of cell division. When a cell's DNA is damaged, the p53 gene senses this abnormality and holds the aberrant cell in S phase of the cell cycle to allow enzymatic repair of the damaged DNA to occur. Thus, mutations of the gene encourage replication of cells with abnormal DNA and increase cell propensity for malignant transformation. Mutations of the p53 gene are found in about 75% of human colon carcinomas, and in a significant percentage of breast carcinomas, hepatomas, and small cell carcinomas. Mutations of the p53 gene are not directly linked to congenital deformities such as micrognathia (choice B), the hereditary disease cystic fibrosis (choice C), the occurrence of pulmonary fibrosis (choice D), and essential hypertension (choice E).

7. **(B)** Chronic alcoholics are prone to many physiological problems due to their poor dietary patterns and the effects of alcohol itself on the gastrointestinal tract, leading to impaired nutrient absorption. The most common problems of chronic alcoholics are neurological in nature, including mental confusion and depression, ataxia, and uncoordinated eye movements. The most severe symptoms are related to those seen in Wernicke–Korsakoff syndrome. Although thiamine deficiency is only one of many nutritional deficiencies seen in chronic alcoholics, administration of thiamine has a dramatic effect on reversing the course of these severe symptoms. None of the other choices (A, C, D, and E) reflect symptoms associated with thiamine deficiency, nor to deficiencies in other vitamins.

8. **(D)** At an early stage of acquired immune deficiency syndrome (AIDS), the patient displays a mononucleosis-like illness, with lethargy, apathy, fever, generalized lymphadenopathy, leukopenia, and maculopapular rashes. All these symptoms are caused by human immunodeficiency virus (HIV), which is an enveloped, single-stranded, positive-polarity RNA virus. The RNA genome of HIV is composed of two identical molecules. The virus also contains protease and an integrase in its nucleocapsid reverse transcriptase. The mumps virus is an enveloped virus with neuraminidase and hemagglutinin spikes, and it has a nonsegmented single-stranded RNA of negative polarity. Mumps is associated with tender swelling of the parotid glands (choice A). Infectious hepatitis is caused by a single-stranded, positive-polarity RNA, non-enveloped virus. The disease is characterized by fever, vomiting, and jaundice (choice B). Lymphocytic choriomeningitis is caused by a single-stranded, circular, segmented RNA, enveloped virus. Lymphocytic choriomeningitis is characterized by vomiting, stiff neck, and changes in mental state (choice C). Pleurodynia is caused by Group B coxsackieviruses. These are non-enveloped viruses, with a single-stranded, positive-polarity RNA genome (choice E).

9. **(E)** The key pathogenic effect of AIDS is destruction of CD4-bearing lymphocytes. Infection of meninges, invasion of spinal fluid, and invasion of bone marrow may occur in AIDS patients, but it is not the key event explaining the pathogenesis of AIDS (choices A, B, and C). Human immunodeficiency virus does not induce any meaningful reduction of plasma cells (choice D).

10. **(A)** The most notable opportunistic neoplasia associated with acquired immunodeficiency disease is Kaposi's sarcoma. It has

been recently published that human herpesvirus 8 may be the etiological agent of Kaposi's sarcoma. Herpes simplex type 1 is the causative agent of oral lesions, not lymphoma (choice B). Burkitt's lymphoma is caused by the Epstein–Barr virus, not AIDS (choice C). Rous sarcoma is caused by the Rous sarcoma virus, a retrovirus isolated by Peyton Rous, who produced tumors in chickens with it (choice D). Herpes simplex type 2 is the causative agent of genital herpetic lesions. Both type 1 and type 2 herpesviruses may produce either local vesicular lesions or severe generalized disease in neonates infected during passage through an infected birth canal (choice E).

11. **(E)** Gastrin infusion stimulates gastric acid secretion. Thus, initially, before peptide x was given, there was high gastric acid concentration. Secretin, sometimes called "nature's antacid," must have been peptide x because it is known to inhibit gastric acid secretion and to stimulate pancreatic bicarbonate production. Peptide x could not have been motilin (choice A), which has mainly to do with motility. Nor could it have been angiotensin II (choice B), which has several functions (e.g., stimulation of aldosterone secretion), none of which is inhibition of gastric acid secretion or stimulation of pancreatic bicarbonate secretion. Nor could it have been CCK (choice C), which mainly stimulates pancreatic enzyme secretion and gallbladder contraction. Somatostatin (choice D) has many inhibitory effects and does not stimulate pancreatic bicarbonate production.

12. **(B)** As its name implies, the calcarine artery courses through the calcarine sulcus to supply the primary visual cortex. Occlusion of this vessel will produce a defect in the contralateral visual field. Lesions involving the lenticulostriate vessels (choice A) typically produce upper motor neuron signs in the contralateral extremities. Occlusion of PICA (choice C) leads to a characteristic somatosensory deficit involving the loss of pain and temperature sensitivity over the ipsilateral half of the face and the contralateral trunk and extremities. Vascular lesions involving the anterior cerebral artery (choice D) or its medial striate (choice E) branch do not lead to visual field defects.

13. **(A)** Tobacco dependence is the most common and most difficult to control drug dependence in the United States. Choice B is incorrect because nicotine is an extremely addicting substance, and sudden cessation of its use results in both physical and psychological withdrawal symptoms. Choice C is incorrect as tobacco dependence usually begins in adolescence. Choice D is incorrect because the relapse rate of smoking cessation programs is 60 to 70%. Choice E grossly underestimates the harmfulness of tobacco because physical complications of chronic tobacco use begin to appear in 20 pack-years.

14. **(B)** The second law of thermodynamics states that in order for a reaction to proceed spontaneously the total entropy of the system must increase. Entropy is a measure of the disorder of a system; therefore, the natural thermodynamically driven tendency is for systems (and the molecules of a system) to tend toward maximum disorder. Some, but not many, reactions proceed spontaneously (choice A); however, the majority require a catalyst. In biological systems the catalysts are enzymes. The total energy of a molecule (choice C) does not impact the second law, but the various entropies of a molecule do. Choice D reflects the first law of thermodynamics, stating that the total energy of a system plus that of its environment must remain constant. Total energy must remain constant, but it can change form (choice E), such as heat energy into work energy.

15. **(B)** Trimethoprim is an inhibitor of dihydrofolate reductase that exhibits great specificity for binding to the bacterial form as opposed to the human form (10^5 higher concentrations are required for inhibition of host dihydrofolate reductase). Trimethoprim is combined with sulfamethoxazole to provide inhibition of sequential steps in bacterial tetrahydrofolate synthesis. Resistance may arise by mutation of bacterial dihydrofolate reductase, although acquisition of a plasmid

encoding altered dihydrofolate reductase is more common for gram-negative bacteria. Expression of β-lactamase activity (choice A) is a mechanism for resistance to the β-lactam antibacterial agents such as the penicillins and cephalosporins. Thickening of the bacterial cell wall (choice C), as well as decreasing activity of pore-forming proteins such as the porins, are mechanisms of resistance for gram-negative bacteria to the protein synthesis inhibitors, since these agents must gain access to the protein synthetic machinery through the cell wall and cell membrane. Expression of altered forms of transpeptidase (choice D) is a mechanism for resistance to the inhibitors of cell wall synthesis, such as the β-lactam penicillins and cephalosporins. Mutation of ribosomal subunits (choice E) is a mechanism for resistance to the protein synthesis inhibitors, such as the tetracyclines and aminoglycosides including streptomycin.

16. **(D)** The quartan fever that accompanies infection with *Plasmodium malariae* is secondary to cyclic release of proliferating merozoites from erythrocytes. The circulating ruptured red cell stroma and free hemoglobin are naturally occurring pyrogens capable of invoking an abrupt febrile episode. Cerebral malaria is a grave prognostic finding. It does not cause cyclic central hypothalamic fever (choice A). Hepatocytes (choice B) serve as a non-lytic reservoir for *Plasmodium malariae* infection. Immune-mediated destruction of the organism (choice C) is a minor feature of malaria infection. It does not produce quartan fever. Cell-mediated cytokines (choice E) are minimally active in *Plasmodium* infections. They do not engender sufficient pyrogenic activity to account for the severe cyclic fevers seen with *Plasmodium malariae* infections.

17. **(D)** Temporary occlusion of the common carotid arteries will decrease vascular pressure within the carotid sinus area. This peripheral baroreceptor responds to changes in pressure and is an important reflex in maintaining relatively constant arterial pressure on a short-term basis. A decrease in pressure will depress the number of impulses that travel from the carotid sinus nerve. Since these impulses normally inhibit the central vasoconstrictor area and excite the vagal center, a decrease in impulses will reflexively cause arterial pressure to rise and heart rate and contractility to increase. The entire circulation will be stimulated to constrict, and thus there will be a reduction in venous capacitance. Increased firing rate of the carotid sinus nerve (choice A) and subsequent vasodilatation (choice B) and decreased heart rate (choice C) would result from an increase in vascular pressure within the carotid sinus area. The venous capacity (choice E) also increases with decreased sympathetic tone as a result of an increased firing rate of the carotid sinus nerve.

18. **(C)** The deoxygenated subunits of the hemoglobin tetramer exist in the T ("tense") conformational state. As erythrocytes enter the capillaries of the lung alveoli the partial pressure of O_2 has increased sufficiently to allow binding to hemoglobin. When one mole of O_2 binds, it causes a shift in the overall conformation of the other subunits to a more R ("relaxed") conformational state. This change in conformation leads to higher affinity of the remaining monomers for O_2. Each deoxygenated monomer has a progressively increased affinity for O_2 as more oxygen binds. This cooperative binding is observed as a sigmoidal saturation curve when plotting the partial pressure of oxygen versus moles of O_2 bound. Oxygen binding shifts the position of the heme group, but not sufficiently to place it on the exterior of any hemoglobin subunit (choices A and E). Binding of oxygen does impact the secondary structure of hemoglobin but only to a minor degree, and, this has no impact on its affinity for CO_2 (choice B). As indicated, oxygen binds cooperatively to hemoglobin, not with equal affinity to each deoxy subunit (choice D).

19. **(C)** The internal laryngeal nerve supplies the laryngeal mucosa above the level of the vocal fold as well as the mucosa of the piriform recess and the epiglottic valleculae.

The pharyngeal plexus (choice A) supplies most of the innervation to the pharynx, including general visceral afferent fibers from the pharyngeal mucosa that are carried in the glossopharyngeal nerve. The glossopharyngeal nerve (choice B) carries afferent fibers from the mucosa of the middle ear, auditory tube, pharynx, palatine tonsils, and posterior one-third of the tongue, but does not supply the laryngeal mucosa. The external laryngeal nerve (choice D) is motor to the cricothyroid muscle and the lowest part of the inferior pharyngeal constrictor muscle. The inferior laryngeal nerve (choice E) is motor to the intrinsic muscles of the larynx except the cricothyroid muscle, and is sensory to the mucosa of the larynx below the level of the vocal fold.

20. (D) Although short-term regulation of arterial blood pressure is primarily affected by the integrated responses of peripheral baroreceptors and the central and sympathetic nervous systems, the primary determinant of regulation of blood pressure in the long run is the relationship of urine output to fluid intake. This system is normally capable of returning blood pressure to normal levels, which is different from the short-term nervous regulation. By adjusting extracellular fluid and blood volumes, renal–body fluid mechanisms alter the venous return. Individual beds then adjust their resistance because of the interplay of local and neuronal factors, and thus arterial pressure is slowly readjusted to control levels. The total peripheral vascular resistance (choice A) is thus altered by those mechanisms rather than being the variable that directly determines blood pressure. The baroreceptor reflex pathway (choice B) involves the autonomic nervous system (choice C) and vital centers in the brainstem portion of the CNS (choice E), but plays little role in long-term regulation of blood pressure.

21. (E) Hyperkeratosis, parakeratosis, acanthosis, club-shaped dermal papillae, and clusters of neutrophils in the upper epidermis (Munro microabscesses) are the defining microscopic features of psoriasis. Clinically, the disease displays erythematous scaly plaques, which preferentially occur over the extensor cutaneous surfaces. Basal cell carcinoma (choice A) is a low-grade cutaneous malignancy and would be characterized by dermal infiltration of small basally oriented tumor cells. The histology of primary malignant melanoma (choice B) would display collections of atypical melanocytes within the epidermis and possibly invading into the dermis. Squamous cell carcinoma (choice C) is defined microscopically by collections of malignant cells with focal squamous differentiation. Pemphigus vulgaris (choice D) is a cutaneous blistering disease. Epidermal bleb formation is the critical histologic observation.

22. (B) By inhibiting entry of calcium into vascular smooth muscle, the calcium channel blockers produce excessive vasodilation with resulting hypotension as an adverse effect in overdose situations. The hypotension results in a reflex increase in sympathetic stimulation to the heart with resultant tachycardia. This effect, along with the systemic hypotension and decreased coronary flow, may exacerbate myocardial ischemia in those patients being treated with calcium channel blockers for angina. Bradycardia has been reported as an adverse effect of nifedipine with intravenous administration and with concurrent β-blocker administration. Clonidine (choice A), an α_2 adrenoreceptor agonist, acts at the level of the vasopressor centers in the brainstem to decrease sympathetic outflow. Cardiac adverse effects, when seen, involve marked bradycardia. The nonselective β-blocker propranolol (choice C) produces bradycardia as a normal aspect of its actions. The cardiac glycosides such as digoxin (choice D) inhibit Na^+-K^+-ATPase. At the level of control of heart rate, the glycosides increase vagal tone and produce a decrease in sympathetic nervous system activity. These effects result in bradycardia. The anticholinesterase pyridostigmine (choice E) is used in the treatment of myasthenia gravis to increase the concentration of acetylcholine at the neuromuscular junction. At the level of the heart, increased acetylcholine levels cause a decrease in heart rate.

23. **(E)** Benzodiazepines are antianxiety agents. They are also muscle relaxants and anticonvulsants as well as sedatives. Because of the sedative action, an elderly patient may develop paradoxical agitation due to the disinhibition of higher cortical function. Benzodiazepines, unlike neuroleptics, do not cause impaired conditioned avoidance learning.

24. **(A)** The primary precursors for gluconeogenesis in the liver are lactate and alanine, which are produced in muscle during intense activity. Alanine is formed from pyruvate by transamination in a reaction catalyzed by alanine aminotransferase. This reaction is the major mechanism of transporting ammonia from nonhepatic tissues to the liver. The liver is the only organ capable of carrying out the urea cycle, the pathway for removal of ammonia waste. Alanine is converted back to pyruvate in the liver and diverted to the gluconeogenesis pathway for the synthesis of glucose. Its function in ammonia transport is the major reason that alanine is the principal glucogenic amino acid. Aspartate (choice B) and glutamate (choice D) are good sources of TCA cycle intermediates through the action of transaminases and as such are glucogenic amino acids. However, they do not supply major sources of carbon for glucose synthesis. Cysteine (choice C) is oxidized to pyruvate, which makes it glucogenic, but like most glucogenic amino acids, it is not the major source of carbon for glucose synthesis. Serine (choice E) is interconvertible with glycine, or can be oxidized to pyruvate, but like other glucogenic amino acids, the latter reaction does not constitute a major source of carbons for glucose synthesis.

25. **(B)** Lesions involving the left lentriculostriate branches result in damage to upper motor neuron axons coursing through the posterior limb of the internal capsule on the left side. This results in motor deficits involving the contralateral extremities, as well as in the musculature innervated by cranial nerves VII, IX, X, XI, and XII, which have been deprived of their motor cortex input. Damage to the left anterior spinal artery (choice A) will produce ipsilateral lower motor neuron signs in the musculature innervated by the damaged levels of the spinal cord. Lesions involving the paramedian branches of the basilar bifurcation on the right (choice C), the right lenticulostriate vessels (choice D), and the right posterior spinal artery (choice E) do not lead to upper motor neuron signs on the right side, or cause the protruded tongue to deviate to the right.

26. **(D)** Malignant mesothelioma is the most common primary malignant tumor of the pleura. The occurrence of this tumor is strongly linked to asbestos exposure, usually after a latency period of several decades. In the past, individuals in the shipbuilding and insulation trades were most likely to develop mesothelioma. Beryllium (choice A) exposure may cause berylliosis, a chronic granulomatous pulmonary disorder. Individuals who work in the production of fluorescent lighting are at greatest risk. Silica (choice B) exposure may cause silicosis, a fibrotic chronic pulmonary disorder unrelated to mesothelioma. Sandblasters, miners, and masons are likely to be exposed to silica. Coal dust (choice C) exposure can cause anthracosis and a severe form of pulmonary fibrosis called black lung disease. Coal dust exposure does not increase the risk of developing mesothelioma. Nitrogen dioxide (choice E) exposure may cause silo-filler's disease, but does not engender mesothelioma.

27. **(C)** Injuries affecting upper cervical segments (above C3) usually quickly cause death from loss of respiratory muscle function. However, transection of the spinal cord between C8 and T1 only severs neural connections between the brainstem and some of the muscles involved in respiration (e.g., intercostal and abdominal muscles), while sparing connections to the diaphragm (phrenic nerves come off spinal neurons in segments C3–C5 ["C three, four, and five keep the diaphragm alive"]). Normal, quiet expiration is passive. However, forced expiration, as in the latter part of vital capacity measurement, requires active participation by expiratory muscles. By definition, functional residual capacity (FRC) is the volume at which the respiratory system stays when all respiratory muscles are inactive. On the other hand, residual volume (RV) is the volume left after maximal expiratory effort (involving intercostal and abdominal muscles). RV is normally about one liter less than FRC. Since this patient has no expiratory muscle function, there cannot be an RV less than FRC, that is, in this patient, FRC = RV. In this patient you might expect a vital capacity (choice A) that is at best only about 50% of normal. In this tetraplegic patient there is essentially complete loss of expiratory muscle function, but only modest loss of inspiratory action (choices B and D) since the diaphragm is the major muscle of inspiration. Since inspiration is less compromised than forced expiration in this patient, any increase in tidal volume during exercise (choice E) would be contributed by the inspiratory reserve volume.

28. (C) The child has celiac disease, a disorder resulting from a hypersensitivity reaction to gluten in the diet. Withdrawal of gluten from the diet is usually curative. Clinically, there is diarrhea, malabsorption, and steatorrhea. Histologically, there is villous atrophy of the small intestinal mucosa. Because the disease is usually cured by dietary measures, the use of antineoplastic drugs (choice A), interferon therapy (choice B), and surgical resection of the small intestine (choice D) would not be appropriate treatment options. A referral to hospice for supportive care (choice E) is unlikely to be necessary since over 95% of patients respond to the removal of gluten from their diet. Recalcitrant cases are rarely life threatening and may be successfully treated with various forms of hyperalimentation which bypass the small intestine.

29. (C) The intravenous anesthetic thiopental shares the property of rapid induction of anesthesia and brief duration of action with propofol because both agents are highly lipid-soluble and are rapidly distributed to the brain. This is followed by redistribution from the brain to skeletal muscle and eventually to adipose tissue as determined by the relative rates of perfusion for these tissues. Thiopental is cleared by hepatic metabolism, but the controlling factor for the duration of action is the redistribution from the brain to other tissues. The serum elimination half-life (choice A) is not the controlling factor for the duration of action of thiopental and propofol as indicated above. Urinary pH (choice B) plays no role in either the duration of action or the systemic clearance of thiopental. Although thiopental reduces hepatic blood flow (choice D), this has no effect on the duration of action for thiopental. The metabolism of thiopental is relatively slow, so induction of metabolism (choice E) may increase the clearance rate, but again this plays no role in the duration of action.

30. (B) One nonallosteric mechanism for regulating the activity of the hepatic form of pyruvate kinase is covalent modification. Both glucagon and epinephrine signal hepatocytes to deliver glucose to the blood. Each of these hormones binds to specific receptors that are coupled to activation of adenylate cyclase, which in turn produces cAMP from ATP. The increased cAMP leads to activation of cAMP-dependent protein kinase (PKA), which phosphorylates numerous substrates. One hepatic substrate is pyruvate kinase. Upon being phosphorylated, the activity of pyruvate kinase is reduced. This prevents any phosphoenolpyruvate (PEP) that is formed during gluconeogenesis from being converted to pyruvate, ensuring its continued entry into glucose production. It is important to distinguish the effects of epinephrine on the activity of hepatic versus muscular pyruvate kinase. In skeletal muscle epinephrine stimulates glycolysis, not gluconeogenesis. The muscular form of pyruvate kinase is not a substrate for PKA. Phosphofructokinase-2 (choice A) does not phosphorylate pyruvate kinase. Its substrate is fructose-6-phosphate yielding fructose-2-6-bisphosphate. Oxaloacetate (choice C) has no allosteric effects on pyruvate kinase. Citrate-mediated polymerization (choice D) occurs with acetyl-CoA carboxylase, but not with pyruvate kinase. Pyruvate kinase is not the target of chymotrypsin (choice E).

31. (C) The abducens nerve is motor to the lateral rectus muscle. Paralysis of this muscle would produce medial deviation of the pupil due the unopposed action of the medial rectus muscle. Damage to the oculomotor nerve would result in a loss of visual accommodation (choice A) due to interruption of the parasympathetic innervation to the sphincter pupillae and ciliary muscles. Ptosis of the upper lid (choice B) can result from damage to the oculomotor muscle supplying the levator palpebrae superioris muscle or from interruption of the sympathetic innervation to the superior tarsal muscle. Lateral deviation of the pupil (choice D) can result from damage to the oculomotor nerve supplying the medial rectus muscle. Lateral deviation of the pupil would result from unopposed action of the lateral rectus muscle. Dilatation of the pupil (choice E) results from interruption of the parasympathetic innervation to the sphincter pupillae muscle carried by the oculomotor nerve.

32. **(B)** Most, except newer atypical antipsychotics like clozapine, are ineffective against the negative symptoms of schizophrenia, such as flat affect and thought blocking. Choice A is incorrect as most neuroleptic antipsychotic agents are dopamine receptor blockers. Choice C is incorrect as serum prolactin levels increase with neuroleptics because of the dopamine blockade in the hypothalamus. Choice D is incorrect as pseudoparkinsonism is a frequent and bothersome side effect of antipsychotic drugs, but it may be effectively managed with anticholinergic agents such as benztropine (Cogentin). Most neuroleptics have some sedative action; therefore, choice E is incorrect.

33. **(B)** The ECG shows atrial fibrillation characterized by an irregularly undulating baseline, absence of P waves, and irregular QRS intervals. Atrial fibrillation is a common arrhythmia that accompanies several forms of chronic heart disease. It probably represents some form of reentry phenomenon in which part of the tissue may be excited at an inappropriately early part of the cardiac cycle. A number of drugs are available to prolong the effective refractory period of selective parts of the heart, and these drugs would be effective in restoring normal atrial contraction. Direct current shock (choice A) is an effective treatment to return the heart to normal rhythm and reverse atrial fibrillation. However, atrial fibrillation per se is not a life-threatening event, and placing the entire myocardium into refractory period usually is not the appropriate course of action. Since the atria do not contract, there are no P waves in this ECG recording (choice C). Activation of conducting tissue in the atrioventricular node becomes variable in time from cycle to cycle, and thus the QRS complex interval becomes less constant (choice D). The strength of ventricular contraction is related to the timing of filling, and thus failure of the atria to effectively contract alters ventricular filling. This produces an irregular pulse (choice E).

34. **(A)** The Negri bodies associated with rabies are large cytoplasmic granules containing rabies viral particles. They are most abundant in the area of the hippocampus known as Ammon's horn. The Negri bodies are best detected by special stains, such as Seller's stain, which reveals the cytoplasmic granules containing the rabies virus in cherry red with dark blue spots; immunofluorescence is another reliable method of identifying these granules. Guarnieri's bodies are seen in poxvirus-infected cells (choice B). Reticulate and elementary bodies are seen in chlamydial infections (choices C and D). There are no bodies known as Ammon's bodies (choice E).

35. **(D)** Cysteine, serine, glycine, and alanine (choices A, B, C, and E) are all converted to pyruvate during amino acid degradation. Thus, each of these amino acids can give rise to glucose via conversion of pyruvate to oxaloacetate and then to phosphoenolpyruvate. In addition, ketone body formation can proceed by conversion of pyruvate to acetyl-CoA. In contrast, leucine can only be converted to potential ketone body precursors. The degradation of leucine leads to the formation of acetyl-CoA and acetoacetate.

36. **(D)** Movement of an individual to a higher altitude (with decreased partial pressure of oxygen) requires greater oxygen-carrying capacity of blood and is thus a stimulus for an increased rate of erythrocyte production. This is reflected by an increased percentage of circulating erythrocytes that are newly developed (reticulocytes). Exposure to infectious agents (choices A and C), vaccines (choice B), or allergens (choice E) will elicit responses involving distinct populations of leukocytes.

37. **(B)** An acute inflammatory reaction typically produces erythema, swelling, pain, and localized heat. There is increased capillary and venous endothelial permeability as their intracellular actin fibers contract and widen intercellular pores. The resultant ultrafiltrate of plasma leaks out through these widened pores into the interstitial tissue and is seen clinically as swelling. Interleukin-5 secretion by T cells (choice A) is useful during a chronic inflammatory reaction for maturation of B cells. Reversible swelling of endoplasmic reticulum (choice C) is the ultrastructural correlate of hydropic change. It is an intracellular phenomenon of reversible cell injury. Pinocytosis (choice D) is a cellular phagocytic process by which extracellular material may be ingested. Margination of neutrophils (choice E) is usually a prominent feature of the acute inflammatory reaction. It is a response to vascular stasis and chemotactic factors, and does not produce edema.

38. **(A)** The femoral head has marked degenerative osteoarthritis. The gradual destruction of articular cartilage can eventually lead to joint compromise through eburnation, osteophyte formation, subchondral cysts, and osteochondral loose body formation. Clinically, these anatomic changes are reflected as joint pain and a restricted range of motion. The photo does not display evidence of a benign neoplasm (choice B), infection (choice C), malignant neoplastic process (choice D), or coagulopathy (choice E).

39. **(D)** The classic complement pathway is usually activated by the antigen–antibody union involving complement components C1q, C4, C2, and C3–C9. The alternate complement pathway proceeds through C3–C9, and it can be activated by aggregated immunoglobulins IgA, IgG_4, IgE, lipopolysaccharides, and endotoxins. Interleukin-1 induces T cells, B cells, neutrophils, fibroblasts, and epithelial cells to grow, differentiate, or elaborate various macromolecules. It also causes fever, but it does not activate the alternate complement pathway (choice A). Interferon is an antiviral substance, and as such is not involved in the activation of the alternate complement pathway (choice B). Lipoproteins have not been shown to be involved in the activation of the alternate complement pathway (choice C). Complement component C1 binds to the antigen–antibody complex and initiates the cascade of the classic complement pathway. It plays no role in the alternate complement pathway (choice E).

40. **(A)** Opioids with μ and κ agonistic properties cause miosis by an excitatory action on the parasympathetic nerve innervating the pupil. Some tolerance develops, but miosis is seen even in addicts. Intestinal spasm and loss of propulsive motion rather than hypermotility (choice B) are seen with opioids. Constipation is a common adverse effect. Respiratory rate is depressed rather than stimulated (choice C). Depression of respiratory drive at the level of the brainstem may lead to respiratory arrest, the most common cause of death in morphine intoxication. Opioids do not relax the lower end of the common bile duct (choice D), but rather constrict the sphincter of Oddi, causing a large increase in bile duct pressure. This may produce symptoms of biliary colic. Opioids depress rather than stimulate the cough reflex (choice E). Codeine is an effective antitussive agent. The antitussive agent dextromethorphan is chemically related to the opioids, but has no actions on opioid receptors and does not possess analgesic or addictive properties.

41. **(D)** The bifunctional enzyme phosphofructokinase-2 (PFK-2) contains a kinase and a phosphatase domain. The kinase domain phosphorylates fructose-6-phosphate (F-6-P)

to yield fructose-2,6-bisphosphate (F-2,6-BP), whereas the phosphatase dephosphorylates F-2,6,-BP yielding F-6-P. F-2,6-BP is a potent allosteric activator of the rate-limiting enzyme of glycolysis, phosphofructokinase-1 (PFK-1), as well as a potent allosteric inhibitor of the gluconeogenic enzyme fructose-1,6-bisphosphatase. The activity of PFK-2 is regulated by cAMP-dependent protein kinase (PKA)-mediated phosphorylation. When phosphorylated, PFK-2 functions as a phosphatase, and as a kinase when dephosphorylated. The PKA-mediated change in activity of PFK-2 allows the level of F-2,6-BP to be regulated by circulating hormones such as glucagon and epinephrine, ultimately controlling the flux through glycolysis. PFK-2 functions as a regulatory enzyme in glycolysis, not the TCA cycle (choice A). As indicated, PFK-2 acts as a phosphatase, not as a kinase, when it itself is phosphorylated. Therefore, when phosphorylated, PFK-2 removes phosphate from its substrate (choice B). The substrate for the kinase activity of PFK-2 is F-6-P (choice C). PFK-2 itself is not an allosteric effector (choice E), but is responsible for regulating the levels of F-2,6-BP, which is an allosteric effector.

42. (A) The muscles of the tongue are innervated by the paired hypoglossal nerves. On protrusion of the tongue, deviation occurs to the side of the damaged nerve and paralyzed muscles. Damage to the left hypoglossal nerve (choice B) results in deviation of the protruded tongue to the left side. Damage to the right lingual nerve (choice C) would have no effect on movement of the tongue, but would produce a loss of general sensation and taste on the right half of the anterior two-thirds of the tongue. Damage to the left lingual nerve (choice D) would have no effect on movement of the tongue, but would produce a loss of general sensation and taste on the left half of the anterior two-thirds of the tongue. Damage to the right glossopharyngeal nerve (choice E) would have no effect on movement of the tongue, but would produce a loss of general sensation and taste on the right half of the posterior one-third of the tongue.

43. (A) All cancers may be associated with depression (choices B, C, D, and E). However, some neoplasms, particularly cancer of the tail of the pancreas, are particularly likely to cause, and often present with, clinical depression.

44. (A) Glaucoma is characterized by increased intraocular pressure with resultant pressure atrophy of the optic disk and decreased visual acuity. Medicinal treatment with pupillary constrictors can provide temporary relief. Definitive surgical correction is successful in about 80% of cases. A cataract (choice B) is an opacity of the lens and is not associated with increased intraocular pressure. Retrolental fibroplasia (choice C) is seen in premature infants exposed to high concentrations of oxygen. Arcus senilis (choice D) is a ring of fatty material in the outer cornea commonly seen in elderly individuals. The ocular pressures and visual acuity are unaffected by this change. Pinguecula (choice E) is an actinically induced growth that does not alter the intraocular pressure.

45. (C) Acute spinal transection causes immediate flaccid paralysis and loss of all sensation and reflex activity below the level of injury. This initial phase is called "spinal shock" and lasts for hours or days. If the spinal cord below the lesion is intact, reflex activity later returns and the flaccid paralysis changes to a spastic paralysis with exaggerated (choice A) or normal (choice B) stretch reflexes. The bladder reflex will also normalize only gradually (choice D), eventually resulting in an automatic bladder since the central control remains lost. All sensation including sense of vibration (choice E) will be absent in parts of the body innervated by spinal cord segments below the lesion.

46. (A) Individuals exposed to acute radiation doses of between zero and 50 cGy do not show any immediate clinical symptoms. However, low-level exposure may increase the likelihood of neoplasia in the future. Exposures between 50 and 200 cGy usually produce acute radiation syndrome (choice B) characterized by fatigue, nausea, and vomiting. Hematopoietic syndrome (choice C) is characterized by leukopenia and thrombocytopenia, in addition to the clinical findings of acute radiation sickness. Exposure dosages are usually between 200 and 600 cGy. The acute mortality rate is between 20 and 50%. Exposures of 600 to 1000 cGy may produce mucosal ulceration, diarrhea, and electrolyte loss as part of the gastrointestinal syndrome (choice D). Acute mortality rates are between 50 and 100%. The cerebral syndrome (choice E) has a 100% mortality rate and is seen with acute doses above 1000 cGy.

47. (B) Fibrinogen is activated by conversion to fibrin monomers through the action of thrombin, which cleaves several peptide bonds in fibrinogen to yield fibrin. The fibrin monomers, thus formed, aggregate with each other to form a clot. Thrombin itself is derived by proteolytic cleavage of its precursor, prothrombin (choice A). Antithrombin III (choice C) is an inhibitor of thrombin activity. It inactivates the enzyme by forming an irreversible complex with it. This inhibition can be enhanced by the presence of heparin (choice E) and is the basis of the latter's anticoagulant properties. Fibrin clots can be dissolved by the action of plasmin (choice D), a serine protease.

48. (C) The best bone marrow donor for this patient is her mother, because the results of the mixed lymphocyte reaction correlate with the degree of dissimilarity of histocompatability (that is, high counts indicate enhanced stimulation suggesting immunologic unrelatedness of tissue tested). Twins who have identical leukocyte antigens do not stimulate mixed leukocyte reactions, indicating that their tissues are mutually transplantable.

49. (B) Cretinism is due to a neonatal lack of thyroxine. Thyroid agenesis, iodine deficiency, ingestion of goitrogens, and hereditary enzymatic deficiencies may all result in a relative lack of biologically active thyroxine. Affected children display lethargy, jaundice, hypothermia, muscular hypotonia, and mental retardation. Medicinal replacement of thyroxine is therapeutic. The mental retardation may not be reversible, however, unless treated early. A lack of vitamin D (choice A) would cause rickets, not cretinism. Treatment with thiamine (choice C) is the appropriate therapy for beriberi, but not cretinism. Antibiotics (choice D) would have no effect in treating cretinism. Growth hormone (choice E) is an effective treatment for pituitary dwarfism. It would have no benefit in cretinism.

50. (A) Tissue plasminogen activator (tPA) directly catalyzes the proteolytic conversion of plasminogen to plasmin. Because tPA binds to fibrin, it is much more effective in activating bound plasminogen than free plasminogen. Although it was originally hoped that the specificity of action at fibrin sites would improve clinical efficacy and safety, studies to date in treating myocardial infarction have shown no great difference in efficacy and safety between tPA, urokinase, and streptokinase. The use of tPA for occlusive strokes offers a great advance in treatment of stroke. The proteolytic breakdown of fibrin (choice B) is the crucial step in thrombolysis that is catalyzed by plasmin. The thrombolytic agents currently in use work at the level of the conversion of plasminogen to plasmin. α_2 Antiplasmin is a naturally occurring inhibitor of plasmin activity. Depletion of α_2 antiplasmin (choice C) is an effect necessary at the site of thrombolysis. Since the binding of α_2 antiplasmin and plasmin is stoichiometric, generation of a large excess of plasmin at the fibrin clot site will deplete the local concentration of α_2 antiplasmin and allow free plasmin to lyse fibrin. The binding of plasminogen to fibrin aids in this localization of effect. Systemic depletion of α_2 antiplasmin would produce a dangerous tendency toward hemorrhage. Formation of an active complex with plasminogen (choice D) is a property of streptokinase. Streptokinase is a protein produced by β-hemolytic streptococci. It has no intrinsic enzymatic activity, but rather forms a stable complex with plasminogen that is enzymatically active in cleaving free plasminogen to plasmin. The streptokinase–plasminogen complex is not inhibited by α_2 antiplasmin. Proteolytic activation of fibrinogen (choice E) to fibrin is a property of thrombin in the formation of the fibrin mesh leading to clot formation.

51. **(B)** The bipolar cells in the retina (and nasal mucosa and spiral ganglion) are first-order sensory neurons and form as true bipolar cells. The first-order sensory neurons in the dorsal root ganglia (choice C) and semilunar ganglia (choice E) are pseudounipolar neurons. Neurons in the spinal cord (choice A) and pyramidal neurons (choice D) are generally regarded as multipolar.

52. **(D)** Dry social kissing is considered to be safe. Unsafe sex and intravenous injection with a contaminated needle are the major causes of dissemination of HIV, and affected individuals should always prevent blood and semen from entering another person's body. Safe sex with a condom, however, need not be prevented. Therefore, choice A is incorrect. Choice B is incorrect because affected individuals should not donate blood whether or not they are receiving treatment. Choice C is incorrect because HIV may cause an encephalopathy with prominent subcortical dementia. Choice E is incorrect because masturbation does not involve body fluids entering another person.

53. **(A)** Phosphofructokinase-1 (PFK-1) is the rate-limiting enzyme of glycolysis catalyzing the phosphorylation of fructose-6-phosphate yielding fructose-1,6-bisphosphate. PFK-1 is under tight allosteric control, being maximally active when energy levels are low and inhibited when energy levels are high. When the level of AMP is rising in the cell, it signals a decrease in overall energy charge. AMP is an allosteric activator of PFK-1. In contrast to AMP, ATP is a potent allosteric inhibitor of PFK-1 by binding to a site distinct from that of the ATP substrate site. As the level of ATP declines there is less allosteric inhibition of PFK-1 and a concomitant increase in allosteric activation by AMP. This allows PFK-1 to "sense" the energy status of the cell and in turn regulate the flux through the glycolytic pathway. PFK-1 is allosterically activated, not inhibited, by fructose-1,6-bisphosphate (choice B). Fructose-1,6-bisphosphatase, a gluconeogenic enzyme, (choice C) has no effect on the activity of PFK-1. Rising NADH levels (choice D) signal that the energy charge of a cell is increasing and would be concomitant with rising ATP levels. ATP is a negative allosteric regulator of PFK-1 activity. PFK-1 does not function in the capacity of substrate level phosphorylation as is characterized by phosphoglycerate kinase and pyruvate kinase (choice E).

54. **(E)** Cerebral blood flow can be calculated by Fick's law in a manner similar to that used for cardiac blood flow if oxygen consumption is known, or oxygen consumption could be calculated if blood flow were known. The Fick principle is derived by applying the law of conservation of mass:

$$\dot{V}O_2 = \dot{Q} \cdot (CaO_2 - CvO_2)$$

where $\dot{V}O_2$ equals O_2 consumption of the organ in question, $\dot{Q}$ is the blood flow through this organ, and CaO_2 and CvO_2 equal the arterial (to the organ) and venous (from the organ) O_2 contents. We calculate by Fick's law (oxygen consumption equals blood flow times arteriovenous oxygen difference):

$$\begin{aligned}\dot{V}O_2 &= \dot{Q} \cdot (CaO_2 - CvO_2)\\ &= 500\ \text{mL/min} \cdot (20\text{–}15)\ \text{mL}\ O_2/100\ \text{mL blood}\\ &= 500\ \text{mL/min} \cdot 5\ \text{mL}\ O_2/100\ \text{mL blood}\\ &= 25\ \text{mL}\ O_2/\text{min}\end{aligned}$$

In practice, cerebral blood flow is more commonly measured from nitrous oxide uptake rather than from O_2 uptake (Kety method).

55. **(C)** This patient has influenza, which is caused by influenza viruses A, B, and C. These viruses are single-stranded RNA microbes. Their genome is segmented into eight moieties, and is surrounded by an envelope that is covered with distinct hemagglutinin and neuraminidase spikes. Antigenic changes in these spikes lead to worldwide epidemics. Influenza virus has hemaggluti-

nating (H) antigen, neuraminidase (N) antigen, and an envelope; thus, choices A, B, and D are incorrect. Influenza virus is a circular virus, not a bullet-shaped virus. The rabies virus is bullet-shaped (choice E).

56. (C) The genetic lack of sphingomyelinase seen with Niemann–Pick disease leads to an accumulation of uncatabolized sphingomyelin within reticuloendothelial cells. This primary pathologic alteration is seen clinically as mental retardation and organomegaly. Tay–Sachs disease (choice A) is also a lysosomal storage disease. The lack of hexosaminidase A leads to an accumulation of ganglioside within neurons. Lesch–Nyhan syndrome (choice B) is a genetic disorder characterized by hyperuricemia, mental retardation and self-mutilating behavior. Pompe's disease (choice D) is a lethal glycogen storage disorder. Fabry's disease (choice E) is a lysosomal storage disorder due to a lack of galactosidase. Ceramide trihexoside is the accumulative product.

57. (C) The most obvious distinctive feature of the simple columnar epithelium that lines the oviduct is that it contains a mixture of two main cell types. The ciliated cells are recognizable by the apical cilia which extend from basal bodies that appear as a row of darkly stained bars underlying the cilia. The secretory cells, which have no cilia, have a tapered shape (narrow at the base and broad at the apex), hence the name peg cell. The apical surfaces of peg cells tend to bulge out into the lumen. The epithelial lining of the small intestine (choice A) is also simple columnar, but the most abundant cell type is an absorptive cell which has a brush border composed of tightly packed microvilli. Microvilli can be distinguished from cilia because microvilli have no basal bodies, and they are much thinner and shorter than cilia. Goblet cells are mucus-secreting cells scattered among the absorptive cells of the epithelium. Like the peg cells of the oviduct, these are tapered cells, but the broad apical portion of the cell is packed with large secretory granules that appear washed out in most histological preparations. The trachea (choice B) is lined by respiratory epithelium, a ciliated, pseudostratified columnar epithelium. As in the oviduct, ciliated cells are the most abundant cell type, but the oviduct does not have the goblet cells and basal cells that are seen in respiratory epithelium. Like the respiratory epithelium of the trachea, the lining of the epididymal duct (choice D) is a pseudostratified columnar epithelium. However, the columnar cells do not have cilia; rather the apical specialization is the presence of extraordinarily long microvilli called stereocilia. The oropharynx (choice E) is lined by a stratified squamous epithelium.

58. (E) Edrophonium is an ultrashort-acting cholinesterase inhibitor because it binds to cholinesterase via ionic interactions rather than forming a covalent complex as do the other clinically used cholinesterase inhibitors. It is used in the diagnosis of myasthenia gravis but, because its duration of action is five minutes, it is not useful for chronic treatment of the disease. Pralidoxime (choice A) is an oxime-type reactivator of organophosphate-inhibited cholinesterase. It is used to treat organophosphate intoxication, but must be administered within a few hours of exposure since chemical rearrangement of the organophosphate–cholinesterase complex is rapid and leads to forms not reactivated by pralidoxime. Isoflurophate (choice B) is an organophosphate irreversible inhibitor of cholinesterase. Its use as a miotic agent in the treatment of glaucoma has been supplanted by the use of echothiophate since the latter compound is stable in aqueous solution and is highly polar, preventing systemic absorption. Physostigmine (choice C) is a tertiary ammonium reversible anticholinesterase with sufficient penetration of the blood–brain barrier to allow its use in treating atropine intoxication. Neostigmine (choice D) is a quaternary ammonium reversible anticholinesterase that is used in the treatment of myasthenia gravis. It does not show specificity for nicotinic or muscarinic synapses. Its limited lipid solubility probably contributes to lack of actions at the ganglionic level.

59. **(C)** Down syndrome occurs in about one of 800 live births. The risk increases with increased maternal age. Mental retardation, epicanthic folds, cardiac abnormalities, and oblique palpebral fissures are commonly observed. The karyotype is trisomy 21. Trisomy 13 (choice A) is also called Patau syndrome. Mental retardation and microcephaly are major features of the disorder. Trisomy 18 (choice B) is also called Edwards' syndrome. Mental retardation, cardiac malformations, and death in infancy usually characterize the disorder. Turner's syndrome has a 45,XO genotype (choice D). Amenorrhea, short stature, cardiac abnormalities, and web neck comprise the syndrome. The XXY genotype (choice E) is also termed Klinefelter's syndrome. Eunuchoid habitus, long legs, atrophic testes, and retarded secondary sexual characteristics are observed.

60. **(C)** The diagram shows a right-sided homonymous hemianopsia, a loss of vision in the right optical field of both left and right eyes (nasal part of left eye and lateral part of right eye). The lesion must be in the left optical tract which carries nerve fibers originating from the lateral retina of the left eye and the nasal retina of the right eye. Note that the lateral visual fields project onto the nasal retinas and the nasal visual fields project onto the lateral retinas. Complete damage to the left optical nerve (choice A) or right optical nerve (choice B) results in total blindness of the left and right eye, respectively. The right optical tract (choice D) carries nerve fibers originating from the lateral retina of the right eye and the nasal retina of the left eye and when damaged would result in a left-sided homonymous hemianopsia. Damage to the optic chiasma (choice E), which is commonly caused by pituitary tumors, results in a bitemporal hemianopsia (loss of the right visual field of the right eye and loss of the left visual field of the left eye). This is because fibers from the nasal portions of the retinas cross over in the chiasm to form the optical tracts.

61. **(C)** Under normal conditions, lactate delivered to the liver is oxidized to pyruvate with the concomitant reduction of NAD^+ to NADH. The pyruvate is then transported to the mitochondria for conversion to oxaloacetate (OAA) catalyzed by pyruvate carboxylase. In the presence of mitochondrial phosphoenolpyruvate (PEP) carboxykinase the OAA is converted to PEP. In cells lacking mitochondrial PEP carboxykinase, OAA is transaminated to aspartate for transport to the cytoplasm. In the cytoplasm the aspartate is converted back to OAA. Cytoplasmic OAA is then converted to PEP by the cytoplasmic PEP carboxykinase. When alcohol is consumed, cytoplasmic alcohol dehydrogenase (ADH) catalyzes the following reaction:

$$\text{Ethanol} + NAD^+ \rightarrow \text{acetaldehyde} + NADH$$

Metabolism of ethanol occurs primarily in the liver and leads to an inhibition of hepatic gluconeogenesis. The large amounts of NADH generated by ADH must be transported to the mitochondria by the malate–aspartate shuttle. The excess cytoplasmic NADH forces the lactate dehydrogenase and cytoplasmic malate dehydrogenase reactions in the direction of lactate and malate production, respectively. The direction of the lactate dehydrogenase reaction inhibits the utilization of lactate as a gluconeogenic substrate. The direction of the cytoplasmic malate dehydrogenase reaction rapidly converts any cytoplasmic OAA to malate preventing its conversion to PEP by PEP carboxykinase. The net effect of the oxidation of ethanol on the direction of these two reactions is that ethanol and OAA are converted to acetaldehyde and malate, respectively. Although the increase in cytoplasmic NADH favorably drives the glyceraldehyde-3-phosphate dehydrogenase reaction in the gluconeogenic direction (choice D), the equilibrium shift in lactate dehydrogenase and malate dehydrogenase reduces the concentrations of pyruvate and OAA for use by the gluconeogenic enzyme pyruvate carboxylase and PEP carboxykinase, respectively. Ethanol metabolism does not activate glycolysis (choice A) at any step (choice B), nor does it signal altered levels of hepatocyte ATP (choice E).

62. **(A)** Degeneration of the substantia nigra is pathognomic for Parkinson's disease and results in progressive rigidity and slowness of movement (bradykinesia) and difficulty initiating movements. On examination, passive movement of the limbs is met with constant resistance. Superimposed tremors give it a "cogwheel"-like quality. Intention tremor (choice B) is characteristic for cerebellar lesions. Hyperkinesia (choice C) is an excess of movement often due to disorders of the basal ganglia. Parkinson's disease is characterized by poverty of movement and a mask-like facial expression. Chorea (choice D)—brief purposeless movements of the distal extremities—and athetosis (choice E)—writhing involuntary movements of the proximal extremities—are examples of hyperkinesias due to dopaminergic overactivity in the basal ganglia.

63. **(C)** This tubular structure has histological features typical of bronchioles. These include a highly corrugated mucosa (a result of smooth muscle contraction) lined by a columnar epithelium and a well-defined layer of circular smooth muscle. The smaller tubular structure to the right is also a bronchiole. The walls of the trachea (choice A) and bronchi (choice B) have some of the same elements as bronchioles, but they are distinguished by the presence of a layer of cartilage. Along with bronchioles, they constitute the conducting portion of the respiratory tree. Respiratory bronchioles, alveolar ducts (choice D), and alveolar sacs constitute the respiratory (gas exchange) component of the respiratory tree. All of these have alveoli as part (respiratory bronchiole) or all (alveolar ducts and sacs) of their lining. Alveoli are lined by a simple squamous epithelium composed of type I and type II pneumocytes. The lining of an arteriole (choice E) may appear corrugated in a histological section; however, the epithelium is simple squamous, not columnar. Moreover, there is no lamina propria of loose connective tissue between the epithelium and the smooth muscle layer that forms the tunica media of an arteriole.

64. **(E)** Colestipol and cholestyramine are bile acid–binding resins. By sequestering bile acids in the intestinal lumen, the bile acid–binding resins decrease negative feedback regulation of the conversion of cholesterol to bile acids within the liver. The resulting lower intracellular cholesterol level allows increased expression and activity of hepatic LDL receptors that mediate endocytosis of LDL particles. Bile acid–binding resins produce less lowering of LDL cholesterol levels than the statins because HMG-CoA reductase activity is also increased with both treatments but this activity is inhibited only by the statins. Gemfibrozil (choice A) and the other fibric acid derivatives reduce plasma triglyceride levels by decreasing the VLDL content of apoprotein CIII which acts as an inhibitor of lipoprotein lipase activity. The resulting increased lipoprotein lipase activity allows more rapid catabolism of VLDL particles in skeletal muscle and adipose tissue vascular beds. Gemfibrozil causes a beneficial increase in HDL cholesterol levels through unknown mechanisms. Probucol (choice B) is an antihyperlipidemic agent that finds use in treating patients with homozygous familial hypercholesterolemia. It may be more important as an indication of future directions for drug development in this area. Probucol functions as an antioxidant to prevent peroxidation of unsaturated fatty acids in lipoprotein particles, a process leading to production of modified forms of LDL that undergo endocytosis by the scavenger receptors of macrophages. These events are currently thought to be involved in the initial stages of atherogenesis. Niacin (choice C) functions as an antihyperlipidemic agent through inhibition of VLDL secretion by an unknown mechanism with subsequent lowering of VLDL and LDL. Etretinate (choice D) is not a lipid-lowering agent, but rather is a retinoic acid analog that is used in the treatment of the inflammatory types of psoriasis.

65. **(C)** The biologic activity of an antibody molecule centers on its ability to specifically bind antigen. The combining site is located on the amino-terminal end of the antibody molecule and is composed of hypervariable

segments within the variable regions of both light and heavy chains. Antibody specificity is a function of both the amino acid sequence and its three-dimensional configuration.

66. **(A)** The kidney in the photo demonstrates severe hydronephrosis characterized by dilation of the renal pelvis at the expense of the subadjacent renal medulla and cortex. Postrenal obstruction, such as a ureteral stone, is the most likely etiology. An acute renal infarct (choice B) would demonstrate a pale wedge-shaped area with its base along the renal capsule. A chronic infarct should show either fibrous scarring or cyst formation. The renal pelvis is usually unaffected with renal infarcts. Hypertension (choice C) mainly affects the blood vessels of the renal cortex, sparing the pelvic region of the kidney. Renal cell carcinoma (choice D) should display a yellowish cortical-based tumor, not hydronephrosis. Abuse of analgesics (choice E) may be associated with necrosis of the renal papillae. The papillae in the photo are not necrotic.

67. **(C)** The stimulation of afferent nerves to salivary gland acini results in the secretion of a solution that resembles plasma. This is accompanied by a loss of cellular potassium ions, which is brought about by a rise in the intracellular concentration of calcium ions. In experiments in which single ionic channels have been recorded directly, it has been demonstrated that the basolateral plasma membranes of salivary gland acinar cells contain calcium-activated potassium channels. It is believed that these account for the efflux of potassium following stimulation. The Na^+-K^+ exchange mechanism (choice A) and voltage-dependent non-specific cation channels (choice B) play little role in the secretory mechanism of salivary gland cells. Na^+-K^+-Cl^- cotransport (choice D) and the ouabain-sensitive Na^+-K^+ pump (choice E) may each contribute to the reuptake of potassium ions by these cells.

68. **(B)** The uncal herniation syndrome includes contralateral hemiplegia and ipsilateral oculomotor nerve signs such as paralysis of the ipsilateral medial rectus muscle. Paralysis of the contralateral (not ipsilateral lower, choice A, or contralateral upper, choice C) lower portion of the facial expression muscles may also be present. Typically, ipsilateral hemiplegia (choices D and E) is not seen, although it is possible for the contralateral cerebral peduncle to be compressed against the tentorial notch and if this occurs, then paralysis might also be present in the extremities ipsilateral to the herniated uncus.

69. **(D)** Clotting factors that are unique to the intrinsic pathway include factors VIII, IX, XI, and XII. The activation of factor X (choice E) represents the point of convergence of the intrinsic and extrinsic pathways. Factors required for clotting that are activated subsequent to activation of factor X are all part of the common pathway. Activated factor X proteolytically cleaves prothrombin (choice C) to thrombin, which in turn cleaves fibrinogen (choice A) to fibrin. Factor V (choice B) stimulates the activation of factor X, and fibrin-stabilizing factor (factor XIII) stabilizes the clot by cross-linking fibrin. The defect in hemophilia A is a deficiency in factor VIII, or the antihemophilic factor. This factor acts at the last step of the intrinsic pathway. Factor VIII, which is activated by minute amounts of thrombin, acts in concert with activated factor IX, a proteolytic enzyme, to activate factor X. (See Figure 8–22.)

70. **(C)** Hyperthyroidism is often characterized by confusion, anxiety, and an agitated depression, combined with fatigue, insomnia, and weight loss despite increased appetite. Choice A, dexamethasone suppression test, may be positive in major depression as well as in Cushing's syndrome, but of questionable clinical value in this case. Psychological tests such as Rorschach and trail making (choices B and E) are unlikely to be of much help. Increased serum calcium level (choice D) may be associated with depressive symptoms, but is of questionable value in this case.

71. **(D)** Psychomotor agitation refers to increased agitated movements with anxiety. It is often seen in depression and seems com-

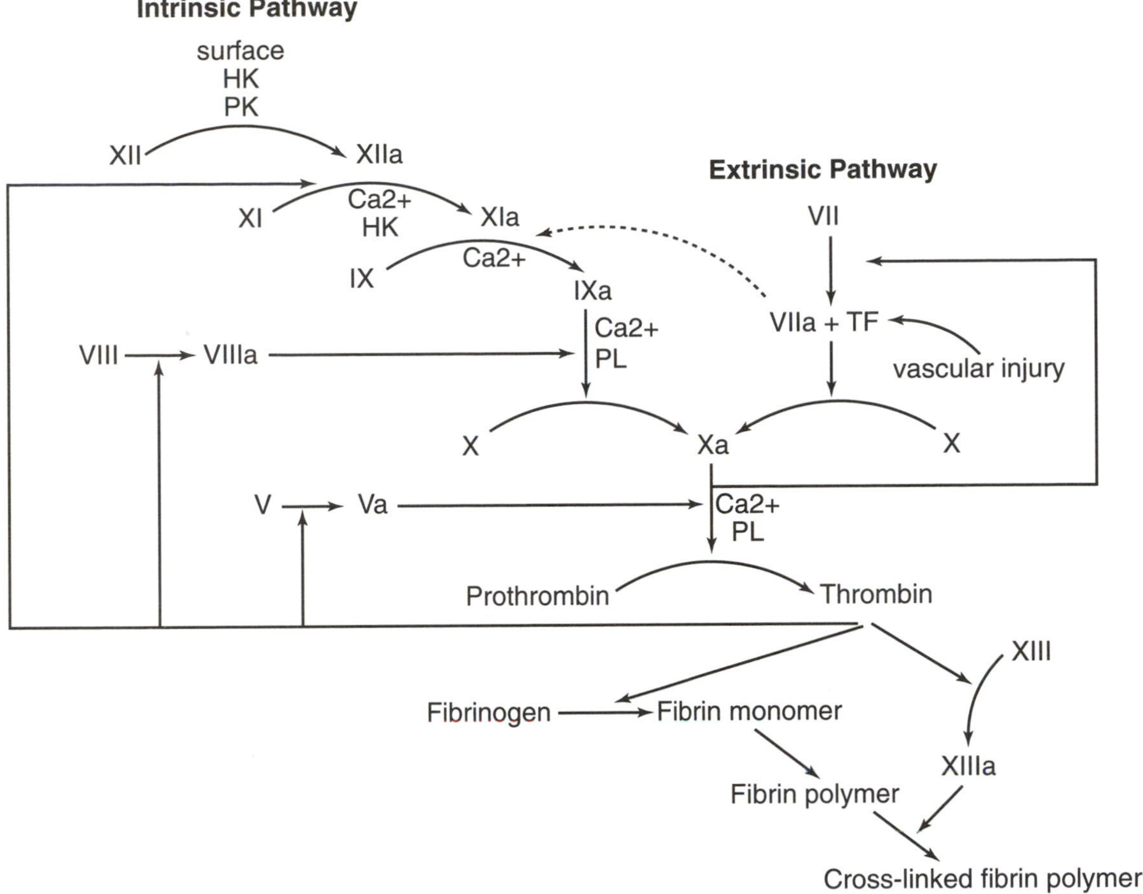

Figure 8–22

patible with the patient's history. Emotional lability may be seen in hysteria and pseudobulbar palsy (choices A and C), but there is no history to support these diagnoses. Psychomotor agitation is a description and not a diagnosis, which seems to fit this patient best. In psychomotor retardation (choice B), there is a slowing of motoric and emotional reactions. Restless leg syndrome (choice E) involves motoric activity not connected with depressive syndrome with agitation.

72. (A) A patient who has suicidal intentions and agitated depression is a very high-risk patient and hospitalization is indicated. Choice B would result in her having in her possession amitriptyline, 1500 mg. If she takes it as prescribed, 50 mg per day, it is probably a subtherapeutic dose. It would be lethal if all 1500 mg are taken together. All other therapies (choices C, D, and E) may be helpful but may not prevent the patient's suicide.

73. (B) Past suicidal attempts increase the risk of suicide. Therefore, coupled with agitated depression, the patient's suicidal intent should be taken very seriously. Choices C and D are therefore incorrect. Whether the patient has a personality disorder (choice E) or whether the mode of previous suicide attempts was by slashing (choice A) bear little relevance to immediate management.

74. (C) Family history of bipolar disorder is most relevant because it may indicate that the patient may be bipolar as well, and one should carefully look for evidence for bipolarity in this patient. Mood stabilizers may be needed if there is an indication that this patient may have bipolar disorder. Family history of all other conditions (choices A, B, D, and E) is important but perhaps not as immediately useful as that of bipolar disorder.

75. **(B)** Nefazodone, a new antidepressant, is sedating and useful for this patient's agitated depression, insomnia, and weight loss, whereas fluoxetine (SSRI) (choice A), while effective, may cause insomnia, increase anxiety, and suppress appetite. Choice C, tranylcypromine, an MAOI, is also stimulating. Choice D, buspirone, an antianxiety agent, is unlikely to treat the depression as is choice E, risperidone, an antipsychotic.

76. **(C)** Bell's palsy is an idiopathic paralysis of the muscles supplied by the facial nerve. Blinking is a function of the orbicularis oculi muscle that is innervated by the facial nerve. This action spreads tears over the surface of the cornea and conjunctiva keeping them moist. Chronic dryness can lead to inflammation and ulceration. A loss of sensory innervation to the cornea and conjunctiva (choice A) would result from interruption of the ophthalmic division of the trigeminal nerve, not from injury to the facial nerve. Reduced secretion of the parotid gland (choice B) would result from an interruption of the parasympathetic fibers originating in the glossopharyngeal nerve. Parasympathetic fibers originating in the facial nerve are secretomotor to the submandibular and sublingual salivary glands and to the lacrimal gland. Unusually warm and dry skin on the face (choice D) is indicative of a loss of sympathetic innervation to the vessels and sweat glands of the skin not involving the facial nerve. Chronic constriction of the pupil (choice E) results from the loss of sympathetic innervation to the dilator pupillae muscle and does not involve the facial nerve.

77. **(A)** The proteolytic blood enzyme thrombin has a specificity for arginine–glycine bonds in a manner similar to trypsin. Thrombin is synthesized as prothrombin, which contains γ-carboxyglutamate residues (*gla*) deriving from vitamin K–dependent, post-translational modification of glutamate. In order to be activated, prothrombin is proteolytically cleaved by factor Xa (*a*ctivated factor X) after being anchored to platelet membranes in a calcium–γ-carboxyglutamate-dependent reaction. The γ-carboxyglutamate end of the prothrombin molecule is removed, leaving an active thrombin. Active thrombin then hydrolyzes fibrinogen to fibrin at four arginine–glycine bonds. The A and B fibrinopeptides that are released spontaneously associate to form a clot of insoluble fibrin fibers. Thrombin does not complex with fibrinopeptides in a clot (choice B), and is a monomeric protein (choice C). The requirement for vitamin K is as a cofactor in the γ-carboxylation of glutamates. The *gla* residues are required for proper localization of prothrombin, but are not required when prothrombin is activated by proteolytic cleavage to thrombin, a process that (as indicated) removes the *gla* residue–containing portion of the protein (choices D and E).

78. **(B)** In cardiogenic shock, an agent that increases myocardial contractility without increasing heart rate and peripheral resistance is required. Particularly in cardiogenic shock resulting from acute myocardial infarction, it is important to select an agent that does not increase the cardiac workload and further extend myocardial damage. Dobutamine, a selective β_1-adrenoceptor agonist, will increase myocardial contractility without producing increases in heart rate or peripheral resistance. Epinephrine (choice A) can increase myocardial contractility but also will increase heart rate and, at doses that produce increased contractility, will also increase peripheral resistance. The result will be an increase in the cardiac workload, an undesirable effect in cardiogenic shock. Propranolol (choice C) is a non-selective β blocker that will decrease contractility. Digoxin (choice D) will produce a positive inotropic effect along with a reduction in heart rate, but its onset of action is not rapid enough to treat this medical emergency. The muscarinic antagonist atropine (choice E) may produce an increase of myocardial contractility under conditions when vagal tone is high, but is not useful in cardiogenic shock where direct stimulation of the myocardium is needed.

79. **(B)** The blood gas data from this patient illustrate chronic respiratory alkalosis with renal compensation. A lowlander at high alti-

tude for two weeks is expected to have low P_{O_2} plus low P_{CO_2} because of hypoxia-induced hyperventilation. Renal compensation in the form of bicarbonate excretion reduces plasma bicarbonate and returns the pH to a nearly normal value. Either severe chronic lung disease (choice A) or an overdose of heroin (choice C) would have caused respiratory acidosis due to abnormally high arterial P_{CO_2} (not the low P_{CO_2} this subject has). Acute aspirin overdose (choice D) in adults usually presents first with a respiratory alkalosis, which includes a low P_{CO_2}, but not a low P_{O_2}. Breathing a low oxygen gas mixture (choice E) is similar to being at high altitude, but if this is only for a few minutes there will be no time for renal compensation.

80. **(A)** In sections of loose connective tissue, active macrophages are relatively large cells with abundant cytoplasm containing phagocytosed material. Sometimes the identity of ingested material (e.g., erythrocytes, carbon particles, bacteria) can be recognized, but often the cytoplasm appears to contain vacuoles of varying size and staining density. The plasma cell (choice B) can be identified by the spherical nucleus with a distinctive clock-face pattern of heterochromatin and by the basophilic cytoplasm. The lymphocyte (choice C) has a small, dense nucleus and a thin rim of basophilic cytoplasm. The distinctive features of the eosinophil (choice D) are the bi-lobed nucleus and the eosinophilic granules that fill the cytoplasm. The cell with the elongated nucleus and scant cytoplasm (choice E) is most likely an inactive fibroblast.

81. **(B)** *Helicobacter pylori* is a small, spiral microbe that produces large amounts of urease. Thus, tests for urease activity have been employed as rapid and useful diagnostic assays. Patients with gastritis caused by *H. pylori* do not show elevation in their IgE levels. Patients with parasitic infections have high IgE levels in their serum (choice A). *H. pylori* does not have any unusual carbohydrate utilization patterns that can be used for the diagnosis of gastritis (choice C). Gram's stains do not provide any reliable information for the diagnosis of gastritis caused by *H. pylori*, because there are many microbes which resemble *H. pylori* (choice D). Culture of gastric contents on blood agar containing metronidazole and bismuth salts will result in the inhibition of growth of *H. pylori*, which is susceptible to metronidazole and bismuth salts (choice E).

82. **(E)** Ascites is a collection of excess fluid in the peritoneal cavity. At least 500 mL has to accumulate before it becomes clinically apparent. Transudative ascites is seen with portal hypertension and certain renal diseases. Exudative ascites may occur with bacterial infections and malignancy. An empyema (choice A) is an abnormal collection of pus within the thoracic cavity. A varicosity (choice B) is an abnormal dilation of a vein. Urticaria (choice C) is a pruritic macular lesion seen on the skin during some allergic reactions. Acantholysis (choice D) is a morphologic alteration of the epidermis characterized by intercellular discohesion with microgap formation.

83. **(D)** Conversion of pyruvate to acetyl-CoA results in the production of 1 mol of NADH. Oxidation of the resultant acetyl-CoA to CO_2 and water via the citric acid cycle yields 3 mol of NADH, 1 mol of $FADH_2$, and 1 mol of guanosine triphosphate (GTP). Oxidation of each mol of NADH during electron transport yields approximately 3 mol of ATP, whereas oxidation of $FADH_2$ results in the formation of approximately 2 mol of ATP. Therefore, beginning with pyruvate, the yield is 12 mol of ATP from 4 mol of NADH, 2 mol of ATP from 1 mol of $FADH_2$, and 1 mol of ATP equivalent (GTP) from substrate-level phosphorylation, giving a total of 15 mol of ATP. No other value of ATP yield is correct (choices A–C, E).

84. **(C)** Filtration pressure (P_{uf}) is calculated from the Starling equation involving four forces:

$$P_{uf} = (P_{GC} - P_{BS}) - (\Pi_{GC} - \Pi_{BS})$$

Normally, the filtrate in Bowman's space has such negligible amounts of protein that Π_{BS} is considered to be zero and is often left out of the Starling equation for glomerular filtration. Choices A, B, and D all give zero P_{uf} (i.e., glomerular filtration equilibrium). Choice E gives a negative filtration pressure of –5 mm Hg, which would favor absorption instead of filtration.

85. (C) Koplik's spots on the buccal mucosa are characteristic of infection with the measles virus. Microscopic examination of these lesions would reveal giant cells containing viral nucleocapsids. Macroscopically, these lesions will appear as small, erythematous macules with white centers. Rubella (German measles) is an acute febrile disease characterized by fever, maculopapular rash, and respiratory symptoms. It does not produce Koplik's spots. Rubella infection during the first trimester of pregnancy leads to congenital malformations (choice A). Herpangina is caused by coxsackie Group A viruses, which are not known to induce Koplik's spot formation (choice B). Thrush is production of white spots due to overgrowth of *Candida albicans* in the oral cavity (choice D). Scarlet fever is a cutaneous rash produced by *Streptococcus pyogenes.* This infection does not include Koplik's spot formation (choice E).

86. (C) The depolarizing blocking agent succinylcholine acts acutely as a nicotinic receptor agonist at the neuromuscular junction to produce depolarization. Succinylcholine is not hydrolyzed by acetylcholinesterase so that a sustained depolarization that prevents impulse transmission is produced. The depolarization blockade is not reversed by anticholinesterases since accumulation of acetylcholine only contributes to the depolarization at the neuromuscular junction. Actions of succinylcholine are eventually terminated by diffusion of the drug from the neuromuscular junction and hydrolysis by plasma pseudocholinesterase. With longer exposure (hrs), the characteristics of the blockade with succinylcholine change from depolarization to a situation resembling antagonist blockade, where anticholinesterases such as edrophonium will overcome the blockade. Pralidoxime (choice E) is a reactivator of cholinesterase inhibited by the irreversible organophosphate anticholinesterases. It does not reactivate cholinesterase inhibited by the reversible agents such as physostigmine or neostigmine.

87. (B) Interactions among antigen-presenting cells, T lymphocytes, and B lymphocytes are necessary for immune responses, and these cellular associations are promoted by the organization of lymph nodes. The deep cortical (paracortical) zone of a lymph node is the T-lymphocyte domain, and it will not develop if the thymus fails in its function of T-lymphocyte production. The presence of germinal centers in the outer cortex indicates that B-lymphocyte responses are underway, precluding a condition of agammaglobulinemia (choice A) or combined immunodeficiency (choice C). An acute bacterial infection (choice D) can lead to enlargement of all zones in lymph nodes. Thrombocytopenia (choice E), a deficiency in platelet numbers, does not change lymph node organization.

88. (B) The photomicrograph depicts a fibroadenoma, a benign tumor of the female breast. The microscopic features of this tumor include compressed benign ducts which are surrounded by non-atypical and normally cellular connective tissue. Medullary carcinoma (choice A) would display syncytial groups of anaplastic epithelial cells with a peripheral lymphoplasmocytic inflammatory reaction. Paget's disease (choice C) is an intraepidermal adenocarcinoma which clinically presents as an ulcerated or scaly lesion of the nipple. Intraductal carcinoma (choice D) would display a proliferation of atypical epithelial cells within the ducts. In most instances, a palpable mass is not present. Scirrhous carcinoma (choice E) is a common form of breast malignancy characterized by anaplastic epithelial cells in a fibrous reactive stroma.

89. (B) Pulmonary arterioles are unique for their ability to constrict under conditions of hypoxia. This results in a local adjustment of perfusion to ventilation. For example, if a bronchiole is obstructed, the lack of O_2 causes contraction of the pulmonary vascular smooth muscle in the corresponding area, shunting blood away from the hypoxic region to better-ventilated regions. Similarly, systemic hypoxia causes an increase in pulmonary artery resistance and increased workload for the right ventricle. Coronary (choice A), renal (choice C), gastrointestinal (choice D), and skeletal muscle (choice E) arteries all dilate under hypoxic conditions, resulting in enhanced blood flow to their respective organs.

90. **(D)** Glucagon-stimulated increases in cAMP levels leads to increased activity of cAMP-dependent protein kinase (PKA). There are numerous hepatic substrates for PKA, including pyruvate kinase, phosphofructokinase-2 (PFK-2) and an inhibitor of protein phosphatases identified as inhibitor-1 (also called protein phosphatase inhibitor-1, PPI-1). The net result of PKA-mediated phosphorylation of these three proteins is a decrease in pyruvate kinase activity (choice A), a decrease in the level of active protein phosphatases by their being bound to PPI-1 (choice E) and an increase in the phosphatase activity of PFK-2, with concomitant decrease in PFK-2 kinase activity (choice C). The phosphatase activity of PFK-2 leads to a decrease in the level of fructose-2,6-bisphosphate which is a potent allosteric activator of phosphofructokinase-1 (PFK-1). Therefore, the activity of PFK-1 will decrease in response to increased hepatic cAMP levels (choice B).

91. **(C)** With the patient seated and the head tilted anteriorly (chin on chest), irrigation of the right ear with warm water produces increased output from the right vestibular sensory apparatus and this leads to activation of the left lateral rectus and right medial rectus muscles. These two muscles then produce slow (not fast, choices B and E) conjugate horizontal movement of the eyes to the left (not right, choices A and D), which is followed immediately by rapid conjugate movement to the right.

92. **(C)** Because of changes in sexual behaviors (practice of safe sex), the percentage of gay and bisexual men with HIV has gradually declined in the United States. Choice A is incorrect as the ratio of men to women who are infected with HIV is estimated to be six to one. Choice B is incorrect as the number of infected women is growing four times faster than the number of infected men. As for choice D, because there is a decrease in the percentage of infected gay and bisexual men, there is an increase in infected heterosexual men. Choice E is incorrect because more women are now being infected through heterosexual intercourse than IV substance abuse.

93. **(D)** The steady state condition means that the input rate equals the output rate. The input rate is 20 mg/hr, so the output rate must equal 20 mg/hr. If 80% of the output is being eliminated by the liver, this means that the liver is handling 20 mg/hr × 0.8, or 16 mg/hr. By the same reasoning, the normal kidney is handling 20 mg/hr × 0.2, or 4 mg/hr. In the patient with 50% renal function, that kidney will be able to clear 4 mg/hr × 0.5, or 2 mg/hr. The patient will be able to clear 16 mg/hr by the liver and 2 mg/hr by the kidney, giving a total capacity of 18 mg/hr. Thus, the infusion rate needs to be 18 mg/hr in the patient with 50% renal function.

94. **(B)** The DiGeorge syndrome is a form of glandular aplasia due to defective embryonic development of the third and fourth pharyngeal pouches, which give rise to the thymus, parathyroid, and thyroid glands. This anomaly results in a depletion of thymic-dependent areas in lymphoid tissues. A depletion of lymph node lymphocytes in both T- and B-dependent areas occurs in combined immunedeficiency disease (SCID), not in DiGeorge syndrome (choice A). In DiGeorge syndrome it is the T cell production that is affected. The number of B cells involved in the production of antibodies, including isohemagglutinins, is not affected (choice C). A defect in the killing of intracellular bacteria by neutrophils occurs in chronic granulomatous disease, but not in DiGeorge's syndrome (choice D). A depletion of B-dependent areas in lymph nodes occurs in Bruton's X-linked agammaglobulinemia, not in DiGeorge's syndrome (choice E).

95. (B) The fine needle biopsy demonstrates a fairly monomorphic population of small mitotically active neoplastic lymphocytes with associated starry sky histiocytes. The morphology of the tumor and the clinical history are typical for endemic Burkitt's lymphoma. There are no parasitic elements (choice A) evident in the photograph. Salivary gland lymphoepithelioma (choice C) is usually seen in an older age group, would contain some remaining epithelial elements, and has larger immunoblastic-type lymphocytes. Chronic lymphocytic leukemia–lymphoma (choice D) is distinctly uncommon in children and would feature mature lymphocytes without a starry sky background. The diagnosis of adenocarcinoma (choice E) is incompatible with the photograph because malignant epithelial elements are not seen.

96. (E) The development of endemic Burkitt's lymphoma is strongly linked to prior infection by the Epstein–Barr virus. Infections with *Wuchereria bancrofti* (choice A) produce an obstructive lymphadenitis called filariasis. This parasitic infection is not related to the development of Burkitt's lymphoma. Sjögren syndrome (choice B) is associated with a higher risk of subsequently developing lymphoma, most often occurring in middle-aged or elderly females. The lymphomas are not of the Burkitt cell type. Aflatoxin (choice C) ingestion increases the risk of hepatoma, not lymphoma. The occurrence of endemic Burkitt's lymphoma is not due to a lack of an essential dietary nutrient (choice D).

97. (D) When lactate enters hepatocytes for conversion to glucose, it is oxidized to pyruvate by lactate dehydrogenase. In this direction lactate dehydrogenase reduces NAD^+ to NADH. The NADH thus generated can be used by glyceraldehyde-3-phosphate dehydrogenase in the gluconeogenic direction converting 1,3-bisphosphoglycerate to glyceraldehyde-3-phosphate. During this reduction reaction NADH is oxidized to NAD^+, completing the cycle between the two enzymes of the gluconeogenesis pathway that require the nicotinamide nucleotide as a cofactor/substrate. Glucose-6-phosphate dehydrogenase requires $NADP^+$ as a cofactor and does not function in the gluconeogenesis pathway (choice A). The primary direction of the glycerol-3-phosphate dehydrogenase-catalyzed reaction is in the transfer of electrons from cytoplasmic NADH to mitochondrial $FADH_2$. The direction of this reaction generates cytoplasmic NAD^+, not NADH (choice B). The cytoplasmic malate dehydrogenase reaction does function in gluconeogenesis and yields cytoplasmic NADH, but is involved in the process when pyruvate is the direct source of carbon (e.g., from amino acids), not lactate (choice C). The phosphoenol pyruvate carboxykinase reaction does not yield any reduced electron carriers (choice E).

98. (B) Sarcoidosis is a multisystem disorder of unknown cause. The characteristic histologic lesion is a poorly formed noncaseating epithelioid granuloma. Fibroblastic proliferations (choice A) are usually seen with the later stages of healing and are not the characteristic histologic feature of sarcoid. A pyogenic abscess (choice C) would be composed of pus, necrotic debris, and neutrophils. Abscesses are not usually present in sarcoidosis. Mucoid cyst (choice D) formation is not a feature of sarcoid. Hyaline membrane formation (choice E) is seen in lungs of neonates with respiratory distress syndrome and the lungs of adults with diffuse alveolar damage. It is not a histologic pattern seen in sarcoidosis.

99. (E) To test the superior oblique muscle, the patient is directed to look far medially and then downward. To test the superior rectus muscle (choice A), the patient is directed to look far laterally and then upward. To test the inferior rectus muscle (choice B), the patient is directed to look far laterally and then downward. To test the medial rectus muscle (choice C), the patient is directed to look far medially. To test the inferior oblique muscle (choice D), the patient is directed to look far medially and then upward.

100. (C) All of the agents listed are in the class of non-steroidal anti-inflammatory drug (NSAID) inhibitors of cyclo-oxygenase, the enzyme responsible for the initial step in the conversion of arachidonic acid to the prostaglandin mediators of inflammation, fever, and pain perception. Anti-inflammatory activity correlates with the ability to inhibit cyclo-oxygenase. In contrast to the other agents listed, acetaminophen is a poor inhibitor of cyclo-oxygenase and possesses little anti-inflammatory activity, while expressing analgesic and antipyretic activity. The reasons for the differences are not clear. The ability of acetaminophen to lower fever and provide analgesia while not suppressing the cytoprotective actions of the prostaglandins in the gastrointestinal system provides a place for its use in antipyresis and analgesia. Indomethacin (choice A) is an NSAID in the indole family of such agents. It is a potent cyclo-oxygenase inhibitor but its use in chronic situations is limited because of the high rate (35 to 50%) of patients experiencing adverse reactions. These include gastrointestinal pains, ulceration, and severe headache. It is used in the treatment of gout and to produce closure of patent ductus arteriosus. Aspirin (choice B) is both the prototype and exception to the NSAIDs. It is the exception in that it causes acetylation of cyclo-oxygenase to produce an irreversible inhibition, whereas the other NSAIDs cause a reversible inhibition. The irreversible inhibition is particularly important for platelet function since platelets, unlike most other cells, are not capable of synthesizing new molecules of cyclo-oxygenase. The result is a loss of ability of the affected platelets to produce thromboxane A_2, a platelet-aggregating agent. This is the basis for the use of low-dose aspirin in prevention of thrombosis and resulting myocardial infarction and occlusive stroke. There are two isoforms of cyclo-oxygenase. Cyclo-oxygenase-1 (COX-1) is the constitutive isoform found in blood vessels, stomach, and kidney. COX-2 is induced under conditions of inflammation. Nabumetone (choice D) is a newer NSAID with selectivity toward COX-2. Such agents offer some promise of treating inflammation with less ulcerogenic activity. Tolmetin (choice E) is an NSAID in the heteroaryl acetic acid class, used in the treatment of osteoarthritis and rheumatoid arthritis.

101. (E) *Bacillus anthracis* is a gram-positive, spore forming microbe. Autoclaving is the best option for killing both the vegetative cells and spores of *B. anthracis* (choices A, B, C, and D).

102. (C) Aromatase is the enzyme that controls the conversion of testosterone to estradiol. It also catalyzes the formation of estrone from androstenedione. The major proportion of circulating estradiol in adult men is formed directly by aromatization of these circulating androgens. Lesser amounts may be secreted by both the Leydig cells (choice A) and the Sertoli cells (choice B) in the testes and by the adrenal cortex (choice D). Estrone and estradiol are the products, not the substrate, of aromatase (choice E).

103. (C) Hypertrophy is the term defining an increase in the size of individual cells without an increase in the actual number of cells. Hypoxia (choice A) is a state of reduced oxygen tension. Shock is an example of tissue hypoxia. Hyperplasia (choice B) refers to an increased number of cells. Endometrial hyperplasia is an example, and it features an increased number of glandular and stromal cells in the endometrium. Metaplasia (choice D) is the exchange of one adult tissue type for another. Squamous bronchial metaplasia due to cigarette smoking is an example. Dysplasia (choice E) is a potentially premalignant change such as that seen in the uterine cervix with human papilomavirus infection.

104. (C) Of the enzymes listed in the question, only glucokinase and glucose-6-phosphatase are found in the liver and not in most other tissues. Hexokinase (choice B) is the glucose phosphorylating enzyme of non-hepatic tissues. A deficiency in glucokinase, which is the hepatic-specific glucose phosphorylating isozyme (choice A), would lead to increased blood sugar levels and hyperglycemia, not hypoglycemia. This would occur because of the liver's decreased ability to phosphorylate free glucose. In contrast, a defect in glucose-6-phosphatase would cause the symptoms observed in von Gierke's disease. This endoplasmic reticulum enzyme catalyzes the dephosphorylation of glucose-6-phosphate, allowing glucose to be released into the blood when levels are low. A lesion at this point would result in massive storage of glycogen in the liver. A deficiency in phosphofructokinase-1 (choice D) also results in a glycogen storage disease. This disease is Tarui's and it is restricted to muscle and erythrocyte involvement leading to exercise-induced cramping and hemolytic anemia. A deficiency in lysosomal α-1,4-glucosidase (choice E), also called lysosomal acid α-glucosidase and acid maltase results in the glycogen storage disease termed Pompe's disease. This disorder leads to glycogen accumulation in most tissues, but the effects are most pronounced in skeletal and cardiac muscle. Affected individuals die at an early age due to massive cardiomegaly.

105. **(A)** Sympathetic stimulation releases the neurotransmitter norepinephrine at the nerve terminals. Norepinephrine acts by increasing membrane permeability to Na^+ and Ca^{2+} ions, resulting in an increased slope of the diastolic depolarization. Therefore, membrane potential reaches the threshold for self-excitation (broken line) earlier, increasing the heart rate. The amplitude of the action potential (curves B and C) is little affected by sympathetic stimulation. Curve D represents the effect of parasympathetic stimulation.

106. **(B)** Not all patients admit to the presence of risk factors, but may request testing. Other indications include being a member of a high-risk group, patients with symptoms of AIDS, women belonging to a high-risk group planning pregnancy, and blood, semen, or organ donors. Homosexuality per se without having had sexual contact with a possibly infected person is not an indication (choice A), nor is being in a psychiatric hospital, medical school, or the military (choices C, D, and E).

107. **(C)** Spasticity is defined as an increase in the resistance to passive movement. Hypertonia (not hypotonia, choice A) is usually associated with spasticity, which is typically the result of damage to an upper motoneuron (not a lower motoneuron, choice B). A hemisection of the spinal cord at C8 would lead to spasticity in the ipsilateral (not contralateral, choice D) lower extremity due to interruption of the corticospinal tract on that side. Spasticity and rigidity are not similar clinical entities as stated in choice E. Spasticity is typically related to pyramidal tract lesions, whereas rigidity is associated with basal ganglia lesions.

108. **(B)** Methimazole is a thioureylene compound that acts within the thyroid gland to inhibit the peroxidase responsible for the incorporation of iodine into thyroglobulin and the coupling of iodotyrosyl residues to form the iodothyronines. It is used to treat hyperthyroidism prior to surgery or radioiodine ablation, or in anticipation of remission of the hyperthyroid state. Hashimoto's thyroiditis (choice A) is an autoimmune disease. It presents as a chronic inflammation of the thyroid gland with lymphocytic infiltration. Goiter is characteristic because the ability of the gland to produce thyroid hormone is decreased and TSH stimulation of the gland increases. Thyroid hormone replacement therapy may decrease the goiter. Occasionally, Hashimoto's thyroiditis and Graves' disease coexist with hyperthyroidism. Thyrotoxicosis factitia (choice C) is a thyrotoxicosis without abnormality of the thyroid gland and arises from inadvertent or deliberate ingestion of thyroid hormone. In adults, it is often attributable to a psychiatric disorder. Hypoparathyroidism (choice D) arises from the lack of parathyroid hormone and is characterized by hypocalcemia with muscle spasms and paresthesias in the extremities. Simple hypothyroidism (choice E) due to inadequate formation of thyroid hormone by the thyroid gland is treated with levothyroxine, the synthetic form of thyroxine.

109. **(A)** In a positive viral hemagglutination test, the virus is the hemagglutinating particle. Antibody specific to the viral hemagglutinin will block this activity and inhibit hemagglutination. The assay is similar to a neutralization test, with the erythrocyte taking the place of a susceptible nucleated host cell. Latex agglutinins are antibodies which will agglutinate antigens bound on the surface of latex spheres. Viral hemagglutination takes places between red blood cells and viruses (choice B). Rh antibody is directed toward the D antigen found on red blood cells (choice C). Hemolysin is a molecule which lyses red blood cells. Staphylococci, streptococci, and other bacteria produce various types of hemolysins (choice D). Certain viruses such as influenza, measles, mumps, and parainfluenza viruses produce hemagglutinins which agglutinate red blood cells, but these viruses promote hemagglutination, they do not inhibit it (choice E).

110. **(D)** Of the conditions listed, only pancreatic head tumors are associated with an increase in conjugated ("direct") bilirubin ("obstructive jaundice"). Increased levels of unconjugated ("indirect") bilirubin result from hemolysis or liver defects that impair uptake or conjugation mechanisms in liver cells (Gilbert's syndrome, choice A). The physiological jaundice of the neonate (choice B) observed during the first week of birth is usually mild and due to relatively immature liver conjugation. Unconjugated bilirubin may cross the immature blood–brain barrier of the newborn and cause kernicterus (choice C). Obstruction of the bile duct by metastatic colon tumors (choice E) could also result in increased blood levels of conjugated ("direct") bilirubin, but is quite rare.

111. **(A)** The double-reciprocal Lineweaver–Burk plot that accompanies the question illustrates a competitively inhibited enzyme. In competitive inhibition, the intercept on the y axis, which is equal to I/V_{max}, does not change. This points out that at significantly high substrate concentration, the inhibition can be overcome. In noncompetitive inhibition (choice B), the V_{max}, and hence the y-axis intercept, does change. Noncompetitive inhibition cannot be overcome by increasing the substrate concentration. Allosteric enzymes (choice C) do not obey Michaelis–Menten kinetics and cannot be plotted as straight lines on double-reciprocal curves. The two depicted lines have, at sufficiently high substrate concentration, the same, not different V_{max} (choice D). Irreversibly inhibited enzymes (choice E) cannot be treated by Michaelis–Menten kinetics.

112. **(C)** Aldosterone is synthesized and secreted by cells of the adrenal cortex. A primary role for mineralocorticoids such as aldosterone is to stimulate the renal reabsorption of sodium ions. After adrenalectomy, the excretion of sodium ions in the urine is significantly increased and plasma sodium ion concentrations fall. At the same time, plasma potassium concentrations increase. If mineralocorticoids are not administered, blood pressure and the volume of plasma decrease and death ensues. Although the loss of glucocorticoids, such as cortisol (choice A) and corticosterone (choice B), may also become lethal in certain circumstances, such as fasting, their loss in adrenalectomy is not as critical as is the loss of aldosterone. Neither are the loss of the androgen dehydroepiandrosterone (choice D), secreted by the adrenal cortex, or the loss of catecholamines (choice E), such as epinephrine, secreted by the adrenal medulla.

113. **(D)** Some individuals exhibit an intolerance to aspirin even at low doses. This tendency is correlated with the presence of nasal polyps and is manifested by a range of symptoms from rhinitis to acute bronchoconstriction, angioedema, and shock. The reaction does not appear to be of immunological origin. The suggestion has been made that the condition arises from inhibition of cyclo-oxygenase and shunting of arachidonic acid into the 5′-lipoxygenase pathway. The efficacy of the leukotriene C_4, D_4, and E_4 antagonist zafirlukast in the prophylaxis of bronchial asthma lends credence to this hypothesis. Infertility (choice A) is not associated with the use of aspirin. Hepatotoxicity (choice B) is associated with chronic aspirin therapy and usually occurs with plasma concentrations maintained at 150 μg/ml or greater. Elevation of liver enzyme activity in the plasma is the usual sign of hepatotoxicity, although hepatomegaly may also be seen. Nephrotoxicity (choice C) is rarely seen with aspirin used alone, but may occur in chronic therapy when salicylates are combined with compounds such as acetaminophen. Aspirin may produce mild hemolysis (choice E) in individuals with a deficiency in erythrocytic glucose-6-phosphate dehydrogenase activity.

114. **(D)** Complement-fixation procedures are performed in two stages. The test system consists of antigen and antibody (one of which is unknown) plus complement. The indicator system consists of sheep erythrocytes and hemolysin (an antisheep–RBC serum), which will sensitize the cells to the lytic action of complement. If complement is fixed in the test system, it is effectively bound (or consumed) in the antigen–antibody complexes there and is not free to participate in the lysis of the sensitized erythrocytes present in the indicator system. In an influenza virus complement-fixation test, the indicator system consists of complement, unlabeled sheep red blood cells, and antibody to sheep red blood cells. Thus, ^{51}Cr-labeled sheep RBCs are not used (choice A). The indicator system does not need antibody to influenza virus, fluorescent-tagged virus, or neuraminidase (choices B, C, and E).

115. **(C)** Each organ site has specific rules by which to stage the extent of tumor involvement. The colon invasion of the tumor into, but not through, the muscularis propria is T2. The presence of pericolic lymph nodes with metastatic carcinoma is N1. The absence of distal non-nodal metastases, such as in the liver, is M0. T1, N0, M0 (choice A) is incorrect because the tumor is T2 and the nodal status is N1. The M status is correct as M0. T2 N0 M1 (choice B) is incorrect because the nodal status is N1 and distant metastatic status is M0. The tumor is correct as T2. T3 N0 M1 (choice D) has all three items coded incorrectly. T4 N0 M1 (choice E) also has all three items coded incorrectly.

116. **(E)** Activity in the sympathetic afferent nerves to the pancreas results in the enhanced secretion of glucagon from the α cells within the pancreatic islets. The stimulation of sympathetic afferents also inhibits insulin secretion from the β cells. The increase in glucagon secretion is a β-adrenergic response that uses a cyclic AMP second messenger mechanism. Agents that elevate cyclic AMP promote rather than inhibit (choice A) glucagon secretion. Inhibitory α-adrenergic receptors are also present, but the β-adrenergic response usually is dominant under sympathetic stimulation. The secretion of glucagon is enhanced, not inhibited, by elevated amino acid concentrations (choice B) in plasma and is inhibited by glucose (choice C) and insulin (choice D).

117. **(B)** Lyme disease is due to a systemic infection by the spirochete *Borrelia burgdorferi.* Infections are usually transmitted to humans through a tick bite. Campers, hikers, and outdoor enthusiasts are at risk, particularly in the northeastern United States. A transient rash followed by migratory arthritis is the typical clinical course. Antibiotics are curative. Rheumatoid arthritis (choice A) should demonstrate an elevated serum rheumatoid factor, not antibodies against *B. burgdorferi.* Achondroplasia (choice C) is an autosomal dominant genetic disorder characterized by dwarfism and arthritis. Osteoarthritis (choice D) would be uncommon in a person only 36 years old. Antibodies directed against *Borrelia* species are not a feature of osteoarthritis. Ochronosis (choice E) is an autosomal recessive disorder characterized by early arthritis, pigmented cartilage, and excess homogentisic acid in the urine.

118. **(B)** Normal catabolism of phenylalanine involves hydroxylation to tyrosine catalyzed by phenylalanine hydroxylase. Mutations in the phenylalanine hydroxylase gene lead to deficiencies in the enzyme and manifest as phenylketonuria (PKU). Patients suffering from PKU have elevated levels of phenylalanine in their blood as well as the transamination product, phenylpyruvate. Phenylpyruvate is converted to phenyllactate and phenylacetate by reduction and oxidation, respectively; all three by-products are excreted in the urine. The standard test for PKU is to test for elevated phenylalanine in the blood of newborns. Hartnup disease (choice A) results from a defect in intestinal and renal transport of neutral amino acids with general neutral aminoaciduria. Maple syrup urine disease (choice C) results from a defect in α-keto acid decarboxylase and leads to elevated levels of the branched-chain amino acids, leucine, isoleucine, and valine, in the blood and urine. Alcaptonuria (choice D) results from a defect in homogentisate oxidase which is involved in tyrosine catabolism. The urine of afflicted individuals darkens upon exposure to air due to the presence of homogentisic acid. Hepatorenal tyrosinemia (choice E) is a form of tyrosinemia, all forms of which lead to elevated levels of tyrosine, or its various metabolites, in the blood.

119. (B) Heterochromatin is a highly condensed form of chromatin in which the DNA is inaccessible to transcription. In light microscopy, heterochromatin stains intensely with basic stains, and the amount and distribution pattern of heterochromatin in the nucleus is a useful feature in identifying both normal and abnormal cells in tissue sections. Euchromatin (choice A) stains less intensely than heterochromatin because the chromatin is in a more dispersed form, and consequently the DNA is accessible to transcription. Cells that are active in either protein synthesis or division tend to have large nuclei containing mostly euchromatin. The nucleolus (choice C) is the site of ribosomal RNA production. Nuclear pores (choice D) provide a regulated portal for movement of material between the nucleus and the cytoplasm. The rough endoplasmic reticulum (choice E) is the site of translation and initial posttranslational modification of proteins destined for export, sequestration within vesicles such as lysosomes, or incorporation into membranes. Those mRNAs coding for such proteins contain a sequence of bases at the 5′ end that codes for a signal sequence of mostly hydrophobic amino acids. This leads to docking of the ribosome-mRNA complex on the membrane of the endoplasmic reticulum. As the newly synthesized protein is inserted into the lumen of the rER, the signal sequence is enzymatically removed by the signal peptidase.

120. (C) The oral anticoagulants exert their effects by inhibiting the reduction of the epoxide of vitamin K formed during the carboxylation of glutamate residues in prothrombin and coagulation factors VII, IX, and X. Formation of gamma-carboxyglutamate residues in these factors is necessary for their activity. Conditions that decrease vitamin K will contribute to anticoagulant activity. Broad-spectrum antibiotics such as cefotaxime, by killing intestinal flora that synthesize vitamin K, will decrease its dietary availability. Cephalosporins with heterocyclic side chains, such as cefotaxime, inhibit the same enzyme as the oral anticoagulants, further contributing to the anticoagulation activity. Phenobarbital (choice A) is an inducer of the hepatic metabolism of the oral anticoagulants. Induction of cytochrome P450 activity will decrease anticoagulant activity. Rifampin (choice B) is also an inducer of the cytochrome P450-dependent metabolism of oral anticoagulants. The bile acid–binding resin cholestyramine (choice D) binds the oral anticoagulants and inhibits their absorption from the gut. This results in decreased anticoagulant activity for a given oral dose. The H_2-blocker ranitidine (choice E) should have no effect on the activity of the oral anticoagulants. It is devoid of the P450-inhibiting property seen with cimetidine, a less potent H_2 blocker.

121. (C) The graft-versus-host reaction occurs when immunocompetent lymphoid cells are transferred to a histoincompatible recipient who is unable to reject them. The donor cells then mount an immune response against the foreign histocompatibility antigens of the recipient and attempt to reject them. This usually occurs in bone marrow transplantation performed as a therapeutic modality in patients with certain leukemias or other blood diseases, such as aplastic anemia. Contamination of the graft with gram-negative bacteria is not known to be a key factor in the graft-versus-host reaction (choice A). Graft-versus-host reactions can occur with any type of tissue grafting, of both neoplastic and non-neoplastic origin (choice B). A graft-versus-host reaction does not occur because the graft has histocompatibility antigens not found in the recipient, but instead occurs when immunocompetent lymphoid cells are transferred to a histoincompatible recipient unable to reject the immunocompetent lymphoid cells (choice D). For the reasons stated above, a graft-versus-host reaction does not occur when a histocompatible graft is irradiated before use (choice E).

122. (C) The colon segment demonstrates ulcerative colitis. The disease is limited to the colon and preferentially involves in continuity the rectum, sigmoid, and descending colon. The affected colon demonstrates a red, granular mucosa with occasional pseudopolyp formation. Deep fissures, skip lesions with alternating areas of diseased and normal colon, and strictures do not typically occur. Pseudomembranous colitis (choice A) is usually an acute colitis occurring after antibiotic therapy. White custard-like debris that partially coats the mucosal surface is the characteristic gross observation of pseudomembranous colitis. Amebic colitis (choice B) is usually limited to the right colon and displays multiple, scattered, separate ulcerations. In collagenous colitis (choice D) the colon appears grossly normal. Gangrenous colitis (choice E) would have an acute clinical course. Grossly, the colon would demonstrate a transmural area of blackened, thinned tissue.

123. (E) Chronic ulcerative colitis carries an increased risk for developing adenocarcinoma. Most patients are followed by annual endoscopies with histologic evaluation of random colonic biopsies. The presence of high-grade dysplasia usually is an indication for prophylactic pancolonic resection. There is no increased risk to develop melanoma (choice A) with ulcerative colitis. A liver abscess (choice B) is a known complication of amebic colitis. It is not observed with ulcerative colitis. Amyloidosis (choice C) does not occur with increased frequency in ulcerative colitis. Strictures (choice D) are not a typical feature of ulcerative colitis. Most strictures are focal lesions capable of being treated by a local resection rather than a pancolectomy.

124. (D) Much progress has been made in the past 10 years in elucidating signal-transduction mechanisms, and this has become a popular topic in the medical board exams. Endothelial cells produce both vasodilator substances (e.g., nitric oxide), and potent vasoconstrictor substances (e.g., endothelins). The vascular smooth muscle ET-1 receptor is coupled via a G protein to phospholipase C, catalyzing the hydrolysis of PIP_2 to IP_3 and DAG. IP_3 in turn releases Ca^{2+} from intracellular stores and causes smooth muscle contraction. Increased cAMP (choice A) and increased cGMP (choice B) result in vascular smooth muscle relaxation and are due to β receptor activation and nitric oxide, respectively. Tyrosine kinase (choice C) mediates the action of insulin and growth factors. Examples of hormones that act via regulation of gene expression (choice E) include steroids, vitamin D, and thyroid hormones. However, direct effects of these hormones on vascular smooth muscle have not been described.

125. (A) Although in bacteria a continuous sequence of triplet codons encode for each protein, genes may be discontinuous in eukaryotic cells. Non-coding intervening sequences of DNA that split genes in eukaryotes are called introns. The coding sequences of split genes are called exons. Mature mRNA translated from such DNA does not contain the sequences of the intron(s). However, all genes that contain introns are transcribed into a primary RNA (termed heteronuclear RNA, hnRNA) that contains the sequences of the introns. These intervening sequences in the primary transcripts are specifically removed and the ends of the exons ligated together (a process termed RNA splicing), so the mature mRNA contains no introns. The non-coding spaces between different genes can be of variable type, but are not referred to as intronic sequences (choice B). Only the non-coding regions between exons of genes are termed introns (choice C). Any untranslated regions (choices D and E) of mRNAs are found at the 5′ end and 3′ end of the message and are sequences contained within exons of the gene.

126. (C) The stylopharyngeus muscle is the only muscle innervated by the glossopharyngeal nerve. The pharyngeal plexus (choice A) includes fibers derived from the vagus nerve that are distributed to the muscles of the pharynx, except the stylopharyngeus, and of the palate, except the tensor veli palatini. The vagus nerve (choice B) contributes fibers to the pharyngeal plexus that are distributed to the muscles of the pharynx, except the stylopharyngeus, and of the palate, except the tensor veli palatini. The facial nerve (choice D) innervates the muscles of facial expression, the posterior belly of the digastric muscle, the stylohyoid muscle, and the stapedius muscle, but not the stylopharyngeus muscle. The mandibular nerve (choice E) innervates the muscles of mastication, the anterior belly of the digastric muscle, the mylohyoid muscle, the tensor tympani muscle, and the tensor veli palatini muscle, but not the stylopharyngeus muscle.

127. (E) The β-blocker propranolol, by blocking cardiac β_1 adrenoceptors, prevents the sympathetic nervous system from increasing heart rate and contractility in response to exertion. This prevents the normal increase in cardiac workload and reduces or maintains the myocardial oxygen demand at a lower level than would otherwise be the case. This effect is prophylactic. Propranolol does not dilate capacitance vessels (choice A). In contrast, the nitrovasodilators such as nitroglycerin dilate capacitance vessels, an effect that reduces cardiac preload. This effect reduces the workload and results in a decrease in myocardial oxygen demand, thus terminating an anginal attack. There is no net change in coronary blood flow (choice B) with propranolol, although there may be some redistribution of flow to ischemic areas. Propranolol does not increase oxygen delivery (choice C). Propranolol does inhibit the release of renin (choice D) from the juxtaglomerular apparatus. This effect may be important in its antihypertensive actions, but does not contribute to the prevention of anginal attacks.

128. (A) *Pseudomonas* infections often occur in patients suffering from cystic fibrosis or burns. These infections are most frequently caused by *Pseudomonas aeruginosa,* which produces a characteristic blue-green pigment. *Legionella pneumophila* and *Mycoplasma pneumoniae* do not produce pigments. *Staphylococcus aureus* and *Staphylococcus epidermidis* produce yellow and white pigments, respectively (choices B, C, D, and E).

129. (C) While all the other items (choices A, B, D, and E) are components of personality, choice C is most comprehensive.

130. (B) Wernicke's area, located at the posterior end of the superior temporal gyrus, is believed to play an important role in the understanding of language, either written or spoken. Patients with lesions in this area have a form of fluid aphasia in which the ability to vocalize is not impaired, but the subject matter of speech is not intelligible. Moreover, the ability to understand either speech or writing is impaired. This is in contrast to lesions of Broca's area, in which understanding is preserved, but the ability to vocalize speech is impaired (choice A). Deficits in the processing of visual information (choice C), dyslexia (choice D), or disorders of short-term memory (choice E) may each result from cerebral lesions, but are not specifically associated with Wernicke's area.

131. (B) Erythroblastosis fetalis can occur when an Rh_0-positive child is being carried by an Rh_0-negative mother. If the mother makes antibodies against the Rh_0(D) antigen, these may cross the placenta and destroy fetal erythrocytes. The induction of this immune response can be blocked if an antibody specific for the Rh_0 antigen is injected into the mother at the time of her first exposure to the fetal RBCs, which usually occurs at parturition. Rh_0 immune globulin (RhoGAM) is a human γ-globulin preparation rich in antibodies specific for the Rh_0 antigen. It is used to prevent the sensitization of the mother, which will then protect a subsequent antigenically incompatible fetus from this disease. Antiinflammatory agents, antilymphocyte antibodies, antiallergen antibodies and enhancing antibodies are not the components of Rh_o-specific immunoglobulin (RhoGAM) (choices A, C, D, and E).

132. (E) Heparin is an important glycosaminoglycan (GAG) involved in the regulation of the clotting cascade. Abundant levels of heparin are found in granules of mast cells lining the blood vessels. In response to injury mast cells release the contents of their granules. Release of heparin inhibits the clotting cascade by complexing with and activating antithrombin III, which in turn inhibits the serine proteases of the clotting cascade. It is this function of the naturally occurring GAG heparin that has been exploited in the use of injected synthetic heparin for anticoagulation therapies. Hyaluronate (choice A) predominates in synovial fluid and vitreous humor. Chondroitin sulfates (choice B) predominate in cartilage and are also found in bone and heart valves. Dermatan sulfates (choice C) are found in skin, heart valves, and vessels. Keratan sulfates (choice D) are found in cornea and bone and in aggregates with chondroitin sulfates in cartilage.

133. (B) The photomicrograph depicts endometrium in the proliferative phase, which spans days 5 to 14 of the idealized menstrual cycle. This is an interval of rebuilding of the stratum functionalis. The tubular endometrial glands are narrow and either straight or coiled, and there is no indication that active secretion has begun. The menstrual phase of the menstrual cycle spans days 1 to 4 (choice A). During this interval, the endometrium is characterized by obvious disruptions of the stratum functionalis. At day 16 of the cycle (choice C), the endometrium is at an early point in the secretory phase. The stratum functionalis is much thicker, and the epithelial cells of the endometrial glands have nuclei displaced from the base by a temporary accumulation of glycogen. At day 21 (choice D), the endometrium is at the peak of the secretory phase, in preparation for implantation if fertilization has occurred and a blastocyst has developed. The lumens of endometrial glands are distended with secretions, giving the glands a tortuous, serrated appearance. At day 26 (choice E), the endometrium has begun to degenerate as a result of declining endocrine support from the involuting corpus luteum.

134. (A) Epinephrine is the agent of choice in the treatment of anaphylaxis because it provides a pressor response through α_1-adrenoceptor actions, cardiac stimulation through β_1-adrenoceptor actions, and bronchodilation and prevention of mast cell release of histamine and leukotrienes through actions on β_2 adrenoceptors. Norepinephrine (choice B) provides pressor activity to treat shock, but does not inhibit mast cell release of mediators of shock. Isoproterenol (choice C) will inhibit mast cell release of mediators and will provide cardiac stimulation, but will not provide needed pressor activity. Phenylephrine (choice D), like norepinephrine, will provide pressor activity, but not the cardiac stimulation or inhibition of mast cell function. The actions of dopamine (choice E) on the cardiovascular system are complex since dopamine exerts effects on renal, mesenteric, and myocardial vascular D_1 receptors (vasodilation), cardiac β_1 receptors (positive inotropic effect) and vascular α_1 receptors (vasoconstriction), depending on the dopamine concentration. Dopamine also causes release of norepinephrine from sympathetic nerve terminals, but it does not inhibit mast cell release of mediators of shock. Dopamine is useful in hypovolemic and cardiogenic shock in maintaining renal perfusion.

135. (A) Individuals with testicular feminization are genetically male with the normal male karyotype of 46,XY. Development of feminine external secondary sexual characteristics at puberty is due to an inherited lack of normal male cellular androgen receptors. 46,XX (choice B) is a normal female karyotype. Although individuals with testicular feminization syndrome appear female externally, they have the usual male karyotype and lack a uterus. 45,XO (choice C) defines Turner syndrome. Short stature, web neck, cardiac anomalies, streak gonads, and amenorrhea comprise the syndrome. 47,XXY (choice D) is the Klinefelter syndrome. Individuals have a tall, eunuchoid male appearance. 47,XX (choice E) is the multi-X female syndrome. Most individuals are physiologically normal females.

136. **(D)** The envelope of hepatitis B virus (HBV) contains an antigen known as HBsAg (hepatitis B surface antigen). This antigen is of importance because production of antibodies to HBsAg indicates immunity against hepatitis B virus, resulting either from infection, or vaccination with HBsAg. Treatment of HBV with nonionic detergent removes the envelope and exposes and viral core, which contains the hepatitis B core antigen (HbcAg). Antibodies to HBcAg are not protective (choice C). Treatment of the viral core with strong detergents results in the release of a soluble core antigen called hepatitis virus antigen e (HBeAg). Production of antibody to HBeAg signals active disease during which the patient is infectious (choice E). The RNA genome of HBV (choice A) and the nucleocapsid proteins of HBV (choice B) are not protective.

137. **(C)** Afferents from muscle spindles in the upper extremity terminate in the lateral cuneate nucleus of the medulla after entering the spinal cord in dorsal roots from C5 to T1. Upper limb muscle spindle afferents do not terminate in the dorsal horn from C3 to C5 (choice A), the nucleus dorsalis (choice B) at any level where this nucleus is present, or in the ipsilateral nucleus gracilis (choice E), which is reserved for lower extremity sensory input. Some muscle spindle afferents from the upper limb may reach the ipsilateral, but not the contralateral (choice D), nucleus cuneatus.

138. **(B)** The description of the symptoms is indicative of B_{12} deficiency. Definitive diagnosis requires the measurement of plasma vitamin B_{12} levels. Plant sources of food lack vitamin B_{12}. Macrocytic megaloblastic anemia arises from derangements in DNA metabolism and is a symptom of both vitamin B_{12} and folate deficiency (choice A). Diagnosis of the underlying cause of the anemia must precede the treatment since folate administration will correct the anemia but allow neurological damage associated with B_{12} deficiency to progress. Neurological problems and even psychotic states may result from demyelination that takes place with B_{12} deficiency. The use of folic acid (choice A) is discussed above. Ferrous sulfate (choice C) is the agent of choice for treating simple iron deficiency anemia. Iron deficiency results in a microcytic, hypochromic anemia. Intrinsic factor (choice D) is a secreted glycoprotein involved in intestinal absorption of vitamin B_{12}. The absence of intrinsic factor will lead to B_{12} deficiency. Alcoholism is the most common cause of deficiency of thiamine (choice E) in the United States. The deficiency may lead to neurological problems and Wernicke's syndrome, sometimes manifested as a global confusion. This condition is treated with oral thiamine. Anemia is not a feature of thiamine deficiency.

139. **(B)** The order of a chemical reaction refers to the number of molecules involved in forming a reaction complex that is competent to proceed to the generation of product(s). In order to determine the order of a given reaction it is necessary to sum the exponents of each concentration term of the substrates in a reaction. The reaction in this question is composed of two substrates, each with concentration exponents of one; therefore, the sum of these exponents is two and the reaction is said to be second order. An example of a first order reaction (choice A) would be of a single substrate being converted to one or more products. Third order reactions (choice C) contain three substrates or two moles of one substrate and one mole of a second substrate or three moles of a single substrate. Pseudo-first order reactions (choice D) are those that involve water, or those in which one reactant is in a much larger quantity than the others, and thus appears to be first order. Zero order reactions (choice E) can only refer to catalyzed reactions and occur when the concentration of substrate is so large that the catalytic site(s) is saturated at all times. In this situation adding more substrate does not increase reaction rate.

140. (E) The arrangement of the conidiospores in strings arising from the columella is characteristic of the genus *Aspergillus.* The organism represented in the illustration is septate (note the divisions, or cross-walls) in the hypha. This observation rules out any of the phycomycetes, since these organisms are cyanoacytic (choice A). The dermatophytes that are the causative agents of the tinea infections usually have single conidiospores and are characterized by their macroconidial forms (choices B, C, and D).

141. (C) Studies of autopsy samples from Alzheimer's disease patients indicate a loss of cholinergic neurons such as those in the nucleus basalis of Maynert. Following the model of enhancing dopamine to treat the loss of dopaminergic neurons in Parkinson's disease, anticholinesterase treatment has been used to treat Alzheimer's patients. Tacrine is an aminoacridine inhibitor of cholinesterase. Use of tacrine appears to slow the decline in cognitive function, but does not arrest the underlying neurodegenerative process. Reversible hepatotoxicity is the most important adverse effect. Although its use has not been reported in the treatment of Alzheimer's disease, the muscarinic antagonist atropine (choice A) would be expected to exacerbate the loss of cognitive function. The H_2-blocker cimetidine (choice B) should have no direct effect in Alzheimer's disease. Atracurium (choice D) is a competitive antagonist at the nicotinic receptor of the neuromuscular junction. Because of the drug's high polarity, it does not gain access to the CNS and would not be expected to exert any actions there. Ipratropium (choice E) is a muscarinic antagonist used in treatment of asthmatic bronchoconstriction. Because of its polarity, it does not enter the CNS.

142. (E) Cervicofacial actinomycosis (lumpy jaw) is an endogenous infection that is usually preceded by a tooth extraction or some other traumatic injury to the mouth. The lesion commonly drains to the cheek or submandibular area. The presence of sulfur granules is of great diagnostic importance. These are actually small (≈1 mm in diameter) colonies of the organism in a calcium phosphate matrix. Each consists of a central filamentous mass of branching bacilli surrounded by radially oriented, club-shaped structures. Amebiasis, mucormycosis, histoplasmosis, and candidiasis (choices A, B, C, and D) are caused by a protozoan and fungi, and none produce sulfur granules.

143. (D) When cardiac muscle contracts, it squeezes blood vessels that course through it, and this extravascular compression has a significant effect on coronary blood flow. In early systole, there is an actual reversal of blood flow, and although coronary blood flow increases during systole, it is not until the ventricle relaxes that maximal left coronary artery blood flows are obtained. Peak flows are obtained in early diastole, when the ventricle is relaxed and aortic pressure has not declined to its diastolic level. During systole (choices A, B, and C) the ventricular muscle contraction impedes coronary blood flow. During late diastole (choice E) coronary blood flow decreases because of the lower aortic blood pressure compared to early diastole.

144. (A) Precise tactile discriminative sensations from the right side of the face (including the teeth) travel via the ipsilateral trigeminal nerve to the ipsilateral principal (chief) sensory trigeminal nucleus (not the spinal trigeminal nucleus, choice B). Sensation from the maxillary teeth is carried to the chief sensory nucleus in the ipsilateral (not contralateral, choice C) spinal trigeminal tract. Somatosensory information from the face travels across the midline via the contralateral ventral trigeminothalamic tract to eventually reach the contralateral (not ipsilateral, choice D) ventral posteromedial thalamic nucleus. The ventral trigeminothalamic tract originates (not terminates, choice E) in the contralateral chief sensory and spinal trigeminal nuclei.

145. (C) Individuals with sickle trait are healthy and not anemic. A hemoglobin electrophoresis will demonstrate a minor proportion of hemoglobin S and a major proportion of hemoglobin A. Fetal hemoglobin and A2 hemoglobin are usually normal. Sickle trait confers the benefit of protecting erythrocytes from some forms of malarial infection. About 9% of blacks in the United States have sickle trait. Thalassemia minor (choice A) and thalassemia major (choice B) would not demonstrate hemoglobin S on electrophoresis. In sickle cell disease (choice D) almost all the hemoglobin would be hemoglobin S. No hemoglobin A would be detected and the patient would have a clinical history of severe anemia. Sickle thalassemia minor (choice E) would present as a chronic microcytic anemia with a major hemoglobin S component and an elevated hemoglobin A2.

146. (D) Mucopolysaccharidoses are a family of diseases collectively termed "lysosomal storage diseases." These diseases result from the inability of cells to effectively degrade complex membrane glycolipids and glycoproteins. The defects in these degradative pathways result from the loss of production of specific lysosomal enzymes. This leads to an accumulation of undegraded membrane components within lysosomes eventually leading to cell death. Of particular clinical significance is the presence of large amounts of complex glycolipids in the myelin sheaths of nerve cells. Genetic defects leading to the inability to degrade these lipids during normal membrane remodeling results in accelerated neuronal cell death. Other characteristic symptoms reflect the multi-organ involvement in these disorders such as the liver, spleen, and heart, as well as the skeletal system. None of the other choices (A, B, C, and E) are reflective of specific disease states related to glycolipid metabolism.

147. (A) Competitive antagonists shift the log dose-response curve for an agonist to the right, maintaining the same shape and maximum response. The equation for the effects of a competitive antagonist is:

$$\text{Response} = \frac{[\text{agonist}]\ \text{Response}_{max}}{[\text{agonist}] + K_D\,(1 + i/K_I)}$$

where K_D is the dissociation constant for the agonist-receptor complex, i is the concentration of the competitive antagonist and K_I is the dissociation constant for the antagonist-receptor complex. The term $[K_D\ (1 + i/K_I)]$ is the new "apparent" dissociation constant for agonist-receptor complex in the presence of the antagonist. When $i = 0$, this term is equal to the true K_D, but as i becomes larger, the apparent dissociation constant becomes greater than K_D. When $i = 9 \times K_I$, the ratio i/K_I is equal to 9, making the new apparent K_D equal to $(1 + 9)$ or 10 times greater than the true K_D. Curve A shows a dose-response curve with all of its concentration values at equal response levels increased by a factor of 10.

148. (E) Unlike other types of hypersensitivity (types I to III) associated with antibodies, histamine, and antigen–antibody complexes, delayed-type hypersensitivity reactions are initiated by antigen-specific T cells. Delayed-type hypersensitivity can be transferred in vivo with sensitized T cells alone. Grass pollens, molds, dust, and dandruff are the usual allergens which induce type I or immediate hypersensitivity, not delayed-type hypersensitivity (choice A). Anaphylaxis and allergic rhinitis are caused by type I hypersensitivity due to IgE absorbed on mast cells. IgE is not involved in delayed (type IV) hypersensitivity (choice B). The destruction of lung tissue seen in tuberculosis, histoplasmosis, and blastomycosis is believed to be associated with delayed type hypersensitivity; therefore this allergy causes tissue damage (choice C). Immediate-type allergy is suppressed by antihistaminic drugs, but delayed-type hypersensitivity is not (choice D).

149. (D) Production of red blood cells is under the control of differentiation inducers that promote differentiation of uncommitted pluripotent stem cells into committed stem cells (colony-forming units), along with growth inducers that promote maturation, but not differentiation, of the cells. Erythropoietin, the principal factor that stimulates red blood cell production, promotes both differentiation of stem cells to proerythroblasts and their maturation. Several other factors including androgens also stimulate bone marrow cells and enhance production of erythrocytes, resulting in higher hematocrit and hemoglobin values in the male. There is little difference in erythrocyte half-life time (choice A), number (choice B), and responsiveness (choice C) of bone marrow stem cells between males and females. Blood loss during a menstrual period (choice E) averages only 30 to 60 mL and cannot explain the difference in hemoglobin values between males and females.

150. **(B)** The maintenance infusion rate (D/T) is calculated using the formula (D/T) = (Target) × CL where D/T is the infusion rate, Target is the desired steady state plasma concentration for which we use the effective plasma concentration and CL is the systemic clearance. After we multiply the clearance (6 L/hr) times the effective plasma concentration (5 mg/L), the resulting product is 30 mg/hr. Note that the units for clearance and Target concentration must be consistent with respect to volume.

REFERENCES

Aidley DJ. *The Physiology of Excitable Cells,* 4th edition. Cambridge, England: Cambridge University Press, 1998

Berne RM, Levy MN. *Physiology,* 4th edition. St. Louis: Mosby-Year Book, 1998

Chandrasoma P, Taylor CR. *Concise Pathology,* 3rd edition. Appleton & Lange, 1998

Davenport HW. *The ABC of Acid-Base Chemistry,* 6th edition. Chicago: University of Chicago Press, 1974

Devlin TM. *Textbook of Biochemistry: With Clinical Correlations,* 4th edition. New York: John Wiley & Sons, 1997

Fauci AS, Braunwald E, Isselbacher KJ, et al. *Harrison's Principles of Internal Medicine,* 14th edition. New York: McGraw-Hill, 1998.

Ganong WF. *Review of Medical Physiology,* 19th edition. Stamford, CT: Appleton & Lange, 1999

Guyton AC, Hall JE. *Textbook of Medical Physiology,* 9th edition. Philadelphia: WB Saunders, 1996

Hall-Craggs ECB. *Anatomy as a Basis for Clinical Medicine,* 3rd edition. Baltimore: Williams & Wilkins, 1995

Hardman JG, Limbird LE, Molinoff PB, et al. *Goodman & Gilman's The Pharmacological Basis of Therapeutics,* 9th edition. New York: McGraw-Hill, 1996

Isselbacher KJ, et al. *Harrison's Principles of Internal Medicine,* 13th edition. New York: McGraw-Hill, 1994

Johnson LR. *Gastrointestinal Physiology,* 5th edition. St. Louis: Mosby-Year Book, 1997

Kandel ER, Schwartz JH, Jessel TM. *Principles of Neural Science,* 3rd edition. Stamford, CT: Appleton & Lange, 1993

Katzung BG. *Basic & Clinical Pharmacology,* 7th edition. Stamford, CT: Appleton & Lange, 1998

Leigh H, Reiser MF. *The Patient: Biological, Psychological, and Social Dimensions of Medical Practice,* 3rd edition. New York: Plenum Press, 1992

McArdle WD, Katch FI, Katch VL. *Exercise Physiology: Energy, Nutrition, and Human Performance,* 4th edition. Philadelphia: Lea & Febiger, 1996

Mountcastle VB. *Medical Physiology,* 14th edition. St. Louis: Mosby-Year Book, 1980

Rose DB. *Clinical Physiology of Acid-base and Electrolyte Disorders,* 4th edition. New York: McGraw-Hill, 1994

Vander AJ. *Renal Physiology,* 5th edition. New York: McGraw-Hill, 1995

West JB. *Best and Taylor's Physiological Basis of Medical Practice,* 12th edition. Baltimore: Williams & Wilkins, 1991

West JB. *Pulmonary Pathophysiology–The Essentials,* 5th edition. Baltimore: Williams & Wilkins, 1998

Subspecialty List: Practice Test I

Question Number and Subspecialty

1. Biochemistry
2. Anatomy
3. Pharmacology
4. Pharmacology
5. Behavioral sciences
6. Pathology
7. Biochemistry
8. Microbiology
9. Microbiology
10. Microbiology
11. Physiology
12. Anatomy
13. Behavioral sciences
14. Biochemistry
15. Pharmacology
16. Pathology
17. Physiology
18. Biochemistry
19. Anatomy
20. Physiology
21. Pathology
22. Pharmacology
23. Behavioral sciences
24. Biochemistry
25. Anatomy
26. Pathology
27. Pathology
28. Pathology
29. Pharmacology
30. Biochemistry
31. Anatomy
32. Behavioral sciences
33. Physiology
34. Microbiology
35. Biochemistry
36. Physiology
37. Pathology
38. Pathology
39. Microbiology
40. Pharmacology
41. Biochemistry
42. Anatomy
43. Behavioral sciences
44. Pathology
45. Physiology
46. Pathology
47. Biochemistry
48. Microbiology
49. Pathology
50. Pharmacology
51. Anatomy
52. Behavioral sciences
53. Biochemistry
54. Physiology
55. Microbiology
56. Pathology
57. Anatomy
58. Pharmacology
59. Pathology
60. Anatomy
61. Biochemistry
62. Physiology
63. Anatomy
64. Pharmacology
65. Microbiology
66. Pathology
67. Physiology
68. Anatomy
69. Biochemistry
70. Behavioral sciences
71. Behavioral sciences
72. Behavioral sciences
73. Behavioral sciences
74. Behavioral sciences

75. Behavioral sciences
76. Anatomy
77. Biochemistry
78. Pharmacology
79. Physiology
80. Anatomy
81. Microbiology
82. Pathology
83. Biochemistry
84. Physiology
85. Microbiology
86. Pharmacology
87. Anatomy
88. Pathology
89. Physiology
90. Biochemistry
91. Anatomy
92. Behavioral sciences
93. Pharmacology
94. Microbiology
95. Pathology
96. Pathology
97. Biochemistry
98. Pathology
99. Anatomy
100. Pharmacology
101. Microbiology
102. Physiology
103. Pathology
104. Biochemistry
105. Physiology
106. Behavioral sciences
107. Anatomy
108. Pharmacology
109. Microbiology
110. Physiology
111. Biochemistry
112. Physiology
113. Pharmacology
114. Microbiology
115. Pathology
116. Physiology
117. Pathology
118. Biochemistry
119. Anatomy
120. Pharmacology
121. Microbiology
122. Pathology
123. Pathology
124. Physiology
125. Biochemistry
126. Anatomy
127. Pharmacology
128. Microbiology
129. Behavioral sciences
130. Physiology
131. Microbiology
132. Biochemistry
133. Anatomy
134. Pharmacology
135. Pathology
136. Microbiology
137. Physiology
138. Pharmacology
139. Biochemistry
140. Microbiology
141. Pharmacology
142. Microbiology
143. Physiology
144. Anatomy
145. Pathology
146. Biochemistry
147. Pharmacology
148. Microbiology
149. Physiology
150. Pharmacology

CHAPTER 9

Practice Test II

Questions

DIRECTIONS: (Questions 1 through 150): Each of the numbered items or incomplete statements in this section is followed by answers or by completions of the statement. Select the ONE lettered answer or completion that is BEST in each case.

1. A comatose patient is admitted with carbon monoxide (CO) poisoning. The toxicity of CO is primarily due to

    (A) reaction with mitochondrial cytochromes
    (B) reaction with hemoglobin
    (C) bone marrow suppression
    (D) cardiac arrhythmia
    (E) suppression of respiratory centers

2. A 47-year-old man has radiographic evidence of a pulmonary abnormality. A photomicrograph of his sputum is shown in Figure 9–1. What is the likely pulmonary disorder?

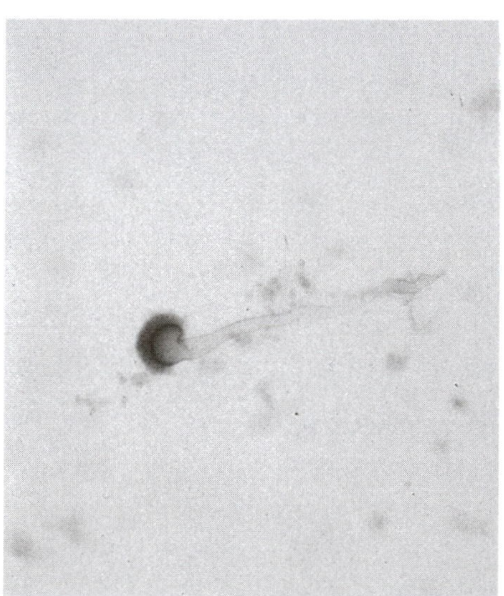

Figure 9–1 (see also Color Insert)

    (A) asbestosis
    (B) tuberculosis
    (C) histoplasmosis
    (D) aspergillosis
    (E) blastomycosis

3. A protozoan disease transmitted by the sandfly *Phlebotomus* is

    (A) leishmaniasis
    (B) trichinosis
    (C) diphyllobothriasis
    (D) toxoplasmosis
    (E) clonorchiasis

4. Imaging studies conducted in the emergency room indicate that a young accident victim has a skull fracture involving the posterior cranial fossa. A fracture involving the posterior cranial fossa is most likely to injure

    (A) the temporomandibular joint
    (B) cranial nerve VIII as it enters the internal acoustic meatus
    (C) the abducens nerve in the cavernous sinus
    (D) the mandibular division of the trigeminal nerve
    (E) the temporal lobe of the cerebral hemisphere

5. Your inpatient is being overly exacting and controlling, complaining if his medication is only five minutes late. One likely reason the patient may be so concerned about exactness is that the patient is

(A) anxious
(B) delusional
(C) depressed
(D) demented
(E) drug seeking

6. The pathway of creatine phosphate synthesis is shown in Figure 9–2. Which amino acid is required in this pathway as indicated by the letter A?

(A) arginine
(B) aspartate
(C) glutamate
(D) asparagine
(E) glutamine

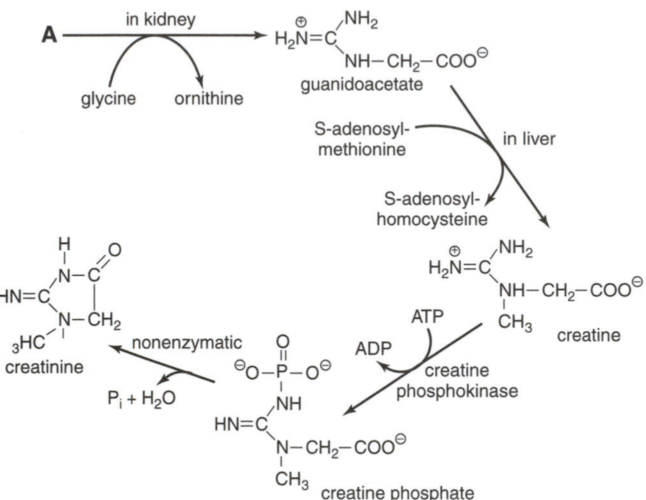

Figure 9–2

7. A 3-month-old baby has been immunized with the poliomyelitis vaccine. Biochemical analysis of the baby's serum six days following immunization indicates the presence of the immunoglobulin shown in Figure 9–3. This immunoglobulin is

(A) IgA
(B) IgE
(C) IgD
(D) IgM
(E) IgG

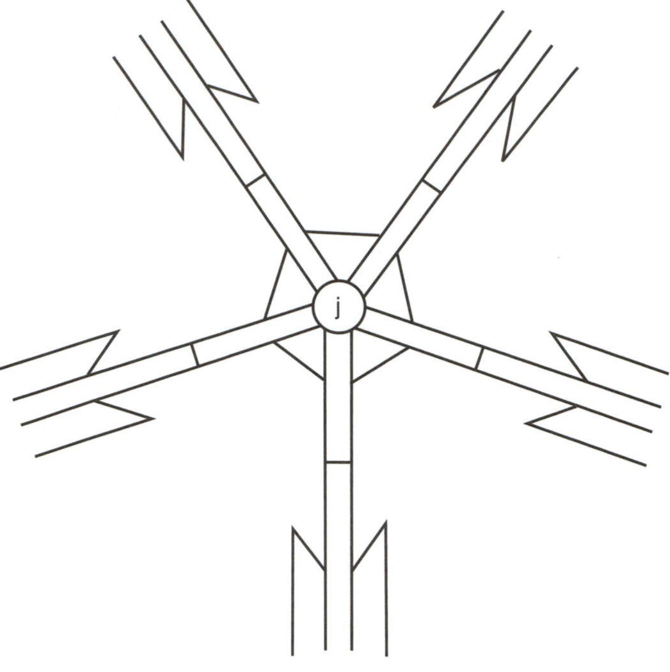

Figure 9–3

8. A 55-year-old male has symptomatic coronary atherosclerosis. Which statement is true about this condition?

(A) increased incidence with low LDL cholesterol
(B) increased incidence with Type B personality
(C) decreased incidence with elevated HDL cholesterol
(D) more common in females than in males
(E) hypertension exerts a beneficial effect

9. A virus which is devoid of hemagglutinating antigens is

(A) rubeola virus
(B) influenza virus
(C) parainfluenza virus
(D) measles virus
(E) papovavirus

10. A 24-year-old nullipara primigravida comes in for her routine obstetric checkup at 18 weeks of gestation. Her serum human chori-

onic gonadotropin (hCG) is 8 U/mL (normal 20 U/mL at 18 weeks' gestation). Which of the following is a possible cause of her abnormally low hCG levels?

(A) twin pregnancy
(B) threatened abortion
(C) trisomy 21
(D) hydatidiform mole
(E) choriocarcinoma

11. Which portion of the heart is most likely to suffer late fibrotic complications with chronic rheumatic heart disease?

(A) coronary arteries
(B) epicardium
(C) mitral valve
(D) pulmonary valve
(E) right ventricle

12. Occlusion of branches of the posterior spinal artery that irrigate the dorsomedial portion of the left side of the caudal medulla might result in damage to a pathway conveying somatosensory signals. If this is the case, which of the following symptoms might be observed?

(A) loss of position sense in the left upper extremity
(B) loss of pain and temperature sensation in the left upper extremity
(C) hyperactive reflexes in the left upper extremity
(D) loss of vibratory sensation in the right upper extremity
(E) hemiplegia involving the right side

13. You are attending a 66-year-old obese female with type 2 non–insulin-dependent diabetes mellitus (NIDDM). Which of the following statements about this patient is correct?

(A) Siblings of this patient are more likely to develop diabetes than siblings of a patient with IDDM.
(B) This patient most likely has HLA type DR3 or DR4.
(C) This patient probably has a higher density of insulin receptors in her tissues compared to non-obese persons.
(D) The affinity of insulin receptors to insulin in this patient is probably higher than in non-obese persons.
(E) Plasma insulin levels in this patient are likely lower than normal.

Questions 14 and 15

A 45-year-old black female complains of gradually increasing fatigue. On physical examination she is noted to have obesity, hypertension, a buffalo hump deformity of her back, moon facies, abdominal striae, and muscle weakness. Radiographic imaging studies identify an abnormality of her right adrenal gland.

14. The right adrenal gland is surgically resected. The intact specimen weighed 24 grams. A hemisection of the gland is displayed in Figure 9–4. What is the diagnosis?

(A) pheochromocytoma
(B) multifocal infarction
(C) adrenal cortical adenoma
(D) Krukenberg tumor
(E) neuroblastoma

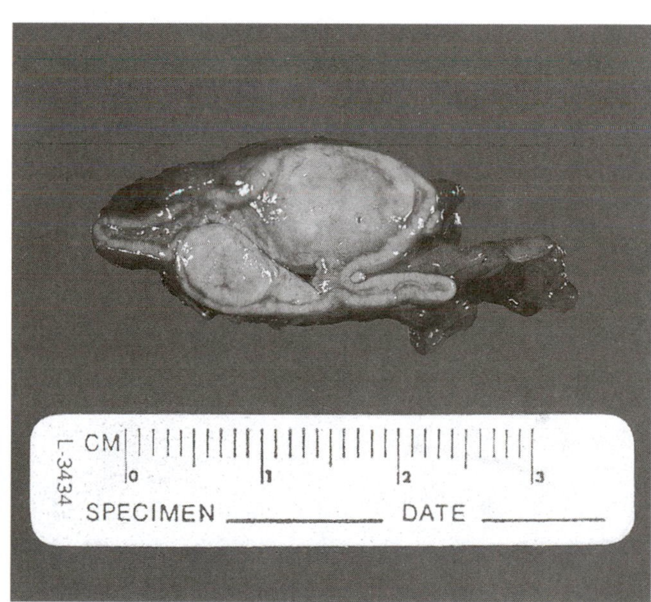

Figure 9–4 (see also Color Insert)

15. Tests on this patient's serum are likely to reveal an elevation of which analyte?

(A) norepinephrine
(B) carcinoembryonic antigen
(C) cortisol
(D) CA-125
(E) neuron-specific enolase

16. Mental depression, dementia, diarrhea, and dermatitis are all associated with a prolonged deficiency in which vitamin?

(A) thiamine
(B) riboflavin
(C) niacin
(D) vitamin C
(E) vitamin A

17. A physician wishes to isolate *Mycoplasma pneumoniae* from a clinical specimen. This can be accomplished by incorporating into the culture medium

(A) erythromycin
(B) penicillin
(C) doxycycline
(D) oxytetracycline
(E) minocycline

18. In treating an elderly male patient with mild congestive heart failure, which of the following agents would be most likely to increase myocardial contractility without producing a concomitant increase in heart rate?

(A) glucagon
(B) digoxin
(C) epinephrine
(D) nitroglycerin
(E) propranolol

19. A 22-year-old white male is found dead at home. Urine obtained at autopsy contains benzoylecgonine. What conclusion can be drawn from this result?

(A) the decedent was taking chemotherapy for cancer
(B) the decedent had recently used cocaine
(C) death was due to status asthmaticus
(D) a congenital deformity of the lower limb is likely
(E) a chromosomal abnormality was present

Questions 20 through 24

A patient with a history of unexplained polydipsia is admitted for evaluation of possible diabetes insipidus. After several hours of fluid deprivation, the following measurements are made:

Plasma osmolarity:	300 mosm/L
Urine osmolarity:	150 mosm/L
Urine solute output:	900 mosm/day

20. The rate of urine production in this patient is

(A) 1.5 L/day
(B) 2.0 L/day
(C) 3.0 L/day
(D) 6.0 L/day
(E) cannot be calculated unless plasma volume is also known

21. Solute clearance in this patient is

(A) 1.5 L/day
(B) 2.0 L/day
(C) 3.0 L/day
(D) 6.0 L/day
(E) cannot be calculated unless plasma volume is also known

22. Free water clearance in this patient is

(A) −3.0 L/day
(B) −1.5 L/day
(C) +1.5 L/day
(D) +3.0 L/day
(E) cannot be calculated unless insulin clearance is also known

23. Since this patient's urine concentration was less than expected after water deprivation, additional tests are performed. Figure 9–5 shows several relationships between urine flow and urine solute excretion. Which of these relationships would support a diagnosis of diabetes insipidus in this patient?

(A) line A
(B) line B
(C) line C
(D) line D
(E) line E

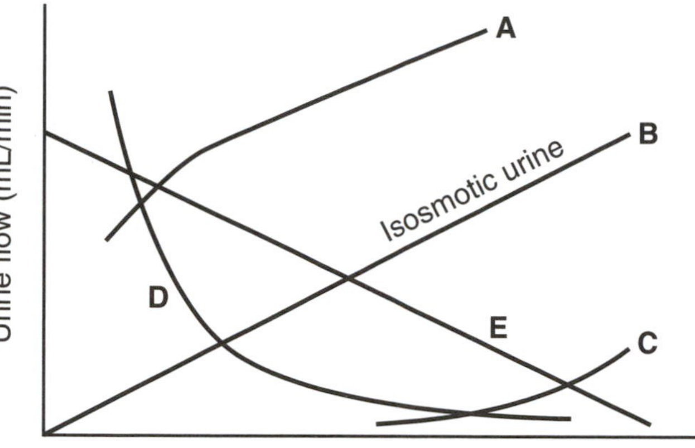

Figure 9–5

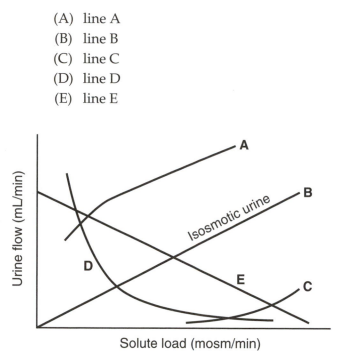

24. Following water deprivation, vasopressin is injected intravenously into the patient (arrow in Figure 9–6) and urine osmolarity is monitored. Based on the graph in Figure 9–6, the patient most likely has

(A) renal diabetes insipidus
(B) central diabetes insipidus
(C) diabetes mellitus
(D) psychogenic polydipsia
(E) no abnormality

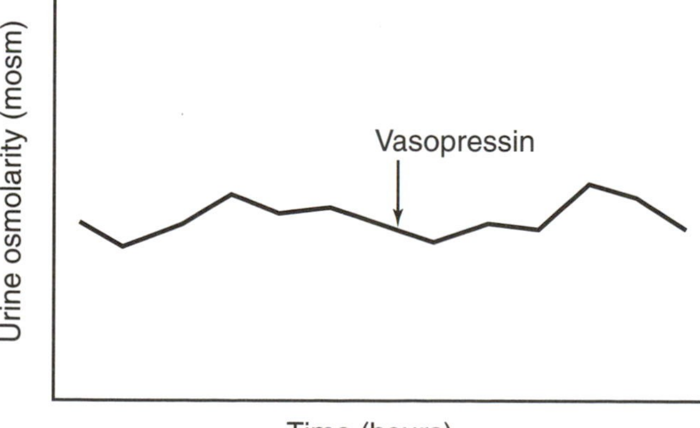

Figure 9–6

25. Exposure to benzidine or naphthylamine is associated with an increased risk to develop carcinoma at which site?

(A) stomach
(B) liver
(C) skin
(D) bladder
(E) oral cavity

Questions 26 through 32

An 18-year-old student is brought to the hospital because she had not come out of her room for three days, missing school. She would eat only when a tray was brought in.

26. If the patient looks disheveled and responds in monosyllables, a possible diagnosis is

(A) schizophrenia
(B) unipolar depression
(C) bipolar depression
(D) substance abuse
(E) all of the above

27. Upon further examination, you find that it is difficult to understand what the patient is saying because she tends to move from one thought to another without much connection. This phenomenon is called

(A) circumstantiality
(B) folie à deux
(C) loose association
(D) thought blocking
(E) autistic thinking

28. While you are trying to understand her, she suddenly seems to be looking past you, and starts a conversation that seems to be with another person, but no one else is present. She probably has

(A) illusion
(B) delusion
(C) ambivalence
(D) hallucination
(E) negativism

29. All of a sudden, she stands up, becomes rigid, and fails to respond to any verbal commands. This phenomenon is called

(A) mutism
(B) catatonia
(C) cataplexy
(D) hebephrenia
(E) coma

30. A useful immediate treatment for the condition described in question 29 would be

(A) electroencephalogram
(B) hypnosis
(C) supportive psychotherapy
(D) psychoanalysis
(E) injection of lorazepam

31. Further history reveals that the patient had been socially withdrawn since her menarche at age 13, and had been preoccupied with the thought that her blood was impure. There seems to be no history of substance abuse. Family history reveals that her maternal grandmother had died in a state hospital. The most likely diagnosis for this patient is

(A) bipolar disorder, type I
(B) folie à deux
(C) schizophrenia
(D) delusional disorder
(E) psychosis secondary to a general medical condition

32. For this patient, an effective drug to treat many of her symptoms is likely to be

(A) benztropine
(B) chlordiazepoxide
(C) lithium chloride
(D) haloperidol
(E) fluoxetine

33. A elderly male complains of flank pain and red-colored urine. Radiographic studies indicate an increased size of his left kidney. The kidney is surgically resected and displayed in Figure 9–7. Why is the kidney enlarged?

(A) infectious process
(B) due to abnormality of ureter or bladder
(C) stone formation
(D) congenital abnormality
(E) neoplastic process

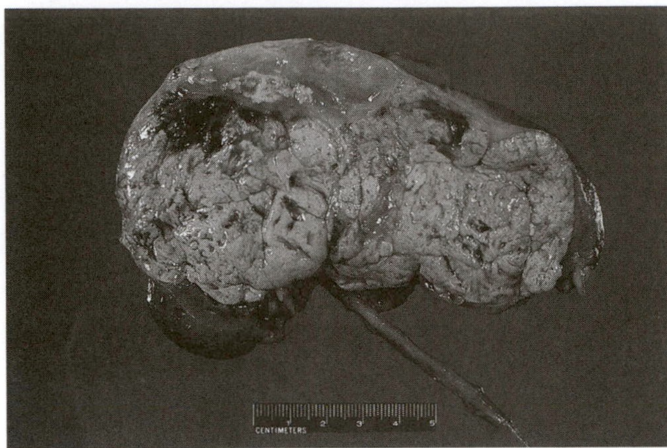

Figure 9–7 (see also Color Insert).

34. Which statement concerning the sympathetic nervous system is most correct?

(A) Postganglionic cell bodies can be found in sympathetic chain ganglia or in prevertebral (preaortic) ganglia.
(B) Sympathetic innervation of the heart originates from preganglionic neurons in the lateral horn of the spinal cord from T6 to T9.
(C) Sensory fibers signaling an increase in vascular carbon dioxide concentration are carried to the spinal cord via branches of sympathetic fibers.
(D) Descending projections to the spinal cord from the hypothalamus have little influence on the sympathetic nervous system.
(E) The enteric nervous system is modulated by parasympathetic, but not sympathetic, fibers.

35. Staphylococcal enterotoxin

(A) is produced by over 90% of the strains of *Staphylococcus epidermidis*
(B) disrupts the stratum granulosum in the epidermis
(C) disrupts the cytoplasmic membrane

(D) blocks release of acetylcholine
(E) resists boiling for 10 minutes

36. Chronic arsenic poisoning may arise from ingestion of well water contaminated with arsenic. The treatment for chronic arsenic poisoning is

(A) deferoxamine
(B) folic acid
(C) calcium disodium edetate
(D) dimercaprol
(E) thiosulfate

37. A 3-year-old girl who has not been immunized against the usual childhood viral diseases has fever, running nose, conjunctivitis, rash, a hacking cough, and red-based, blue-white centered lesions in her mouth. The virus responsible for this girl's symptoms most likely is

(A) coronavirus
(B) adenovirus
(C) hantavirus
(D) measles virus
(E) orthomyxovirus

38. A 57-year-old female dies after a four-month history of increasingly severe dementia. An examination of the brain demonstrates Creutzfeldt–Jakob disease. What causes this disorder?

(A) protozoan infection
(B) hereditary lysosomal storage disease
(C) increased neurofibrillary tangles
(D) acquired or inherited prion
(E) repeated exposure to a chemical toxin

Questions 39 and 40

39. The electron micrograph in Figure 9–8 illustrates a section of

(A) cerebral cortex
(B) red nucleus
(C) gray matter of the spinal cord
(D) nerve fiber tract in the central nervous system
(E) peripheral nerve

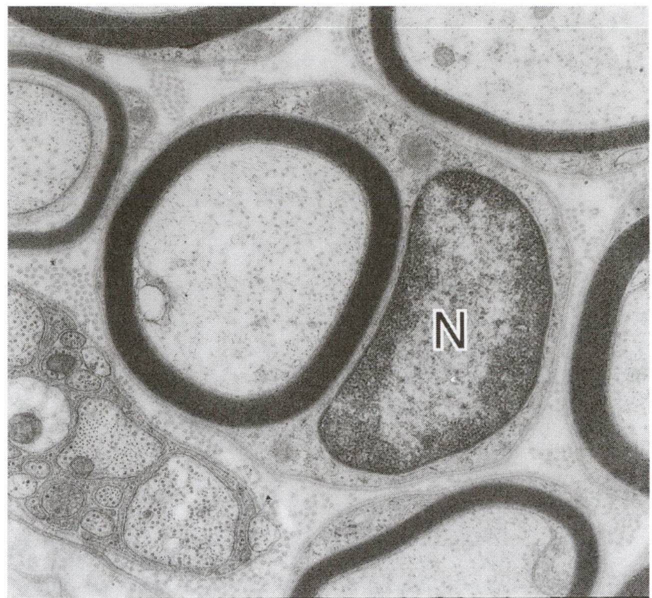

Figure 9–8

40. The label N indicates the nucleus of

(A) an oligodendrocyte
(B) a Schwann cell
(C) a sensory neuron
(D) a somatic motor neuron
(E) a microglial cell

41. A sewer worker arrives at the emergency room with intense headache, stiff neck, hepatitis, and nephritis. Examination of centrifuged urine by dark-field microscopy reveals many small spirochetes with thin, tightly coiled turns and hooks at both ends. The most likely presumptive diagnosis is

(A) relapsing fever
(B) yaws
(C) pinta
(D) leptospirosis
(E) legionellosis

42. Which of the following structures is directly associated with the vestibular system?

(A) stria vascularis
(B) tunnel of Corti
(C) external cuneate nucleus
(D) zone of Lissauer
(E) Scarpa's ganglion

43. A 45-year-old male has recently noticed that he regurgitates his food. Radiographic studies show a dilated lower esophagus. The probable diagnosis is achalasia. What pathologic abnormality is consistently present with this disorder?

(A) *Helicobacter pylori* infection
(B) decreased ganglion cells in the myenteric plexus
(C) fibrous stricture
(D) hiatal hernia
(E) formation of one or more diverticula

44. High plasma levels of the lipoprotein particle identified as lipoprotein(a) [Lp(a)] have been shown to be a primary risk factor for coronary heart disease and stroke. Lp(a) is a unique lipoprotein assembled from LDL and a single glycoprotein called apolipoprotein(a) or apo(a). Apo(a) is associated with LDL via a disulfide linkage to which other apolipoprotein?

(A) apo C-II
(B) apo B-100
(C) apo B-48
(D) apo A-I
(E) apo E

45. An eruption of shingles over the cutaneous distribution of the opthalmic nerve (herpes zoster ophthalmicus) is a common and often painful affliction. Your patient has involvement over the dorsum of the nose extending to the tip. Which of the following cutaneous branches of the ophthalmic nerve is involved?

(A) external nasal nerve
(B) supratrochlear nerve
(C) supraorbital nerve
(D) lacrimal nerve
(E) zygomaticotemporal nerve

46. The health benefits of regular exercise are well recognized and it is important to understand the cardiovascular changes normally occurring during exercise. With different levels of aerobic exercise under steady state conditions,

(A) cardiac output is almost linearly related to oxygen uptake
(B) stroke volume is linearly related to oxygen uptake up to maximal oxygen consumption
(C) arterial diastolic blood pressure decreases substantially
(D) blood perfusion of the skin decreases
(E) blood pressure in the pulmonary artery approaches that of the systemic arteries

47. When used in standard dosing regimens, which of the following agents may accumulate to toxic or lethal levels in patients with a genetic deficiency in the enzyme dihydropyrimidine dehydrogenase?

(A) nifedipine
(B) 5-fluorouracil
(C) acyclovir
(D) isoniazid
(E) acetaminophen

48. The lesion shown in Figure 9–9 is characteristic of

(A) an abscess
(B) a granuloma
(C) a keloid
(D) an infarct
(E) a thrombus

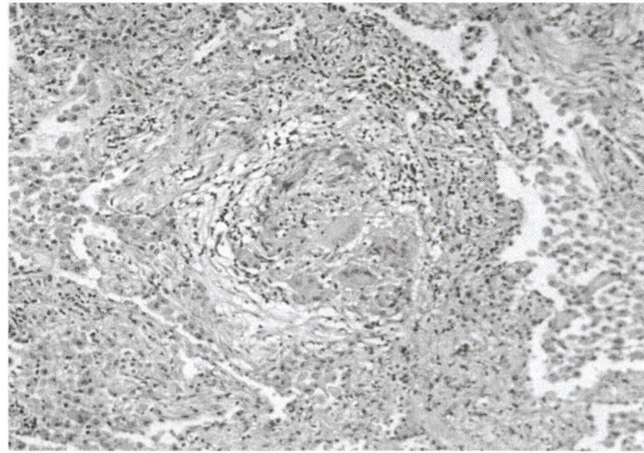

Figure 9–9 (see also Color Insert)

49. B cell receptors play a significant role in the development of immune responses. Which one of the following statements about B cell antigen specific receptors is correct?

(A) Surface immunoglobulin synthesized by a B cell clone does not serve as an antigen receptor for that clone.
(B) Surface immunoglobulin is dimeric and contains only two heavy chains.
(C) It appears that different receptor isotypes do not have different functions on the same cell.
(D) The surface immunoglobulin of the immature B cells is IgM.
(E) The mature B cell has IgE on its surface.

50. A 12-month-old female exhibits severe developmental delay with associated macrocephaly, dysmorphic facies, hypotonia, and hepatosplenomegaly. Clouding of the corneas is not evident. A pebbly ivory-colored lesion is present over the infant's back. The activity of iduronate sulfatase in the plasma is not detectable. These symptoms are indicative of which mucopolysaccharidosis?

(A) Morquio B
(B) Hunter
(C) Maroteaux–Lamy
(D) Sanfilippo A
(E) Hurler

Questions 51 and 52

A 67-year-old white female complains of gradually increasing fatigue. On physical examination she is found to be anemic and has a peripheral neuropathy characterized by loss of position and vibratory sense. Laboratory studies document an anemia which is found to be macrocytic in character. In addition, her white blood cell count and platelets are both decreased.

51. What pathologic mechanism would account for these findings?

(A) myelodysplastic sideroblastic anemia
(B) a diet deficient in folate
(C) autoantibodies against parietal cells or intrinsic factor
(D) diabetes mellitus
(E) chronic blood loss

52. If this condition persists, which organ is at most risk for developing carcinoma?

(A) pancreas
(B) lung
(C) central nervous system
(D) genital tract
(E) stomach

53. Symptoms such as resting tremor, akinesia, and bradykinesia are associated with Parkinson's disease. Which of the following is currently thought to be related to the primary neural substrate of this disease?

(A) loss of GABA neurons in the ventrolateral nucleus of the thalamus
(B) facilitation of pyramidal tract neurons in the primary motor cortex
(C) degeneration of neurons in the pars compacta of the substantia nigra
(D) vascular infarct in the subthalamic nucleus
(E) loss of cholinergic interneurons in the caudate nucleus

54. A 62-year-old man developed a temperature of 101°F and bacteremia seven days following the insertion of a mitral prosthesis. He was also fitted with intravenous catheters. Following the operation this patient was treated for five days with penicillin, streptomycin, and methicillin. When his temperature rose to 101°F on the seventh postoperative day, antibiotic treatment was changed to ampicillin. A blood culture yielded *Escherichia coli* sensitive to ampicillin. The most important initial step is

(A) removal of the intravenous catheters
(B) culture of the patient's urine
(C) treatment with gentamicin
(D) avoid disturbing the mitral valve
(E) continue treatment with ampicillin

55. The dural reflection that separates the occipital lobe of the cerebrum from the cerebellum is the

(A) diaphragma sellae
(B) tentorium cerebelli
(C) falx cerebri
(D) falx cerebelli
(E) crista galli

56. The activity of pyruvate dehydrogenase is regulated by both allosteric effectors and phosphorylation. The level of phosphorylation is increased by an elevation in the concentration of

(A) pyruvate
(B) NAD^+
(C) ADP
(D) acetyl-CoA
(E) NADPH

57. Which of the following hormones has its primary effect via regulation of gene expression?

(A) angiotensin II
(B) epinephrine acting on α_1 receptors
(C) epinephrine acting on β receptors
(D) thyroid hormones
(E) insulin

58. The most rapid rate of recovery for inhalational general anesthetics correlates with the smallest value for the

(A) oil:gas partition coefficient
(B) onset of hepatic metabolism
(C) organ system distribution from the blood
(D) blood:gas partition coefficient
(E) minimum alveolar concentration (MAC)

59. If food poisoning is assumed to be due to enterotoxin produced by *Clostridium perfringens*, final confirmation will rest upon

(A) enterotoxin production in food and neutralization by its antiserum
(B) the presence of many gram-positive rods in food
(C) demonstration of spores in suspected food
(D) growth of gram-positive bacilli in thioglycolate broth
(E) presence of antibodies against *C. perfringens* in the patient's serum

60. Which of the following is useful in treating severe chemotherapy-induced emesis?

(A) diphenhydramine
(B) metoclopramide
(C) diphenoxylate
(D) scopolamine
(E) ipecac

61. Patients who exhibit a prolonged mucocutaneous bleeding time with a normal coagulation time, clot retraction, and platelet count, and have normal levels of the coagulation factor VIII, will exhibit a deficiency in which protein involved in hemostasis?

(A) fibrinogen
(B) thrombin
(C) von Willebrand factor
(D) tissue factor
(E) factor IX

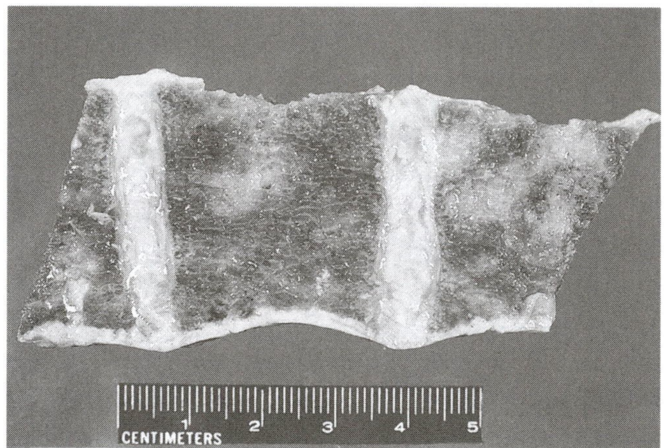

Figure 9–10 (see also Color Insert)

62. A 63-year-old male has a two-month history of back pain. An autopsy specimen of his spine is displayed in Figure 9–10. What abnormal process is evident?

(A) trauma
(B) ischemia
(C) degeneration

(D) neoplasia
(E) infection

63. The cell bodies of postganglionic parasympathetic neurons are located in the

(A) ciliary ganglion
(B) geniculate ganglion
(C) superior cervical ganglion
(D) nucleus of Edinger–Westphal
(E) celiac ganglion

64. Your patient has abdominal pain, distention, and a temperature of 100°F. Exploratory surgery is conducted and a portion of the colon is removed. However, during surgery the contents of the large bowel were spilled into the peritoneal cavity, giving rise to peritonitis. The microbe that is likely to be involved in the development of peritonitis is

(A) *Escherichia coli*
(B) *Bacteroides fragilis*
(C) *Enterococcus faecalis*
(D) *Fusobacterium nucleatum*
(E) all of the above

65. Your patient is being overly controlling and exacting about his care, and complains about "sloppy" treatment. If he turns out to have a newly diagnosed serious medical condition, you should

(A) withhold the information from the patient
(B) tell the patient about the diagnosis in very general terms, with a cheerful attitude
(C) tell the patient about the diagnosis in great detail
(D) ask the patient if he would like to hear the bad news
(E) tell the family about the diagnosis, and tell the patient he should discuss it with the family

66. A 4-month-old female presents with frequent hypoglycemia with associated seizures and lactic acidosis following a short fast. In addition, the infant has hepatomegaly, a protuberant abdomen, thin extremities, short stature, and xanthomas over the upper and lower extremities. Assay for enzymes of glucose and glycogen metabolism show a severe deficiency in glucose-6-phosphatase. These symptoms and clinical findings are indicative of

(A) Pompe disease
(B) McArdle disease
(C) Tarui disease
(D) Anderson disease
(E) von Gierke disease

67. Patient H.D. has been diagnosed with *Pseudomonas aeruginosa* septicemia. The current treatment of choice is

(A) tetracycline
(B) chloramphenicol
(C) nafcillin + kanamycin
(D) sulfamethoxazole + trimethoprim
(E) ticarcillin + tobramycin

68. A 27-year-old man has schistosomiasis. Which of the following statements concerning this disease is correct?

(A) Its incidence cannot be significantly reduced by proper disposal of human fecal waste.
(B) It is not likely to induce high eosinophil counts.
(C) It is not usually diagnosed by the demonstration of ova in clinical specimens.
(D) It may cause blockage of the portal venous system.
(E) It is caused by a microbe that has a head with hooks and suckers.

69. Which of the following is an agent used to terminate an episode of reentrant supraventricular arrhythmia and possesses a serum half-life of less than one minute?

(A) amiodarone
(B) digoxin
(C) phenylephrine
(D) adenosine
(E) propafenone

Questions 70 through 72

A patient with multiple rib fractures following an automobile accident is brought to the emergency room.

70. Which of the following arterial blood gas values would you expect in this patient?

	pH	Bicarbonate [mmol/L]	P_{CO_2} [mm Hg]
(A)	7.25	26	60
(B)	7.35	31	60
(C)	7.35	18	33
(D)	7.50	22	30
(E)	7.45	19	30

71. Which of the following statements about renal handling of bicarbonate (HCO_3^-) in this patient is correct?

(A) Most of the HCO_3^- filtered through the glomeruli is lost with the urine.
(B) Most of the filtered HCO_3^- is recovered by the distal tubular cells.
(C) Filtered HCO_3^- enters tubular cells by a HCO_3^-/Cl^- exchange mechanism.
(D) For each HCO_3^- recovered by the renal tubular cells, one H^+ is secreted.
(E) This patient's kidneys generate less net HCO_3^- than kidneys from a healthy subject.

72. After several days of chronic acidosis, the main route of renal H^+ excretion in this patient is as

(A) non-titratable acid
(B) uric acid
(C) phosphoric acid
(D) bicarbonate
(E) free protons (urine pH < 5)

73. Shown in Figure 9–11 are the sequences that constitute the consensus sequences for eukaryotic mRNA splicing. The nucleotides depicted by Xs are invariant in all introns sequenced (i.e., these sequences appear 100% of the time at the indicated locations). What are the invariant sequences found at the 5′ and 3′ ends, respectively, of all mRNA introns?

(A) AT and GT
(B) GT and AG
(C) GC and AG
(D) CT and TA
(E) GG and AA

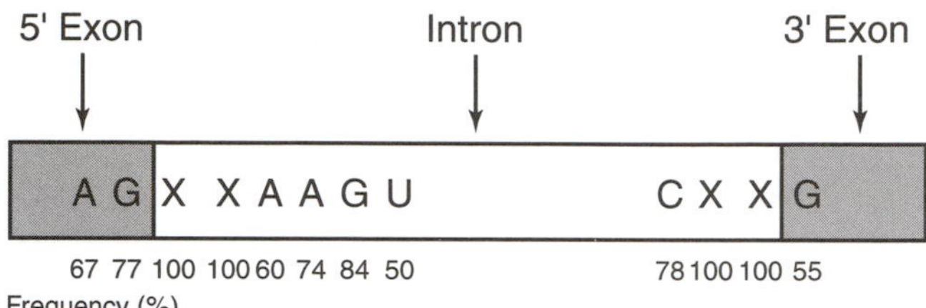

Figure 9–11

74. Acquired immune deficiency syndrome is caused by a virus which

(A) has a double-stranded genome
(B) is a member of the adenovirus group
(C) lacks reverse transcriptase
(D) destroys T4 lymphocytes
(E) lacks a viral envelope

Questions 75 and 76

"Alternating hemiplegia" is the result of damage to descending corticospinal fibers in combination with a cranial nerve. Typically, hemiplegia is present contralateral to the lesion side while cranial nerve signs are observed ipsilateral to the lesion. Three varieties have been described and they include superior, middle, and inferior alternating hemiplegia. The following two questions pertain to the clinical entity known as inferior alternating hemiplegia.

75. The cranial nerve involvement associated with inferior alternating hemiplegia affects which of the following muscles or muscle groups?

(A) extraocular muscles
(B) muscles of mastication

(C) muscles of facial expression
(D) laryngeal musculature
(E) tongue musculature

76. The alternating hemiplegias are typically the result of vascular infarcts. The vessel(s) most commonly involved in inferior alternating hemiplegia is

(A) lenticulostriate arteries
(B) thalamoperforating vessels
(C) vertebral artery
(D) penetrating branches of anterior spinal artery
(E) posterior inferior cerebrellar artery

Questions 77 and 78

Shortly after birth a neonate was diagnosed as having a meconium ileus. Laboratory tests indicate an abnormally high content of sodium chloride in the infant's sweat. Genetic testing confirms an abnormality of chromosome 7.

77. What disorder does the child have?

(A) cystic fibrosis
(B) hemophilia
(C) Wilson's disease
(D) alkaptonuria
(E) phenylketonuria

78. Damage to which organ system accounts for most deaths with this disorder?

(A) intestine
(B) lung
(C) brain
(D) pancreas
(E) liver

79. As a medical examiner, you are investigating a suspected homicide. The victim gives the appearance of having been poisoned with strychnine. You wish to confirm the presence of the poison in the victim. If a steady state concentration of strychnine had been present in the systemic circulation and equilibration between the systemic circulation and tissue compartments had been achieved before death, which of these fluid compartments would have the largest total fluid:blood concentration ratio for the weak base strychnine (pKa = 6)?

(A) urine in bladder at pH 6.0
(B) cerebrospinal fluid at pH 7.35
(C) synovial fluid at pH 7.3
(D) jejunum and ileum contents at pH 7.6
(E) stomach contents at pH 2.0

80. A 24-year-old male has a long history of an obsessive personality disorder. Which pain-control technique may be most efficacious for this patient?

(A) patient-controlled analgesia (PCA)
(B) hypnosis
(C) as needed pain medication (prn medication)
(D) placebo
(E) general anesthesia

81. A 21-year-old student has been informed by his physician that he is suffering from allergic rhinitis. Which of the following statements concerning his allergy is correct?

(A) His type of allergy does not lead to IgE production.
(B) Administration of sodium cromolyn will increase the release of histamine.
(C) His allergic antigen–antibody reactions do not neutralize the toxicity of the antigen.
(D) The mast cells in his circulation do not possess any immunoglobulin on their surface.
(E) His immunological responses are highly unspecific.

82. Muscles which arise from the second pharyngeal arch mesoderm include the

(A) mylohyoid muscle
(B) stapedius muscle
(C) stylopharyngeus muscle
(D) masseter muscle
(E) superior pharyngeal constrictor muscle

83. The current drug of choice for treatment of pinworm (*Enterobius*) infections is

(A) mebendazole
(B) ivermectin
(C) praziquantel
(D) niclosamide
(E) diethylcarbamazine

84. A newborn male (2 days old) delivered by normal labor (with no known prenatal risk factors) has become lethargic and requires stimulation for feeding. When vomiting and hyperventilation ensued, routine laboratory results showed BUN was less than 1 mg/dL. The infant quickly lapsed into a coma and was placed on a ventilator. Bulging of the fontanel suggested an intracranial hemorrhage, but a CT scan revealed only cerebral edema. Within several hours the infant died. Death was ascribed to sepsis; however, a postmortem analysis of the plasma samples taken at admission showed dramatically elevated serum ammonia and citrulline levels 100 times normal. The enzyme deficiency found to be associated with these severe neonatal symptoms is

(A) medium-chain acyl-CoA dehydrogenase
(B) 3-hydroxy, 3-methylglutaryl CoA lyase
(C) argininosuccinate synthetase
(D) pyruvate carboxylase

85. Patient F.K. has had a persistent cough for 10 days. He experiences spasms of coughing in which thre are multiple coughs per expiration. Nasopharyngeal swab cultures show the presence of *Bordetella pertussis.* The treatment of choice for this patient and for prophylaxis of exposed, susceptible family members is

(A) tetracycline
(B) chloramphenicol
(C) erythromycin
(D) gentamicin
(E) cefoxitin

86. Undifferentiated progenitor cells develop into lymphocytes in

(A) the thymus
(B) lymph nodes
(C) the white pulp of the spleen
(D) all lymph nodules that have germinal centers
(E) mucosa-associated lymphoid tissue (MALT)

Questions 87 and 88

87. The function of the cell in the electron micrograph in Figure 9–12 is most likely

(A) endocrine secretion of polypeptide hormones
(B) synthesis and secretion of immunoglobulins
(C) regulated exocrine secretion of digestive enzymes
(D) endocrine secretion of steroid hormones
(E) contraction

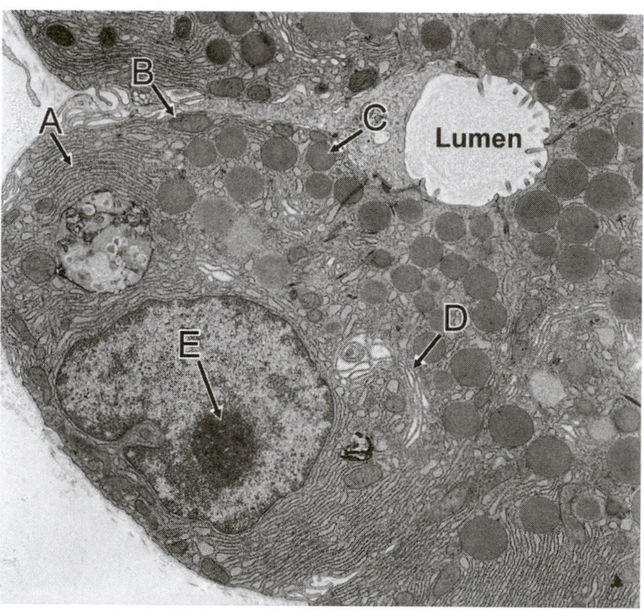

Figure 9–12

88. Which label (A through E) indicates a mitochondrion?

89. When exposed to air the urine of persons with alkaptonuria will turn dark. Late in the course of the disease patients exhibit increased pigmentation of the connective tissues and develop a form of arthritis. Alkaptonuria results from a defect in

(A) phenylalanine hydroxylase
(B) tyrosine transaminase
(C) tryptophan oxygenase
(D) α-keto acid decarboxylase
(E) homogentisate oxidase

90. The plateau phase of the cardiac myocyte action potential is most closely associated with which of the following phases of the ECG?

(A) P wave
(B) QRS complex
(C) ST segment
(D) T wave
(E) QT interval

91. A 46-year-old female complains of abdominal pain in the right upper quadrant after eating fatty foods. A photograph of her opened gallbladder is displayed in Figure 9–13. What abnormal process is evident?

(A) neoplasia
(B) infection
(C) stone formation
(D) thrombosis
(E) congenital malformation

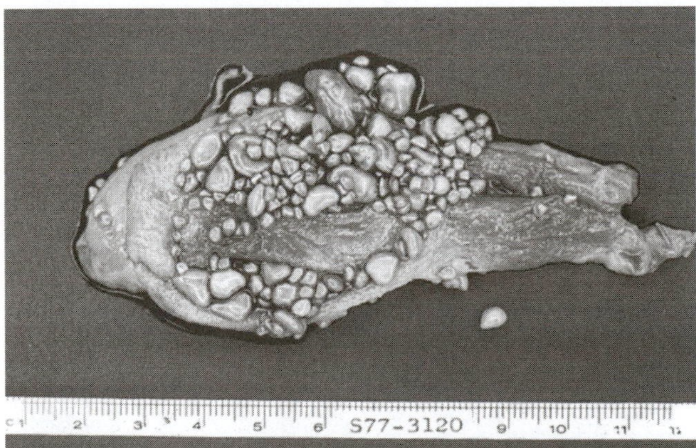

Figure 9–13 (see also Color Insert)

92. Which of the following is a correct statement regarding the relative actions of clozapine and haloperidol in treating schizophrenia?

(A) Clozapine has greater affinity for D_2 receptors than does haloperidol.
(B) Unlike clozapine, haloperidol binds to 5-HT_2 receptors.
(C) Clozapine produces extrapyramidal symptoms to the same extent as haloperidol.
(D) Clozapine improves negative symptoms whereas haloperidol does not.
(E) Unlike haloperidol, clozapine does not produce orthostatic hypotension.

93. A 17-year-old boy with influenza has a hemagglutination inhibition titer of 1:400. Which one of the following statements is correct?

(A) A 400-fold dilution of his serum will prevent agglutination of red blood cells.
(B) There are 400 viral particles per mL of serum.
(C) There are 400 hemagglutinins on each red blood cell.
(D) Each red blood cell can bind 400 viral particles.
(E) A 400-fold dilution of serum will have no effect in a hemagglutination inhibition assay.

94. Following a tonsillectomy, your patient reports numbness on the back of the tongue and a reduced awareness of taste. After examination, you confirm a loss of general sensation and taste from the posterior third of the tongue. You suspect injury to the

(A) lingual nerve
(B) hypoglossal nerve
(C) facial nerve
(D) vagus nerve
(E) glossopharyngeal nerve

95. The insulin receptor belongs to a class of receptor proteins that possess intrinsic enzymatic activity. The intrinsic enzymatic activity of the insulin receptor is

(A) guanylate cyclization
(B) tyrosine dephosphorylation
(C) serine/threonine phosphorylation
(D) GTPase activation
(E) tyrosine phosphorylation

96. A 34-year-old female has an ovarian tumor surgically excised. The pathologic examination shows that the tumor is derived from ovarian germ cells. Which neoplasm is compatible with this observation?

(A) serous papillary carcinoma
(B) endometrioid adenocarcinoma
(C) mature cystic teratoma
(D) Brenner tumor
(E) mucinous cystadenoma

97. Which of the following correctly matches an antiepileptic agent with its mechanism of action?

(A) lamotrigine: activation of potassium channels
(B) carbamazepine: blockade of sodium channels
(C) tiagabine: inhibition of GABA aminotransferase
(D) ethosuximide: activation of chloride channels
(E) vigabatrin: competitive blockade of $GABA_A$ receptor

98. A 12-year-old boy without diabetes exhibited extensive eruptive xanthomas, hepatosplenomegaly, and milky plasma. The milky plasma was due to a massive accumulation of chylomicrons and triglycerides. Upon switching to a fat-free diet, the lipemia and all other symptoms disappeared. A deficiency in which apolipoprotein would account for the observed symptoms of hyperlipoproteinemia?

(A) apo E
(B) apo D
(C) apo C-II
(D) apo B-100
(E) apo A-I

99. Which one of the following diseases is transmitted by ingestion of the etiological agent?

(A) African trypanosomiasis
(B) malaria
(C) amebiasis
(D) leishmaniasis
(E) loiasis

100. Figure 9–14 represents five left ventricular pressure-volume loops, each labeled by a letter (A through E). Loop D shows the normal pressure-volume loop of a healthy adult at rest. Which curve represents a patient with mitral stenosis?

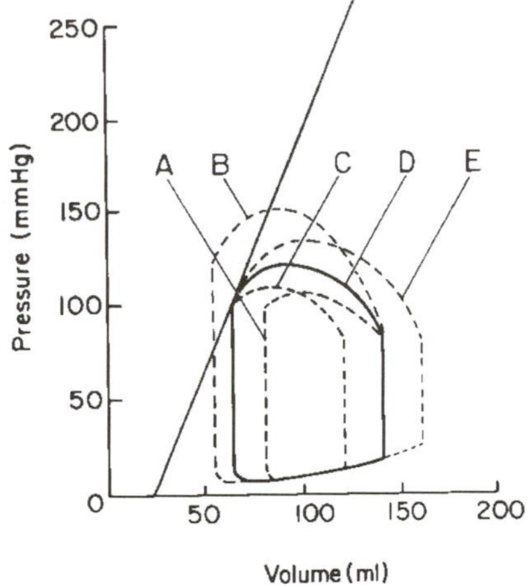

Figure 9–14

101. Immunohistochemistry may be used in an attempt to characterize a biopsy from a tumor in order to identify the cell type from which the tumor originated. Neoplastic cells that are of epithelial origin would be expected to stain selectively with antibodies against

(A) keratins
(B) nuclear lamins
(C) desmin
(D) actins
(E) β tubulins

102. Neurotransmitters are stored in secretory vesicles in the terminal buttons of nerve cells. Which of the following is the chemical trigger leading to the release of stored neurotransmitters?

(A) Ca^{2+}
(B) inositol-1,4,5-trisphosphate (IP_3)
(C) cAMP
(D) cGMP
(E) diacylglycerol (DAG)

103. The sensory (somatosensory) decussation occurs at the level of the

(A) posterior limb of internal capsule
(B) thalamus
(C) midbrain
(D) pons
(E) medulla

104. A 27-week-old male fetus is delivered prematurely and subsequently dies of respiratory distress syndrome. What pathologic process lead to his demise?

(A) in utero viral infection
(B) inadequate conjugation of bilirubin
(C) congential pulmonary malformation
(D) inadequate humoral immunity
(E) inadequate pulmonary surfactant

Questions 105 through 107

A 47-year-old man is brought to the clinic for evaluation of a movement disorder.

105. If the patient is observed to have a resting tremor, an important part of history taking would be

(A) history of exposure to Von Economo's disease
(B) history of alcoholism
(C) history of treatment with an anxiolytic drug
(D) history of treatment with an antipsychotic drug
(E) family history of seizure disorder

106. In addition to the resting tremor, the patient shows slow, rhythmic movements of the lips. A useful test to perform would be

(A) Babinski test
(B) Hoover test
(C) ask the patient to open his mouth, then protrude his tongue
(D) ask the patient to run
(E) ask the patient to close his eyes and smile

107. If the patient also exhibits choreiform movements of the arms and legs, the most likely diagnosis is

(A) multiple sclerosis
(B) vascular dementia
(C) Creutzfeldt–Jakob disease
(D) tardive dyskinesia
(E) Sydenham's chorea

108. The graph shown in Figure 9–15 shows a viral multiplication curve. Which of the following statements is correct?

(A) The viral growth curve is similar to bacterial growth curve.
(B) The time period of 6 to 8 hours represents the uncoating of the viral particle.
(C) During the time period of 0 to 6 hours the virus retains its infectivity.
(D) The period of 0 to 6 hours represents the eclipse period.
(E) The time period of 6 to 8 hours represents the appearance of immature virus.

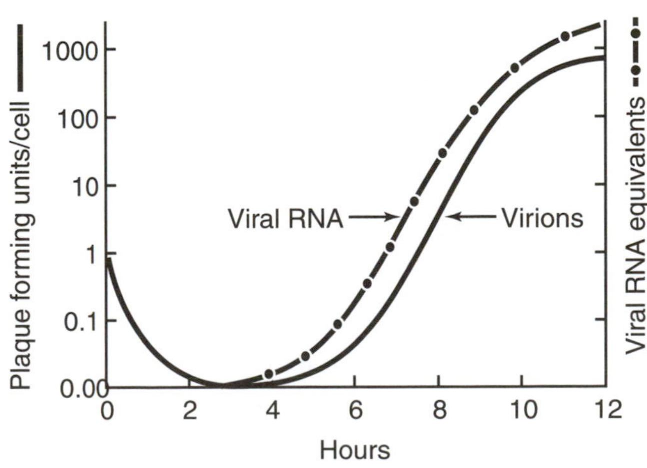

Figure 9–15

109. The primary mechanism for resistance to saquinavir in the treatment of HIV is

(A) mutations in the sequence of reverse transcriptase
(B) mutations in the sequence of viral protease
(C) mutations in the sequence of viral DNA polymerase
(D) deletion of thymidine kinase
(E) deletion of thymidylate synthase

110. Which statement is true concerning hepatitis A infection?

(A) increased incidence of infection with higher socioeconomic class
(B) viral genome is DNA
(C) spread mainly by parenteral route
(D) no vaccine is yet available
(E) carrier state does not exist

111. Shown in Figure 9–16 is a ring structure which constitutes the backbone of the purine nucleotides. Which of the numbered atoms are derived from the amino acid glycine during the synthesis of the purine ring?

(A) 1, 2, and 6
(B) 4, 5, and 7
(C) 2, 3, and 4
(D) 7, 8, and 9
(E) 4, 8, and 9

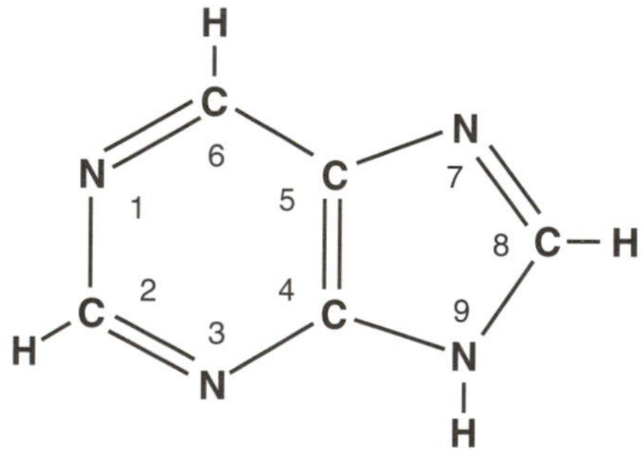

Figure 9–16

112. Osteopetrosis is an inherited disease characterized by defective osteoclasts that lack the ruffled border characteristic of this cell type. An expected consequence of osteoclast inactivity would be

(A) elevation in blood Ca^{++} levels
(B) enlarged marrow spaces
(C) overgrowth and thickening of bones
(D) abnormal deposits of calcium in arterial walls and the kidneys
(E) low concentration of circulating parathyroid hormone

113. A drug with a half-life of two hours is administered by continuous intravenous infusion. How long will it take for the drug to reach 94% of its final steady state level?

(A) 2 hr
(B) 4 hr
(C) 8 hr
(D) 16 hr
(E) 48 hr

114. A postoperative patient with a febrile episode is carefully monitored. Temperatures measured are rectal and given in degrees Centigrade in Figure 9–17. At which point or period does the patient begin to behave as if in a hot environment (sweats and complains of "burning up")?

(A) Period A
(B) Point B
(C) Point C
(D) Period D

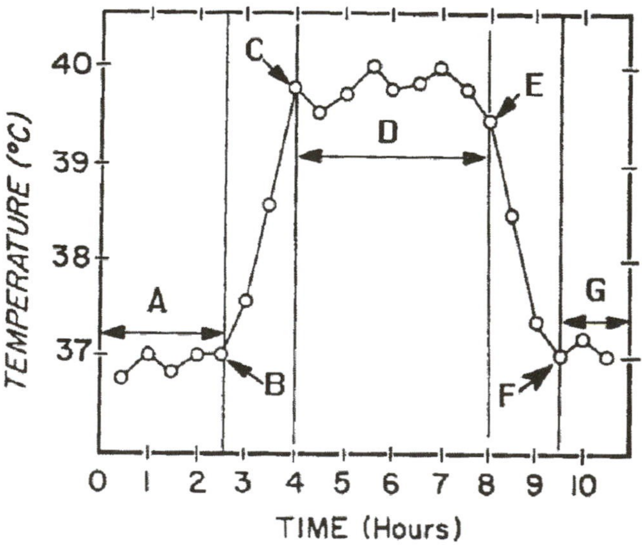

Figure 9–17

(E) Point E
(F) Point F
(G) Period G

115. Adenosine deaminase (AD) deficiency is associated with severe combined immunodeficiency. The immune dysfunction occurs because the enzyme deficiency

(A) leads to an inability of immune cells to salvage ATP from inosine, resulting in their death from lack of energy production
(B) causes lysis of T and B lymphocytes due to their extreme sensitivity to the increased levels of inosine which accompany the enzyme deficiency
(C) leads to elevations in uric acid, which is toxic to T and B lymphocytes
(D) leads to elevations in dATP levels which inhibits ribonucleotide reductase, thereby limiting production of deoxynucleotides for DNA synthesis in T and B lymphocytes
(E) prevents the generation of inosine required for the rapid salvage of thymidine nucleotides needed for DNA replication in T and B lymphocytes

116. Which item best describes the histology of granulation tissue from a healing wound site?

(A) irregular dense collagen and sparse fibroblasts
(B) central necrotic debris with peripheral multinucleate giant cells and histiocytes
(C) newly formed capillaries, proliferating fibroblasts, and a few inflammatory cells
(D) coagulative necrosis and many neutrophils
(E) extravasated erythrocytes, fibrin, and serous fluid

117. You are undertaking a surgical dissection of the posterior triangle of the neck to remove a small tumor mass. Which of the following structures is at risk in the posterior triangle?

(A) accessory nerve
(B) vertebral artery
(C) vagus nerve
(D) superior thyroid artery
(E) thoracic duct

118. A 50-year-old woman appears to be infected with a fungus which causes cutaneous mycosis. Which one of the following tests is likely to be of extremely little value for the diagnosis of this fungus?

(A) examination of the fungal colonies
(B) agglutination assays
(C) microscopic examination of skin scrapings, hair, and nails
(D) growth on Sabouraud's agar plates at a temperature of 25°C
(E) cultivation on Sabouraud's medium at pH 5.5

119. An internist tells the psychiatric consultant that she is having difficulty with a patient. The patient is very upset about the "sloppiness" of the hospital personnel. He insists on having all medicine administered exactly at the scheduled minute, on the dot. He complains if his medicine is only five minutes late. The patient most likely has traits of

(A) narcissistic personality
(B) depressive personality
(C) borderline personality
(D) obsessive personality
(E) antisocial personality

120. Which enzyme catalyzes the following reaction?

$$Fe^{2+} + O_2 + 4H^+ \rightarrow 2H_2O + Fe^{3+}$$

(A) cytochrome oxidase
(B) catalase
(C) ferrochetalase
(D) superoxide dismutase
(E) peroxidase

121. A 55-year-old female with lobular carcinoma of the breast underwent radical mastectomy and chemotherapy four years ago. Two out of 14 axillary lymph nodes at the time were positive for malignant cells. She now presents with bone metastases, and during her lab workup a peptide with PTH-like activity is found in her plasma. The physiologic effects of this substance would be to

(A) stimulate bone resorption
(B) decrease metabolism of vitamin D to the 1,25-OH form
(C) decrease serum calcium
(D) decrease renal phosphate excretion
(E) decrease serum calcitonin levels

122. The graph in Figure 9–18 shows the blood pressure responses to an intravenous infusion of epinephrine followed by infusion of Drug X. The top of the bars indicate the systolic pressure, the bottom the diastolic pressure, and the filled circles the mean pressure. Heart rate increased from 70 to 105 per minute during the infusion of Drug X. Identify Drug X.

(A) atenolol
(B) phenylephrine
(C) labetalol
(D) norepinephrine
(E) isoproterenol

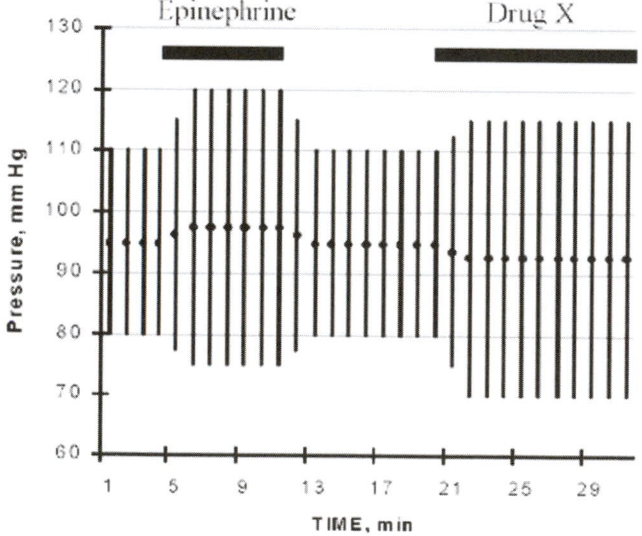

Figure 9–18

123. A morphologic change seen only with cell death is

(A) cloudy swelling
(B) pyknosis
(C) steatosis
(D) lipofuscin accumulation
(E) hydropic change

124. A loss of gastric parietal cells (oxyntic cells) as a result of atrophic gastritis would most likely result in a deficiency in

(A) pepsinogen secretion
(B) neutralization of chyme by bicarbonate
(C) the mucus coating of the gastric lining
(D) absorption of vitamin B_{12}
(E) secretion of gastrin

125. A 10-year-old girl exhibiting the following symptoms is suffering from which disease? Marked hepatomegaly, variceal bleeding, chronic bilateral pulmonary infiltrates, chronic liver disease, hepatic encephalopathy, and only 5% of normal sphingomyelinase activity in peripheral blood leukocytes.

(A) Krabbe disease
(B) Tay–Sachs disease
(C) Fabry disease
(D) Gaucher disease
(E) Niemann–Pick type B disease

126. Which of the following statements regarding systemic hemodynamics is correct?

(A) The greatest cross-sectional area is within the small veins.
(B) The velocity of blood flow is highest in the capillaries.
(C) The greatest drop in pressure occurs in the arterioles rather than in the large arteries.
(D) The compliance of the venous circulation is less than that of the arterial circulation.
(E) The greatest percentage of blood volume is in the capillaries.

127. This agent is used in combination therapy for squamous carcinoma. Its most serious toxicity is pulmonary fibrosis.

(A) bleomycin
(B) 5-fluorouracil
(C) paclitaxel
(D) cisplatin
(E) cyclophosphamide

128. A 65-year-old male is admitted to a neurosurgical unit due to rapidly worsening dementia. Radiology studies reveal multiple lesions in the cerebral cortex. A stereotactic biopsy of one of the lesions is obtained. A touch imprint cytology of the biopsy is shown in Figure 9–19. What is the nature of this man's cerebral lesions?

(A) viral infection
(B) malignant neoplasm
(C) chronic demyelinating disorder
(D) parasitic infection
(E) deficient in an essential nutrient

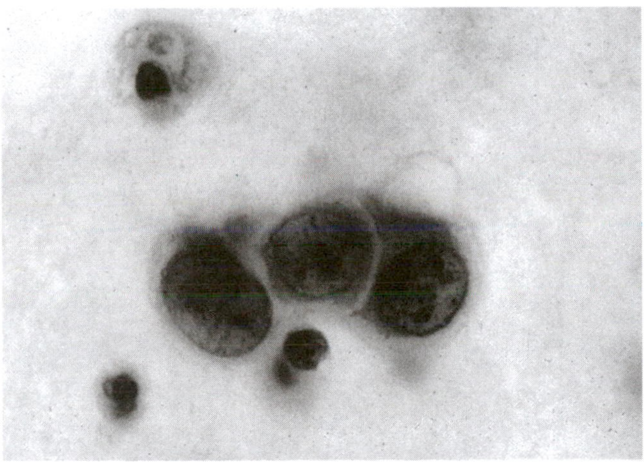

Figure 9–19 (see also Color Insert)

129. Microbial spores play an important role in the transmission of diseases. Which one of the following statements is accurate concerning bacterial spores?

(A) They are destroyed upon heating at 80°C for 10 to 15 minutes.
(B) They require iron as an effector molecule for germination.
(C) They are formed under optimal growth conditions.
(D) They contain calcium dipicolinate.
(E) They are important constituents of gram-negative bacteria.

130. Which of the following is a predictable adverse effect of treatment with a butyrophenone such as haloperidol?

(A) nausea and vomiting
(B) Tourette's syndrome
(C) excessive salivation
(D) hyperprolactinemia
(E) diarrhea

131. Anastomoses between which of the following vessels could potentially provide collateral circulation to the brain in the event of a blockage of the internal carotid artery?

(A) angular artery and dorsal nasal artery
(B) lingual artery and facial artery
(C) superficial temporal artery and middle meningeal artery
(D) superficial temporal artery and occipital artery
(E) superior thyroid artery and inferior thyroid artery

132. Tumors of the adrenal medulla that are actively producing catecholamines are called pheochromocytomas. Patients with these tumors experience sudden, periodic increases in catecholamine blood levels. During such an episode, patients may experience

(A) decreased blood pressure
(B) decreased heart rate
(C) decreased blood glucose
(D) decreased sweat secretion
(E) cardiac ischemia

133. Which of the following correctly matches an immunosuppressive agent with its mechanism of action?

(A) tacrolimus: inhibition of activation of T-cell transcription factors for cytokine expression
(B) cyclosporine: prevention of clonal expansion of T and B lymphocytes
(C) cyclophosphamide: inhibition of antigen presentation
(D) azathioprine: negative regulation of T-cell expression of lymphokines
(E) prednisone: inhibition of IMP dehydrogenase

134. A 72-year-old male with a known history of chronic essential hypertension dies unattended at home. The medical examiner determines the cause of death to be a hypertensive intracerebral hemorrhage. At which site is the hemorrhage most likely?

(A) cerebellum
(B) basal ganglia or thalamus
(C) occipital lobe
(D) pons
(E) frontal lobe

135. Which of the following viruses produces a rash and has an RNA genome?

(A) variola virus
(B) herpesvirus
(C) molluscum contagiosum virus
(D) papovavirus
(E) measles virus

136. Cushing's syndrome results from chronic glucocorticoid therapy. The symptoms of Cushing's syndrome are similar to those of Cushing's disease, which is caused by pituitary tumors that secrete excess amounts of which hormone?

(A) follicle-stimulating hormone (FSH)
(B) thyroid-stimulating hormone (TSH)
(C) adrenocorticotropic hormone (ACTH)
(D) prolactin (PRL)
(E) growth hormone (GH)

137. A lung autopsy specimen with an abnormality of the vasculature is depicted in Figure 9–20. What is the most likely associated clinical finding?

(A) sudden death due to occlusive embolus
(B) chronic idiopathic thrombocytopenic purpura
(C) disseminated intravascular coagulation
(D) hemoptysis due to aneurysmal rupture
(E) hemoptysis due to tumor eroding into blood vessel

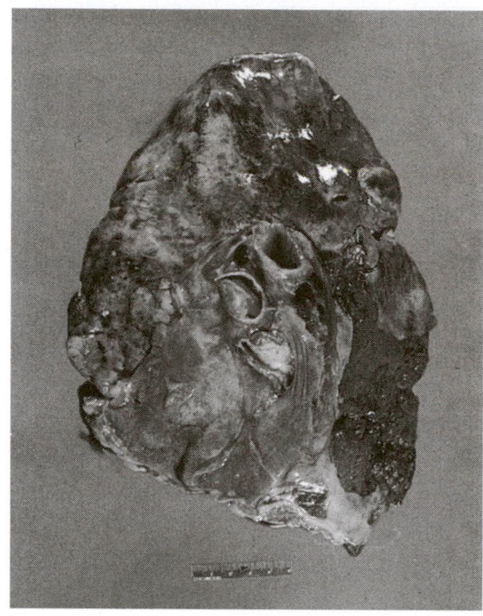

Figure 9–20 (see also Color Insert)

138. Which of the following is associated with secondary hyperaldosteronism?

(A) Conn's syndrome
(B) heart failure
(C) buffalo hump
(D) truncal obesity
(E) skin striae

139. Which of these drugs is used in treatment of gouty arthritis to increase the urinary excretion of uric acid?

(A) allopurinol
(B) piroxicam
(C) probenecid
(D) colchicine
(E) indomethacin

140. Azidothymidine (AZT), also called zidovudine (ZDV), is used as a treatment for infection by HIV. The function of AZT is to

(A) induce the synthesis of interferon which prevents replication of HIV
(B) bind to the RNA genome of HIV and prevent reverse transcription from occurring
(C) block the packaging of replicated HIV, preventing the infection of other cells
(D) interfere with the reverse transcriptase of HIV through its action as an antimetabolite
(E) selectively poison cells infected with HIV, thereby preventing growth of the virus

141. The electroencephalogram (EEG) during a petit mal epileptic attack is characterized by

(A) generalized high-voltage spikes
(B) 3-per-second "spikes and domes"
(C) REM onset sleep
(D) irregular spikes limited to the temporal lobes
(E) no consistent EEG abnormalities

142. A 32-year-old male has a four-month history of glomerulonephritis and recurrent pulmonary hemorrhage. His serum contains an antibody directed against basement membrane. What disorder does he suffer from?

(A) fibrosing alveolitis
(B) Wegener's granulomatosis
(C) Goodpasture's syndrome
(D) Kartagener's syndrome
(E) systemic lupus erythematosus

143. Severe anion-gap metabolic acidosis and retinal destruction from formic acid is characteristic of intoxication by

(A) methanol
(B) ethanol
(C) isopropanol
(D) methylene chloride
(E) ethylene glycol

144. Membrane-spanning receptors that are coupled to the ligand-induced activation of intracellular G-proteins are defined by a structure that includes

(A) seven transmembrane spanning domains
(B) cysteine-rich extracellular domains
(C) immunoglobulin-like extracellular domains
(D) heterodimers linked through disulfide bonds
(E) a domain for binding lipophilic hormones

145. The graph in Figure 9–21 shows the response of retinal photoreceptors as a function of light wavelength. Which of the following statements is correct?

(A) A green sensation is elicited by maximally stimulating the Green cone (arrow c).
(B) A red sensation is elicited by maximally stimulating the Red cone (arrow e).
(C) A yellow sensation is elicited by about equal stimulation of the Green cone and Red cone (arrow d).
(D) There are four receptor types in the retina corresponding to the primary colors (red, green, blue, and yellow).
(E) Color is a subjective sensation and cannot be measured objectively.

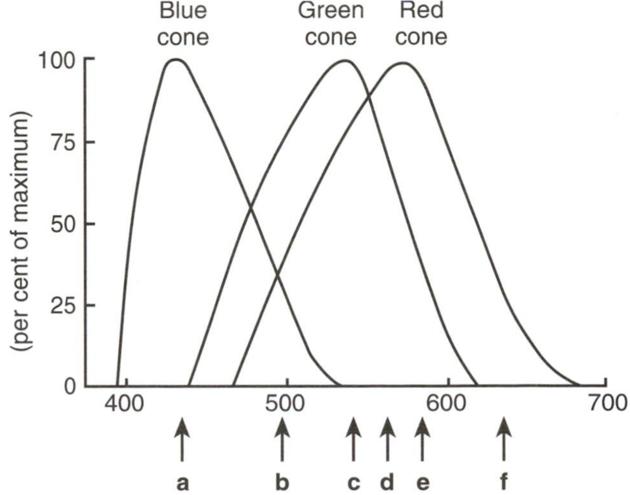

Figure 9–21. *(Reprinted with permission from Guyton & Hall.* Textbook of Medical Physiology. *9th ed. W.B. Saunders Co.; 1995.)*

146. Patient J.M. is a 23-year-old African American male who is working as a construction laborer. Because he was suffering from wheezing and difficulty in breathing with exertion, he was first treated with theophylline. Because of a complaint of palpitations, cromolyn sodium was substituted for theophylline. The change in medication brought on two episodes of angioedema and severe headache. Which of the following agents offers a choice for prophylaxis without the risk of palpitations, drug allergy, or adverse metabolic effects?

(A) terbutaline
(B) aminophylline
(C) zafirlukast
(D) ipratropium
(E) nedocromil

147. A 59-year-old man has pneumonia caused by *Streptococcus pneumoniae.* The virulence of this microbe is associated with the presence of

(A) cell wall teichoic acid
(B) pneumolysin
(C) polysaccharide capsule
(D) M protein
(E) peptidoglycan

148. Which of the following represents the correct pathway in the conversion of tyrosine to the various neurotransmitters?

(A) tyrosine → norepinephrine → dopamine → dopa → epinephrine
(B) tyrosine → dopa → dopamine → norepinephrine → epinephrine
(C) tyrosine → dopamine → dopa → epinephrine → norepinephrine
(D) tyrosine → dopamine → dopa → norepinephrine → epinephrine
(E) tyrosine → epinephrine → dopa → norepinephrine → dopamine

149. A 65-year-old male complains of difficulty swallowing. A mass in the lower esophagus is found on endoscopic examination and biopsied. A photomicrograph of the biopsy is displayed in Figure 9–22. Which statement concerning this esophageal mass is true?

(A) It usually arises in Barrett's metaplasia.
(B) Its development is associated with alcoholism and smoking.
(C) This disorder is rare in males but common in females.
(D) The prognosis is excellent with a high cure rate.
(E) Dysphagia is an uncommon symptom of this disorder.

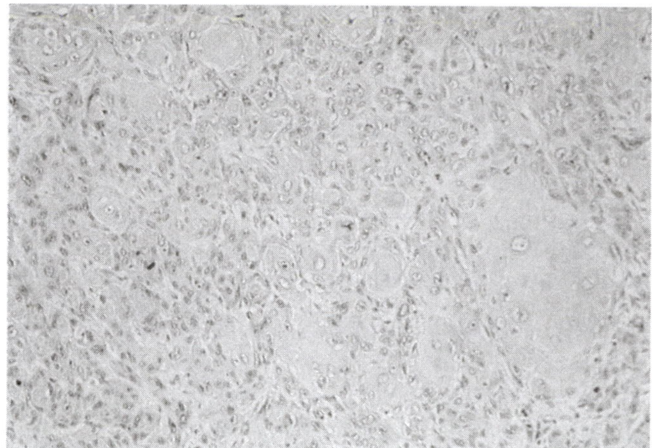

Figure 9–22 (see also Color Insert)

150. In cases of acute cyanide poisoning, cyanide binds to the Fe^{3+} of a cytochrome. Which statement best describes this cytochrome?

(A) It directly oxidizes cytochrome b.
(B) It is found in complex II of the respiratory chain.
(C) It is found in complex I of the respiratory chain.
(D) It binds carbon monoxide.
(E) It directly reduces cytochrome c_1.

Answers and Explanations

1. **(B)** Carbon monoxide (CO) reacts with hemoglobin to form carboxyhemoglobin which gives blood a cherry-red appearance. The affinity of CO to hemoglobin is more than 200 times larger than the affinity of O_2 to hemoglobin. Therefore a small CO partial pressure is sufficient to replace most of the O_2 and cause acute tissue hypoxia. CO also inhibits mitochondrial cytochromes (choice A), but the concentrations required are much larger than the lethal dose. Bone marrow suppression (choice C), cardiac arrhythmias (choice D), and direct suppression of the respiratory centers (choice E) are not primary causes of CO toxicity.

2. **(D)** The photomicrograph displays the distinctive fruiting head structure diagnostic for *Aspergillus* species. Pulmonary infections by these organisms may include allergic bronchopulmonary aspergillosis, cavity-occupying aspergilloma, or invasive aspergillosis. Asbestosis (choice A) should display iron-encrusted, baton-shaped asbestos bodies. Microscopic examination of sputum from individuals with tuberculosis (choice B) may reveal multinucleate giant cells. Fungal bodies are not seen. Histoplasmosis (choice C) may demonstrate small yeast-shaped organisms or multinucleate giant cells. Blastomycosis (choice E) could be diagnosed if large, encapsulated budding yeasts were evident.

3. **(A)** *Leishmania* species are 1- to 3-μm protozoa that are transmitted to humans by bites of infected sandflies of the genera *Phlebotomus* and *Lutzomyia.* Following infection, *Leishmania* circulates freely in the blood and lives inside the macrophages of liver, spleen, and bone marrow. Leishmaniasis (or kala-azar) caused by *Leishmania donovani* is characterized by spleen and liver enlargement, undulant fever, loss of weight, visible pulsation of carotid arteries, anemia, and bleeding of the nose, gums, intestine, and lips. Trichinosis is transmitted by eating infected undercooked meat, usually pork, not by bites of the sandfly *Phlebotomus* (choice B). Diphyllobothriasis is acquired by eating infected raw fish (choice C). Toxoplasmosis is transmitted by the ingestion of meat infected with cysts of *Toxoplasma gondii* (choice D). Clonorchiasis is transmitted by eating raw or undercooked fish infected with metacercariae of *Clonorchis sinensis* (choice E).

4. **(B)** The internal acoustic meatus is a feature of the posterior cranial fossa. It transmits cranial nerves VII and VIII. The temporomandibular joint (choice A) is the joint between the head of the mandible and the mandibular fossa of the squamous part of the temporal bone. The mandibular fossa is related superiorly to the middle cranial fossa. The abducens nerve in the cavernous sinus (choice C) lies in the middle cranial fossa along the body of the sphenoid bone. The mandibular division of the trigeminal nerve (choice D) exits the middle cranial fossa through the foramen ovale. The temporal lobe of the cerebral hemisphere (choice E) occupies the middle cranial fossa.

5. **(A)** Hospitalization increases anxiety, and the patient tends to exaggerate his or her personality traits to reduce the heightened

anxiety. Therefore, in this patient, the exacting, obsessive traits are exaggerated. From the known history, choices B, C, D, and E are not supported.

6. **(A)** Creatine and the energy reserve form phosphocreatine are present in skeletal muscle, brain, and blood. Creatine synthesis begins in the kidney from arginine and glycine. The products of the first reaction are ornithine and guanidoacetate. Guanidoacetate is transported to the liver where it is converted to creatine by methylation from S-adenosylmethionine. Phosphorylation of creatine is carried out by creatine kinase, CK. CK plays an important role in the reversible transfer of phosphate from ATP to creatine when energy levels are high, and then from creatine to ADP when energy levels fall and demand for energy is high. Creatine can spontaneously cyclize to creatinine. Creatinine clearance by any given individual is amazingly constant from day to day and is proportional to muscle mass. None of the other amino acid choices (B, C, D, and E) are involved in creatine synthesis.

7. **(D)** Of the five immunoglobulin classes, only IgM has a pentameric configuration as displayed in Figure 9–3. IgM is the first immunoglobulin to appear in the serum upon initial exposure of an antigen to the immune system. Peak levels of IgM occur about one week after initial exposure to the sensitizing antigen. IgA (choice A) may be encountered as either a monomer or dimer, but not as a pentamer. IgE (choice B), IgD (choice C), and IgG (choice E) only exhibit a monomer configuration.

8. **(C)** Coronary atherosclerosis is a major cause of premature death in industrialized nations. Elevations of HDL cholesterol exert a protective effect against the development of coronary atherosclerosis. A decreased LDL cholesterol level (choice A) would discourage the development of coronary atherosclerosis. Type B personality (choice B) is less likely to sustain coronary atherosclerosis than are Type A individuals. Female gender (choice D) exerts a relative protective effect against the development of coronary atherosclerosis. Hypertension (choice E) exacerbates the deleterious effects of coronary atherosclerosis.

9. **(E)** The human papovavirus is a naked DNA virus which does not possess hemagglutinin, and cannot attach to human cells. The envelopes of rubeola, influenza, parainfluenza, and measles viruses all have hemagglutinins, which enable them to attach to human cells (choices A, B, C, and D).

10. **(B)** Human chorionic gonadotropin (hCG) is a glycoprotein similar in structure and function to LH from the anterior pituitary gland. hCG is produced by the syncytial trophoblast and it prevents involution of the corpus luteum during pregnancy. Measurement at 16 to 18 weeks is recommended for all pregnant women as part of the triple screen. Ectopic pregnancy and trisomy 18 are associated with low serum hCG levels. Low levels of hCG also frequently indicate a threatened abortion. Twin pregnancy (choice A), trisomy 21 (choice C), hydatidiform mole (choice D), and choriocarcinoma (choice E) are all associated with elevated levels of plasma hCG.

11. **(C)** Fibrosis is the major pathologic feature seen with chronic rheumatic heart disease. The mitral valve is almost always involved by this fibrotic process. Valvular stenosis is the usual late clinical sequela. The coronary arteries (choice A) are rarely affected by fibrotic chronic rheumatic heart disease. The epicardium (choice B) may sustain some degree of adhesive pericarditis with chronic rheumatic heart disease, but it is seen far less frequently than mitral valve fibrosis. The pulmonary valve (choice D) is also less likely to be deranged than are the mitral or aortic valves. The right ventricle (choice E) is infrequently involved by endocardial fibrosis with chronic rheumatic heart disease.

12. **(A)** The vascular infarct in this case would affect the left dorsal columns and dorsal column nuclei resulting in a loss of position sense in the left upper and lower extremities, but no involvement of dorsal column modali-

ties on the right side (choice D). Pain and temperature sensibility (choice B) would not be affected, nor would there be hyperactive reflexes in the left upper extremity (choice C). Damage to the dorsal medulla would not involve the pyramidal tract, and thus no hemiplegia (choice E) would be expected.

13. **(A)** Both type 1 and type 2 diabetes tend to run in families, but the mechanism of inheritance is unclear. Identical twin concordance is over 80% for NIDDM, but less than 40% for IDDM. Most patients with IDDM express either DR3 or DR4 or both (choice B). In contrast, a strong HLA association has not been described for NIDDM. Patients with NIDDM are almost always obese and have resistance to insulin. This is due to a lower density (choice C) of insulin receptors in their tissues and a lower affinity of the receptor for insulin (choice D). Plasma insulin levels (choice E) are low to absent in patients with IDDM, but normal or high in patients with NIDDM.

14. **(C)** The adrenal gland contains a cortical adenoma. Grossly, these neoplasms appear as a well demarcated round to oval, yellowish solitary nodule arising within the adrenal cortex. The surrounding non-neoplastic cortex is thinned and atrophic. The underlying medulla is normal. The associated clinical findings suggest Cushing's syndrome due to excessive secretion of cortisol by the adenoma. A pheochromocytoma (choice A) appears as a hemorrhagic red-tan medullary tumor. Clinically, there may be signs of excessive norepinephrine secretion. Adrenal infarcts (choice B) may be associated with certain bacterial infections and shock. The gland would appear diffusely hemorrhagic and necrotic, without the formation of a discrete tumor nodule. Krukenberg tumor (choice D) is an enlarged ovary due to metastatic carcinoma. Neuroblastoma (choice E) is an adrenal tumor of infancy. The typical gross appearance is a large, tan hemorrhagic mass. Hypercortisolemia is not seen.

15. **(C)** The clinical and gross anatomic findings suggest a diagnosis of Cushing's syndrome due to a functioning adrenal cortical adenoma. Cortisol is the most likely analyte to be elevated. Norepinephrine (choice A) may be elevated episodically with pheochromocytomas. Carcinoembryonic antigen (choice B) is usually elevated with carcinomas of the breast, lung, or gastrointestinal tract. Elevations of CA-125 (choice D) can be seen with serous carcinomas of the ovary. Neuron-specific enolase (choice E) may be elevated with neuroblastoma.

16. **(C)** Niacin is required for conversion to the nicotinamide nucleotide coenzymes required for numerous redox reactions. Symptoms seen early in a dietary deficiency of niacin include glossitis of the tongue. Severe deficiency leads to pellagra, characterized by dermatitis, diarrhea, dementia, mental depression, digestive disorders, and weight loss. Thiamine (choice A) is required for oxidative decarboxylation reactions (e.g., the pyruvate dehydrogenase and α-ketoglutarate dehydrogenase reactions) and in the transketolase reactions of the pentose phosphate pathway. Early symptoms of a deficiency in thiamin are peripheral neuropathy, exhaustion, and anorexia. Progressive deficiency results in edema and muscular, neurological, and cardiovascular degeneration. Wernicke–Korsakoff syndrome is associated with thiamine deficiency. Beriberi is caused by a carbohydrate-rich, low-thiamine diet. Riboflavin (choice B) is required for conversion to the flavin nucleotide coenzymes involved in numerous redox reactions. Deficiencies in riboflavin are rarely seen in the United States due to adequate dietary amounts in eggs, milk, meat, and cereals, and are therefore usually seen only in patients with a poor diet such as chronic alcoholics. Characteristic symptoms of riboflavin deficiency include angular stomatitis and chelitis, glossitis, scaly dermatitis (seborrhea), and photophobia. Vitamin C (choice D) is important as a reducing agent in numerous hydroxylation reactions. The principle reaction requiring ascorbate is the hydroxylation of proline and lysine residues in procollagen. A deficiency in vitamin C leads to scurvy, characterized by subcutaneous hemorrhaging; anemia; muscle weakness; soft, swollen gums; loose teeth;

poor wound healing; and loss of mineralized bone. Vitamin A (choice E) has numerous functions in the body, including promoting early development through the control of gene expression. Its function in vision leads to night blindness with dietary insufficiency. Prolonged deficiency leads to keratinization of the epithelial tissue of the eye, lungs, and gastrointestinal and genitourinary tracts, and reductions in mucus production. The keratinization of the eye is termed xerophthalmia, a condition that leads to blindness.

17. **(B)** *Mycoplasma pneumoniae* is a microorganism that lacks a cell wall, and therefore it is resistant to penicillin, which inhibits cell wall synthesis, hence the use of penicillin in a culture medium designed to isolate *M. pneumoniae.* Erythromycin, doxycycline, oxytetracycline, and minocycline are effective antibiotics for the treatment of mycoplasmal infections (choices A, C, D, and E).

18. **(B)** The cardiac glycosides such as digoxin inhibit Na^+-K^+-ATPase at the plasma membrane. Inhibition of the sodium pump causes an elevation of intracellular sodium ion concentrations and a resultant decrease in sodium–calcium exchange. The increased intracellular calcium concentration at the contractile machinery produces the therapeutic increase in cardiac contractility needed in congestive heart failure (CHF). The cardiac glycosides produce a decrease in heart rate by enhancing baroreceptor sensitivity and producing a reflex withdrawal of the elevated sympathetic tone associated with heart failure. Glucagon (choice A) exerts both positive inotropic and chronotropic effects on the heart by acting through glucagon receptors that couple to the heterotrimeric G_s protein that stimulates adenylyl cyclase activity in a fashion similar to the β_1 adrenoceptor. Epinephrine (choice C) exerts both positive inotropic and chronotropic effects on the heart by acting on β_1 adrenoceptors. Nitroglycerin (choice D) is a nitrovasodilator that does not increase contractility, but will lower total peripheral resistance and may produce a reflex tachycardia. Propranolol (choice E) is a β blocker. Because increased sympathetic drive to the heart is a compensatory mechanism in heart failure, the use of β-blockers was considered to be contraindicated in CHF. Recently, some clinical trials have given an indication that the use of the β_1-selective antagonist metoprolol decreases the necessity of cardiac transplantation as compared with placebo. The use of β blockers in the treatment of CHF is being re-evaluated.

19. **(B)** Benzoylecgonine is the urinary metabolite of cocaine. It is detectable in urine for about 24 hours after the last episode of cocaine use. If the decedent was taking chemotherapy for cancer (choice A) either residual neoplasm or chemotherapeutic metabolites should have been noted at necropsy. Status asthmaticus (choice C) is an occasional cause of sudden death in young males. Autopsy findings of bronchial mucous plugs and distended lungs are the usual correlates. There is no evidence of a congenital deformity (choice D) or a chromosomal abnormality (choice E) from the given history.

20. **(D)** Remember that concentration equals amount of substance divided by volume. Therefore,

urine volume = urine solute output/urine osmolarity
= 900 mosm/day/150 mosm/L
= 6.0 L/day.

Plasma volume (choice E) is not required for this calculation.

21. **(C)** Clearance is the amount of plasma that contained the solute excreted. Since in this patient the urine solute concentration is half the plasma concentration, the amount of plasma concentration, the amount of plasma that contained this solute must be half the urine volume per day. Alternatively, you can calculate clearance from the usual equation:

Clearance = urine flow · [urine concentration]/[plasma concentration]
= 6.0 L/day · 150 mosm/L/300 mosm/L
= 3.0 L/day

Plasma volume (choice E) is not required for this calculation. Clearance is the fraction of plasma volume that contained the excreted amount of solutes (per day or minute).

22. **(D)** Free water clearance (C_{H_2O}) is the gain or loss of water by excretion of concentrated or diluted urine. In dilute urine it equals the amount of water lost that did not contribute to excretion of solutes. In other words:

$$\begin{aligned} C_{H_2O} &= \text{urine flow} - \text{solute clearance} \\ &= 6.0\ \text{L/day} - 3.0\ \text{L/day} \\ &= +3.0\ \text{L/day} \end{aligned}$$

Choices A and B: Negative values indicate water conservation while positive values indicate water loss. If the urine were more concentrated than the plasma, free water clearance would be < 0 (antidiuresis). Calculation of free water clearance requires knowledge of solute clearance, but not knowledge of inulin clearance (choice E).

23. **(A)** Generally speaking, the urine flow should increase with solute load (amount of solutes excreted). Patients with diabetes insipidus are unable to concentrate their urine and require a larger urine volume to excrete the solute load. Therefore, relationship A would support a diagnosis of diabetes insipidus. Line B indicates excretion of urine that is isosmotic to plasma. Line C indicates urine production in the presence of maximal vasopressin effect. Lines D and E are false, since urine flow should increase with solute load.

24. **(A)** Vasopressin should increase urine concentration and result in antidiuresis. Patients with renal diabetes insipidus have defective vasopressin receptors and intravenous injection of vasopressin fails to increase urine osmolarity. These patients already have a high level of circulating vasopressin. In central diabetes (choice B) the posterior pituitary gland fails to produce adequate amounts of vasopressin. However, the kidneys would respond normally (i.e., concentrating the urine) when vasopressin is injected intravenously. Patients with diabetes mellitus (choice C) often are in a state of osmotic diuresis because of the high plasma and urine glucose concentration. Vasopressin would increase urine osmolarity in these patients. Therefore, water deprivation tests should not be performed in patients with diabetes mellitus because of severe risk of hyperosmolar coma. Patients with psychogenic polydipsia (choice D) should have concentrated urine following water deprivation. Since the patient's kidneys do not respond to vasopressin, choice E must be false.

25. **(D)** Exposure to benzidine or naphthylamine is known to increase the risk of developing transitional cell carcinomas of the bladder. The bladder may be particularly susceptible because these compounds are converted to carcinogenic metabolites which are preferentially concentrated in urine. Leather, chemical, dye, and rubber workers can be exposed to these agents. Nitrosamines are the chemical most closely linked to stomach cancer (choice A). Aflatoxin is the chemical most closely linked to liver carcinoma (choice B). Skin cancers (choice C) may develop after exposure to arsenic. Oral cancers (choice E) may be seen after exposure to tobacco products, alcohol, and betel nut.

26. **(E)** Both psychosis and depression could present this picture. Substance abuse may cause either psychosis or depression.

27. **(C)** Loose association is characterized by loosening of the associative (thought process) linkages. Circumstantiality (choice A) is an inability to get to the point without laborious elaborations. Folie à deux (choice B) is delusion shared by two people, thought blocking (choice D) is sudden absence of thought, and autistic thinking (choice E) is a more generic term denoting psychotic thinking.

28. **(D)** Responding to a percept without apparent sensory input indicates hallucination (probably visual and auditory in this case). An illusion (choice A) is a misperception of sensory stimulus, a delusion (choice B) is a belief not based on reality, ambivalence (choice C) is having strong opposing feelings

at the same time, and negativism (choice E) is persistent negative response.

29. **(B)** Catatonia is characterized by rigid muscle tone, immobility, and mutism. Choice A, mutism, simply refers to absence of verbal communication. Choice C, cataplexy, is sudden loss of muscle tone. Choice D, hebephrenia, is a disorganized type of schizophrenia. In coma (choice E), there is loss of consciousness, whereas in catatonia, consciousness is intact.

30. **(E)** For immediate treatment of catatonia to induce responsiveness, parenteral use of lorazepam has been effective. Any other talking therapy (choices B, C, and D) cannot work without the patient's being responsive. EEG (choice A) in catatonia without an organic lesion usually shows an arousal pattern, but is of no therapeutic value.

31. **(C)** The patient has loosening of association, catatonic rigidity, and delusions, making schizophrenia the most likely diagnosis. The onset of symptoms in her teens supports this diagnosis. Bipolar disorder (choice A) is not impossible, but there is no evidence of mania or severe depression. There is no evidence of a general medical condition (choice E) that may cause psychosis, and she has more symptoms of schizophrenia than just a delusion (choice D). Folie à deux involves two people (choice B).

32. **(D)** An antipsychotic drug such as haloperidol is likely to be effective for the hallucinations, delusions, loosening of association, and catatonia. Benztropine (choice A), an anticholinergic, may be useful if she develops neuroleptic-induced pseudoparkinsonism. Lithium chloride (choice C) is useful for manic symptoms. Fluoxetine (choice E) is an antidepressant. Chlordiazepoxide (choice B), a benzodiazepine, is usually ineffective as a primary drug for psychosis.

33. **(E)** The kidney contains a large renal cell carcinoma. These malignant tumors are more frequent in the elderly, and may first become apparent as flank pain or hematuria. Grossly, there is a large, solitary cortical mass whose surface displays a variegated red, yellow, and tan coloration. Necrosis is usually evident. The tumor may erode through the renal capsule or into the renal vein. In the photograph there is no evidence of an infectious process (choice A), postrenal process (choice B), calculi (choice C), or congenital anomaly (choice D).

34. **(A)** Postganglionic neuronal somata are found in two locations, the sympathetic chain ganglia and the prevertebral or preaortic ganglia. Sympathetic innervation of the heart arises from preganglionic sympathetic neurons located in the lateral horn between T1 and T5 (not T6 to T9 as in choice B). Vascular carbon dioxide concentration is carried over fibers of cranial nerves IX and X (not via sympathetic fibers as in choice C). Descending projections from the hypothalamus do influence the sympathetic nervous system (not the contrary as indicated in choice D) and the enteric nervous system is modulated through both parasympathetic and sympathetic inputs (not the contrary as indicated in choice E).

35. **(E)** The enterotoxins are considered to be quite heat resistant since after boiling crude solutions for 30 min, some toxicity remains. They are also resistant to proteolytic enzymes such as trypsin, chymotrypsin, rennin, and papain. Approximately 30% of strains of *S. aureus* isolated from patients produce enterotoxins. Synthesis of enterotoxins by *S. epidermidis* is doubtful. Six antigenically distinct types of enterotoxins—A, B, C, C_2, D, and E—are produced by *S. aureus*. Enterotoxin A has been most frequently implicated in food intoxication in the United States (choice A). Disruption of the stratum granulosum in the epidermis is due to the action of exfoliative toxins, which are produced by some strains of *S. aureus*. The exfoliative toxins A and B are responsible for the development of the staphylococcal scalded skin syndrome (choice B). Disruption of the cytoplasmic membrane is due to the action of the various hemolysins elaborated by *S. aureus* (choice C). Botulinum toxin is responsible for the

blockage of the release of acetylcholine at the neuromuscular junction (choice D).

36. (D) Arsenic exists naturally in both inorganic and organic forms with various valence states. Arsenate can substitute for phosphate in oxidative phosphorylation to form an unstable ATP analog that spontaneously hydrolyzes, thus essentially uncoupling oxidative phosphorylation. The trivalent forms readily react with sulfhydryl compounds including enzymes and lipoic acid. Pyruvate dehydrogenase is particularly sensitive to this inhibition. Arsenic poisoning is treated with chelation therapy using dimercaprol, succimer (2,3-dimercaptosuccinic acid), or penicillamine. Deferoxamine (choice A) is an iron-chelating agent used in the treatment of toxicity from iron. This may arise from ingestion of iron supplements (as with children swallowing adult preparations), or diseases such as thalassemia. Folic acid (choice B) is a necessary dietary constituent that functions in synthesis of purines and pyrimidines. Calcium disodium edetate (choice C) will bind any available divalent or trivalent metal that has a greater affinity for EDTA than calcium. In lead poisoning for example, the calcium ion in calcium disodium edetate is readily displaced by lead, forming a lead chelate that is excreted in the urine. Thiosulfate (choice E) is an agent used to treat cyanide toxicity. The mitochondrial enzyme rhodanese will combine cyanide and thiosulfate to form thiocyanate, which is excreted by the kidney.

37. (D) The infection caused by measles virus is characterized by hacking cough, fever, runny nose, conjunctivitis, rash, and the presence of the red based, blue-white centered oral lesions known as Koplik's spots. Coronavirus, adenovirus, or orthomyxovirus produces influenza-like infections without rash or Koplik's spots (choices A, B, and E). Hantavirus is the etiological agent of Korean hemorrhagic fever. This disease causes petechial hemorrhages, renal failure, fever, and shock, but it does not produce Koplik's spots (choice C).

38. (D) Creutzfeldt–Jakob disease is caused by a prion which may either be inherited or acquired during life. Prions are composed of protein only and behave like a slow viral infection. Human prion disease has recently become more prominent with the outbreak of "mad cow disease" in England due to human consumption of beef tainted with prions. Creutzfeldt–Jakob disease is not known to be caused by protozoan infections (choice A) or to be inherited as a lysosomal storage disease (choice B). Increased neurofibrillary tangles (choice C) are seen with Alzheimer's disease, not Creutzfeldt–Jakob disease. Repeated exposure to chemical toxins (choice E) can cause dementia. Alcohol is a common example. However, the histology of chemical dementia usually differs in character and distribution from the cortical spongiform changes seen in Creutzfeldt–Jakob disease.

39. (E) Sections of all of the listed structures would be expected to have myelinated and unmyelinated axons, but only in the peripheral nervous system is there an investment of unmyelinated axons by the cytoplasm of Schwann cells (lower left). In the center of the micrograph, a Schwann cell has formed a myelin sheath around a segment of a single axon. The cerebral cortex (choice A), red nucleus (choice B), spinal cord gray matter (choice C), and nerve fiber tracts (choice D) are all constituents of the central nervous system (CNS). Unmyelinated axons in these locations would have no ensheathment by cytoplasm of support cells. Moreover, the cerebral cortex, red nucleus, and spinal cord gray matter contain neuronal cell bodies (also called somas or perikarya) which are not evident in this electron micrograph.

40. (B) Schwann cells are the glia of the peripheral nervous system. Larger axons in peripheral nerves are myelinated by Schwann cells through development of multiple layers of Schwann cell membrane. The counterpart of the Schwann cell in the CNS is the oligodendrocyte (choice A), which generally provides myelin sheaths for segments of several axons. An additional distinction is the presence of a basal lamina on each Schwann cell as seen in the micrograph. Oligodendrocytes have no basal lamina. The perikaryon (soma) of either a sensory neuron (choice C) or a motor neuron (choice D) has a large spherical nucleus and extensive cytoplasm with abundant rough endoplasmic reticulum seen as Nissl bodies in light microscopy. The sensory neuron has a single process, and the motor neuron has multiple processes (an axon and several dendrites), but neither would have a myelinated axon embedded within its cytoplasm. Microglia (choice E) are the counterparts within the central nervous system of macrophages located in peripheral tissues. Inactive microglia are small cells with few distinctive morphological features. Active microglia have characteristics similar to active macrophages (i.e., abundant cytoplasm containing primary and secondary lysosomes).

41. **(D)** The clinical features of leptospirosis (Weil's disease) include intense headache, stiff neck, hepatitis, and nephritis. This disease is caused by *Leptospira interrogans,* a spirochete. The germ has tightly coiled spirals with hooks at its ends that serve to differentiate it from spirochetes belonging to genera *Treponema* and *Borrelia.* Relapsing fever is caused by *Borrelia recurrentis.* This spirochete is twice as big as *Leptospira interrogans,* it has large spirals, and lacks hooks at its ends. Relapsing fever begins with a high fever of 100 to 102°C, headache, muscle spasms, and splenomegaly. It has a characteristic spiking curve due to emergence of various antigenic variants (choice A). Yaws is characterized by the development of cauliflower-like lesions and it is caused by *Treponema pertenue.* This spirochete has acute spiral curves and pointed ends. It is a non-venereal disease transmitted by direct contact with infected persons (choice B). Pinta is caused by *Treponema carateum,* a spirochete similar to *T. pertenue* and *T. pallidum.* Pinta is another non-venereal disease characterized by hyperpigmentation of the skin (choice C). Legionellosis is caused by *Legionella pneumophila,* a gram-negative rod. This organism causes an influenza-like illness which can progress to severe pneumonia, mental confusion, diarrhea, proteinuria, and microscopic hematuria (choice E).

42. **(E)** Scarpa's ganglion contains the cell bodies of the primary afferent neurons whose peripheral processes form synaptic contact with hair cells of the vestibular sensory end organs. The stria vascularis (choice A) and tunnel of Corti (choice B) are parts of the auditory system, whereas the external cuneate nucleus (choice C) and zone of Lissauer (choice D) are parts of the somatosensory system.

43. **(B)** Achalasia is an esophageal disorder due to inadequate peristalsis. The most consistent feature is a decreased number of ganglion cells in the myenteric plexus. Clinically, there is regurgitation, chest pain, and odynophagia. *Helicobacter pylori* infections (choice A) are not related to the development of achalasia. These infections are usually seen in the stomach and predispose to ulcer formation. Fibrous strictures (choice C) of the esophagus may be congenital or occur after damage to the submucosa. Hiatal hernia (choice D) is a herniation of the stomach through the diaphragm. Diverticula formation (choice E) is not a consistent feature of achalasia.

44. **(B)** Apo(a) is a large glycoprotein with a striking degree of homology to the clotting factor plasminogen, in that apo(a) contains numerous kringle IV domains. There are more than 30 size alleles of apo(a) due to differing numbers of kringle IV domains, which in turn yield more than 500 potential different phenotypes of the protein. The apo(a) protein is disulfide bonded to apo B-100 of LDLs, generating a lipoprotein particle identified as Lp(a). The size of apo(a) allows it to occupy the exterior surface of the resultant Lp(a) particle, exposing its kringle IV domains to the vasculature. The presence of the plasminogen-like kringle domains in apo(a) suggests that it interferes with the normal process of thrombosis at the endothelial cell surface by inducing a prothrombotic state, and evidence indicates that this does indeed occur. This leads to the deposition of fibrin clots and atherosclerotic plaque formation. Apo C-II (choice A) is required in chylomicrons, VLDLs, LDL, and IDLs for the activation of endothelial cell-associated lipoprotein lipase, but is not linked to apo(a). Apo B-48 (choice C) is exclusively associated with chylomicrons and therefore is not found in association with apo(a). Apo A-I (choice D) is a major component of HDLs necessary for the activation of lecithin-cholesterol acyltransferase (LCAT) and is not associated with apo(a). Apo E (choice E) is necessary for chylomicron remnant and LDL interaction with the hepatic LDL receptor and is not associated with apo(a).

45. (A) The external nasal nerve is the terminal cutaneous branch of the anterior ethmoidal nerve (from the nasociliary branch of the ophthalmic nerve). It emerges from the inner surface of the nasal bone to be distributed to the skin down the dorsum of the nose. The supraorbital nerve (choice C) is a cutaneous branch of the frontal nerve (from the ophthalmic nerve) and is distributed to the skin of the forehead, scalp, and upper eyelid. The supratrochlear nerve (choice B) is a cutaneous branch of the frontal nerve (from the ophthalmic nerve) and is distributed to the skin of the lower medial forehead. The lacrimal nerve (choice D) is a branch of the ophthalmic nerve that supplies the lacrimal gland and then becomes cutaneous to supply the conjunctiva and skin of the upper eyelid. The zygomaticotemporal nerve (choice E) is a cutaneous branch of the maxillary nerve.

46. (A) In dynamic (isotonic) aerobic exercise, workload and body oxygen consumption are directly related (indeed it is often easier to calculate the workload from the oxygen consumption than to measure it directly). With increased workload (or increased oxygen consumption), there is an almost perfectly linear increase in heart rate, whereas the curve for stroke volume (choice B) increases at first, but then levels off (plateau) at about half maximal workload (or half maximal oxygen consumption). Thus, for strenuous exercise, the increased levels of cardiac output depend almost entirely on increases in heart rate (at essentially a constant stroke volume). Although mean arterial blood pressure and systolic arterial blood pressure rise with increasing levels of dynamic exercise, the diastolic blood pressure (choice C) remains virtually constant. With increasing levels of exercise, blood flow to the skin (choice D) decreases at first, but then as heat production from the exercising muscles begins to increase, the blood flow to the skin also increases to aid in temperature regulation. Blood pressures in the pulmonary circulation (choice E) are much lower than in the systemic circulation. Even if the cardiac output were to increase fourfold during exercise, there would be only about a doubling of the pulmonary arterial blood pressure (e.g., from 12 to 24 mm Hg), which would be nowhere near systemic arterial pressures.

47. (B) Dihydropyrimidine dehydrogenase activity is present in the intestinal mucosa and liver. This enzyme converts 5-fluorouracil (5-FU) to a fluoro-dihydrouracil form that is subsequently converted to fluoro-β-alanine. Patients with an inherited deficiency of this enzyme were found to be extremely sensitive to 5-FU. Inhibition of this enzyme by co-administration of compounds such as eniluracil allows oral 5-FU to be used effectively for treatment of a variety of cancers. Nifedipine (choice A) is a dihydropyridine calcium channel blocker that is metabolized by cytochrome P4503A4. Acyclovir (choice C) is an antiherpesvirus agent that causes irreversible inhibition of viral DNA polymerase and chain termination. It is cleared primarily by renal excretion of the parent compound. Isoniazid (choice D) is an antitubercular agent that appears to act by inhibiting mycolic acid synthesis. It is cleared by metabolism through acetylation and hydrolysis. Acetaminophen (choice E) is an antipyretic and analgesic agent that is cleared by metabolism. The primary route of metabolism is through glucuronide formation. In overdose situations, a highly reactive cytochrome P450 metabolite is formed that depletes glutathione levels and leads to hepatotoxicity.

48. (B) The lesion shown in the photo is a pulmonary granuloma. A granuloma is a localized collection of multinucleate giant cells, histiocytes, lymphocytes, plasma cells, and a few fibroblasts. The center of the granuloma may be necrotic or non-necrotic. An abscess (choice A) would be composed of abundant neutrophils in a sea of liquefied necrotic debris. Histologically, a keloid (choice C) would display irregular dense collagen bands with a few fibroblasts. It is a form of abnormal healing with excessive matrix formation. An infarct (choice D) would contain abundant necrotic cellular elements with or without an inflammatory component. A thrombus (choice E) would appear as a segment of clotted blood within a vessel.

49. **(D)** The surface immunoglobulin of the immature B cell is IgM. The surface immunoglobulin synthesized by a B cell clone serves as an antigen receptor for that clone (choice A). The surface immunoglobulins are not dimeric. They also contain a kappa or lambda chain (choice B). It is generally believed that different receptor isotypes have been generated to perform diverse functions on the same cells (choice C). The mature B cells have IgD on their surface, not IgE (choice E).

50. **(B)** Although multiorgan involvement, liver and spleen enlargement, and skeletal abnormalities are common to all the mucopolysaccharidotic (MPS) diseases, each encompasses specific and unique features. Each different MPS is caused by defects in different enzymes which allows for specific diagnosis. Hunter syndrome is characterized by progressive multiorgan failure and premature death. Hallmark features include enlargement of the spleen and liver, severe skeletal deformity, and coarse facial features (which are associated with the constellation of defects referred to as dystosis multiplex). Unlike Hurler syndrome, whose symptoms are similar (but more severe), Hunter syndrome does not cause corneal opacities. Hunter syndrome results from a defect in iduronidate sulfatase activity and this activity can be measured in the plasma. Morquio's syndrome (choice A) comprises two related disorders (Morquio A and B), both of which are characterized by short-trunk dwarfism, fine corneal deposits, and a skeletal dysplasia (spondyloepiphyseal) distinct from other MPS. Morquio B results from a defect in β-galactosidase. Maroteaux–Lamy syndrome (choice C) encompasses symptoms similar to Hurler, but with normal mental development. Maroteaux–Lamy syndrome results from a defect in *N*-acetylgalactosamine-4-sulfatase (also called arylsulfatase B). Sanfilippo syndrome (choice D) comprises four recognized types (A, B, C, and D), all of which result from defects in the degradation of heparan sulfates. Sanfilippo syndromes are characterized by severe central nervous system degeneration with only mild involvement of other organ systems. Symptoms do not appear until 2 to 6 years of age. Sanfilippo A is the result of defects in α-*N*-acetyl-D-glucosaminidase. Hurler syndrome (choice E) has features similar to Hunter, but with the added symptom of corneal clouding. Hurler syndrome results from a defect in α-L-iduronidase.

51. **(C)** The clinical and laboratory findings suggest a diagnosis of pernicious anemia. Almost all cases are due to autoantibodies against parietal cells or intrinsic factor. These autoantibodies disrupt the normal absorption of vitamin B_{12}. The inability to absorb vitamin B_{12} leads to a macrocytic pancytopenia and peripheral neuropathy. Myelodysplastic sideroblastic anemia (choice A) may present hematologically with a macrocytic pancytopenia. A peripheral neuropathy is not seen. A diet deficient in folate (choice B) can cause a macrocytic anemia. In folate deficiency there are no concomitant neuropathic findings. Anemia and peripheral neuropathy commonly occur with diabetes mellitus (choice D). However, the anemia is normocytic and the neuropathy is sensory. Chronic blood loss (choice E) will usually result in a microcytic hypochromic anemia due to iron deficiency.

52. **(E)** There is an increased risk to develop adenocarcinoma of the stomach with pernicious anemia. Before developing carcinoma, the stomach mucosa usually displays metaplastic or dysplastic changes for a variable time period. Carcinomas of the pancreas (choice A), lung (choice B), central nervous system (choice C), and genital tract (choice D) are not statistically increased in patients with pernicious anemia.

53. (C) Degeneration of dopaminergic neurons of the substantia nigra pars compacta is thought to be the primary defect in Parkinson's disease, whereas loss of GABA neurons in the VL thalamus (choice A) and facilitation of pyramidal tract neurons (choice B) might be secondary or indirect factors in this disease. Vascular lesions involving the subthalamic nucleus (choice D) lead to the condition known as hemiballism, while Huntington's disease might involve loss of cholinergic interneurons in the caudate nucleus and putamen (choice E).

54. (A) It is not possible to determine if the bacteremia was caused by *Escherichia coli,* an intravenous catheter infection, or endocarditis. A reculture of blood after the intravenous catheters have been removed could be of value in differentiating between these possibilities. Bacteremia induced by infected intravenous catheters is not an uncommon phenomenon. The infection is usually localized and removal of the catheter, which tends to be infected with *Staphylococcus aureus,* suppresses bacteremia. When bacteremia persists following the removal of catheters, there is either infection in the vein, or in some other location. At any rate, in the absence of knowledge concerning antibiotic sensitivity of the etiological agent of bacteremia, blind antibiotic treatment is of little if any value.

55. (B) The tentorium cerebelli is a tent-like partition that covers the posterior cranial fossa and the cerebellum and supports the occipital lobes of the cerebral hemispheres. The diaphragma sellae (choice A) is a horizontal projection of dura that forms the roof of the hypophyseal fossa. The falx cerebri (choice C) is a sickle-shaped, midline fold that extends into the median fissure between the cerebral hemispheres attaching anteriorly to the crista galli and the frontal crest and posteriorly to the tentorium cerebelli. The falx cerebelli (choice D) is a small sickle-shaped projection between the cerebellar hemispheres that attaches above to the tentorium cerebelli and below to the internal occipital crest of the occipital bone. The crista galli (choice E) is the superior project of the ethmoid bone that gives attachment to the falx cerebri. It is not a dural reflection.

56. (D) The activity of pyruvate dehydrogenase (PDH) kinase is affected both positively and negatively by numerous allosteric effectors, of which acetyl-CoA is the only one listed that has a positive effect on its activity. An increase in the activity of PDH kinase leads to an increase in the phosphorylation of PDH, which in turn has the effect of decreasing the activity of PDH towards pyruvate. Pyruvate (choice A), NAD^+ (choice B), and ADP (choice C) all have a negative impact on the activity of PDH kinase. NADPH (choice E) has no effect on the activity of PDH kinase.

57. (D) The thyroid hormones T3 and T4 bind directly to nuclear receptors that control the function of gene operators regulating DNA transcription. Angiotensin II (choice A) and adrenergic α_1 receptors (choice B) activate phospholipase C, which catalyzes the hydrolysis of PIP_2 to IP_3 and DAG, resulting in Ca^{2+} release from intracellular stores. In contrast, adrenergic β receptors (choice C) are coupled via a stimulatory G protein to adenylate cyclase and increase production of cAMP, which then binds to the regulatory subunit of protein kinase A, activating its catalytic activity. The insulin receptor (choice E) is a complex molecule consisting of an α subunit that binds insulin and a membrane-spanning β subunit that phosphorylates tyrosine residues. Thus, the primary action of insulin is via tyrosine kinase. However, among the many proteins activated by tyrosine kinase is the ras → raf → MAP kinase cascade, which in turn modulates gene expression and is responsible for some of the long-term effects of insulin.

58. (D) The blood:gas partition coefficient is a measure of the solubility of the inhalation anesthetic in the blood. Blood provides the means of delivery to the brain. The solubility of the agent in blood determines how rapidly the partial pressure will rise in the blood. Agents with high solubility (large blood:gas partition coefficients) require large amounts of the anesthetic to be put into the blood before the partial pressure will increase enough to effectively deliver the agent to the brain. Thus agents with lower blood solubilities (small blood:gas partition coefficients) will have more rapid rates of onset of anesthesia. The rate of recovery also depends on the amount of agent dissolved in blood. The lower the blood:gas solubility, the less agent will be in the blood, thus allowing more rapid recovery from anesthesia. Desirable properties for inhalation anesthetic agents include high potency and low blood solubility. The halogenated hydrocarbons such as desflurane and sevoflurane fit these criteria and are extensively used. The oil:gas partition coefficient (choice A) is a measure of the lipid solubility of the anesthetic agent. This correlates with the potency as measured by the MAC, the minimum alveolar concentration required for anesthesia. Hepatic metabolism (choice B) plays no role in onset of action or rate of recovery, but may be important in terms of possible liver and kidney damage resulting from the production of toxic metabolites from some of the halogenated inhalational anesthetic agents. The organ system distribution from the blood (choice C) does not play a role in the rate of onset or recovery for inhalational general anesthetic agents since body tissues do not act as depots for the inhalational anesthetics. This is unlike the situation with thiopental and propofol, where high lipid solubility and relative tissue perfusion rates cause distribution and redistribution to be primary determinants of rates of onset and recovery. The MAC value (choice E) is a measure of the potency of the agent, but does not give an indication of the rate of onset or rate of recovery for an agent.

59. **(A)** In bacterial food poisoning caused by *Clostridium perfringens,* final confirmation rests upon toxin production by *C. perfringens* and its neutralization by specific antiserum. Demonstration of the presence of large gram-positive rods or spores in the suspected food is not very helpful for the identification of *C. perfringens* because of possible confusion with other clostridia or other large bacilli. Growth in thioglycolate broth will also not allow classification of the various anaerobic large gram-positive rods (choices B and D). Demonstration of spores in food indicates that a spore-forming organism contaminates the food, but it does not prove that *Clostridium perfringens* caused food poisoning (choice C). Demonstration of antibodies against *C. perfringens* in the patient's serum indicates exposure of the patient to *C. perfringens,* but does not prove that *C. perfringens* caused food poisoning (choice E).

60. **(B)** Metoclopramide is a D_2-receptor antagonist with properties that include blocking emesis induced by apomorphine and producing hyperprolactinemia. It does not possess useful antipsychotic activity, but high doses may produce extrapyramidal symptoms that are controlled with antimuscarinic agents such as diphenhydramine and benztropine. Metoclopramide is effective against severe chemotherapy-induced emesis. It is also used to treat gastric atony. CNS adverse effects including drowsiness, dizziness, and anxiety are common. Diphenhydramine (choice A) is an antihistamine (H_1 blocker) with antimuscarinic activity that is useful in treating extrapyramidal symptoms of dopamine receptor blockers as indicated above. Diphenhydramine itself possesses weak antiemetic activity but may be used effectively in combination with other agents such as metoclopramide to reduce the dosage, and therefore the adverse effects, of the other agent. Diphenoxylate (choice C) is a congener of meperidine that is used to control gastrointestinal hypermotility. At its therapeutic dose levels, no morphine-like effects are observed. Scopolamine (choice D) is a muscarinic antagonist that has weak antiemetic activity. It is not useful in treating severe emesis. Syrup of ipecac (choice E) is a household emetic agent useful in treating poisonings by oral ingestion. It acts by producing local irritation of the enteric tract and stimulating the chemoreceptor trigger zone in the area postrema of the medulla. Emesis should not be induced in poisonings involving corrosive chemicals or

petroleum distillates, or if the patient is comatose.

61. **(C)** Von Willebrand disease (vWD) is the most common bleeding disorder that occurs in man. The disorder is due to a deficiency in the protein (von Willebrand factor, vWF) named after Erik von Willebrand who described the bleeding disorder in 1926 which also bears his name. vWF is a complex multimeric glycoprotein found in plasma, platelet α granules, and subendothelial connective tissue. vWF binds to specific receptors on the surface of platelets (identified as GPlb/IX) and in the collagen of subendothelial connective tissue to form a bridge between the platelet and areas of vascular damage. vWF also binds to and stabilizes coagulation factor VIII, an interaction that is necessary to increase the survival of factor VIII in the circulation. Loss of vWF leads to defective platelet adhesion and activation in response to tissue injury. In contrast to classical hemophilia, where bleeding occurs primarily in the joints and deep tissues, bleeding associated with vWD is primarily mucocutaneous. Loss of fibrinogen (choice A) and thrombin (choice B) would have dramatic effects on coagulation time. Loss of tissue factor (choice D) would affect the extrinsic clotting cascade which is the pathway of clotting initiated in response to loss of vascular integrity from an injury such as a cut. Loss of factor IX (choice E) is associated with hemophilia B.

62. **(D)** The spine demonstrates several discrete white abnormal nodules of metastatic carcinoma within the cancellous bone compartment. The nodules are white because the tumor is a prostatic carcinoma, which invokes an osteoblastic response. Most lytic bony metastases are red and soft on gross inspection. The joint space and bony confines show no evidence of trauma (choice A) in the photograph. Ischemic changes (choice B) are rare in the spine. Those that do occur are thromboembolic in nature and heal without significant anomaly. Degeneration (choice C) is common in the spine. Grossly, there is either collapse of the intervertebral disk or the vertebral body. In the photo the disk space and vertebral height both appear normal. Infection (choice E) in the spine is usually due to either hematogenous spread in septicemia or from the outside as with a postoperative wound infection. Osteomyelitis usually demonstrates pus formation on gross examination.

63. **(A)** The ciliary ganglion is one of the four parasympathetic ganglia of the head. It receives preganglionic parasympathetic fibers from the oculomotor nerve and gives rise to postganglionic fibers to the sphincter pupillae and ciliary muscles. The geniculate ganglion (choice B) is the sensory ganglion of the facial nerve and contains no parasympathetic cell bodies. The superior cervical ganglion (choice C) contains the cell bodies of postganglionic sympathetic neurons. The nucleus of Edinger–Westphal (choice D) is the parasympathetic nucleus of the oculomotor nerve. It contains preganglionic parasympathetic cell bodies. The celiac ganglion (choice E) is a prevertebral sympathetic ganglion containing the cell bodies of postganglionic sympathetic neurons.

64. **(E)** *Fusobacterium nucleatum, Escherichia coli, Bacteroides fragilis,* and *Enterococcus faecalis* act synergistically in the pathogenesis of peritonitis following rupture of the large colon and spilling of these microorganisms into the peritoneum.

65. **(C)** Exacting, orderly, controlling personalities gain a sense of control and mastery by having exact information. Detailed explanation about the diagnosis, although initially upsetting, may enhance the collaboration between the patient and the physician, and lead to more effective management plans. Choice A will result in a mistrustful patient, with choice B, the patient's idea that the hospital and physician are incompetent and sloppy is likely to increase, choice D will sound patronizing, and choice E will tend to increase the level of distrust of the patient about the physician and the hospital, in addition to being patronizing.

66. **(E)** Von Gierke disease is caused by a deficiency in glucose-6-phosphatase activity in the liver, kidney, and intestinal mucosa leading to excessive glycogen deposition in these tissues. The lack of glucose-6-phosphatase greatly impairs the ability of the liver to deliver glucose to the blood via the gluconeogenic pathway as would be necessary during periods of fasting. Clinical manifestations of von Gierke disease include growth retardation, hepatomegaly, hypoglycemia, lactic acidemia, hyperuricemia, and hyperlipidemia. Pompe disease (choice A) is caused by a defect in lysosomal acid α-glucosidase, also called acid maltase. It is a rapidly progressing fatal disorder of infancy characterized by cardiomegaly, macroglossia, progressive muscle weakness, and hypotonia. McArdle disease (choice B) is caused by a deficiency in muscle phosphorylase. Symptoms usually appear in adulthood and are characterized by exercise intolerance and muscle cramps. Tarui disease (choice C) is caused by a deficiency in muscle phosphofructokinase-1 leading to symptoms similar to those of McArdle disease. Anderson disease (choice D) results from a deficiency in glycogen branching activity which leads to the accumulation of glycogen with long, unbranched outer chains.

67. **(E)** *Pseudomonas aeruginosa* is an aerobic gram-negative bacterium that is frequently associated with septicemia. *P. aeruginosa* infections are treated with a broad-spectrum β-lactam cell wall synthesis inhibitor such as ticarcillin in combination with a broad-spectrum aminoglycoside such as tobramycin. Tetracycline (choice A) is a bacteriostatic protein synthesis inhibitor. When first introduced, tetracycline was effective in treating *Pseudomonas,* but now all strains are resistant. Chloramphenicol (choice B) is a bacteriostatic protein synthesis inhibitor. *P. aeruginosa* is resistant to chloramphenicol. Nafcillin + kanamycin (choice C) is a combination of a penicillinase-resistant penicillin plus a limited spectrum aminoglycoside. Nafcillin is useful in treating penicillinase-producing staphylococcal infections, but does not possess a broad enough antibacterial spectrum to treat *P. aeruginosa.* Kanamycin is not effective against *P. aeruginosa.* Sulfamethoxazole + trimethoprim (choice D) is a combination of a folate synthesis inhibitor plus a dihydrofolate reductase inhibitor effective in treating urinary tract infections. *P. aeruginosa* is resistant to this combination.

68. **(D)** The larvae of *Schistosoma mansoni* penetrate human skin and are then transported by veins into the arterial circulation. The schistosomes that enter the superior mesenteric artery are introduced into the portal circulation, where they can cause blockage of the portal venous system. Control of schistosomiasis is directed toward proper disposal of human waste, which may contain ova of *S. mansoni.* The ova hatch into miracidia and infect snails. An individual is infected when the free-swimming larvae of *S. mansoni* penetrate the human skin (choice A). Schistosomiasis produces eosinophilia and this symptom is taken into consideration in the diagnosis of this disease (choice B). Schistosomiasis can be diagnosed by the demonstration of ova of *S. mansoni,* which have a characteristic lateral spine (choice C). Head suckers and hooks are the cytological features of *Taenia solium* and *Taenia saginata,* not *S. mansoni* (choice E).

69. **(D)** The naturally occurring nucleoside adenosine activates cardiac adenosine receptors that are coupled to the heterotrimeric G_i protein. Activation of G_i inhibits cyclic AMP accumulation and activates a hyperpolarizing K^+ channel. The slowing of automaticity and reduction in calcium currents increase AV nodal refractoriness and inhibit delayed afterdepolarizations, thereby producing antiarrhythmic effects. Adenosine must be given as a rapid bolus dose through a central intravenous line since it is rapidly taken up by endothelial cells and undergoes deamination. Its serum half-life is measured in seconds. The short half-life is advantageous in that the actions of adenosine are terminated immediately after the reentrant ventricular arrhythmia is terminated. Amiodarone (choice A) is a structural analog of thyroid hormone. The molecular mechanisms for its antiarrhythmic actions are unclear. It prolongs refractoriness in cardiac tissues by blocking Na^+ channels, blocking delayed repolarizing K^+ channels and inhibiting cell–cell coupling. The most serious adverse effect of amiodarone is pulmonary fibrosis. The cardiac glycoside digoxin (choice B) may be used chronically to treat atrial tachycardia, but it is not a drug of choice in an acute situation because of its slow onset of action. Digoxin has a half-life of 39 hours. Cautious intravenous administration of the α_1-adrenoceptor agonist phenylephrine (choice C) will activate constriction of arteriolar smooth muscle, thereby raising total peripheral resistance in this hypotensive patient. The resulting rise in blood pressure will increase vagal tone, causing release of acetylcholine at the heart to terminate the arrhythmia. Carotid sinus pressure is sometimes used in combination with phenylephrine. The serum half-life for phenylephrine is 2 to 3 hours. Propafenone (choice E) is a Na^+ channel blocker with a slow recovery rate from blockade. It slows conduction in fast-response tissues and is used to treat supraventricular arrhythmias. It is cleared by hepatic cytochrome P450 2D6, for which there is a polymorphism, and by renal elimination. It has a serum half-life of 5.5 hours.

70. (A) Patients with multiple rib fractures or flail chest are likely to develop respiratory acidosis due to the pain and insufficient rib cage movements. In the acute phase, immediate tissue buffering elevates plasma bicarbonate only slightly, by about 1 mmol/L for each increase of 10 mm Hg in P_{CO_2}. Any increase in plasma bicarbonate beyond this expected value would be due to renal compensation. Choice B represents a respiratory acidosis with renal compensation. Bicarbonate reabsorption in the kidneys is increased due to enhanced excretion of acid. Over a period of several days, plasma bicarbonate rises up to 3.5 mmol/L for each increase of 10 mm Hg in P_{CO_2}. Choice C is typical for a metabolic acidosis; the decrease in pH stimulates respiration and P_{CO_2} is lowered. Typically, each 1 mmol/L decrement in plasma bicarbonate results in a decrease of P_{CO_2} of about 1.2 mm Hg. Choice D represents an acute respiratory alkalosis. In acute hypocapnia, plasma bicarbonate falls approximately 2 mmol/L for each decrease in 10 mm Hg in P_{CO_2}. Choice E is typical for a compensated respiratory alkalosis, with a 4 to 5 mmol/L fall in plasma bicarbonate for each decrease of 10 mm Hg in P_{CO_2}.

71. (D) Kidneys regulate plasma pH by regulating the concentration of HCO_3^-. Almost all of the filtered HCO_3^- must be reabsorbed and this is accomplished by secretion of H_2CO_3-derived H^+. The secreted H^+ combines with HCO_3^- in the urine and the resulting H_2CO_3 is "lost." However, in the process of generating each H^+ within the tubular epithelium cells, one HCO_3^- is also produced. As a result, for each H^+ secreted, one HCO_3^- is "recovered" by the kidneys. More than 99.9% of the filtered HCO_3^- (choice A) is recovered by this mechanism occurring predominantly in the proximal, not the distal tubules (choice B). The HCO_3^-/Cl^- exchange mechanism (choice C) is important in red blood cells, but not in renal tubular cells. Tubular fluid HCO_3^- combines with H^+ to form H_2CO_3 which then dissociates into H_2O and CO_2. The CO_2 diffuses passively through cell membranes and does not require active transport mechanisms. Since this patient is in respiratory acidosis, his kidneys generate more, not less, HCO_3^- than kidneys from a healthy subject (choice E). This renal compensation happens by excess H^+ secretion of the tubular cells, resulting in net generation of HCO_3^-.

72. (A) Body metabolism produces about 80 mEq of non-volatile (i.e., not CO_2) acid per day. The majority of net H^+ excreted by the kidneys is bound to non-titratable acid (i.e., NH_4^+, pK > 7.4) and various titratable acids (i.e., buffers with pK < 7.4). Under normal conditions, about 50% of H^+ eliminated by the kidneys is in the form of NH_4^+. Under conditions of chronic acidosis, this amount can increase more than 10-fold, making the ammonia buffer quantitatively the most important route of renal H^+ excretion. Uric acid (choice B) and phosphoric acid (choice C) are the main titratable acids and together account for the remaining 50% of the total H^+ excreted. For each bicarbonate (choice D) secreted, one H^+ has been reabsorbed by the kidneys, and net H^+ excretion equals NH_4^+ excretion plus urinary titratable acids minus bicarbonate excretion. Less than 0.1 mEq is excreted as free H^+ (choice E) since urine contains only up to $10^{-4.5}$ Eq/L = 0.03 mEq/L H^+ at pH = 4.5.

73. **(B)** Sequencing of thousands of eukaryotic cDNAs and their corresponding genes has led to the identification of sequences that are required for accurate and efficient splicing of introns from precursor mRNAs. Sequences at the 5′ and 3′ ends of every intron analyzed show characteristic invariance. These sequences are GT at the 5′ end and AG at the 3′ end of each intron. Alteration in these sequences leads to aberrant or non-functional splicing. No other combination of dinucleotides (choices A, C, D, and E) can substitute for the invariant sequences of the intron boundaries.

74. **(D)** The HIV multiplies in CD4 lymphocytes and this multiplication leads to severe lymphopenia due to the lysis of $CD4^+$ lymphocytes. The human immunodeficiency virus (HIV) is a member of the retrovirus group that contains single-stranded RNA viruses and an enzyme that synthesizes DNA from RNA (reverse transcriptase). It also has an envelope (choices A, B, C, and E).

75. **(E)** Inferior alternating hemiplegia involves cranial nerve XII which innervates the intrinsic musculature of the tongue. Superior and middle alternating hemiplegia involve extraocular musculature (choice A) innervated by cranial nerves III and VI, respectively. The muscles of mastication (choice B) and facial expression (choice C), as well as the laryngeal musculature (choice D), are not involved in alternating hemiplegia syndromes.

76. **(D)** Branches of the anterior spinal artery supply the medullary pyramid and the laterally adjacent fibers of the hypoglossal nerve. The lenticulostriate (choice A), and thalamoperforating vessels (choice B), and vertebral artery (choice C) are not associated with alternating hemiplegia syndrome. The posterior inferior cerebellar artery (PICA, choice E) is associated with the lateral medullary (Wallenberg's) syndrome.

77. **(A)** Meconium ileus is a very common early clinical expression of cystic fibrosis. An increased sweat sodium chloride level confirms the diagnosis. About 70% of children with cystic fibrosis have a deletional abnormality of chromosome 7. Pancreatic insufficiency, recurrent pulmonary infections, and biliary obstruction may complicate the disorder. Hemophilia (choice B) is an X-linked hereditary disease caused by a relative lack of coagulation factors VIII or IX. Wilson's disease (choice C) is an autosomal recessive disorder of copper accumulation that principally affects the liver and brain. Alkaptonuria (choice D) is an autosomal recessive disease that causes abnormal pigmentation and degeneration of cartilage. Phenylketonuria (choice E) is due to a hereditary lack of the enzyme phenylalanine hydroxylase. Mental retardation is the major clinical finding.

78. **(B)** The abnormal pulmonary mucus seen with cystic fibrosis leads to recurrent pulmonary infections. Eventually the lung becomes fibrotic and the majority of deaths are due to a failure of these organs. Only a fraction of cystic fibrosis deaths are due to abnormalities of the intestine (choice A). Those rare deaths occur in the neonatal period because of intestinal perforation secondary to undiagnosed meconium ileus. The major abnormality in cystic fibrosis is the production of abnormal mucus. Since the brain (choice C) does not synthesize mucus it is not affected by this disorder. The exocrine pancreas (choice D) usually fails sometime during the disease. However, excellent oral medicines are available to replace most of the missing pancreatic agents. The liver (choice E) is minimally affected by cystic fibrosis. Hepatic failure is not a feature of the disorder.

79. **(E)** Strychnine is a weak base with a pKa value of 6.0. The unprotonated form (or the "free base") will be uncharged and will be

the permeant species that crosses biological membranes. At equilibrium the concentration of the permeant species will be the same on both sides of the membrane, but the total amount (base + protonated form) present in each compartment will depend on the pH of the compartment. For a weak base, the total amount will be the highest in the most acidic compartment. This is because lower pH values will cause protonation of the base to the protonated form that then becomes trapped in the compartment since the charged protonated base cannot cross the membrane. The lower the pH value for the compartment, the greater the total amount present. Stomach contents at pH 2.0 has the lowest pH value. The value for the total amount at any pH may be calculated using the Henderson–Hasselbalch equation [pH = pKa + log (unprotonated form/protonated form)].

80. (A) Because being in control is important to this orderly, controlling personality, patient-controlled analgesia is especially effective for this type of patient (it is effective in almost all types of patients). As needed medication (prn) schedule (choice C) will tend to be troublesome since the patient may become dissatisfied with the lag time between the request and delivery. Hypnosis (choice B) may be seen by the patient as loss of control, as would general anesthesia (choice E). Use of a placebo (choice D) with this type of patient is likely to be discovered, increasing his level of suspicion.

81. (C) In contrast to a classical antigen–antibody reaction, allergic reactions do not result in the neutralization of toxicity or antigen. For example, in type I hypersensitivity, IgE binds to the surface of mast cells. Upon subsequent contact with the specific antigen to which an individual has been sensitized, mast cells release histamine and other vasoactive substances. This leads to anaphylaxis, or other type I hypersensitivity reactions. In type I hypersensitivity, IgE binds to the surface of mast cells, thus IgE is produced in a type I allergy such as allergic rhinitis (choice A). Administraton of sodium cromolyn prevents release of histamine from mast cells, and it is used to treat type I allergy (choice B). Type I allergy begins with the formation of IgE which then binds to the mast cells. Therefore, mast cells in circulation have IgE on their surface (choice D). The reaction of IgE with its allergen is highly specific (choice E).

82. (B) The stapedius, posterior digastric, and stylohyoid muscles and the muscles of facial expression arise from the mesoderm of the second pharyngeal arch, and all are innervated by the facial nerve. The mylohyoid muscle (choice A), the anterior belly of the digastric muscle, the tensor tympani muscle, the tensor veli palatini muscles, and the muscles of mastication all develop from the mesoderm of the first pharyngeal arch, and are all innervated by the trigeminal nerve. The stylopharyngeus muscle (choice C) is derived from the mesoderm of the third pharyngeal arch and is innervated by the nerve of the third arch, the glossopharyngeal nerve. The muscles of mastication, including the masseter muscle (choice D), the anterior belly of the digastric, the mylohyoid, the tensor tympani, and the tensor veli palatini muscles are all derived from the mesoderm of the first pharyngeal arch, and all are innervated by the trigeminal nerve. The superior pharyngeal constrictor muscle (choice E) is derived from the mesoderm of the fourth pharyngeal arch and is innervated by the nerve of the fourth to sixth arches, the vagus nerve.

83. (A) Mebendazole is a broad-spectrum antihelmintic that is effective against a variety of nematodes, including hookworm (*Necator, Ancylostoma*), whipworm (*Thichuris*), threadworm (*Stronglyloides*), and pinworm (*Enterobius*). Adverse effects are rare. Ivermectin (choice B) is used to treat *Onchocerca volvulus,* the agent responsible for river blindness in west and central Africa. Praziquantel (choice C) is an agent of choice for the treatment of beef tapeworm (*Taenia saginata*), pork tapeworm (*Taenia solium*), and dwarf tapeworm (*Hymenolepis nana*). it is also effective in treating flukes (*Schistosoma haematobium, Schistosoma mansoni, Fasciola hepatica,* and others). Niclosamide (choice D) shows an antihelmintic spectrum similar to praziquantel and is considered a second-choice drug for many of the same indications. It should not be used, however, in the treatment of *Taenia solium,* since it does not kill ova that are liberated following digestion of dead adult segments. Diethylcarbamazine (choice E) was developed in a search during World War II for a treatment for filariasis. Because of adverse effects that include nausea, vomiting, headache, leukocytosis, and proteinuria, its use today has been largely supplanted by other antifilarial agents, except in the case of *Loa loa,* where it remains the drug of choice.

84. **(C)** The clinical presentation of patients with defects in several enzymes of urea synthesis are virtually identical. These enzymes are carbamoyl phosphate synthetase (CPS), ornithine transcarbamoylase (OTC), argininosuccinate synthetase (AS), and argininosuccinase. The hallmark of these urea cycle enzyme defects is a normal birth with no known prenatal risk factors. Within 24 to 72 hours after birth the infant becomes lethargic and requires stimulation for feeding. Additional symptoms develop within hours, including vomiting, increased lethargy, hypothermia, and hyperventilation. The hyperventilation is often misdiagnosed as pulmonary disease. Sepsis is often suspected. Routine blood work indicates a reduced BUN (blood urea nitrogen). Lack of proper intervention will lead to coma and death. Correct analysis of hyperammonemia is paramount to proper treatment as this is indicative of a urea cycle defect when presenting in the newborn. Analysis of plasma amino acids can aid in the differentiation of which enzyme is defective. Elevated citrulline (to 100 times normal levels) results from a deficiency in argininosuccinate synthetase. Several other inborn errors are associated with neonatal hyperammonemia, such as medium-chain acyl-CoA dehydrogenase (MCAD) deficiency (choice A), 3-hydroxy, 3-methylglutaryl CoA (HMG CoA) lyase deficiency (choice B), and pyruvate carboxylase (choice D) deficiency. Careful clinical assessment accompanying appropriate laboratory studies (e.g., plasma pyruvate and lactate levels and urinalysis) can distinguish these disorders. In MCAD deficiency, fatty acid oxidation and gluconeogenesis are impaired, whereas they would not be in an infant with a urea cycle defect. HMG CoA lyase deficiency is associated with an increase in 3-hydroxy-3-methylglutaric, 3-methylglutaconic, and 3-hydroxyisovaleric acids in the urine.

85. **(C)** Persistent cough is responsible for approximately 20% of all visits to primary care physicians. *Bordetella pertussis* is increasingly the causative agent, even in adults. In a recent study of college students with persistent cough lasting one week or longer, 26% had serologic evidence of pertussis infection. The reasons for the increase are probably increased prevalence of *B. pertussis* in the community and declining immunity in previously vaccinated adults. Although erythromycin is the drug of choice, unless administered early it does not alter the course of the disease. Exposed infants and small children should be evaluated if cough develops, with prophylaxis using erythromycin considered for those who are unvaccinated and thus at greatest risk for serious disease. Tetracycline (choice A) is a bacteriostatic protein synthesis inhibitor. The tetracyclines exhibit a broad spectrum of activity, but their widespread use has led to increased bacterial resistance, thus limiting their usefulness. Tetracyclines are agents of choice in treating rickettsial, mycoplasma, and chlamydial infections. Chloramphenicol (choice B) is a bacteriostatic protein synthesis inhibitor and is the agent of choice for typhoid fever. Its general use is limited because of the rare occurrence of aplastic anemia. Gentamicin (choice D) is an aminoglycoside that is a bactericidal protein synthesis inhibitor. The aminoglycosides are used in treating infections caused by aerobic gram-negative bacteria. Cefoxitin (choice E) is a second-generation cephalosporin that is used in treating anaerobic or mixed aerobic–anaerobic infections such as lung abscess.

86. **(A)** New lymphocytes differentiate in the two primary lymphoid organs. The bone marrow is the site of production of new (naive) B lymphocytes, and the thymus is the site of differentiation of new T lymphocytes. Lymph nodes (choice B) are secondary lymphoid organs. Although lymph nodes are sites of expansion of both T- and B-lymphocyte clones, the new cells arise by proliferation of stimulated pre-existing lymphocytes. The white pulp of the spleen (choice C) is another secondary lymphoid tissue where clonal selection and expansion occurs. Again, new lymphocytes are produced only by proliferation of stimulated functional lymphocytes, and there is no differentiation of lymphocytes from progenitor cells. Although terminology of lymph nodules (follicles) is not used uniformly, most authors designate lymph nodules (choice D) that have germinal centers as secondary nodules or secondary follicles. These are found in lymph nodes, the spleen, and widely distributed as part of the mucosa-associated lymphoid tissue (choice E). Secondary lymph nodules are organized foci of B lymphocyte stimulation, proliferation, and differentiation into plasma cells and memory cells. Thus, they contain mostly B lymphocytes, but there are smaller numbers of helper T lymphocytes, macrophages, antigen-presenting cells, and reticular cells. When a lymphocyte is stimulated, both the nucleus and cytoplasm become enlarged and the cell stains less densely than a small unstimulated lymphocyte. The aggregation of stimulated "blast" lymphocytes in the center of a lymph nodule results in paler staining of the germinal center. The periphery of the lymph nodule consists of a mantle of mostly small, dark lymphocytes.

87. (C) This pancreatic acinar cell contains several adaptations that indicate its function of synthesis of proteins and their regulated secretion into a lumen. These include the extensive rough endoplasmic reticulum in the basal portion of the cell, the prominent Golgi apparatus, and the large number of granules adjacent to an apical (lumenal) surface. Cells that secrete peptide hormones (choice A) share some features with this cell, but there are also distinct differences. With some exceptions (e.g., enteroendocrine cells), endocrine cells have no contact with an exocrine duct. Moreover, the granules of endocrine cells are generally smaller and they are oriented toward the interface of the cell with connective tissue (which is the location of the nearest capillaries). The cells that secrete immunoglobulins (choice B) are plasma cells, which are located within connective tissue rather than epithelia. Like pancreatic acinar cells, plasma cells have extensive rough endoplasmic reticulum and well developed Golgi complexes. However, plasma cells secrete immunoglobulin as rapidly as it is synthesized and packaged. Thus, accumulations of secretory granules are not seen in plasma cells. Cells that secrete steroid hormones (choice D) have no secretory granules and only moderate amounts of rough endoplasmic reticulum. They are characterized by their content of smooth endoplasmic reticulum, lipid droplets, and specialized mitochondria that have tubular cristae. The essential feature of contractile cells (choice E) is the predominance of contractile filaments (actin and usually myosin) in the cytoplasm.

88. (B) Mitochondria assume a variety of sizes and shapes, but the organization of their membranes distinguishes them from other cellular organelles. In electron micrographs, it is possible to see that there is both an outer membrane and an inner membrane. The inner mitochondrial membrane is highly folded to form cristae, shelf-like or tubular projections that extend into the interior of the mitochondrion. Note that mitochondria in this cell are concentrated near the basal membrane, a common adaptation of epithelial cells that are engaged in membrane transport processes with a high energy demand at the interface with the underlying connective tissue. The rough endoplasmic reticulum (choice A), which is extremely abundant in exocrine secretory cells, is composed of flattened membranous cisternae studded with ribosomes. This is the site of translation of the nucleic acid sequences of mRNAs into the amino acid sequences of polypeptides. A secretory granule (choice C) consists of secretory product delimited by a single membrane. The secretory product in the granules of this pancreatic acinar cell appears homogeneous and moderately electron dense. Golgi complexes (choice D) are also well developed in protein-secreting cells. These are recognizable as stacks of membranous cisternae that typically have a convex and a concave face. The nucleolus (choice E) is located within the nucleus. It is the site of synthesis of ribosomal RNA and assembly of ribonucleoprotein particles, so nucleoli are prominent in cells specialized for synthesis and secretion of proteins.

89. **(E)** Alkaptonuria results from a defect in the enzyme homogentisate oxidase which is required for the catabolism of tyrosine. Increased homogentisic acid is found in the urine and when exposed to the air it oxidizes to a brownish-black color. A deficiency in phenylalanine hydroxylase (choice A), an enzyme required for the conversion of phenylalanine to tyrosine, is associated with phenylketonuria (PKU). Tyrosine transaminase (choice B) deficiency leads to type II tyrosinemia (Richner-Hanhart syndrome), which results in elevated plasma tyrosine levels, eye and skin lesions, and moderate mental retardation. No deficiencies in tryptophan oxygenase (choice C) are known. Deficiencies in α-keto acid decarboxylase (choice D) leads to maple syrup urine disease (branched chain ketonuria), characterized by the burnt sugar odor of the urine of affected individuals.

90. **(C)** The sustained depolarization of the plateau phase is represented by the ST interval (which is not normally associated with any voltage deflection). The depolarization observed in the P wave (choice A) signals the onset of atrial contraction, whereas the QRS complex (choice B) is associated with the initiation of ventricular contraction. The T wave (choice D) is associated with the onset of ventricular repolarization. The QT interval (choice E) comprises not only the plateau phase, but also the rapid upstroke (phase 0) and partial repolarization (phase 1) of the cardiac action potential.

91. **(C)** The gallbladder contains numerous stones. Gallstone formation is frequently seen in middle aged, overweight females. An elevated biliary cholesterol may be conducive to stone formation. Potential complications of gallstones include obstructive jaundice, acute cholecystitis, and perforation. There is no evidence of a neoplastic process (choice A) in the opened gallbladder. Although infection (choice B) may be a later complication of cholelithiasis, in the photo there is no evidence of an infection. The gallbladder does not show any evidence of a thrombotic process (choice D). The gallbladder does not display a congenital malformation (choice E).

92. **(D)** Unlike the typical neuroleptic agents such as haloperidol, clozapine has a weak affinity for the D_2 receptor (choice A). This accounts for the lower incidence of extrapyramidal side effects with this drug (choice C). Clozapine binds to D_4, α_1, and 5-HT_2 receptors with higher affinity than D_2 receptors, whereas haloperidol does not (choice B). Unlike the neuroleptics, it improves negative symptoms (emotional blunting, social withdrawal, lack of motivation) as well as positive symptoms, has minimal effects on serum prolactin levels, and is effective for treatment-resistant schizophrenia. Because clozapine also antagonizes adrenergic, cholinergic, and histaminergic receptors, it produces sedation, orthostatic hypotension (choice E), hypersalivation, and can also produce agranulocytosis.

93. **(A)** A hemagglutination inhibition titer of 400 means that when a patient's serum is diluted 400-fold it will prevent agglutination of the assay red blood cells.

94. **(E)** The glossopharyngeal nerve conducts the general sensation (GVA) and taste (SVA) from the posterior one-third of the tongue. The lingual nerve (choice A) provides general sensation to the anterior two-thirds of the tongue and distributes to the same area taste fibers that communicate from the facial nerve to the lingual nerve via the chorda tympani. The hypoglossal nerve (choice B) provides motor innervation to the muscles of the tongue. It has no sensory component. The facial nerve (choice C) has no general sensory

distribution to the mucosa of the tongue, but does provide taste fibers to the anterior two-thirds of the tongue via the chorda tympani and lingual nerve. The vagus nerve (choice D) has no sensory distribution to the mucosa of the tongue, but does provide taste fibers over the epiglottis.

95. (E) Numerous cell surface receptors possess intrinsic enzymatic activity. Receptors that have intrinsic enzymatic activities include tyrosine kinases. The insulin receptor belongs to this class of receptor, a class that also includes the platelet-derived growth factor (PDGF), epidermal growth factor (EGF), and fibroblast growth factor (FGF) receptors. Receptors with intrinsic enzymatic activity also include those with guanylate cyclase activity (choice A), such as the natriuretic peptide receptors, tyrosine phosphatase activity (choice B), such as the CD45 [cluster determinant-45] protein of T cells and macrophages, and serine/threonine kinase activity (choice C), such as the activin and transforming growth factor-β (TGF-β) receptors. Several receptors are coupled to intracellular proteins with a GTPase activating function (choice D), but are not themselves capable of this activity.

96. (C) Mature cystic teratoma (dermoid cyst) is a benign ovarian tumor that arises from germ cells. It occurs most frequently in young and middle-aged females. A mixture of hair, sebaceous debris, soft tissue, and teeth may be grossly evident. Microscopically, these mixed elements appear mature. Serous papillary carcinoma (choice A) is the most common type of ovarian malignancy. It arises from ovarian epithelium, not germ cells. Endometrioid adenocarcinoma (choice B) is an infrequently seen ovarian malignancy arising from ovarian epithelium. Brenner tumor (choice D) is an uncommon benign ovarian tumor. Transitional epithelial nests within a fibrous stroma characterize this tumor, which is derived from ovarian epithelium. Mucinous cystadenoma (choice E) is a benign ovarian neoplasm that originates from epithelial cells, not germ cells.

97. (B) The mechanisms of action for the antiepileptic agents that are effective in treating partial and secondarily generalized tonic-clonic seizures fall into two primary areas: (a) promoting the inactive state of voltage-dependent sodium channels to inhibit sustained repetitive neuronal firing and (b) enhancing gamma-amino butyrate (GABA) inhibition of synaptic transmission. The mechanism of action for agents effective against absence seizures involves limiting the activation of T-type voltage-dependent calcium channels. Carbamazepine slows the rate of recovery of inactivated sodium channels. It is a primary drug for the treatment of partial and tonic-clonic seizures. Carbamazepine is cleared by hepatic metabolism and induces its own metabolism. Adverse effects include drowsiness, vertigo, ataxia, and double vision. Lamotrigine (choice A), like phenytoin and carbamazepine, inhibits sodium channel function to inhibit high-frequency repetititive neuronal firing. Lamotrigine does this by promoting the voltage- and use-dependent inactivation of the sodium channel. It is effective against partial, absence, and generalized seizures. Adverse effects include dizziness, ataxia, double vision, nausea, and vomiting. GABA is the most abundant inhibitory neurotransmitter in the brain. Tiagabine (choice C) was designed as an inhibitor of uptake of GABA, thereby enhancing its actions in inhibiting synaptic function. It is effective against both partial and generalized tonic-clonic seizures. Its adverse effects include dizziness, tremor, and nervousness. Ethosuximide (choice D) inhibits T-type calcium channels involved in the thalamic 3-Hz spike rhythm of absence seizures. Adverse effects include nausea, vomiting, drowsiness, dizziness, and headache. Vigabatrin (choice E) is an irreversible inhibitor of GABA aminotransferase, the enzyme responsible for metabolic inactivation of GABA. It is effective against partial seizures. Adverse effects include drowsiness, dizziness, and weight gain.

98. (C) Apolipoprotein C-II is required to activate the enzyme lipoprotein lipase, present on the surfaces of vascular endothelial cells.

The function of lipoprotein lipase is to hydroize fatty acids from the triglycerides present in chylomicrons and VLDLs. Therefore, a lack of this enzyme results in the inability to remove the dietary fatty acids packaged in chylomicrons. Afflicted individuals exhibit extremely elevated plasma levels of both chylomicrons and triglycerides. A deficiency in apo C-II is one type of a family of three related inherited disorders that lead to chylomicronemia and triglyceridemia. The other two related disorders are due to a deficiency in lipoprotein lipase and a familial inhibitor of lipoprotein lipase. The restriction to a fat-free diet prevents elevations in plasma chylomicrons and triglycerides. Apo E (choice A) is required for LDL interaction with the LDL receptor. Familial dysbetalipoproteinemia results in persons with a mutant form of apo E (apo E-2). Symptoms include hypercholesterolemia and hypertriglyceridemia. Apo D (choice B) is also called cholesterol ester transfer protein (CETP) and is found associated with HDLs. No identified disorders are associated with apo D. Apo B-100 (choice D) is found associated with VLDLs and LDLs and is required in conjunction with apo E for LDL receptor recognition of LDLs. Abetalipoproteinemia is due to loss of apo B, whereas familial hypobetalipoproteinemia is due to mutant forms of apo B. The former disorder is characterized by the virtual absence of VLDLs and LDLs from the plasma, and the liver and intestine accumulate triglycerides, and erythrocytes exhibit a thorny appearance (acanthocytosis). The latter disorder is characterized by dramatically reduced levels of plasma VLDLs and LDLs. Apo A-I (choice E) is a major protein of HDLs and is required for the activation of lecithin:cholesterol acyltransferase (LCAT). Deficiency in apo A-I results in Tangier disease, characterized by a severe deficiency in HDLs in the plasma. This leads to the accumulation of cholesteryl esters in tissues throughout the body.

99. **(C)** Transmission of amebiasis is via the oral–fecal route during which cysts of *Entamoeba histolytica* enter the intestinal tract. The cysts transform into trophozoites that cause intestinal ulcers, or they may migrate to the liver and produce liver abscesses. The vectors of African trypanosomiasis, malaria, leishmaniasis, and loiasis are tsetse flies, anopheles mosquitoes, sandflies (*Phlebotomus*, or *Lutzomyia*), and deer flies, respectively (choices A, B, D, and E).

100. **(C)** Mitral stenosis impedes the filling of the left ventricle, resulting in decreased end-diastolic filling volume. The actual preload on myocardial fibers is the stretch placed on them at the end of diastole just before the beginning of systole. This stretch determines the resting length of the fibers prior to contraction. For practical purposes, the end-diastolic volume is used as a convenient index of preload (the greater the end-diastolic volume, the greater the stretch). The pressure-volume loop with the lowest end-diastolic volume, and therefore the lowest preload, is loop C. Choice A represents a negative inotropic effect (parasympathetic stimulation). Note that the stroke volume is reduced and the end-systolic volume (blood left in ventricle after systole) is increased. The other two curves (choices B and E) have stroke volumes greater than normal, but only one of these shows increased contractility. Which of the two has increased contractility can be determined from the location of the end-systolic pressure-volume point. The end-systolic pressure-volume point for loop E is on the same line as for the normal individual (diagonal line in illustration). In contrast, loop B has an end-systolic pressure-volume point at a higher level (falls on an end-systolic pressure-volume line that begins at about the same intercept with the abscissa, but has a steeper slope than for normal contractility). Thus loop B represents a pressure-volume loop for increased contractility. Loop E most closely resembles the pressure-volume loop one might expect if the venous return were increased, resulting in a larger filling volume of the ventricle.

101. **(A)** The keratins (choice A) are a diverse family of cytoskeletal proteins that form intermediate filaments in epithelial cells. Specific sets of keratins are associated with specific epithelial tissues, so immunostaining for keratin variants can be useful in determining the precise origin of carcinomas (epithelial cancers). Nuclear lamins (choice B) form the meshwork of intermediate filaments that supports the nuclear envelope of all cells. Desmin (choice C), one of many proteins that form intermediate filaments, is limited in distribution to smooth muscle and striated muscle cells. Desmin is a member of the vimentin family of intermediate filament proteins, which also includes vimentin (many cells of mesenchymal origin), glial fibillary acidic protein (astrocytes), and peripherin (neurons). Actins (choice D) form microfilaments (thin filaments) that, along with intermediate filaments and microtubules, constitute the cell cytoskeleton. Although actin filaments are constituents of all eukaryotic cells, they are most prominent in cells specialized for contraction (e.g., smooth and striated muscle). Microtubules are formed from α and β tubulins (choice E). Microtubules are another ubiquitous component of the cytoskeleton of eukaryotic cells.

102. **(A)** Ca^{2+} is the key to the release of neurotransmitters from synaptic vesicles. When an action potential reaches the presynaptic terminal it triggers the opening of a voltage-gated Ca^{2+} channel. The channel opening results in an influx of Ca^{2+} which triggers fusion of the vesicles with the plasma membrane and release of their contents. Inositol trisphosphate (choice B) and diacylglycerol (choice E) are the products of ligand-receptor-mediated activation of G-proteins that in turn activate phospholipase C-γ (PLC-γ) which hydrolyzes membrane phosphoinositides. Cyclic AMP (choice C) is produced by ligand-receptor-mediated activation of a G-protein that in turn activates adenylate cyclase. Cyclic GMP (choice D) is produced by guanylate cyclases in a ligand-receptor–mediated process similar to that for cAMP production.

103. **(E)** The medial lemniscus which contains decussated (crossed) ascending somatosensory fibers originating in the dorsal column nuclei, is formed in the caudal medulla just rostral to the levels of the motor (pyramidal) decussation. The somatosensory fibers of the dorsal column–medial lemniscal system that ascend through the pons (choice D), midbrain (choice C), thalamus (choice B), and internal capsule (choice A) have crossed at medullary levels and are contralateral to their origin at these levels.

104. **(E)** Surfactant serves to reduce surface tension within the alveoli and prevents atelectasis. In premature infants the lack of adequate surfactant predisposes to the development of respiratory distress syndrome. Several in utero viral infections (choice A) may prove deleterious to neonates. However, these infections do not cause a lack of surfactant in premature infants. Neonates have a reduced capacity to conjugate bilirubin (choice B) which may lead to hyperbilirubinemia or kernicterus. The pulmonary surfactant is not altered. Congenital pulmonary malformations (choice C) would not affect the secretion of surfactant. Infants have a reduced humoral immunity capacity (choice D). The production of surfactant is related to gestational age and is not linked to immune status.

105. **(D)** Neuroleptic-induced pseudoparkinsonism, including pill-rolling tremor, should be ruled out since it can be treated effectively with anticholinergic drugs. Von Economo's encephalitis (choice A), pandemic in 1917 to 1918, often resulted in Parkinsonism, but this patient's age makes it unlikely. The other items (choices B, C, and E) are of importance in history taking, but not as important as history of neuroleptic drugs.

106. **(C)** When tardive dyskinesia is suspected, the abnormal involuntary movement scale (AIMS) is useful. A part of the test includes asking the patient to open his mouth and observe his tongue (it may have slow movements), and to protrude the tongue (it may show movements, or there may be quick withdrawal of the tongue). All the other tests (choices A, B, D, and E) are unlikely to document involuntary movements associated with tardive dyskinesia.

107. (D) Choreoathetoid movements coupled with pseudoparkinsonism is diagnostic of tardive dyskinesia associated with neuroleptic use. There is no evidence of dementia (choices B and C). Multiple sclerosis (choice A) is associated with intention tremor and other neurologic signs, and Sydenham's chorea (choice E) is predominantly a disease of childhood not associated with athetoid movements.

108. (D) The time interval of 0 to 6 hours is called the eclipse period. During this period of the viral growth cycle, the virus is absorbed to the host cell, enters the host cell, and the viral nucleic acid is separated from its capsid. The bacterial growth curve is bell-shaped and composed of the lag phase, in which the cell population is constant, the logarithmic phase of growth, in which the number of cells increases in a geometric fashion (1-2-4-8-16, etc.), the stationary phase, in which the cell population remains constant, and the phase of decline, in which the cells die in an exponential fashion (choice A). The time period 6 to 8 hours represents a portion of the rise period, which marks the appearance of mature virus (choices B and E). The time period of 0 to 6 hours is the eclipse period, and represents events which lead to loss, not retention, of viral infectivity (choice C).

109. (B) Saquinavir is an HIV protease inhibitor. The current HIV protease inhibitors are not sufficient for monotherapy because of the rapid emergence of resistance due to mutations in the HIV protease sequence. Combination therapy using saquinavir with two of the reverse transcriptase inhibitors such as zidovudine, lamivudine, or didanosine is currently effective in making patients virus-free. The HIV protease inhibitors are expensive and generally unavailable in underdeveloped countries. The nucleosides zidovudine (AZT), didanosine (ddI), lamivudine (3TC), and zalcitabine (ddC) produce inhibition of viral reverse transcriptase. These nucleosides are metabolized to the triphosphate forms that competitively inhibit reverse transcriptase. Combinations of agents are used since resistance arising from mutations in the reverse transcriptase sequence (choice A) frequently arises with monotherapy. Mutations in the sequence of viral DNA polymerase (choice C) are a mechanism of resistance for the antiherpesvirus nucleosides acyclovir, valacyclovir, famciclovir, and ganciclovir. These agents are metabolized to their nucleotide triphosphate forms that competitively inhibit the herpesvirus DNA polymerase. Acyclovir and valacyclovir also cause DNA chain termination. Deletion of thymidine kinase (choice D) is another mechanism for resistance of herpesvirus to acyclovir. Although thymidylate synthase is a target of 5-fluorouracil action, deletion of the enzyme (choice E) is not a mechanism for resistance, since thymidylate synthase is an essential activity.

110. (E) There is no known carrier state with hepatitis A viral infection. A single infection usually results in lifelong immunity. There is an increased incidence of infection seen in lower, not higher (choice A), socioeconomic classes. Crowding and inadequate sanitation contribute greatly to the spread of the virus. The viral genome is RNA, not DNA (choice B). Hepatitis A virus is mainly spread by oral ingestion of material which has been fecally contaminated with the virus. The parenteral route (choice C) accounts for less than 5% of hepatitis A infections. There is a vaccine available for hepatitis A (choice D). Nonimmune adults traveling out of the country and infants are the principal candidates for vaccination.

111. (B) De novo synthesis of the purine nucleotides requires atoms from aspartate, respiratory CO_2 (as bicarbonate), glutamate, tetrahydrofolate, and glycine. The atoms of the ring that are derived from glycine are 4,5, and 7. None of the other combinations (choices A, C, D, and E) of ring atoms are derived from a single source. Atom 6 is derived from CO_2, atom 1 from aspartate, atoms 2 and 8 from tetrahydrofolate, and 3 and 9 from glutamate.

112. (C) The normal function of osteoclasts is removal of bone matrix, a process that is crucial both in regulation of circulating $Ca^{+}+$ concentration and in modeling and remodeling of bones. Congenital failure of osteoclast function results in development of thick, abnormally dense bones. The regulation of calcium concentration in plasma and tissue fluid depends on a dynamic system of hormone-mediated calcium removal and deposition in bone. Activity of osteoclasts is an important component of the system, and failure of osteoclast function would tend to reduce rather than increase (choice A) calcium in circulation. During bone development, osteoclasts are required for replacement of the initial spongy core of the bone by a marrow cavity. Thus, failure of osteoclast function results in reduced, not enlarged (choice B) marrow cavities. The consequences of this include deficient hematopoietic capacity. Individuals with osteopetrosis typically suffer from anemia and increased susceptibility to infections. Abnormal deposition of calcium in sites such as the kidney and vessel walls (choice D) is a consequence of excessive calcium release from bone into circulation. This is a condition associated with inappropriately high activity of osteoclasts as a result of their stimulation by excessive parathyroid hormone. Low levels of circulating calcium stimulates release of parathyroid hormone, which stimulates calcium release from bone by osteoclasts. Failure of osteoclasts to respond and the consequent failure of circulating calcium levels to return to normal would more likely result in increased, rather than decreased, parathyroid hormone levels (choice E).

113. (C) The kinetics for the approach to the steady state concentration are controlled by the elimination half-life. The concentration will traverse half of the remaining distance to the steady state in each half-life. In this case, after 2 hr or one half-life, the concentration will be 50% of the steady state level. After 4 hr or two half-lives, the concentration will be at 75% of steady state. After 8 hr or four half-lives, the concentration will be at 93.75% of the steady state level.

114. (E) Endogenous and exogenous pyrogens, resulting from the presence of infecting pathogenic microorganisms, raise the hypothalamic set point and thereby cause a rise in body temperature (fever). If the factors originally responsible for the fever are gone (successfully eliminated by the body's immune system), the hypothalamic set point returns to normal. For a while, the body's core temperature is above the now normal set point. This has the same effect as if the individual were too hot. The patient begins sweating and complains of "burning up" because of his hot skin (due to vasodilation). During period A the patient is comfortable because his body temperature matches his set point. When the set point is first raised due to pyrogens (point B), the body temperature is temporarily below the new, higher set point, just as if the body were too cool. The hypothalamus stimulates the usual responses to produce additional heat (shivering) and to conserve the heat present (skin vasoconstriction and lack of sweating). The patient subjectively feels chilled and seeks to raise his body temperature until he is more comfortable (piles on blankets, sits by the fire, or gets a heating pad). Once the patient's temperature has risen to match the newer, higher set point (choices C and D), the patient is comfortable and his new, higher temperature is well regulated around the new set point. Similarly, when the patient reaches his normal temperature at the end of the febrile episode (choices F and G), he once again feels comfortable since his body temperature matches his set point.

115. (D) Adenosine deaminase (ADA) is required for the catabolism of adenosine to inosine. In the absence of ADA, deoxyadenosine is phosphorylated to yield levels of dATP that are 50-fold higher than normal. The levels are especially high in lymphocytes, which have abundant amounts of the salvage enzymes, including nucleoside kinases. High concentrations of dATP inhibit ribonucleotide reductase, thereby preventing other dNTPs from being produced. The net effect is to inhibit DNA synthesis. Since lymphocytes must be able to proliferate dramatically in response to antigenic challenge, the inability to synthesize DNA seriously impairs the immune responses, and the disease is usually fatal in infancy unless special protective measures are taken. ADA deficiency does not impair salvage of ATP (choice A). There is no increase in inosine levels in ADA deficiency (choice B). Loss of adenosine catabolism would not lead to increased uric acid production (choice C). Inosine (a purine) cannot be used to salvage thymidine (a pyrimidine) nucleotides for DNA synthesis (choice E).

116. **(C)** Granulation tissue is composed of newly formed capillaries, proliferating fibroblasts, and a few inflammatory cells. Grossly, it appears as pink to red colored soft tissue with a granular surface. It serves as an intermediary tissue during wound healing. Irregular dense collagen and sparse fibroblasts (choice A) describes a mature cicatrix, hypertrophic scar, or keloid. Central necrotic debris with peripheral multinucleate giant cells and histiocytes (choice B) is the morphology observed with granulomatous inflammation. Coagulative necrosis and many neutrophils (choice D) describes an abscess or acute necrotizing inflammation. Extravasated erythrocytes, fibrin, and serous fluid (choice E) would define an area of hemorrhage.

117. **(A)** The accessory nerve emerges from deep in the sternocleidomastoid muscle and passes posteriorly across the posterior triangle to supply the trapezius muscle. The vertebral artery (choice B) arises from the first part of the subclavian artery in the root of the neck and under cover of the sternocleidomastoid muscle. It is not related to the posterior triangle of the neck. The vagus nerve (choice C) descends in the neck within the carotid sheath. Superiorly it lies in the carotid triangle, and inferiorly it lies under cover of the sternocleidomastoid muscle. The superior thyroid artery (choice D) arises from the external carotid artery in the carotid triangle and descends through the neck in the anterior triangle. The thoracic duct (choice E) enters the root of the neck on the left side under cover of the sternocleidomastoid muscle and empties at the junction of the internal jugular and subclavian veins.

118. **(B)** Serological tests, such as agglutination reactions, are of little, if any value, for the diagnosis of dermatophytes because they tend to have common antigens and they generally grow in clumps. Thus homogeneous fungal cell suspensions are extremely difficult to produce and use in proper agglutination reactions.

119. **(D)** The patient is an exacting, orderly, controlling person who is very conscious of punctuality. The other personalities (choices A, B, C, and E) do not explain his preoccupation with exactness.

120. **(A)** The reaction shown is that catalyzed during the final step of oxidative phosphorylation, which requires cytochrome oxidase (cytochrome a, a_3) of complex IV. Catalase (choice B) is responsible for the destruction of hydrogen peroxide to water. Ferrochetalase (choice C) catalyzes the conversion of protoporphyrin IX to iron protoporphyrin IX, the heme prosthetic group of hemoglobin. Superoxide dismutase (choice D) catalyzes the conversion of superoxide radicals to hydrogen peroxide and O_2. Peroxidases (choice E) reduce peroxides such as hydrogen peroxide to water using various electron acceptors.

121. **(A)** PTH-like peptides are most commonly produced by massive squamous lung carcinomas, renal malignancies, and some breast cancers. Parathyroid hormone and PTH-like substances stimulate bone resorption and vitamin D conversion (choice B), thereby elevating serum calcium levels (choice C). Serum calcitonin would consequently be expected to rise. A PTH-like effect on the kidneys would increase calcium absorption while markedly increasing phosphate excretion (choice D). Calcitonin levels (choice E) are expected to increase secondary to the elevated blood Ca^{2+} concentration. Hypercalcemia due to malignancy is common, often severe, and difficult to treat.

122. (E) With the infusion of epinephrine, we observe an increase in systolic pressure indicative of an increase in cardiac output. Increased cardiac output is a result of an increase in cardiac function from an agent exhibiting positive inotropicity. Epinephrine acts on cardiac β_1 adrenoceptors to stimulate inotropicity. The decrease in diastolic pressure indicates that peripheral resistance has decreased. Epinephrine acts on β_2 adrenoceptors in skeletal muscle to relax vascular smooth muscle. Since skeletal muscle constitutes a large percentage of body mass, total peripheral resistance will decrease even though epinephrine also acts on α_1 adrenoceptors in arterioles throughout the body to produce vasoconstriction. The large pulse pressure (the difference between systolic and diastolic) and small effect on mean pressure are characteristic of epinephrine. With the infusion of Drug X, we observe a larger decrease in diastolic pressure than that seen with epinephrine. This is consistent with either antagonism of vasoconstricting α_1-adrenoceptors or vasodilation through activation of β_2 adrenoceptors. The systolic pressure has increased to a lesser extent than that seen with epinephrine. The increase in systolic pressure indicates a stimulation of cardiac output over the decrease in diastolic pressure. This is consistent with β_1-adrenoceptor stimulation. Mean pressure is seen to have decreased slightly. The increase in heart rate from 70 to 105 per minute is perhaps greater than might be expected as a reflex response to decreased diastolic pressure. All of the observations are consistent with injection of an agent such as isoproterenol that possesses β_1- and β_2-adrenoceptor agonistic properties. Atenolol (choice A) is a β_1-selective antagonist that is used in the treatment of hypertension. In a normal individual, atenolol infusion would produce little change in resting systolic and diastolic pressures and would certainly not raise heart rate. Phenylephrine (choice B) is an α_1-adrenoceptor agonist. It would increase diastolic pressure by increasing total peripheral resistance. It should have little direct effect on the heart, but the increase in diastolic pressure will cause a reflex bradycardia and negative inotropicity. Labetalol (choice C) has both α_1- and β-adrenoceptor blocking activity. Labetalol infusion would be expected to produce a decrease in diastolic pressure with α_1-blockade and the β-blocking activity would prevent reflex tachycardia and positive inotropicity. Norepinephrine (choice D) will stimulate the heart to cause an increase in systolic pressure, but it also produces a large increase in total peripheral resistance, thereby raising diastolic pressure. Norepinephrine is bound by β_2 receptors with poor affinity so that β_2 effects are not evident in its actions.

123. (B) Morphologic observations of cell death include pyknosis, karyorrhexis, and rupture of the nuclear membrane. Pyknosis appears as a marked shrinkage of the nucleus with loss of intranuclear details, and with most histologic stains, a dramatic nuclear darkening (basophilia). Cloudy swelling (choice A) is a reversible morphologic marker of cell injury due to the abnormal accumulation of fluid within the endoplasmic reticulum and other organelles. Steatosis (choice C) is a reversible accumulation of fat within the cytoplasm. Hepatic steatosis is a common finding with alcoholism and diabetes. Lipofuscin (choice D) is a degradative brown pigment that may harmlessly accumulate in certain cell types. Hydropic change (choice E) is another term for cloudy swelling.

124. (D) The major products of parietal cells are hydrochloric acid and intrinsic factor. Intrinsic factor is a glycoprotein that combines with vitamin B_{12} to form a complex that is absorbed by enterocytes of the ileum. Although atrophic gastritis results in decreased pepsin in gastric juice, pepsinogen (choice A) is secreted by chief cells, the other major cell type of fundic glands of the stomach. Neutralization of the highly acidic chyme (choice B) that passes from the stomach into the jejunum is mainly a function of bicarbonate secretion by the pancreas in response to signaling by the peptide hormone secretin, a product of enteroendocrine cells in the duodenum. The protective mucous coat of the gastric lining (choice C) is mainly a product of the cells of the surface epithelium. Acid secretion by parietal cells is stimulated by gastrin (choice E), but these cells do not produce this polypeptide hormone. Gastrin is secreted by enteroendocrine cells of the stomach and duodenum.

125. **(E)** Niemann–Pick disease (NPD), comprises three types of lipid storage disorder, two of which (Type A and B NPD) result from a defect in acid sphingomyelinase. Type A is a disorder that leads to infantile mortality. Type B is variable in phenotype and is diagnosed by the presence of hepatosplenomegaly in childhood and progressive pulmonary infiltration. Pathological characteristics of Niemann–Pick are the accumulation of histiocytic cells that result from sphingomyelin deposition in cells of the monocyte-macrophage system. Krabbe disease (choice A), also called globoid-cell leukodystrophy, results from a deficiency in galactosylceramidase (galactocerebroside β galactosidase). This disease progresses rapidly and invariably leads to infantile mortality. Tay–Sachs disease (choice B) results from a defect in hexosaminidase A leading to the accumulation of G_{M2} gangliosides, particularly in neuronal cells. This defect leads to severe mental retardation, progressive weakness, and hypotonia which prevents normal motor development. Progression of the disease is rapid and death occurs within the second year. Fabry disease (choice C) is an X-linked disorder that results from a deficiency in α-galactosidase A. This leads to the deposition of neutral glycosphingolipids with terminal α-galactosyl moieties in most tissues and fluids. Most affected tissues are heart, kidneys, and eyes. With increasing age the major symptoms of the disease are due to increasing deposition of glycosphingolipid in the cardiovascular system. Indeed, cardiac disease occurs in most hemizygous males. Three types of Gaucher disease (choice D) have been characterized and are caused by defects in lysosomal acid β glucosidase (glucocerebrosidase). Defects in this enzyme lead to the accumulation of glucosylceramides (glucocerebrosides) which leads primarily to central nervous system dysfunction, and also hepatosplenomegaly and skeletal lesions.

126. **(C)** Resistance to blood flow primarily occurs in arterioles with smooth muscle, and thus this is the site of the largest pressure drop. Although the capillaries are the smallest vessels, by virtue of their large number and parallel arrangement, their effective cross-sectional area is very large, larger than that of small veins (choice A). Since velocity is inversely related to cross-sectional area, the velocity in the capillaries is very low (choice B). This large surface area and low velocity promote exchange of substances between blood and tissue. Compliance (stretchability) of veins is much larger than that of arteries due to their lack of elastic fibers and thinner walls (choice D). Blood volume is greatest not in the capillaries (choice E), but in the small veins, which serve as a blood reservoir by nature of their high compliance (low elasticity).

127. **(A)** Bleomycin is a *Streptomyces* fermentation product that binds to DNA and acts as a ferrous oxidase in using cellular reducing equivalents to generate reactive oxygen species that produce single and double strand breaks. It is highly useful in combinations since it produces little myelosuppression, but it does produce cutaneous toxicity. The most serious toxicity involves the lung, where damage can result in life-threatening pulmonary fibrosis. 5-Fluorouracil (choice B) is used to treat a wide variety of carcinomas. Toxicity from 5-fluorouracil is expressed as GI disturbances (anorexia, nausea, stomatitis, and diarrhea) and myelosuppression. Paclitaxel (choice C) is a natural product isolated from the bark of the Western yew tree. It is a mitotic inhibitor by promoting microtubule formation. This drug is particularly useful in treating metastatic breast and ovarian cancer. The primary toxicity of paclitaxel is bone marrow suppression. Cisplatin (choice D), an inorganic platinum-containing complex, becomes hydrated and binds to DNA where it forms intra- and interstrand crosslinks. Cisplatin is particularly effective in testicular and ovarian cancers in combination with other antitumor agents. Cisplatin exerts a renal toxicity that may be prevented by the infusion of 1 to 2 liters of saline prior to administration. Ototoxicity involving high frequency hearing loss is a toxicity that is not prevented by hydration. Cyclophosphamide (choice E) is metabolized by the cytochrome P450 CYP2A isoform to the phosphoramide mustard that acts as the alkylating agent. This agent is widely used in combination regimens. Nausea and vomiting are the most common toxicities. Hemorrhagic cystitis attributable to the acrolein also produced from cyclophosphamide metabolites may be minimized by hydration and frequent voiding of the bladder.

128. **(B)** The touch imprints show a metastatic carcinoma. The cells demonstrate cytologic features of malignancy such as anaplasia, molding, wrinkled nuclear membranes, and hyperchromatism. The finding of large, atypical cohesive epithelial cells in a cerebral biopsy would be diagnostic of a malignant process. The displayed cells do not demonstrate any cytologic features of viral infection (choice A) such as inclusion bodies or multinucleation. A chronic demyelinating disorder (choice C) would not contain atypical epithelial cells on touch imprint. The cells do not show any cytologic features of parasitic infestation (choice D) such as inclusion body formation, eggs, or cysts. The displayed cells are malignant epithelial cells. The lack of an essential nutrient (choice E) is not pertinent to the observed cells.

129. **(D)** Bacterial spores contain 10 to 15% calcium dipicolinate, which is thought to play a role in the resistance of spores to heat. Heating bacterial spores at 80°C for 15 to 30 minutes actually is used to initiate spore germination, not to kill bacterial spores (choice A). Spores do not require iron for germination. The presence of L-alanine or adenosine facilitates germination (choice B). Bacterial spores are formed when spore-forming bacteria multiply in culture media that lack the necessary nutrients to sustain growth (choice C). Spores are important constituents of such gram-positive bacteria as *Bacillus anthracis, Clostridium tetani,* and others (choice E).

130. **(D)** Prolactin secretion from the anterior pituitary is under negative regulation by dopamine released by the hypothalamus. Blockade of dopamine receptors by the neuroleptic agents will increase prolactin secretion. Hyperprolactinemia may cause galactorrhea, amenorrhea, and infertility in women and infertility, impotence, and galactorrhea in men. Nausea and vomiting (choice A) are common effects with many drugs, but the neuroleptic agents have antiemetic actions through their effects on the chemoreceptor trigger zone. Gilles de la Tourette's syndrome (choice B) consists of chronic multiple motor and phonic tics of unknown etiology. The motor tics commonly affect the face and may consist of repetitive blinking or closing of the eyes. The phonic tics may involve grunts or coughs or coprolalia (involuntary swearing). Although the cause is unknown, the symptoms are often controlled with haloperidol treatment, suggesting excess dopamine activity in a brain region. The butyrophenones possess weak antimuscarinic activity that causes decreased salivation (choice C). The weak antimuscarinic activity of the butyrophenones may cause constipation rather than diarrhea (choice E).

131. **(A)** The angular artery, a branch of the facial artery, anastomoses with the dorsal nasal artery, a branch of the ophthalmic artery, providing a potentially significant anastomosis between the external carotid and internal carotid arteries. The lingual artery and the facial artery (choice B) are both branches of the external carotid artery. The superficial temporal artery is a branch of the external carotid artery and the middle meningeal artery arises from the maxillary artery, a branch of the external carotid (choice C). The superficial temporal artery and the occipital artery (choice D) are both branches of the external carotid artery. The superior thyroid artery is a branch of the external carotid artery and the inferior thyroid artery arises from the thyrocervical trunk, a branch of the subclavian artery (choice E).

132. **(E)** Catecholamines produced by the healthy adrenal medulla are epinephrine and, to a lesser extent, norepinephrine. However, many pheochromocytomas produce predominantly norepinephrine, resulting in α-adrenergic effects. Cardiac ischemia results from increased cardiac oxygen demand and coronary artery spasm. Systemic actions of catecholamines include increased blood pressure (choice A) and heart rate (choice B) and increased glucose levels (choice C) through insulin suppression and enhanced gluconeogenesis. Sweat glands (choice D) are innervated by sympathetic fibers utilizing acetylcholine as the transmitter substance and are not directly stimulated by circulating catecholamines. However, the paroxysmal release of catecholamines precipitates a generalized activation of the sympathetic nervous system, and episodic profuse sweating is common in these patients.

133. **(A)** Tacrolimus, formerly known as FK506, is used in liver transplantation. It acts intracellularly by binding to a cytoplasmic FK506-binding protein, FKBP12, to form a complex that inhibits the calcium-stimulated phosphoprotein phosphatase calcineurin. Calcineurin is involved in translocation and activation of a T cell transcription factor, NFAT, involved in the expression of the genes for cytokines including IL-2, *c-myc* and H-*ras*, and the IL-2 receptor. The result is that tacrolimus prevents T cell activation. Cyclosporine (choice B) works in much the same manner as tacrolimus, except that its cytoplasmic binding protein is cyclophilin. The cyclosporine–cyclophilin complex also inhibits calcineurin from activating translocation of NFAT, thus preventing T cell activation. Cyclosporine produces nephrotoxicity in 75% of patients treated. Cyclophosphamide (choice C) is an antineoplastic alkylating agent that affects both T and B cells, but the primary effect is on suppression of humoral immunity, since the B cell population is slower to recover. Its toxicities include hemorrhagic cystitis, cardiotoxicity, and pancytopenia. Azathioprine (choice D) is converted to 6-mercaptopurine, which is metabolized to 6-mercaptopurine nucleotides that inhibit purine synthesis and purine salvage pathways. It is also metabolized to 6-thio-GTP which damages DNA after incorporation. Azathioprine exerts toxicity on bone marrow and gastrointestinal cells. Prednisone (choice E) is a glucocorticoid used in immunosuppression. The glucocorticoids inhibit T-cell proliferation and the expression of cytokines. The mechanism listed, inhibition of IMP dehydrogenase, is the mechanism by which mycophenolic acid exerts its immunosuppressive actions.

134. **(B)** About 65% of hypertensive intracerebral hemorrhages occur within the basal ganglia or thalamus. Chronic hypertension predisposes to weakening of arteriole walls with subsequent production of Charcot–Bouchard aneurysms. A rupture of these aneurysms frequently results in fatal intracerebral hemorrhage. The cerebellum (choice A) is the site of hypertensive hemorrhage about 8% of the time. Hypertensive hemorrhages are very rare in the occipital lobe (choice C). The pons (choice D) is the site of hypertensive hemorrhage about 15% of the time. Hypertensive hemorrhages are very rare in the frontal lobe (choice E).

135. **(E)** Measles is a highly contagious childhood disease associated with a maculopapular rash, fever, and respiratory symptoms. Measles virus is an enveloped, single-stranded RNA, linear, non-segmented, negative-polarity virus. Variola and some types of herpesvirus (types 1, 3, and 6) are associated with production of a rash. However, both variola and herpesvirus are double-stranded DNA viruses (choice A and B). Molluscum contagiosum virus is an enveloped double-stranded DNA virus which causes small, pink, papular wart-like benign skin tumors (choice C). Papovaviruses are double-stranded DNA viruses which cause lytic and transforming infections, warts, and cervical carcinoma (choice D).

136. **(C)** Cushing's disease results from pituitary tumors that lead to the excess secretion of ACTH. Symptoms include obesity with central fat distribution, hypertension, glucose intolerance, and gonadal dysfunction (amenorrhea or impotence). Additional clinical findings are moon-shaped facies, hirsutism, poor wound healing, acne, proximal muscle weakness, and superficial fungal infections. Other pituitary adenomas have been identified and some synthesize gonadotropins such as FSH (choice A), but they do not lead to elevated levels of secretion, while others do lead to elevated secretion of TSH (choice B). Neither of these pituitary adenoma classes lead to the symptoms of Cushing's disease or syndrome. Excess production of PRL (choice D) or GH (choice E) would not result in Cushing's disease symptoms.

137. (A) The photograph depicts a large occlusive embolus in the pulmonary artery. Clinically, this finding is associated with sudden death in an individual with a hypercoagulable state or peripheral venous thrombi. Chronic idiopathic thrombocytopenic purpura (choice B) is an unlikely milieu to form thromboemboli due to the paucity of platelets. Likewise, with disseminated intravascular coagulation (choice C), there is a lack of both clotting factors and platelets, making thrombus formation improbable. The photo does not display an aneurysm (choice D) or a neoplasm (choice E).

138. (B) Mineralocorticoid excess is either primary, due to hormone-producing tumors of the adrenal cortex or secondary due to activation of the renin–angiotensin system. Conditions of absolute or relative hypovolemia (e.g., pregnancy, heart failure, or shift of vascular volume to the interstitial space as in liver cirrhosis with ascites), as well as dietary sodium restriction, activate the renin–angiotensin system and result in secondary hyperaldosteronism. Conn's syndrome (choice A) is a primary hyperaldosteronism due to hormone-producing tumors of the adrenal cortex. Buffalo hump (choice C), truncal obesity (choice D), and skin striae (choice E) are signs of Cushing's syndrome (an excess of corticosteroids).

139. (C) Probenecid is a uricosuric agent. Renal uric acid excretion is determined by the balance between the amount filtered plus that actively secreted and the amount undergoing passive and active reabsorption. At low doses, probenecid inhibits active secretion and thus promotes retention of uric acid. At higher doses, both active secretion and active reabsorption are inhibited, with the result that excretion is enhanced. The decreased plasma level of uric acid prevents deposition of uric acid crystals or tophi. Combined use with sulfinpyrazone, another uricosuric agent, produces an additive effect and will lower plasma uric acid levels to such an extent that uric acid tophi already present will shrink and disappear. Probenecid was originally designed to inhibit active tubular secretion of penicillin and prolong the half-life of the antibiotic when that drug was in short supply, and it still finds use in this capacity today. Allopurinol (choice A) and its metabolite alloxanthine inhibit xanthine oxidase, thus preventing conversion of xanthine and hypoxanthine to uric acid. Deposition of uric acid crystals in joints leads to acute gout attacks. By slowing the formation of uric acid, allopurinol prevents deposition of uric acid crystals in joints. Allopurinol is not useful in an acute gout attack; it must be used prophylactically. Piroxicam (choice B) is a non-steroidal anti-inflammatory agent with a long half-life that allows once-a-day dosing. Its therapeutic action is probably derived from an ability to inhibit the biosynthesis of prostaglandins, known mediators of inflammation. Piroxicam is used to treat rheumatoid arthritis and osteoarthritis. Colchicine (choice D) is an inhibitor of microtubule function that brings relief in an acute gout attack by inhibiting the motility of granulocytes and preventing the formation of mediators of inflammation of leukocytes. Indomethacin (choice E) is a non-steroidal anti-inflammatory drug (NSAID) that, by inhibiting cyclooxygenase, prevents formation of prostaglandins and eicosanoids involved in the inflammatory process and pain perception in an acute episode of gouty arthritis.

140. (D) Azidothymidine, or AZT (zidovudine, ZDV), is a modified thymidine nucleotide lacking the 3′-hydroxyl, it being replaced by an azido group. When taken up by cells, AZT is phosphorylated to AZT triphosphate. The action of AZT is to inhibit the action of reverse transcriptases such as that of HIV. When incorporated into DNA the presence of AZT blocks further elongation of the replicating DNA. The specificity of AZT for HIV-infected cells stems from the fact that HIV reverse transcriptase is at least 100-fold more sensitive to AZT than the host cell DNA polymerase. AZT does not induce interferon production (choice A), does not bind to the genome of HIV (choice B), does not block HIV packaging (choice C), nor does it selectively poison HIV-infected cells (choice E).

141. **(B)** Absence seizures (petit mal or "blank spells") are generalized seizures characterized by momentary loss of responsiveness, during which patients are unaware of their surroundings, but do not lose muscle tone. The EEG shows a characteristic "spike and dome" pattern with a frequency of 3 per second during these blank spells. Generalized high-voltage spikes (choice A) are characteristic of grand mal seizures. REM onset sleep (choice C) is characteristic of narcolepsy. Partial seizures of the temporal lobe (choice D) manifest complex automatic behaviorisms or may spread to become secondarily generalized grand mal attacks.

142. **(C)** Goodpasture's syndrome consists of antibodies against basement membrane material, recurrent pulmonary hemorrhage, and glomerulonephritis. The pathologic changes are due to a type II hypersensitivity reaction along the basement membranes of the lung and kidney. Steroids, plasmapheresis, and immunosuppresive medicines may help in a minority of cases. Fibrosing alveolitis (choice A) is a pulmonary disorder of unknown etiology. Glomerulonephritis and pulmonary hemorrhage are not observed clinically. Wegener's granulomatosis (choice B) may present clinically with pulmonary hemorrhages and renal insufficiency. There are antibodies against neutrophil components, not basement membrane material. Kartagener's syndrome (choice D) is a hereditary disease of infancy due to a defect in respiratory ciliary action. Systemic lupus erythematosus (choice E) may present with renal insufficiency. Antibodies are directed against nuclear antigens.

143. **(A)** Methanol, a common solvent, is metabolized by alcohol dehydrogenase to formaldehyde and then formic acid. Because the molecular weight is small (32 Da), ingestion of small volumes will generate relatively high concentrations of formic acid, thus producing a profound anion-gap metabolic acidosis. Methanol produces little intoxication, but formic acid will produce blindness. Treatment of the acidosis is essential. Further metabolism of methanol may be slowed by administration of ethanol, producing a competitive substrate inhibition of alcohol dehydrogenase. Dialysis may also be effective in removing methanol and correcting acidosis. Ethanol (choice B) is metabolized to acetaldehyde and acetic acid by alcohol dehydrogenase. Because acetic acid is metabolized to normal cellular constituents, acidosis is not a problem with ethanol. Ethanol intoxication is a major factor in automobile accidents. Isopropanol (choice C) is metabolized slowly to acetone. It is a CNS depressant and does not produce retinal damage or acidosis. Methylene chloride (choice D) is metabolized by cytochrome P450 to carbon monoxide. It prodcues CNS depression. Ethylene glycol (choice E) is metabolized to glycoaldehyde by alcohol dehydrogenase and then to glycolic (hydroxyacetic) acid by aldehyde dehydrogenase. Glycolic acid is further metabolized by α-hydroxyacid oxidase to glyoxylic acid. Glyoxylic acid can then be metabolized by lactate dehydrogenase to oxalic acid. Ethylene glycol is a CNS depressant. Its relatively low molecular weight means that ingestion of small amounts will generate high concentrations of metabolites, thus producing a profound metabolic acidosis. Treatment consists of sodium bicarbonate for the metabolic acidosis and measures to inhibit further metabolism. This may include ethanol as a competitive substrate for alcohol dehydrogenase or 4-methylpyrazole as an inhibitor. Hemodialysis may be useful.

144. **(A)** Receptors that couple ligand binding to intracellular activation of downstream effector proteins that are of the G-protein class (e.g., glucagon, and β adrenergic) possess a structure that contains seven transmembrane spanning domains. This class of receptors are termed the serpentine receptors. Several receptor classes have intrinsic enzymatic activity. Receptors that have enzyme activity have been shown to contain cysteine-rich extracellular domains (choice B), immunoglobulin-like extracellular domains (choice C), and are composed of heterodimeric proteins linked through disulfide bonds (choice D). Receptors that are found intracellularly are those of the steroid/thyroid superfamily of receptors, each of which has a domain for binding the lipophilic ligand (choice E).

145. (C) This question is not meant to make you memorize wavelengths of various light colors, but rather to appreciate the complex relationship between objective wavelength of light and subjective color sensation and the active role the CNS plays in our perception of the world. Based on careful observation of our visual sensations and logical deductions, Helmholtz postulated in the 1860s the existence of three light receptors (blue, green, and red). When these were indeed discovered in 1965, it was found that the light absorption maxima were at 440, 535, and 565 nm, corresponding to blue, yellow-green, and orange. Nevertheless, the old names "blue," "green," and "red" were retained for historical purposes. Further processing of color information in the CNS results in opposition of red and green, as well as yellow and blue, i.e., neurons excited by green are inhibited by red, and so on. Any color of the spectrum can be generated by stimulating the three light receptors in ratios characteristic for each color. For example, yellow sensation is due to 1:1 stimulation of red and green receptors. Green sensation (choice A) is due to stimulation of blue, green, and red receptors at a ratio of 1:2:1 (arrow b) and red sensation is due to stimulation of red cones without simultaneous stimulation of green cones (arrow f). Light waves with a frequency equal to the peak response of red receptors (choice B) would also stimulate green receptors and thereby elicit a sensation of orange. The number of distinct retinal color receptors (choice D) is three, as postulated by Helmholtz, not four. Color perception (choice E), while subjective, can be measured in an objective way using Ishihara charts or through color mixing. When mixing yellow from green and red light, patients with protanomaly (low levels of red pigment) require higher red levels than normal subjects to elicit a yellow sensation.

146. (C) Zafirlukast is an antagonist at the cysteinyl leukotriene LTC_4, LTD_4, and LTE_4 receptors. It provides significant relief from asthmatic symptoms with chronic use. This drug is not a bronchodilator and is not effective in acute episodes. The drug's efficacy in treating bronchial asthma supports the hypothesis that the leukotrienes play a role in asthma. Theophylline is an adenosine receptor antagonist and cyclic AMP phosphodiesterase inhibitor that is used for prophylaxis of asthma. It may produce palpitations in sensitive patients. Cromolyn appears to act by inhibiting mast cell function. It is not a bronchodilator and must be used for prophylaxis. It may produce angioedema and severe headache in sensitive individuals. Headache, nausea, and diarrhea are adverse effects reported with zafirlukast. Inhalational terbutaline (choice A) and other β_2-selective receptor agonists including albuterol, pirbuterol, and bitolterol are the agents of choice for treating bronchoconstriction in an acute asthma attack. The β_2-selective agonists produce bronchial relaxation by stimulating cyclic AMP formation in bronchiolar smooth muscle. β_2-selective agonists may be combined with ipratropium to enhance the bronchiolar relaxation. It is not used in prophylaxis. Aminophylline (choice B) acts in the same manner as theophylline and would be expected to produce similar adverse effects. The use of methylxanthines in asthma has declined with the advent of better and safer drugs. The methylxanthines are not effective in terminating acute bronchoconstriction. Inhalational ipratropium (choice D) produces bronchial relaxation more slowly than the β_2 agonists and should not be the sole agent used to treat acute exacerbations. It may be combined with a β_2 agonist beneficially and it is not used prophylactically. Nedocromil (choice E) is an agent similar to cromolyn and shares the same adverse effects. It is used prophylactically to prevent acute episodes. It is not a smooth muscle relaxing agent. Rather, it appears to prevent release of histamine and other mediators of inflammation from mast cells.

147. **(C)** The importance of the capsule in the virulence of the pneumococcal bacteria is apparent from the observation that only encapsulated strains are virulent, and vaccine efficacy is type specific (the organisms are divided into more than 80 types on the basis of antigenic differences in the capsular carbohydrate composition). Cell wall teichoic acid and peptidoglycan are found in rough pneumococci, and are not involved in the pathogenesis of pneumonia (choices A and E). Pneumolysin is a cytolytic enzyme for pneumococci, not human cells, and plays no documented important role in the pathogenesis of pneumonia (choice B). M protein is a potent antiphagocytic cell wall component of Group A streptococci, not pneumococci (choice D).

148. **(B)** Tyrosine is the precursor for the neurotransmitters dopa, dopamine, norepinephrine, and epinephrine. The order of their synthesis from tyrosine is first to dopa, then to dopamine, then to norepinephrine, and finally to epinephrine. No other choice (A, C, D, and E) reflects the correct order of neurotransmitter synthesis from tyrosine.

149. **(B)** The photograph demonstrates a squamous cell carcinoma, a malignant neoplasm characterized by infiltrating nests of atypical squamous epithelium. The development of esophageal squamous cell carcinoma is closely associated with the risk factors of smoking and alcoholism. Carcinomas that arise in Barrett's metaplasia (choice A) are almost always adenocarcinomas, not squamous cell carcinomas. This disorder is more common in males (choice C) than in females. The 5-year survival rate from esophageal carcinoma is less than 10%. The prognosis is poor (choice D). Dysphagia is a clinical term meaning pain or difficulty swallowing. It is a common finding (choice E) with esophageal carcinoma.

150. **(D)** Cyanide binds to the iron of cytochrome oxidase (cytochrome a, a_3). This is the same target as that of carbon monoxide (CO). Cytochrome oxidase is found in complex IV of the oxidative-phosphorylation pathway, not complex II (choice B) or complex I (choice C). Cytochrome b (choice A) is oxidized when it in turn reduces cytochrome c_1 (choice E).

REFERENCES

Aidley DJ. *The Physiology of Excitable Cells,* 3rd edition. Cambridge University Press, 1991

Berne RM, Levy MN, eds. *Physiology,* 3rd edition. St. Louis: Mosby-Year Book, 1993

Brooks GF, Butel JS, Morse SA. *Jawetz, Melnick, and Adelberg's Medical Microbiology,* 21st edition. Stamford, CT: Appleton & Lange, 1998

Chandrasoma P, Taylor CR. *Concise Pathology,* 3rd edition. Appleton & Lange, 1998.

Davenport HW. *The ABC of Acid-Base Chemistry,* 7th edition. Chicago: University of Chicago Press, 1974

Devlin TM. *Textbook of Biochemistry: With Clinical Correlations,* 4th edition. New York: John Wiley & Sons, 1997

Elkin GD. *Introduction to Clinical Psychiatry.* Stamford, CT: Appleton & Lange, 1998

Fauci AS, Braunwald E, Isselbacher KJ, et al. *Harrison's Principles of Internal Medicine,* 14th edition. New York: McGraw-Hill, 1998

Ganong WF. *Review of Medical Physiology,* 17th edition. Los Altos, CA: Appleton & Lange, 1995

Guyton AC, Hall JE. *Textbook of Medical Physiology,* 9th edition. Philadelphia: WB Saunders, 1995

Hall-Craggs ECB. *Anatomy as a Basis for Clinical Medicine,* 3rd edition. Baltimore: Williams & Wilkins, 1995

Hardman JG, Limbird LE, Molinoff PB, et al. *Goodman & Gilman's The Pharmacological Basis of Therapeutics,* 9th edition. New York: McGraw-Hill, 1996

Isselbacher KJ, et al. *Harrison's Principles of Internal Medicine,* 13th edition. New York: McGraw-Hill, 1994

Ibelgaufts H. *Dictionary of Cytokines.* New York: VCH, 1994

Joklik WK, Willett HP, Amos BD, Wilfert CM. *Zinsser Microbiology,* 20th edition. Norwalk, CT: Appleton & Lange, 1992

Kandel ER, Schwartz JH, Jessel TM. *Principles of Neural Science,* 3rd edition. New York: Elsevier, 1993

Kaplan HI, Sadock BJ. *Comprehensive Textbook of Psychiatry/VI CD-ROM* Teton Data Systems, Jackson, Wyoming, Baltimore: Williams & Wilkins, 1998

Kaplan HI, Sadock BJ. *Kaplan and Sadock's Synopsis of Psychiatry,* 8th edition. Baltimore: Williams & Wilkins, 1998

Katzung BG. *Basic & Clinical Pharmacology,* 7th edition. Stamford, CT: Appleton & Lange, 1998

Leigh H, Reiser MF. *The Patient: Biological, Psychological, and Social Dimensions of Medical Practice,* 3rd edition. New York: Plenum Press, 1992

Levinson WE, Jawetz E. *Medical Microbiology & Immunology,* 5th edition. Stamford, CT: Appleton & Lange, 1998

Lewis WH, Elvin-Lewis MPF. *Medical Botany.* New York: John Wiley & Sons, 1977

Moore KL. *Clinically Oriented Anatomy,* 3rd edition. Baltimore: Williams & Wilkins, 1992

Mountcastle VB. *Medical Physiology,* 14th edition. St. Louis: CV Mosby Co, 1980

Murray PR, Rosenthal KS, Kobayashi GS, Pfaller MA. *Medical Microbiology,* 3rd edition. St. Louis: Mosby-Year Book, 1998

Murray RK, ed. *Harper's Biochemistry,* 24th edition. Stamford, CT: Appleton & Lange, 1996

Roitt I, Brostoff J, Male D. *Immunology,* 5th edition. London, UK: Mosby-Year Book, 1998

Rose DB. *Clinical Physiology of Acid-Base and Electrolyte Disorders,* 4th edition. New York: McGraw-Hill,1994

Rosse C, Gaddum-Rosse P. *Hollinshead's Textbook of Anatomy,* 5th edition. Philadelphia: Lippincott Raven Publishers, 1997

Rubin F, Farber JL. *Pathology,* 2nd edition. Philadelphia: JB Lippincott, 1994.

Vander AJ. *Renal Physiology,* 5th edition. New York: McGraw-Hill, 1995

West JB, ed. *Best and Taylor's Physiological Basis of Medical Practice,* 12th edition. Baltimore: Williams & Wilkins, 1991

West JB. *Pulmonary Pathophysiology—The Essentials,* 4th edition. Baltimore: Williams & Wilkins, 1992

Woodburne RT, Burckel WE. *Essentials of Human Anatomy,* 9th edition. New York: Oxford University Press, 1994

Subspecialty List: Practice Test II

Question Number and Subspecialty

1. Physiology
2. Pathology
3. Microbiology
4. Anatomy
5. Behavioral sciences
6. Biochemistry
7. Microbiology
8. Pathology
9. Microbiology
10. Physiology
11. Pathology
12. Anatomy
13. Pharmacology
14. Pathology
15. Pathology
16. Biochemistry
17. Microbiology
18. Pharmacology
19. Pathology
20. Physiology
21. Physiology
22. Physiology
23. Physiology
24. Physiology
25. Pathology
26. Behavioral sciences
27. Behavioral sciences
28. Behavioral sciences
29. Behavioral sciences
30. Behavioral sciences
31. Behavioral sciences
32. Behavioral sciences
33. Pathology
34. Anatomy
35. Microbiology
36. Pharmacology
37. Microbiology
38. Pathology
39. Anatomy
40. Anatomy
41. Microbiology
42. Anatomy
43. Pathology
44. Biochemistry
45. Anatomy
46. Physiology
47. Pharmacology
48. Pathology
49. Microbiology
50. Biochemistry
51. Pathology
52. Pathology
53. Anatomy
54. Microbiology
55. Anatomy
56. Biochemistry
57. Physiology
58. Pharmacology
59. Microbiology
60. Pharmacology
61. Biochemistry
62. Pathology
63. Anatomy
64. Microbiology
65. Behavioral sciences
66. Biochemistry
67. Pharmacology
68. Microbiology
69. Pharmacology
70. Physiology
71. Physiology
72. Physiology
73. Biochemistry
74. Microbiology

75. Anatomy
76. Anatomy
77. Pathology
78. Pathology
79. Pharmacology
80. Behavioral sciences
81. Microbiology
82. Anatomy
83. Pharmacology
84. Biochemistry
85. Pharmacology
86. Microbiology
87. Anatomy
88. Anatomy
89. Biochemistry
90. Physiology
91. Pathology
92. Pharmacology
93. Microbiology
94. Anatomy
95. Biochemistry
96. Pathology
97. Pharmacology
98. Biochemistry
99. Microbiology
100. Physiology
101. Anatomy
102. Biochemistry
103. Anatomy
104. Pathology
105. Behavioral sciences
106. Behavioral sciences
107. Behavioral sciences
108. Microbiology
109. Pharmacology
110. Pathology
111. Biochemistry
112. Anatomy
113. Pharmacology
114. Physiology
115. Biochemistry
116. Pathology
117. Anatomy
118. Microbiology
119. Behavioral sciences
120. Biochemistry
121. Physiology
122. Pharmacology
123. Pathology
124. Anatomy
125. Biochemistry
126. Physiology
127. Pharmacology
128. Pathology
129. Microbiology
130. Pharmacology
131. Anatomy
132. Physiology
133. Pharmacology
134. Pathology
135. Microbiology
136. Biochemistry
137. Pathology
138. Physiology
139. Pharmacology
140. Biochemistry
141. Physiology
142. Pathology
143. Pharmacology
144. Biochemistry
145. Physiology
146. Pharmacology
147. Microbiology
148. Biochemistry
149. Pathology
150. Biochemistry

Practice Test I

NAME ______________________________
Last First Middle

ADDRESS ______________________________
Street

____
City State Zip

SOC SEC	NUMBER	
S		0 1 2 3 4 5 6 7 8 9
O	N	0 1 2 3 4 5 6 7 8 9
	U	0 1 2 3 4 5 6 7 8 9
C	M	0 1 2 3 4 5 6 7 8 9
	B	0 1 2 3 4 5 6 7 8 9
S		0 1 2 3 4 5 6 7 8 9
	E	0 1 2 3 4 5 6 7 8 9
E	R	0 1 2 3 4 5 6 7 8 9
C		0 1 2 3 4 5 6 7 8 9

DIRECTIONS Mark your social security number from top to bottom in the appropriate boxes on the right.
Use No. 2 lead pencil only.
Mark one and only one answer for each item.
Make each mark black enough to obliterate the letter within the parentheses.
Erase clearly any answer you wish to change.

1. (A) (B) (C) (D) (E)
2. (A) (B) (C) (D) (E)
3. (A) (B) (C) (D) (E)
4. (A) (B) (C) (D) (E)
5. (A) (B) (C) (D) (E)
6. (A) (B) (C) (D) (E)
7. (A) (B) (C) (D) (E)
8. (A) (B) (C) (D) (E)
9. (A) (B) (C) (D) (E)
10. (A) (B) (C) (D) (E)
11. (A) (B) (C) (D) (E)
12. (A) (B) (C) (D) (E)
13. (A) (B) (C) (D) (E)
14. (A) (B) (C) (D) (E)
15. (A) (B) (C) (D) (E)
16. (A) (B) (C) (D) (E)
17. (A) (B) (C) (D) (E)
18. (A) (B) (C) (D) (E)
19. (A) (B) (C) (D) (E)
20. (A) (B) (C) (D) (E)
21. (A) (B) (C) (D) (E)
22. (A) (B) (C) (D) (E)
23. (A) (B) (C) (D) (E)
24. (A) (B) (C) (D) (E)
25. (A) (B) (C) (D) (E)
26. (A) (B) (C) (D) (E)
27. (A) (B) (C) (D) (E)
28. (A) (B) (C) (D) (E)
29. (A) (B) (C) (D) (E)
30. (A) (B) (C) (D) (E)
31. (A) (B) (C) (D) (E)
32. (A) (B) (C) (D) (E)
33. (A) (B) (C) (D) (E)
34. (A) (B) (C) (D) (E)
35. (A) (B) (C) (D) (E)
36. (A) (B) (C) (D) (E)
37. (A) (B) (C) (D) (E)
38. (A) (B) (C) (D) (E)
39. (A) (B) (C) (D) (E)
40. (A) (B) (C) (D) (E)
41. (A) (B) (C) (D) (E)
42. (A) (B) (C) (D) (E)
43. (A) (B) (C) (D) (E)
44. (A) (B) (C) (D) (E)
45. (A) (B) (C) (D) (E)
46. (A) (B) (C) (D) (E)
47. (A) (B) (C) (D) (E)
48. (A) (B) (C) (D) (E)
49. (A) (B) (C) (D) (E)
50. (A) (B) (C) (D) (E)
51. (A) (B) (C) (D) (E)
52. (A) (B) (C) (D) (E)
53. (A) (B) (C) (D) (E)
54. (A) (B) (C) (D) (E)
55. (A) (B) (C) (D) (E)
56. (A) (B) (C) (D) (E)
57. (A) (B) (C) (D) (E)
58. (A) (B) (C) (D) (E)
59. (A) (B) (C) (D) (E)
60. (A) (B) (C) (D) (E)
61. (A) (B) (C) (D) (E)
62. (A) (B) (C) (D) (E)
63. (A) (B) (C) (D) (E)
64. (A) (B) (C) (D) (E)
65. (A) (B) (C) (D) (E)
66. (A) (B) (C) (D) (E)
67. (A) (B) (C) (D) (E)
68. (A) (B) (C) (D) (E)
69. (A) (B) (C) (D) (E)
70. (A) (B) (C) (D) (E)
71. (A) (B) (C) (D) (E)
72. (A) (B) (C) (D) (E)
73. (A) (B) (C) (D) (E)
74. (A) (B) (C) (D) (E)
75. (A) (B) (C) (D) (E)
76. (A) (B) (C) (D) (E)
77. (A) (B) (C) (D) (E)
78. (A) (B) (C) (D) (E)
79. (A) (B) (C) (D) (E)
80. (A) (B) (C) (D) (E)
81. (A) (B) (C) (D) (E)
82. (A) (B) (C) (D) (E)
83. (A) (B) (C) (D) (E)
84. (A) (B) (C) (D)
85. (A) (B) (C) (D) (E)
86. (A) (B) (C) (D) (E)
87. (A) (B) (C) (D) (E)
88. (A) (B) (C) (D) (E)

89. (A) (B) (C) (D) (E)
90. (A) (B) (C) (D) (E)
91. (A) (B) (C) (D) (E)
92. (A) (B) (C) (D) (E)
93. (A) (B) (C) (D) (E)
94. (A) (B) (C) (D) (E)
95. (A) (B) (C) (D) (E)
96. (A) (B) (C) (D) (E)
97. (A) (B) (C) (D) (E)
98. (A) (B) (C) (D) (E)
99. (A) (B) (C) (D) (E)
100. (A) (B) (C) (D) (E)
101. (A) (B) (C) (D) (E)
102. (A) (B) (C) (D) (E)
103. (A) (B) (C) (D) (E)
104. (A) (B) (C) (D)
105. (A) (B) (C) (D) (E)
106. (A) (B) (C) (D) (E)
107. (A) (B) (C) (D) (E)
108. (A) (B) (C) (D) (E)
109. (A) (B) (C) (D) (E)
110. (A) (B) (C) (D) (E)
111. (A) (B) (C) (D) (E)
112. (A) (B) (C) (D) (E)
113. (A) (B) (C) (D) (E)
114. (A) (B) (C) (D) (E) (F) (G)
115. (A) (B) (C) (D) (E)
116. (A) (B) (C) (D) (E)
117. (A) (B) (C) (D) (E)
118. (A) (B) (C) (D) (E)
119. (A) (B) (C) (D) (E)
120. (A) (B) (C) (D) (E)
121. (A) (B) (C) (D) (E)
122. (A) (B) (C) (D) (E)
123. (A) (B) (C) (D) (E)
124. (A) (B) (C) (D) (E)
125. (A) (B) (C) (D) (E)
126. (A) (B) (C) (D) (E)
127. (A) (B) (C) (D) (E)
128. (A) (B) (C) (D) (E)
129. (A) (B) (C) (D) (E)
130. (A) (B) (C) (D) (E)
131. (A) (B) (C) (D) (E)
132. (A) (B) (C) (D) (E)
133. (A) (B) (C) (D) (E)
134. (A) (B) (C) (D) (E)
135. (A) (B) (C) (D) (E)
136. (A) (B) (C) (D) (E)
137. (A) (B) (C) (D) (E)
138. (A) (B) (C) (D) (E)
139. (A) (B) (C) (D) (E)
140. (A) (B) (C) (D) (E)
141. (A) (B) (C) (D) (E)
142. (A) (B) (C) (D) (E)
143. (A) (B) (C) (D) (E)
144. (A) (B) (C) (D) (E)
145. (A) (B) (C) (D) (E)
146. (A) (B) (C) (D) (E)
147. (A) (B) (C) (D) (E)
148. (A) (B) (C) (D) (E)
149. (A) (B) (C) (D) (E)
150. (A) (B) (C) (D) (E)

Practice Test II

NAME ____
Last First Middle

ADDRESS ____
Street

____
City State Zip

SOC SEC	NUMBER									
S	N	0	1	2	3	4	5	6	7	8	9
O	U	0	1	2	3	4	5	6	7	8	9
C	M	0	1	2	3	4	5	6	7	8	9
S	B	0	1	2	3	4	5	6	7	8	9
E	E	0	1	2	3	4	5	6	7	8	9
C	R	0	1	2	3	4	5	6	7	8	9
		0	1	2	3	4	5	6	7	8	9
		0	1	2	3	4	5	6	7	8	9
		0	1	2	3	4	5	6	7	8	9

DIRECTIONS Mark your social security number from top to bottom in the appropriate boxes on the right.
Use No. 2 lead pencil only.
Mark one and only one answer for each item.
Make each mark black enough to obliterate the letter within the parentheses.
Erase clearly any answer you wish to change.

1. (A) (B) (C) (D) (E)
2. (A) (B) (C) (D) (E)
3. (A) (B) (C) (D) (E)
4. (A) (B) (C) (D) (E)
5. (A) (B) (C) (D) (E)
6. (A) (B) (C) (D) (E)
7. (A) (B) (C) (D) (E)
8. (A) (B) (C) (D) (E)
9. (A) (B) (C) (D) (E)
10. (A) (B) (C) (D) (E)
11. (A) (B) (C) (D) (E)
12. (A) (B) (C) (D) (E)
13. (A) (B) (C) (D) (E)
14. (A) (B) (C) (D) (E)
15. (A) (B) (C) (D) (E)
16. (A) (B) (C) (D) (E)
17. (A) (B) (C) (D) (E)
18. (A) (B) (C) (D) (E)
19. (A) (B) (C) (D) (E)
20. (A) (B) (C) (D) (E)
21. (A) (B) (C) (D) (E)
22. (A) (B) (C) (D) (E)
23. (A) (B) (C) (D) (E)
24. (A) (B) (C) (D) (E)
25. (A) (B) (C) (D) (E)
26. (A) (B) (C) (D) (E)
27. (A) (B) (C) (D) (E)
28. (A) (B) (C) (D) (E)
29. (A) (B) (C) (D) (E)
30. (A) (B) (C) (D) (E)
31. (A) (B) (C) (D) (E)
32. (A) (B) (C) (D) (E)
33. (A) (B) (C) (D) (E)
34. (A) (B) (C) (D) (E)
35. (A) (B) (C) (D) (E)
36. (A) (B) (C) (D) (E)
37. (A) (B) (C) (D) (E)
38. (A) (B) (C) (D) (E)
39. (A) (B) (C) (D) (E)
40. (A) (B) (C) (D) (E)
41. (A) (B) (C) (D) (E)
42. (A) (B) (C) (D) (E)
43. (A) (B) (C) (D) (E)
44. (A) (B) (C) (D) (E)
45. (A) (B) (C) (D) (E)
46. (A) (B) (C) (D) (E)
47. (A) (B) (C) (D) (E)
48. (A) (B) (C) (D) (E)
49. (A) (B) (C) (D) (E)
50. (A) (B) (C) (D) (E)
51. (A) (B) (C) (D) (E)
52. (A) (B) (C) (D) (E)
53. (A) (B) (C) (D) (E)
54. (A) (B) (C) (D) (E)
55. (A) (B) (C) (D) (E)
56. (A) (B) (C) (D) (E)
57. (A) (B) (C) (D) (E)
58. (A) (B) (C) (D) (E)
59. (A) (B) (C) (D) (E)
60. (A) (B) (C) (D) (E)
61. (A) (B) (C) (D) (E)
62. (A) (B) (C) (D) (E)
63. (A) (B) (C) (D) (E)
64. (A) (B) (C) (D) (E)
65. (A) (B) (C) (D) (E)
66. (A) (B) (C) (D) (E)
67. (A) (B) (C) (D) (E)
68. (A) (B) (C) (D) (E)
69. (A) (B) (C) (D) (E)
70. (A) (B) (C) (D) (E)
71. (A) (B) (C) (D) (E)
72. (A) (B) (C) (D) (E)
73. (A) (B) (C) (D) (E)
74. (A) (B) (C) (D) (E)
75. (A) (B) (C) (D) (E)
76. (A) (B) (C) (D) (E)
77. (A) (B) (C) (D) (E)
78. (A) (B) (C) (D) (E)
79. (A) (B) (C) (D) (E)
80. (A) (B) (C) (D) (E)
81. (A) (B) (C) (D) (E)
82. (A) (B) (C) (D) (E)
83. (A) (B) (C) (D) (E)
84. (A) (B) (C) (D)
85. (A) (B) (C) (D) (E)
86. (A) (B) (C) (D) (E)
87. (A) (B) (C) (D) (E)
88. (A) (B) (C) (D) (E)

89. (A) (B) (C) (D) (E)
90. (A) (B) (C) (D) (E)
91. (A) (B) (C) (D) (E)
92. (A) (B) (C) (D) (E)
93. (A) (B) (C) (D) (E)
94. (A) (B) (C) (D) (E)
95. (A) (B) (C) (D) (E)
96. (A) (B) (C) (D) (E)
97. (A) (B) (C) (D) (E)
98. (A) (B) (C) (D) (E)
99. (A) (B) (C) (D) (E)
100. (A) (B) (C) (D) (E)
101. (A) (B) (C) (D) (E)
102. (A) (B) (C) (D) (E)
103. (A) (B) (C) (D) (E)
104. (A) (B) (C) (D)

105. (A) (B) (C) (D) (E)
106. (A) (B) (C) (D) (E)
107. (A) (B) (C) (D) (E)
108. (A) (B) (C) (D) (E)
109. (A) (B) (C) (D) (E)
110. (A) (B) (C) (D) (E)
111. (A) (B) (C) (D) (E)
112. (A) (B) (C) (D) (E) (F) (G)
113. (A) (B) (C) (D) (E)
114. (A) (B) (C) (D) (E)
115. (A) (B) (C) (D) (E)
116. (A) (B) (C) (D) (E)
117. (A) (B) (C) (D) (E)
118. (A) (B) (C) (D) (E)
119. (A) (B) (C) (D) (E)
120. (A) (B) (C) (D) (E)

121. (A) (B) (C) (D) (E)
122. (A) (B) (C) (D) (E)
123. (A) (B) (C) (D) (E)
124. (A) (B) (C) (D) (E)
125. (A) (B) (C) (D) (E)
126. (A) (B) (C) (D) (E)
127. (A) (B) (C) (D) (E)
128. (A) (B) (C) (D) (E)
129. (A) (B) (C) (D) (E)
130. (A) (B) (C) (D) (E)
131. (A) (B) (C) (D) (E)
132. (A) (B) (C) (D) (E)
133. (A) (B) (C) (D) (E)
134. (A) (B) (C) (D) (E)
135. (A) (B) (C) (D) (E)

136. (A) (B) (C) (D)
137. (A) (B) (C) (D) (E)
138. (A) (B) (C) (D) (E)
139. (A) (B) (C) (D) (E)
140. (A) (B) (C) (D) (E)
141. (A) (B) (C) (D) (E)
142. (A) (B) (C) (D) (E)
143. (A) (B) (C) (D) (E)
144. (A) (B) (C) (D) (E)
145. (A) (B) (C) (D) (E)
146. (A) (B) (C) (D) (E)
147. (A) (B) (C) (D) (E)
148. (A) (B) (C) (D) (E)
149. (A) (B) (C) (D) (E)
150. (A) (B) (C) (D) (E)

APPLETON & LANGE REVIEW SERIES

HEALTH RELATED

Appleton & Lange's Review of Cardiovascular-Interventional Technology
Vitanza
1995, ISBN 0-8385-0248-2, A0248-3

Appleton & Lange's Review for the Chiropractic National Boards, Part I
Shanks
1992, ISBN 0-8385-0224-5, A0224-4

Appleton & Lange's Review for the Dental Assistant, 3/e
Andujo
1992, ISBN 0-8385-0135-4, A0135-2

Appleton & Lange's Review for the Dental Hygiene National Board Review, 5/e
Barnes and Waring
1998, ISBN 0-8385-0342-X, A0342-4

Appleton & Lange's Review for the Medical Assistant, 5/e
Palko and Palko
1997, ISBN 0-8385-0285-7, A0285-5

Appleton & Lange's Review of Pharmacy, 6/e
Hall and Reiss
1997, ISBN 0-8385-0281-4, A0281-4

Appleton & Lange's Review for the Physician Assistant, 3/e
Cafferty
1997, ISBN 0-8385-0279-2, A0279-8

Appleton & Lange's Review of Physiology for the USMLE Step 1
Penney
1998, ISBN 0-8385-0274-1, A0274-9

Appleton & Lange's Review for the Radiography Examination, 3/e
Saia
1997, ISBN 0-8385-0280-6, A0280-6

Appleton & Lange's Review for the Surgical Technology Examination, 4/e
Allmers and Verderame
1996, ISBN 0-8385-0270-9, A0270-7

Appleton & Lange's Review for the Ultrasonography Examination, 2/e
Odwin
1993, ISBN 0-8385-9073-X, A9073-6

Essentials of Advanced Cardiac Life Support: Program Review & Exam Preparation (PREP)
Brainard
1997, ISBN 0-8385-0259-8, A0259-0

Radiography: Program Review & Exam Preparation (PREP)
Saia
1996, ISBN 0-8385-8244-3, A8244-4

FIRST AID

1998 First Aid for the USMLE Step 1
A Student-to-Student Guide
Bhushan, Le, and Amin
1998, ISBN 0-8385-2603-9, A2603-7

First Aid for the USMLE Step 2, 2/e
A Student-to-Student Guide
Go, Curet-Salim, and Fullerton
1998, ISBN 0-8385-2604-7, A2604-5

First Aid for the Wards
A Student-to-Student Guide
Le, Bhushan, and Amin
1997, ISBN 0-8385-2594-4, A2595-5

First Aid for the Match
A Student-to-Student Guide
Le, Bhushan, and Amin
1996, ISBN 0-8385-2596-2, A2596-3

FLASH FACTS

Flash Facts for USMLE Steps 2 and 3
Kaiser and Kaiser
1998, ISBN 0-8385-2606-3, A2606-0

INSTANT EXAM

The Instant Exam Review for the USMLE Step 2, 2/e
Goldberg
1996, ISBN 0-8385-4328-6, A4328-9

The Instant Exam Review for the USMLE Step 3, 2/e
Goldberg
1997, ISBN 0-8385-4337-5, A4337-0

KAPLAN®

USMLE Step 1 Starter Kit
Kaplan® and Appleton & Lange
1998, ISBN 0-8385-8665-1, A8665-0

USMLE Step 2 Starter Kit
Kaplan® and Appleton & Lange
1998, ISBN 0-8385-8666-X, A8666-8

COMPREHENSIVE A&L REVIEWS

Appleton & Lange's Review for the USMLE Step 1, 2/e
Barton
1996, ISBN 0-8385-0265-2, A0265-7

Appleton & Lange's Review for the USMLE Step 2, 2/e
Catlin
1996, ISBN 0-8385-0266-0, A0266-5

Appleton & Lange's Review for the USMLE Step 3, 2/e
Jacobs
1997, ISBN 0-8385-0305-5, A0305-1

BASIC SCIENCE

Appleton & Lange's Review of Anatomy for the USMLE Step 1, 5/e
Montgomery
1995, ISBN 0-8385-0246-6, A0246-7

Appleton & Lange's Review of Epidemiology & Biostatistics for the USMLE
Hanrahan and Madupu
1994, ISBN 0-8385-0244-X, A0244-2

Appleton & Lange's Review of Microbiology and Immunology, 3/e
Yotis
1996, ISBN 0-8385-0273-3, A0273-1

Appleton & Lange's Review of General Pathology, 3/e
Lewis and Barton
1993, ISBN 0-8385-0161-3, A0161-8

CLINICAL SCIENCE

Appleton & Lange's Review of Internal Medicine, 2/e
Goldlist
1999, ISBN 0-8385-0335-1, A0335-6

Appleton & Lange's Review of Obstetrics and Gynecology, 5/e
Julian, et al.
1995, ISBN 0-8385-0231-8, A0231-9

Appleton & Lange's Review of Pediatrics, 6/e
Lorin
1998, ISBN 0-8385-0303-9, A0303-6

Appleton & Lange's Review of Psychiatry, 5/e
Easson
1994, ISBN 0-8385-0247-4, A0247-5

Appleton & Lange's Review of Surgery, 3/e
Wapnick
1998, ISBN 0-8385-0245-8, A0245-9

SPECIALTY BOARD REVIEWS

The MGH Board Review of Anesthesiology, 5/e
Dershwitz
1999, ISBN 0-8385-6348-1, A6348-5

Specialty Board Review of Family Practice, 6/e
Yen
1999, ISBN 0-8385-8739-9, A8739-3

More on reverse →